Updates in Hypertension and Cardiovascular Protection

Series Editors

Giuseppe Mancia, Milan, Italy
Enrico Agabiti Rosei, Brescia, Italy

The aim of this series is to provide informative updates on both the knowledge and the clinical management of a disease that, if uncontrolled, can very seriously damage the human body and is still among the leading causes of death worldwide. Although hypertension is associated mainly with cardiovascular, endocrine, and renal disorders, it is highly relevant to a wide range of medical specialties and fields – from family medicine to physiology, genetics, and pharmacology. The topics addressed by volumes in the series *Updates in Hypertension and Cardiovascular Protection* have been selected for their broad significance and will be of interest to all who are involved with this disease, whether residents, fellows, practitioners, or researchers.

Adel E. Berbari • Giuseppe Mancia
Editors

Blood Pressure Disorders in Diabetes Mellitus

Springer

Editors
Adel E. Berbari
American University of
Beirut Medical Center
Beirut, Lebanon

Giuseppe Mancia
University of Milano-Bicocca
Milano, Italy

ISSN 2366-4606 ISSN 2366-4614 (electronic)
Updates in Hypertension and Cardiovascular Protection

ISBN 978-3-031-13011-3 ISBN 978-3-031-13009-0 (eBook)
https://doi.org/10.1007/978-3-031-13009-0

This Springer imprint is published by the registered company Springer Nature Switzerland AG
The registered company address is: Gewerbestrasse 11, 6330 Cham, Switzerland

Preface

Hypertension and diabetes mellitus often coexist and are among the most common diseases and cardiorenal risk factors, and their frequency is increasing due to obesity epidemic and aging of the population. Elevated BP values are a common finding in patients with type 2 diabetes mellitus. Development of hypertension in diabetic subjects heightens markedly the risk of macro- and micro-vascular complications. Over the past several years, a wealth of new information has accumulated about the association of this metabolic and hemodynamic disorder.

This book is intended to be an in-depth and up-to-date review of the various aspects of the association between blood pressure disorders and diabetes mellitus. In addition, a unique feature of this work includes discussion of topics infrequently considered and/or acknowledged by clinicians, namely the role of hemodynamic alterations on the vasculature of target organs (retina, kidney, brain, and gravid uterus).

Beirut, Lebanon
Milano, Italy

Adel E. Berbari
Giuseppe Mancia

Contents

Part I

Introduction

Coexistence of Diabetes Mellitus and Hypertension

1

Adel E. Berbari, Najla A. Daouk, and Edgar M. Nasr

1.1 Introduction

Hypertension and diabetes mellitus (DM) are common serious comorbidities which involve 31% and 10%, respectively, of the adult world population [1, 2].

According to the World Health Organization, obesity, arterial hypertension, and diabetes mellitus represent major risk factors for cardiovascular disorders [3]. Due to the obesity epidemic, the prevalence of hypertension and diabetes mellitus has increased significantly worldwide, reaching pandemic proportions [4]. It is estimated that by 2025–2030, the total number of diabetics will rise to 552 million and that of hypertensives will reach 1.56 billion [4].

Hypertension and diabetes mellitus often co-occur in the same individual, a pattern associated with markedly enhanced risk of cardiorenovascular disorders [1–4]. The presence of one of the two conditions increases the risk of developing the other by 1.5–2.0 times [5].

A. E. Berbari (✉) · N. A. Daouk
Department of Internal Medicine, American University of Beirut Medical Center, Beirut, Lebanon
e-mail: ab01@aub.edu.lb

E. M. Nasr
Department of Medicine, St George Hospital University Medical Center, Beirut, Lebanon

A. E. Berbari, G. Mancia (eds.), *Blood Pressure Disorders in Diabetes Mellitus*, Updates in Hypertension and Cardiovascular Protection,
https://doi.org/10.1007/978-3-031-13009-0_1

1.2 Hypertension–Diabetes Mellitus: A Bidirectional Relationship

1.2.1 Definition

Impaired blood pressure (BP) regulation and blunted glucose/insulin metabolism are closely associated [1, 6, 7].

The coexistence of a dual diagnosis of hypertension and diabetes mellitus represents a serious comorbid cardiorenometabolic disorder characterized by a persistent nonphysiologic BP elevation and a dysglycemic state and a two- to threefold increased risk of macro-/microangiopathic complications and premature cardiorenal mortality [7, 8]. In the context of the hypertension–diabetes mellitus coexistent syndrome, it has been reported that 25% of the cardiorenal events is attributed to hypertension, while diabetes mellitus confers 30% of death [9].

1.2.2 Epidemiology

The association of a dual diagnosis of hypertension and diabetes mellitus is highly prevalent and is increasing worldwide because of the global obesity epidemic and ageing of the population [4, 10].

Several studies indicate that glycemia, BP, renal function, body weight, and genetic susceptibility appear to be the most relevant risk factors for the development of the hypertension/diabetes mellitus coexistent syndrome [10]. The relationship between hypertension and diabetes mellitus is substantial and bidirectional [5]. Both disorders overlap in the population and predict each other [3, 11–13]. About 50% of patients with noninsulin-dependent diabetes mellitus (NIDDM) (type 2 diabetes mellitus) are hypertensive, while about 20% of subjects with hypertension have NIDDM [3, 5].

Hypertension is very frequent in the diabetic population globally, with an estimated prevalence of over 50% [4, 14]. However, at a national level, occurrence rates of the association of hypertension and diabetes mellitus vary widely in different populations. In the Hong Kong Cardiovascular Risk Factor Prevention study, 46% of diabetic Chinese subjects were hypertensive [15]. Higher association rates were reported in other populations [5]. Prevalence close to 50% was noted in four Japanese studies and in the Honolulu Heart Study and Strong Heart Study [5]. Of note, the population of the Honolulu Heart Study was of Japanese ancestry [5]. Further, 70% of a cohort of Korean elderly diabetic subjects exhibited high BP levels [16, 17]. In addition, in a national cross-sectional survey, 80% of Jordanian diabetic patients were hypertensive [18].

Epidemiologic surveys indicate that the relationship between diabetes mellitus and hypertension is influenced by physiologic parameters. Gender and duration of diabetes mellitus appear to be determinant factors [5, 19].

The prevalence of hypertension in diabetes mellitus and its relationship to the duration of diabetes was assessed in 702 subjects aged 18–74 years who have been selected as a representative sample of patients with diabetes mellitus diagnosed between 1939 and 1965 [20]. Analysis of data of the study conducted in 1964–1965 revealed that (i) the prevalence rates of hypertension were higher in diabetic women than in diabetic men, that is, 36% versus 26%, respectively [20]. These rates were higher than those in the US general population in 1962 [20]. Diabetic men and women had prevalence rates of 1.7, 1.9, and 2.1 times higher than those of the US general population 1962 census [20]. (ii) Further, diabetic women tend to develop hypertension at an earlier decade, that is, 45–54 years old versus 55–64 years old than their nondiabetic counterparts [21]. These observations suggest that diabetic women are more prone to disturbed BP control. (iii) There is a direct relation between the duration of diabetes mellitus and the prevalence of hypertension [20]. The increasing prevalence of hypertension associated with the increasing duration of diabetes was independent of ageing. The mechanisms by which the duration of diabetes mellitus relates to BP elevation could not be elucidated from the data of the study [20]. However, it has been postulated that obesity and microvascular complications may have contributed to the short-term and long-term relation between hypertension and the duration of diabetes mellitus [20].

Age also impacts the hypertension–diabetes mellitus relationship [21, 22]. In a study which assessed various features of hypertension in 662 diabetics and an equal number of matched nondiabetic subjects of the Dupont Company, the prevalence rates of hypertension, defined as a BP ≥150/95 mmHg, were greater in diabetic men younger than 45 years of age, with an excess of 54% [21]. On the other hand, in a community survey performed in Rancho Bernardo, California, in 1972–1974, which includes a population of 3456 of primarily white middle-aged class subjects, aged 50–79 years, excess hypertension in diabetic patients tends (i) to decrease with age and (ii) to disappear in men older than 70 years [22]. Two factors have been postulated to explain the age-related effects in the hypertension–diabetes mellitus association: (i) prior mortality leading to selective removal of older diabetic men and (ii) weakening predisposition to diabetes mellitus with ageing [22].

Although it is well established that diabetes mellitus is a strong predictor of incident hypertension, the rate of progression from normotension to hypertension remains unclear. The rate of BP changes during the development of hypertension in subjects with and without diabetes mellitus have been evaluated, using data from the MCDS (Mexico City Diabetes Study, a population-based study of diabetes mellitus in Hispanic whites) and in the FOS (Framingham Offspring Study, a community-based study in non-Hispanic whites) during a 7-year follow-up [23]. Analysis of data of these studies revealed that (i) diabetes mellitus at baseline was a significant predictor of hypertension. Conversely hypertension at baseline was an independent predictor of incident diabetes. (ii) In MCDS, in over 60% of converters, progression from normotension to hypertension was characterized by a steep rather than a progressive increase in BP values, with an average of about 20 mmHg for systolic BP within 3.5 years; (iii) conversion to diabetes or hypertension was associated with a metabolic syndrome phenotype [23].

A similar pattern has been reported in the progression to overt diabetes mellitus [23, 24]. In about 70% of subjects with normoglycemia or impaired glucose intolerance in the MCDS study, the development to overt diabetes mellitus was characterized by an abrupt increase in plasma glucose values by about 50 mg/dL within 3.5 years [23, 24]. The diabetic converters exhibited features of the metabolic syndrome [23].

1.3 Classification of Hypertension–Diabetes-Associated Phenotypes

1.3.1 Hypertension in Diabetes Mellitus

1.3.1.1 Type 2 Diabetes Mellitus

Hypertension is very common in both type 1 and type 2 diabetes mellitus, being twice as frequent in subjects with the metabolic disorder as in those without [25, 26].

Although diabetes mellitus is etiologically classified into two main types, type 2 diabetes mellitus (type 2 DM) accounts for over 85% of the diabetic population globally [27].

Several studies have established that type 2 DM increases the risk of hypertension development. In the treatment options for Type 2 Diabetes Mellitus in Adolescents and Youth study (TODAY) which recruited 699 adolescents, aged 10–17 years with diabetes of less than 2 years' duration, the prevalence of hypertension increased from 11.6% to 33.8% after a follow-up of 3.9 years [28]. Further, in a retrospective study of 5016 adults without a history of diabetes mellitus or hypertension, an approximate twofold higher risk of incident hypertension was reported in patients with prediabetes compared to normoglycemic subjects [29].

Estimates of hypertension in diabetes mellitus depend upon the definition of hypertension and population studied.

Earlier studies have applied a higher BP threshold as an indicator of hypertension. In the Dupont Study, considering hypertension as BP ≥150/95 mmHg, Pell and DiAllonzo reported that employees with diabetes mellitus exhibited a 54% greater prevalence of hypertension compared to the nondiabetic controls [21]. In a nationwide survey of diabetic subjects performed in England in 1991–1994 for cardiovascular risk assessment, a prevalence of hypertension of 51% was demonstrated with BP criterion >160/90 mmHg [30].

By shifting to lower BP targets, recent investigations suggest that hypertension appears to be much more prevalent among subjects with diabetes mellitus than documented by previous evaluations [31, 32].

A recent analysis of data of US adults with diabetes mellitus in the US National Health and Nutrition Survey (NHANES), 2011–2016, demonstrated high hypertension prevalent rates of 77% and 66% according to whether BP targets of >130/80 mmHg or >140/90 mmHg based on guidelines of the American Heart Association (AHA) and American Diabetes Association (ADA) were applied [31]. Further, a retrospective chart analysis of 2227 patients with type 2 DM confirmed that a downward shift of BP targets to 130/80 mmHg was associated with increasing rates of hypertension, with values of 60.2%, 76.5%, and 85.8% at BP thresholds of

140/90 mmHg, 130/85 mmHg, and 130/80 mmHg, respectively [32]. Moreover, the data suggested that hypertension also affects elderly diabetic subjects reaching prevalence rates of over 94% at age of 80 years [32].

1.3.1.2 Type 1 Diabetes Mellitus

Type 1 diabetes mellitus (T1DM) affects about 10%–15% of the diabetic population, involving more commonly children and young adults [33]. The incidence of T1DM is increasing at an alarming rate, as it is estimated that about 90000 children are diagnosed yearly [33, 34].

In T1DM, hypertension is quite prevalent and more common than in the general population [35]. In a series of 900 patients with T1DM admitted to the Joslin clinic, Christlieb et al. reported that the prevalence of hypertension, defined as SBP/DBP >160/90 mmHg was significantly higher in diabetic subjects than in nondiabetic controls, with the relative risk of high BP greater among diabetic women than diabetic men counterparts [36]. Further, in a study which included 10202 Danish subjects representing a sample of Danish population, Norgaard et al. reported that hypertension was more prevalent in T1DM patients than in the general population, with rates of 14.7% and 4.4%, respectively [37]. The excess of hypertension in T1DM was attributed to diabetic nephropathy as evidenced by increased urinary albumin excretion [37]. However, some patients with T1DM develop hypertension with no evidence of clinical and laboratory diabetic nephropathy, but exhibit a strong family history of hypertension [37]. These patients are categorized as having essential hypertension [37].

In T1DM, hypertension is generally not present at the time of diagnosis of the metabolic disorder [25]. BP remains normal for the first 5–10 years but expresses subtle altered patterns which are apparent only by ambulatory BP monitoring (ABPM) [38, 39]. Lurbe et al. examined the circadian pattern of BP by ABPM and urinary albumin excretion in 45 patients with T1DM who were completely normotensive by standard criteria and the same number of age-/sex-matched controls [39]. They demonstrated that many patients with T1DM displayed a blunted nocturnal fall in BP, elevation in nocturnal systolic and diastolic BP, and often nocturnal hypertension [39]. These BP changes antedated albuminuria and might lead to progression to diabetic nephropathy [39]. Similarly, Mateo-Gavita et al. evaluated, in a prospective observational study, the circadian BP pattern by ABPM of 85 clinically normotensive and normoalbuminuric patients with T1DM [40]. They reported a high prevalence of altered BP patterns, defined as masked hypertension and non-dipping nocturnal pattern and after a long-term follow-up development of microvascular complications [40]. In most patients with T1DM, BP elevation often coincides with the development of incipient or overt nephropathy [37, 41]. In T1DM of over 30 years, hypertension develops in 50% of subjects with incipient or overt nephropathy, while BP remains normal in subjects who escape the renal disease-caused damage [41].

There is limited information about the overall prevalence of elevated BP in youth with diabetes mellitus [33, 35]. Although quite frequent, hypertension and BP disorders are poorly recognized and often in T1DM undertreated, especially in the pediatric age group [33, 42]. In a retrospective cohort study, about 70% of hypertensive disorders in children with T1DM remained untreated for over one year after diagnosis [33].

Epidemiologic surveys and clinical studies reported variable estimates of elevated BP in children and young adults with T1DM [33]. The prevalence of hypertension varies between 4% and 16% [35]. In the SEARCH for Diabetes in Youth Study, a large multicenter study in North America which included 3691 youths aged 3–17 years with T1DM, the prevalence of elevated BP was 5.9% [43]. However, other clinical studies reported that, in T1DM, the occurrence rates of hypertension were higher in older patients [33, 44]. The EURODIAB IDDM Complications study, a cross-sectional study which enrolled 3250 randomly selected type 1 diabetic patients with a mean age of 32.7 years and a mean duration of diabetes mellitus of 14.7 years, revealed a 24% hypertension prevalence, with only 11.3% of those with high BP treated and controlled [42]. Further, in the Coronary Artery Calcification in Type I Diabetes Mellitus (CACTI) study, a population of an overwhelming non-Hispanic white type 1 adult diabetes, the mean hypertension prevalence was 43%, which was much higher than that in age-/sex-matched nondiabetic controls [44].

1.3.2 Diabetes Mellitus in Hypertension

Glucose intolerance and diabetes mellitus are highly prevalent in hypertensive subjects [13, 45]. Different occurrence rates of diabetes mellitus in hypertensive patients have been reported in various studies conducted in Japan and Western countries [5, 46]. Among the Japanese studies, the prevalence rates of diabetes mellitus in hypertension varied between 10% and 20% [5, 46, 47]. In contrast, studies performed in Western countries revealed higher prevalence rates. In the San Antonio Heart Study and in the Framingham Study, over 50% of hypertensive subjects experienced impaired glucose tolerance or diabetes mellitus [5, 9, 48]. Further, the Strong Heart Study, whose participants were American Indians living in Arizona, reported a still higher prevalence of 53.5% [5, 49]. In addition, the Jackson Heart Study, which involved blacks, also reported a relatively high association rates [50].

The differences in the prevalence rates between Japanese and Western studies have been attributed to older age of participants in the Framingham Study and to ethnic background (Puma Indians) in the Strong Heart Study and race in the Jackson Heart Study [5, 47, 50].

Several prospective studies have documented a relationship between elevated BP levels/hypertension and the development of impaired glucose tolerance/diabetes mellitus [3, 5, 8, 51]. In a meta-analysis of 30 cohort studies, each 20 mmHg of higher systolic BP was associated with a 77% higher risk of type 2 diabetes mellitus [52].

Several factors have been shown to predict incident diabetes mellitus in hypertension. Race, altered BP phenotype patterns, baseline BP levels, and body mass index (BMI) appear to be associated with increased risk of new-onset diabetes mellitus and/or disturbed glucose homeostasis [19].

Analysis of combined data from several studies (Atherosclerosis Risk in Communities [ARIC] study, Coronary Artery Risk Development in Young Adults (CARDIA) study, and the Framingham Heart Study Offspring Cohort), which include a large cohort of 10843 middle-aged African-Americans and white Americans, with a follow-up of 8.9 years, revealed that compared to normotensive subjects, the risk of developing new-onset diabetes mellitus was higher in hypertensive African-Americans than in white hypertensive Americans with occurrence rates of 14.6% versus 7.9%, respectively [19]. Further, in addition to hypertension, prehypertension was associated with incident diabetes mellitus only in white subjects and not in African Americans [19].

In a cohort of 1412 subjects of the Pressione Arteriosa Monitorate e Loro Associazon (PAMELA) study, the incidence of impaired glucose tolerance and new-onset diabetes mellitus was examined in white coat hypertension and masked hypertension with BP phenotypes identified by out-of-office BP and ambulatory BP monitoring [53]. Over a period of 10 years, the incidence of glucose intolerance and diabetes mellitus was significantly greater in both white coat hypertension and masked hypertension, compared to truly normotensive subjects, with age-/sex-adjusted risk of 2.9 and 2.7, respectively, similar to sustained hypertension [53]. Further, the most important independent predictors of new-onset diabetes mellitus or impaired fasting blood glucose state were baseline blood glucose, BMI, and 24-hour mean or home diastolic BP [53].

The onset of new-onset diabetes mellitus associated with increasing baseline BP categories classified as optimal (≤120/75 mmHg), normal (120–129/75–84 mmHg), high normal (130–139/85–89 mmHg), and established hypertension (≥140/90 mmHg), progression to higher BP levels, and increasing BMI were assessed in the Women's Health Study [54]. This study which represents a prospective cohort study of 38172 middle-aged women free of diabetes mellitus and cardiovascular disease at baseline revealed that, after a follow-up of 10 years, 1.4%, 2.9%, 5.7%, and 9.4% of women across the baseline BP categories developed type 2 diabetes mellitus [54]. The risk of incident diabetes mellitus was sevenfold greater in women with established hypertension at baseline compared to those with optimal BP at baseline [54].

Further, this study demonstrated that changes across BP categories was associated with a significant trend of increasing incidence of new-onset diabetes mellitus [54]. Compared to women with stable normal or lower BP levels, in women progression to higher BP levels but within the normotensive range induced a 26% increase, while progression to hypertension was associated with a 64% increased risk of incident diabetes mellitus [54].

Obese women tend to have the highest event rate across all BP categories [54]. The risk of incident diabetes mellitus is 25-fold higher in women with increased BMI (≥30 kg/m^2) compared to those with normal BMI (<25 kg/m^2) [54]. However, BP remains a strong predictor of incident diabetes mellitus within each category of BMI [54].

Several recent reports and clinical studies suggest that inadequately controlled BP in nondiabetic hypertensive patients on antihypertensive medication is a predictor of incident diabetes mellitus [55]. In a large cohort of 1754 nondiabetic hypertensive patients, free of cardiovascular disease, suboptimal BP control was associated with a twofold increased risk of incident diabetes mellitus, independent of age, BMI, baseline BP, or fasting blood glucose [56]. However, the results of the recent SPRINT randomized trial appear to challenge this notion [57]. In this study, the incidence of altered glucose homeostasis (impaired fasting glucose/new-onset diabetes mellitus) was higher in the intensive BP strategy (SBP <120 mmHg) compared with the standard BP strategy (SBP <140 mmHg) [57].

1.4 New-Onset Diabetes Mellitus and Antihypertensive Medications

New-onset diabetes mellitus represents a form of diabetes, usually of the type 2 phenotype, which develops during therapy of different disorders such as hypertension [58]. The natural incidence of new-onset diabetes mellitus in untreated hypertensive patients varies widely across various trials extending from 0.8% to 3.9% [59].

Common major currently clinically used antihypertensive medications fall into four classes: (a) diuretics with all their different target sites, (b) beta-adrenergic receptor blockers (beta blockers), (c) calcium channel antagonists, and (d) renin–angiotensin aldosterone system (RAAS) inhibitors [58].

Numerous studies indicate that the major classes of antihypertensive medications appear to exert differing effects in glycemic control and incidence of diabetes mellitus [58, 60, 61]. Thiazide diuretics and beta blockers are potentially diabetogenic, and calcium channel antagonists appear neutral, while RAAS inhibitors are associated with improvement on glycemic control and may even lower diabetes incidence [61]. The risk of new-onset diabetes mellitus has been reported to be lower with calcium channel antagonists than with beta blockers and thiazide diuretics but higher than with RAS inhibitors [61, 62]. The ALLHAT study evaluated the incidence of new-onset diabetes mellitus in patients randomized to chlorthalidone, amlodipine, and lisinopril. At 4 years, the cumulative incidence of new-onset diabetes mellitus was 11.6% for the chlorthalidone group, as compared with 9.8% for the amlodipine group and 8.1% for patients randomized to lisinopril [63].

Several large-scale clinical trials have demonstrated that thiazide diuretics and beta blockers adversely impair glucose homeostasis predisposing to the development of new-onset diabetes mellitus [62, 63].

In a long-term observational study which involves three large cohorts, Nurses Health Studies I/II and Health Professionals Follow-Up study, the relative risk for incident diabetes mellitus in subjects taking a thiazide diuretic compared to those taking none was 20% higher in older women, 45% higher in younger women, and 36% higher in men [64, 65]. Further, the relative risk of new-onset diabetes mellitus in subjects taking a beta blocker compared to those taking none was 32% greater in older women and 20% greater in men [64, 65].

The risk of incident diabetes mellitus with beta blockers and nondiuretic antihypertensive medications (calcium channel antagonists and RAAS inhibitors) was evaluated in a meta-analysis of 94292 hypertensive subjects [66]. Compared to placebo, beta blockers induced a 33% increase in incidence of new-onset diabetes mellitus [66]. In contrast, compared to beta blockers, calcium channel antagonists and RAAS inhibitors reduced by 21% and 23%, respectively, new-onset diabetes mellitus [66].

Calcium channel antagonists and RAAS inhibitors are considered to have minimal or even no impact on glucose homeostasis [65, 67]. Several clinical studies and trials have demonstrated that administration of these classes of antihypertensive medications are associated with decreased new-onset diabetes mellitus and with RAAS inhibitors, even with improvement in glucose metabolism [68]. In the Intervention as a Goal in Hypertension Treatment (INSIGHT) trial, new-onset diabetes mellitus was slightly but significantly lower in hypertensive patients receiving long-acting nifedipine than in those receiving a low dose of the diuretic co-amilozide (4.3% versus 5.6%) [69].

Increasing evidence suggests that RAAS inhibitors provide a potentially beneficial effect at the incidence of diabetes mellitus [65]. In a meta-analysis, of 72128 nondiabetic subjects at baseline, angiotensin-converting enzyme inhibitor therapy was associated with reduced incidence of new-onset diabetes mellitus compared to controls (OR 0.80 [0.71, 0.91]) irrespective of achieved BP levels at follow-up and compared with beta blockers/diuretics (OR 0.78 [0.65, 0.93]), calcium channel antagonists (OR 0.85 [0.73, 0.99]), and patients with hypertension (OR 0.8 [0.68, 0.93]) [58, 70].

Similarly, in the Heart Outcomes Prevention Evaluation (HOPE) study, in which about 50% of participants had high BP, ramipril, an angiotensin-converting enzyme inhibitor, reduced the incidence of new-onset diabetes mellitus from 5.4% to 3.6%, a 34% decrease, compared to placebo [71].

Angiotensin receptor blockers (ARBs) have also been reported to reduce the occurrence of new-onset diabetes mellitus in hypertensive subjects. In the Candesartan in Heart Failure Assessment of Reduction in Mortality and Morbidity (CHARM) study, candesartan, an ARB, was associated with a reduction in new-onset diabetes mellitus from 7% to 6% (RR 0.78 [0.64–0.95]) [72].

A large cohort of 134967 nondiabetic subjects conducted at the Kaiser Permanente Northwest examined the atherogenic potential of combination antihypertensive medications [73]. This study revealed that exposure to a combination of thiazide diuretic/beta blockers (TD/BB) and thiazide diuretic/calcium channel blockers (TD/CCBs) was associated with a diabetogenic risk of diabetes mellitus with adjusted risks of 1.99 (1.80–2.20) and 1.52 (1.28–1.82), respectively. In contrast, treatment with a combination of a thiazide diuretic/renin–angiotensin system inhibitor (TD/RASI) or beta blockers/renin–angiotensin system inhibitor (BB/RASI) resulted in a negative diabetogenic influence with adjusted risks of diabetes mellitus of 1.08 (0.97–1.20) and 0.98 (0.89–1.09), respectively, suggesting that RASI might inhibit or reduce the diabetogenic risk of thiazide diuretics or beta blockers [73].

Not all antihypertensive medications within the same class possess a similar influence on glycemic control [74, 75].

All loop diuretics have similar efficacy in the treatment of hypertension, but in equipotent doses, they are less effective than thiazides and thiazide-like diuretics. Further, spironolactone, a potassium-sparing diuretic and an aldosterone antagonist, is an effective antihypertensive agent [74]. Both loop diuretics and spironolactone have minimal adverse reactions on glucose metabolism [74].

Some beta-adrenergic agents appear to have minimal deleterious effects on glucose homeostasis [75]. B_1-selective beta blockers with B_2 agonist properties, beta blockers with intrinsic sympathomimetic effects (e.g., acebutolol), and beta blockers with alpha-blocking activity (e.g., carvedilol) are reported not to be associated with incident diabetes mellitus [75].

1.5 Gestational Diabetes Mellitus and Pregnancy-Induced Hypertension Association

Gestational diabetes mellitus and gestational hypertension are the most frequent obstetric disorders during pregnancy [76]. Coexistence of both disorders is associated with significant maternal and fetal complications and poor outcome [76, 77].

Several studies have evaluated the relationship between gestational diabetes mellitus and gestational hypertension. In a study which comprised 215 successive pregnancies in Danish women demonstrated that the frequency of gestational hypertension (defined as SBP ≥140/90 mmHg) was higher in women with gestational diabetes mellitus than in nondiabetic pregnant women (28% versus 10%) [78]. Increased body mass index enhanced the risk of gestational diabetes mellitus and hypertension [76].

A large population-based case control study, using data drawn from electronic records of women who delivered in 1992–1998 and conducted in Washington State, explored the relation between gestational diabetes mellitus and subtypes of gestational hypertension [77]. Gestational diabetes mellitus was associated with a significant 1.5-fold increased risk of severe and mild preeclampsia and 1.4-fold increase in gestational hypertension with a prevalence of 3.9% in women with eclampsia, 4.5% in women with severe preeclampsia, and 4.4% in both women with mild preeclampsia and women with gestational hypertension compared with 2.7% in controls [77]. Afro-American ethnicity and increased body mass index enhanced the risk of gestational diabetes mellitus/hypertension association [77, 79].

1.6 Hypertension—Diabetes Mellitus Coexistence and COVID-19 Relationship

Coronavirus disease 2019 (COVID-19) caused by the novel coronavirus (SARS-CoV-2) is a major global health threat [80, 81]. Mortality and severe outcomes from SARS-CoV-2 have been associated with cardio-cerebrovascular disease, hypertension, and diabetes mellitus [81]. The incidences of hypertension, cardio-cerebrovascular disease, and diabetes mellitus are twofold, threefold, and twofold higher, respectively, in intensive care unit (ICU)/severe cases of COVID-19 than in their non-ICU/severe counterparts [82]. Similarly, in a cohort of COVID-19 cases hospitalized in New York, the most common comorbidities were hypertension (56%), obesity (41.7%), and diabetes mellitus (33.8%) [83].

Data from the onset of the COVID-19 pandemic in China demonstrated that while mortality without comorbidities was 0.9%, it increased to 10.5% with cardio-cerebrovascular disease, to 7.5% with diabetes mellitus, and to 6% with systemic hypertension [83]. In the Lombardy cohort of severe cases of COVID-19 admitted to the ICU, systemic hypertension, diabetes mellitus, and cardiovascular disease were reported with frequencies of 49%, 17%, and 21%, respectively [83].

Several investigations have demonstrated that age, hypertension, diabetes mellitus, and cardiorenal disease aggravate the course and increase the risk of mortality of COVID-19 infection [83, 84]. However, there is no evidence that any class of antihypertensive drugs portends an increase risk or worsening of COVID-19 infection [80]. Conversely, inhibitors of the renin–angiotensin system may be protective [85, 86].

1.7 Conclusion

Coexistent hypertension/diabetes mellitus represents a common serious vasculo-metabolic disorder with a wide occurrence rate. This disorder is multifactorial and is associated with significant risk of macro-/microangiopathic complications and premature mortality. Maintenance of appropriate body weight, achievement of adequate BP, and glycemic control reduce the incidence and may even prevent the development of this disorder in hypertension, diabetes, pregnancy, and COVID-19 infection. Further, inhibitors of RAS may improve the prognosis of COVID-19-infected patients.

References

1. Mancia G. The Association of hypertension and diabetes: prevalence, cardiovascular risk, and protection by blood pressure reduction. Acta Diabetol. 2005;42:S17–25.
2. Ferrannini E, Cushman WC. Diabetes and hypertension: the bad companions. Lancet. 2012;380:601–10.
3. Colussi G, Porto DA, A, Cavarape A. Hypertension and type 2 diabetes: lights and shadows about causality. J Human Hypertens. 2020;34:91–3.
4. Lago RM, Singh PP, Nesto RW. Diabetes and hypertension. Nat Clin Pract Endocrinol Metab. 2007;3:667.
5. Tatsumi Y, Ohkubo T. Hypertension with diabetes: significance from an epidemiologic perspective for Japanese. Hypertens Res. 2017;40:795–806.
6. Kannel WB, Wilson PWF, Zhang TJ. The epidemiology of impaired glucose tolerance and hypertension. Am Heart J. 1991;121:1266–73.

7. Libianto R, Batu D, MacIsaac RJ, Cooper ME, Ekinc EI. Pathophysiological links between diabetes and blood pressure. Can J Cardiol. 2018;34:585–94.
8. Petrie JR, Guzik TJ, Touyz RM. Diabetes, hypertension and cardiovascular disease: clinical insights and vascular mechanisms. Can J Cardiol. 2018;34:575–84.
9. Chen G, McAlister FA, Walker RL, Hemmelgarn BR, Campbell NRC. Cardiovascular outcomes in framingham participants with diabetes: the importance of blood pressure. Hypertension. 2011;57:891–7.
10. Yildiz M, Esenboğa K, Oktay AA. Hypertension and diabetes mellitus: highlights of a complex relationship. Curr Opin Cardiol. 2020;35:397–404.
11. Lai T-S, Curhan GC, Forman JP. Insulin resistance and risk of incident hypertension among men. J Clin Hypertens (Greenwich). 2009;11:483–90.
12. Goff DC Jr, Zaccaro DJ, Haffner SM, Saad MF. Insulin Resistance Atherosclerosis Study. Insulin sensitivity and the risk of incident hypertension: insights from the Insulin Resistance Atherosclerosis Study. Diabetes Care. 2003;26:805–9.
13. Emdin CA, Anderson SG, Woodward M, Rahimi K. Usual blood pressure and risk of new-onset diabetes: evidence from 4.1 million adults and a meta-analysis of prospective studies. J Am Coll Cardiol. 2015;66:1552–62.
14. Lastra G, Syed S, Kurukulasuriya L, Manrique C, Sowers JR. Type 2 diabetes mellitus and hypertension: an update. Endocrinol Metab Clin North Am. 2014;43:103–22.
15. Cheung BMY. The hypertension-diabetes continuum. J Cardiovasc Pharmacol. 2010;55:333–9.
16. Lee H-S, Lee S-S, Hwang I-Y, Park Y-J, Yoon S-H, Han K, et al. Prevalence, awareness, treatment and control of hypertension in adults with diagnosed diabetes: the Fourth Korea National Health and Nutrition Examination Survey (KNHANES IV). J Hum Hypertens. 2013;27:381–7.
17. Shu J, Matarese A, Santulli G. Diabetes, body fat, skeletal muscle, and hypertension: The ominous chiasmus? J Clin Hypertens (Greenwich). 2019;21:239–42.
18. Al-Azzam N, Al-Azzam S, Elsalem L, Karasneh R. Hypertension prevalence and associated factors among patients with diabetes: A retrospective cross-sectional study from Jordan. Ann Med Surg. 2021;61:126–31.
19. Wei GS, Coady SA, Goff DC Jr, Brancati FL, Levy D, Selvin E, et al. Blood pressure and the risk of developing diabetes in African Americans and whites: ARIC, CARDIA, and the Framingham heart study. Diabetes Care. 2011;34:873–9.
20. Krolewski AS, Warram JH, Cupples A, Gorman CK, Szabo AJ, Christlieb AR. Hypertension, orthostatic hypotension and the microvascular complications of diabetes. J Chronic Dis. 1985;38:319–26.
21. Pell S, D'Alonzo CA. Some aspects of hypertension in diabetes mellitus. JAMA. 1967;202:104–10.
22. Barret-Connor E, Criqui MH, Klauber MR, Holdbrook M. Diabetes and hypertension in a community of older adults. Am J Epidemiol. 1981;113:276–84.
23. Tsimihodimos V, Gonzalez-Villalpando C, Meigs JB, Ferrannini E. Hypertension and diabetes: co-prediction and time trajectories. Hypertension. 2018;71:422–8.
24. Ferrannini E, Nannipieri M, Williams K, Gonzales C, Haffner SM, Stern MP. Mode of onset of type 2 diabetes from normal or impaired glucose tolerance. Diabetes. 2004;53:160–5.
25. Simonson DC. Etiology and prevalence of hypertension in diabetic patients. Diabetes Care. 1988;11:821–7.
26. El-Atat F, McFarlane SI, Sowers JR. Diabetes, hypertension, and cardiovascular derangements: pathophysiology and management. Curr Hypertens Rep. 2004;6:215–23.
27. Haratz S, Tanne D. Diabetes, hyperglycemia and the management of cerebrovascular disease. Curr Opin Neurol. 2011;24:81–8.
28. TODAY Study Group. Rapid rise in hypertension and nephropathy in youth with type 2 diabetes: the TODAY clinical trial. Diabetes Care. 2013;36:1735–41.
29. Geva M, Shlomai G, Berkovich A, Maor E, Leibowitz A, Tenenbaum A, et al. The association between fasting plasma glucose and glycated hemoglobin in the prediabetes range and future development of hypertension. Cardiovasc Diabetol. 2019;18:53. https://doi.org/10.1186/s12933-019-0859-4.

30. Colhoun HM, Dong W, Barakat MT, Mather HM, Poulter NR. The scope for cardiovascular disease risk factor intervention among people with diabetes mellitus in England: a population-based analysis from the Health Surveys for England 1991-94. Diabet Med. 1999;16:35–40.
31. Muntner P, Whelton PK, Woodward M, Carey RM. A comparison of the 2017 American College of Cardiology/American Heart Association Blood Pressure guideline and the 2017 American Diabetes Association Diabetes and Hypertension Position Statement for U.S. adults with diabetes. Diabetes Care. 2018;41:2322–9.
32. Kabakov E, Norymberg C, Osher E, Koffler M, Tordjman K, Greenman Y, et al. Prevalence of hypertension in type 2 diabetes mellitus: impact of the tightening definition of high blood pressure and association with confounding risk factors. J Cardiometab Syndr. 2006;1:95–101.
33. Katsimardou A, Imprialos K, Stavropoulos K, Sachinidis A, Doumas M, Athyros VG. Treatment strategies for hypertension in patients with type 1 diabetes. Expert Opin Pharmacother. 2020;21:1241–52.
34. Diaz-Valencia PA, Bougnères P, Valleron A-J. Global epidemiology of type 1 diabetes in young adults and adults: a systematic review. BMC Public Health. 2015;15:255.
35. Downie ML, Ulrich EH, Noone DG. An update on hypertension in children with type 1 diabetes. Can J Diabetes. 2018;42:199–204.
36. Christlieb AR, Warram JH, Krolewski AS, Busick EJ, Ganda OP, Asmal AC, et al. Hypertension: The major risk factor in juvenile-onset insulin-dependent diabetics. Diabetes. 1981;30(Suppl 2):90–6.
37. Nørgaard K, Feldt-Rasmussen B, Borch-Johnsen K, Saelan H, Deckert T. Prevalence of hypertension in type 1 (insulin-dependent) diabetes mellitus. Diabetologia. 1990;33:407–10.
38. Holl RW, Pavlovic M, Heinze E, Thon A. Circadian blood pressure during the early course of type 1 diabetes. Analysis of 1,011 ambulatory blood pressure recordings in 354 adolescents and young adults. Diabetes Care. 1999;22:1151–7.
39. Lurbe A, Redón J, Pascual JM, Tacons J, Alvarez V, Batlle DC. Altered blood pressure during sleep in normotensive subjects with type I diabetes. Hypertension. 1993;21:227–35.
40. Mateo-Gavira I, Vílchez-López FJ, García-Palacios MV, Carral-San Laureano F, Jiménez-Carmona S, Aguilar-Diosdado M. Nocturnal blood pressure is associated with the progression of microvascular complications and hypertension in patients with type 1 diabetes mellitus. J Diabetes Complications. 2016;30:1326–32.
41. Sampanis C, Zamboulis C. Arterial hypertension in diabetes mellitus: from theory to clinical practice. Hippokratia. 2008;12:74–80.
42. Collado-Mesa F, Colhoun HM, Stevens LK, Boavida J, Ferriss JB, Karamanos B, et al. Prevalence and management of hypertension in type 1 diabetes mellitus in Europe: the EURODIAB IDDM Complications Study. Diabet Med. 1999;16:41–9.
43. Rodriguez BL, Dabelea D, Liese AD, Fujimoto W, Waitzfelder B, Liu L, et al. Prevalence and correlates of elevated blood pressure in youth with diabetes mellitus: the SEARCH for diabetes in youth study. J Pediatr. 2010;157:245–51.
44. Maahs DM, Kinney GL, Wadwa P, Snell-Bergeon JK, Dabelea D, Hokanson J, et al. Hypertension prevalence, awareness, treatment, and control in an adult type 1 diabetes population and a comparable general population. Diabetes Care. 2005;28:301–6.
45. García-Puig J, Ruilope LM, Luque M, Fernández J, Ortega R, Dal-Ré R, et al. Glucose metabolism in patients with essential hypertension. Am J Med. 2006;119:318–26.
46. Ohkubo T, Kikuya M, Metoki H, Asayama K, Obara T, Hashimoto J, et al. Prognosis of "masked" hypertension and "white-coat" hypertension detected by 24-h ambulatory blood pressure monitoring 10-year follow-up from the Ohasama study. J Am Coll Cardiol. 2005;46:508–15.
47. Kadowaki S, Okamura T, Hozawa A, Kadowaki T, Kadota A, Murakami Y, et al. Relationship of elevated casual blood glucose level with coronary heart disease, cardiovascular disease and all-cause mortality in a representative sample of the Japanese population. NIPPON DATA80. Diabetologia. 2008;51:575–82.
48. Mitchell BD, Stern MP, Haffner SM, Hazuda HP, Patterson JK. Risk factors for cardiovascular mortality in Mexican Americans and non-Hispanic whites. San Antonio Heart Study. Am J Epidemiol. 1990;131:423–33.

49. de Simone G, Devereux RB, Chinali M, Lee ET, Galloway JM, Barac A, et al. Diabetes and incident heart failure in hypertensive and normotensive participants of the Strong Heart Study. J Hypertens. 2010;28:353–60.
50. Diaz KM, Veerabhadrappa P, Brown MD, Whited MC, Dubbert PM, Hickson DA. Prevalence, determinants, and clinical significance of masked hypertension in a population-based sample of African Americans: the Jackson Heart study. Am J Hypertens. 2015;28:900–8.
51. Mancusi C, Izzo R, di Gioia G, Losi MA, Barbato E, Morisco C. Insulin resistance the hinge between hypertension and type 2 diabetes. High Blood Press Cardiovasc Prev. 2020;27:515–26.
52. Lin J, Thompson TJ, Cheng YJ, Zhuo X, Zhang P, Gregg E, et al. Projection of the future diabetes burden in the United States through 2060. Population Health Metrics. 2018;16:9. https://doi.org/10.1186/s12963-018-0166-4.
53. Mancia G, Bombelli M, Facchetti R, Madotto F, Quarti-Trevano F, Grassi G, et al. Increased long-term risk of new-onset diabetes mellitus in white-coat and masked Hypertension. J Hypertens. 2009;27:1672–8.
54. Conen D, Ridker PM, Mora S, Buring JE, Glynn RJ. Blood pressure and risk of developing type 2 diabetes mellitus: the Women's Health Study. Eur Heart J. 2007;28:2937–43.
55. Arcucci O, de Simone G, Izzo R, Rozza F, Chinali M, Rao M-A-E, et al. Association of suboptimal blood pressure control with body size and metabolic abnormalities. J Hypertens. 2007;25:2296–300.
56. Izzo R, de Simone G, Chinali M, Iaccarino G, Trimarco V, Rozza F, et al. Insufficient control of blood pressure and incident diabetes. Diabetes Care. 2009;32:845–50.
57. Roumie CL, Hung AM, Russell GB, Basile J, Kreider KE, Nord J, et al. Blood pressure control and the association with diabetes mellitus incidence: results from SPRINT randomized trial. Hypertension. 2020;75:331–8.
58. Li Z, Li Y, Liu Y, Xu W, Wang Q. Comparative risk of new-onset diabetes mellitus for antihypertensive drugs: a network meta-analysis. J Clin Hypertens (Greenwich). 2017;19:1348–56.
59. Verdecchia P, Angeli F, Reboldi GP, Gattobigio R. New onset of diabetes in treated hypertensive patients. Curr Hypertens Rep. 2005;7:174–9.
60. Vasisht KP, Bakris G. New onset diabetes: can it be delayed? J Hum Hypertens. 2008;22:517–9.
61. Asfaha S, Padwal R. Antihypertensive drugs and incidence of type 2 diabetes: evidence and implications for clinical practice. Curr Hypertens Rep. 2005;7:314–22.
62. Elliott WJ, Meyer PM. Incident diabetes in clinical trials of antihypertensive drugs: a network meta-analysis. Lancet. 2007;369:201–7.
63. ALLHAT Officers and Coordinators for the ALLHAT Collaborative Research Group. Major outcomes in high-risk hypertensive patients randomized to angiotensin-converting enzyme inhibitor or calcium channel blocker vs diuretic: The Antihypertensive and Lipid-Lowering Treatment to Prevent Heart Attack Trial (ALLHAT). JAMA. 2002;288:2981–97.
64. Taylor EN, Hu FB, Curhan GC. Antihypertensive medications and the risk of incident type 2 diabetes. Diabetes Care. 2006;29:1065–70.
65. Sarafidis PA, Bakris GL. Antihypertensive therapy and the risk of new-onset diabetes. Diabetes Care. 2006;29:1167–9.
66. Bangalore S, Parkar S, Grossman E, Messerli FH. A meta-analysis of 94,492 patients with hypertension treated with beta blockers to determine the risk of new-onset diabetes mellitus. Am J Cardiol. 2007;100:1254–62.
67. Lithell HO. Effect of antihypertensive drugs on insulin, glucose, and lipid metabolism. Diabetes Care. 1991;14:203–9.
68. Abuissa H, Jones PG, Marso SP, O'Keefe JH Jr. Angiotensin-converting enzyme inhibitors or angiotensin receptor blockers for prevention of type 2 diabetes: a meta-analysis of randomized clinical trials. J Am Coll Cardiol. 2005;46:821–6.
69. Brown MJ, Palmer CR, Castaigne A, de Leeuw PW, Mancia G, Rosenthal T, et al. Morbidity and mortality in patients randomised to double-blind treatment with a long-acting calcium-channel blocker or diuretic in the International Nifedipine GITS study: Intervention as a Goal in Hypertension Treatment (INSIGHT). Lancet. 2000;356:366–72.

70. Geng DF, Jin DM, Wu W, Liang WD, Wang JF. Angiotensin converting enzyme inhibitors for prevention of new-onset type 2 diabetes mellitus: a meta-analysis of 72,128 patients. Int J Cardiol. 2013;167:2605–10.
71. Yusuf S, Sleight P, Pogue J, Bosch J, Davies R, Dagenais G; Heart Outcomes Prevention Evaluation Study Investigators. Effects of an angiotensin-converting-enzyme inhibitor, ramipril, on cardiovascular events in high-risk patients. N Engl J Med. 2000;342:145–53.
72. Pfeffer MA, Swedberg K, Granger CB, Held P, McMurray JJV, Michelson EL, et al. Effects of candesartan on mortality and morbidity in patients with chronic heart failure: the CHARM-Overall programme. Lancet. 2003;362:759–66.
73. Cooper-DeHoff RM, Bird ST, Nichols GA, Delaney JA, Winterstein AG. Antihypertensive drug class interactions and risk for incident diabetes: a nested case-control study. J Am Heart Assoc. 2013;2:e000125. https://doi.org/10.1161/JAHA.113.000125.
74. Houston MC. The effects of antihypertensive drugs on glucose intolerance in hypertensive nondiabetics and diabetics. Am Heart J. 1988;115:640–56.
75. Karnes JH, Cooper-DeHoff RM. Antihypertensive medications: benefits of blood pressure lowering and hazards of metabolic effects. Expert Rev Cardiovasc Ther. 2009;7:689–702.
76. Sibai BM, Ross MG. Hypertension in gestational diabetes mellitus: pathophysiology and long-term consequences. J Matern Fetal Neonatal Med. 2010;23:229–33.
77. Bryson CL, Ioannou GN, Rulyak SJ, Critchlow C. Association between gestational diabetes and pregnancy-induced hypertension. Am J Epidemiol. 2003;158:1148–53.
78. Kvetny J, Poulsen HF. Incidence of gestational hypertension in gestational diabetes mellitus. Arch Gynecol Obstet. 2003;267:153–7.
79. Kuller LH, Catov J. Invited commentary: Gestational hypertension and diabetes – a major public health concern. Am J Epidemiol. 2017;186:1125–8.
80. Bauer AZ, Gore R, Sama SR, Rosiello R, Garber L, Sundaresan D, et al. Hypertension, medications, and risk of severe Covid-19: a Massachusetts community-based observational study. J Clin Hypertens (Greenwich). 2021;23:21–7.
81. Richardson S, Hirsch JS, Narasimhan M, Crawford JM, McGinn T, Davidson KW, et al. Presenting characteristics, comorbidities, and outcomes among 5700 patients hospitalized with COVID-19 in the New York City área. JAMA. 2020;323:2052–9.
82. Tascioglu D, Yalta K, Yetkin E. Hypertension and diabetes mellitus in patients with COVID 19: a viewpoint on mortality. Cardiovasc Endocrinol Metab. 2020;9:108–9.
83. Sanchez CMC, Roque JCG, Rodriguez LGG, Leon LAG, Velazquez JMG, Escanaverino IA, et al. Arterial hypertension and diabetes mellitus as risk factors in the evolution of patients with COVID-19. Am J Lab Medicine. 2021;6:22–6.
84. Shah H, Khan MSH, Dhurandhar NV, Hegde V. The triumvirate: why hypertension, obesity, and diabetes are risk factors for adverse effects in patients with COVID-19. Acta Diabetol. 2021;58:831–43.
85. Zhang P, Zhu L, Cai J, Lei F, Qin JJ, Xie J, et al. Association of inpatient use of angiotensin-converting enzyme inhibitors and angiotensin II receptor blockers with mortality among patients with hypertension hospitalized with COVID-19. Circ Res. 2020;126:1671–81.
86. Kjeldsen SE, Narkiewicz K, Burnier M, Oparil S. Potential protective effects of antihypertensive treatments during the Covid-19 pandemic: from inhibitors of the renin-angiotensin system to beta-adrenergic receptor blockers. Blood Press. 2021;30:1–3.

Part II

Epidemiological Aspects

Blood Pressure Disorders in Diabetic Children and Adolescents

2

Empar Lurbe

2.1 Characteristics of Blood Pressure Measurement in the Pediatric Age

Although evolving technology can offer the means to measure complex functions of cardiovascular (CV) physiology, it is worth emphasizing that the basic phenotype remains blood pressure (BP). According to the Guidelines on Hypertension in Children and Adolescents [1, 2], office BP is the basis for hypertension (HTN) screening and diagnosis in type 1 diabetes mellitus (T1DM) and type 2 diabetes mellitus (T2DM), and despite the increasing use of out-of-office BP, the former remains indispensable for defining BP phenotypes. Office BP is widely available, permitting universal and regular screening for HTN in the pediatric age, which is recommended from the age of 3 years [1–3]. Hypertension has been defined in childhood as systolic and/or diastolic BP ≥95th percentile of age-, sex-, and height-adjusted normative BP data [4], due to the absence of data on future adverse outcomes such as heart failure, stroke, or kidney failure in the pediatric age. The definition of HTN in children and adolescents by current guidelines [1, 2, 5] are shown in Table 2.1.

Office BP, despite its persistence as the main reference for BP classification and HTN management, may offer limited insights into the variability and patterns of BP under normal living conditions, and then ambulatory blood pressure monitoring (ABPM) needs to be considered. The role of ABPM over 24 h in T1DM and

E. Lurbe (✉)
Pediatric Department, Consorcio Hospital General, University of Valencia, Valencia, Spain

CIBER Fisiopatología Obesidad y Nutrición (CB06/03), Instituto de Salud Carlos III, Madrid, Spain
e-mail: empar.lurbe@uv.es

A. E. Berbari, G. Mancia (eds.), *Blood Pressure Disorders in Diabetes Mellitus*, Updates in Hypertension and Cardiovascular Protection,
https://doi.org/10.1007/978-3-031-13009-0_2

Table 2.1 Definition of arterial hypertension in children and adolescents by current guidelines

Guidelines	Year	Method	Hypertension threshold
European Society of Hypertension [1]	2016	Age–sex–height nomograms (based on the Fourth Report)[a]	≥95th percentile (≥16 years) ≥140/90 mmHg
American Academy of Pediatrics [2]	2017	New age–sex–height nomograms (includes only normal-weight children from the Fourth Report)	≥95th percentile (≥13 years) ≥130/80 mmHg
Hypertension Canada Guidelines [5]	2020	New age–sex–height nomograms (includes only normal-weight children from the Fourth Report)	≥95th percentile ≥120/80 mmHg (6–11 years) ≥130/85 mmHg (12–17 years)

[a]National High Blood Pressure Education Working Group on High Blood Pressure in Children and Adolescents. The fourth report on the diagnosis, evaluation, and treatment of high blood pressure in children and adolescents. Pediatrics. 2004;114:555–76. [19]

T2DM subjects has been increasingly recognized and further reinforced by the latest pediatric guidelines [1, 2]. It offers a more representative observation of BP levels, not only allowing for a large number of measurements in a regular life environment, both day and night, during activity and while at rest, and furthermore assesses the circadian profile [6]. There is a consensus that the diagnosis of HTN by office BP should be confirmed by ABPM to avoid treatment for white coat HTN [1, 2, 5].

According to the reference values of ABPM for children [7], the 95th percentile is the threshold to define ambulatory HTN. However, using the 95th percentile, values will be higher than ABPM thresholds for adults. Considering this, it is not reasonable for ABPM to establish higher thresholds for children than for adults, and therefore, it makes sense to use the lower of either the 95th percentile from normative ABPM data or the accepted criteria for adults (24-h mean 130/80 mmHg; daytime mean 135/85 mmHg; nocturnal mean 125/75 mmHg) [1, 8].

The prognostic value of ABPM in T1DM was first demonstrated in a cohort of normotensive type 1 diabetics in whom an increase in systolic BP during nighttime antedated the development of persistent microalbuminuria, indicating an early stage of diabetic nephropathy [9]. Ambulatory BP monitoring is now considered a predictive tool in the risk assessment of nephropathy in T1DM [1, 2]. Abnormal circadian variability has been associated with diabetes, both T1DM and T2DM [1, 2, 6].

The role of home BP monitoring in T1DM and T2DM during the process of HTN diagnosis is not currently supported. However, it is recommended for follow-up when strict BP control is mandatory [1, 2]. This finding supports the recommendations for its use in T1DM and T2DM hypertensive patients as a complementary tool for pharmacological treatment dose titration, assessment of BP control, and timing of repeated ABPM.

2.2 Type 1 Diabetes Mellitus

2.2.1 Introduction

Type 1 diabetes mellitus in children and adolescents is a chronic disease which has been on the rise, with an increase in the number of diagnosed children. In 2002–2003, the incidence of youth-onset T1DM in the USA was 19.5 cases/100,000 youths per year, increasing to 21.7 cases/100,000 youths per year in 2011–2012 [10]. This trend has also been observed in other parts of the world [11], and recent estimates from the International Diabetes Federation indicate that worldwide there are over 1 million individuals younger than 19 years living with T1DM, with around 100,000 new cases every year in this age group [12]. Therefore, T1DM has consistently remained one of the most common chronic diseases affecting children and adolescents and represents a substantial clinical and public health burden.

Concern has been raised about the increasing incidence of T1DM in very young children [11] as this can lead to higher rates of long-term complications such as retinal and kidney disease, neuropathy, and cardiovascular disease (CVD). People with early-onset T1DM have up to a 30 times higher probability of severe cardiovascular outcomes as compared to healthy individuals, being the leading cause of morbidity and mortality [13–15]. Overall, those diagnosed with T1DM before 10 years of age die an average of 16 years earlier, and the lives of those diagnosed at age 26–30 years are shortened by an average of 10 years [16].

Despite guidelines recommendation on the importance of screening for abnormalities in BP, this is still suboptimal, remaining both underdiagnosed and perhaps also undertreated [17]. The relevance is based on the importance of early detection and treatment of BP abnormalities that together with adequate glycemic control is paramount to prevent further micro- and macrovascular complications [18].

2.2.2 Prevalence of Hypertension and Risk Factors

Hypertension in childhood is not an uncommon condition, with a prevalence of approximately 4% [4]. Alarmingly, the prevalence of HTN in patients with T1DM is higher than in the general population. Several studies have assessed the prevalence of HTN in T1DM; however, important discrepancies exist due to different methodologies, normative data, and thresholds applied to define HTN. Recently, the prevalence of HTN in pediatric patients with T1DM in Germany, Austria, and Luxemburg according to different criteria has been assessed. The prevalence largely differs, applying the references of the Fourth Report [19], those corresponding to the German Health Interview and Examination Survey for Children and Adolescents (KIGGS) [20] or the American Academy of Pediatrics [2]. The AAP criteria result in a significant increase in HTN prevalence in older adolescents with T1DM, more evident in boys [21].

Data coming from the SEARCH study including T1DM subjects aged 3–17 years reflects the prevalence of office HTN at 5.9% [22]. Similarly, 4% of patients were hypertensive in a Norwegian study where the mean age was 13 years [23]. This prevalence increased up to 10% in a large cohort of youth [24] and it was even higher in a study performed in Australian children and adolescents where it was documented at 16% [25].

It is relevant to identify the presence of HTN not only because it is a risk factor for CVD [26] but also due to the impact on diabetes-related micro- and macrovascular complications [27]. Starting at an early age, these complications can have an even greater detrimental impact. Hypertension was linked to arterial stiffness [28] and elevated carotid intima media thickness (CIMT) [29] in the SEARCH study. Applying 24-h ABPM, an increment in CIMT was associated with loss of nighttime systolic BP dipping [30]. The most recent studies assessing the prevalence of office HTN [21, 31–36] are shown in Table 2.2.

Risk factors for HTN in youths with T1DM have been identified including poor glycemic control, overweight and obesity, and genetic predisposition to HTN. In the Diabetes Prospective Follow-up DPV study [21], the increase in nocturnal BP was related to insulin dosage, female sex, body mass index (BMI), glycated hemoglobin (HbA1c), and diabetes duration.

Obesity is a well-known risk factor for the development of HTN. The prevalence of pediatric overweight and obesity is increasing globally, from 4% in 1975 to 18% in 2016, an estimated 340 million youth [37]. A similar trend has been observed in youth with T1DM and is likely related to factors such as decreased physical activity and sleep and increased high-calorie food consumption and aggressive insulin management to target euglycemia [38–40]. Weight gain is a concern in patients with T1DM and may be associated with an increased risk of HTN and vascular complications.

The Diabetes Control and Complications Trial (DCCT) demonstrated that weight gain and obesity were associated with intensive insulin management. Excess weight gain in DCCT is associated with sustained increase in central adiposity, insulin resistance, progressive rise in BP, and dyslipidemia [41]. Based on these results, efforts should be made to limit excess weight gain that accompanies intensive glucose treatment in T1DM patients. Not only obesity, but also body fat distribution needs to be taken into consideration. In fact, results from the SEARCH study indicated that waist-to-height ratio as a marker of central obesity may be an important factor for HTN in youths and young adults with T1DM [36]. Despite the ever-increasing prevalence of obesity in youth and its potential additive effect on early markers of CV and kidney health in T1DM, only a few studies have evaluated its impact. Among these studies, a higher prevalence of HTN, dyslipidemia, and microalbuminuria in obese as compared to nonobese have been identified [39, 42].

Additional risk factors for HTN should be considered including family history of HTN, high sodium intake, smoking, other drugs used, obstructive sleep apnea, and the presence of renal impairment in addition to microalbuminuria [1, 2].

Table 2.2 Hypertension in children and adolescents with type 1 and type 2 diabetes mellitus

Reference	Design	Subjects	Results	Conclusions
Type 1 diabetes				
Ahmadizar F [31]	Retrospective Clinical Practice Research Datalink 1988–2014	3728 youth <19 years and 18 513 healthy children age-/gender-matched	HTN was present in 35% T1DM vs 11% controls 20 years after the onset of diabetes.	Annual prevalence rates of HTN in T1DM was significantly higher as compared to controls.
Urbina EM [32]	The SEARCH for Diabetes in Youth Study	1809 youth <20 years At onset and after 5 years	Higher BP, adiposity, and lipid levels (CVRFs) were related to T1DM.	In T1DM, persistent poor glycemic control and higher levels of traditional CVRFs are independently associated with arterial aging.
Stankute I [33]	Joint Lithuanian-Swiss project "Genetic Diabetes in Lithuania	883 patients <25 years of age	HTN more prevalent in overweight and obese T1DM and associated with microvascular complications.	The frequency of cardiovascular risk factors is high in youth with T1DM and associated with diabetes duration, obesity, and metabolic control.
Dost A [21]	Prospective	74,677 children and adolescents 5–20 years	HTN was seen in 44.1%, 29.5%, and 26.5% by AAP 2017, KiGGS, and fourth report guidelines, respectively.	Use of AAP 2017 results in a significant increase in the prevalence of HTN in teenagers.
Krepel Volsky S [34]	Retrospective 1998–2013	170 T1DM <18 years	HTN 25%, overweight/obesity 40%, and dyslipidemia 60% at the last visit.	Clustering of CM risk factors was more prominent in young adults diagnosed with T1DM in early childhood.
Type 1 vs type 2 diabetes				
Tommerdahl [35]	Cross-sectional	284 youth 12–21 years T1DM, T2DM, and controls	HTN prevalence in T1DM and obese.	Youth with T1DM and obesity correlates with a less favorable cardiovascular and kidney risk profile, nearly approximating the phenotype of youth with T2DM.
Koebnick C [36]	The SEARCH for Diabetes in Youth Study	1518 (T1DM) 177 (T2DM)	HTN in youths with T2DM was 35.6% vs 14.8% in T1DM.	Increasing central obesity was a major risk factor for incident HTN.

HTN Hypertension, *T1DM* Type 1 diabetes mellitus, *BP* Blood pressure, *CVRF* Cardiovascular risk factors, *AAP* American Academy of Pediatrics, *CM* Cardiometabolic, *T2DM* Type 2 diabetes mellitus

2.2.3 Pathophysiology of HTN

There are several pathophysiologic mechanisms involved in the development of HTN in T1DM patients driven by hyperglycemia, low-grade inflammation, endothelial dysfunction, and activation of both the sympathetic nervous system and the renin–angiotensin-aldosterone system (RAAS) [43].

The mechanisms underpinning endothelial dysfunction are still not entirely understood and likely multifactorial [44], with hyperglycemia being considered a primary mediator. According to the DCCT, after age, hyperglycemia was the major factor responsible for the increase in CVD. An increment on the production of reactive oxygen species reduces the bioavailability of nitric oxide, thereby leading to endothelial dysfunction, vasoconstriction, and increased peripheral resistance [45] contributing to the increase in BP.

Activation of the RAAS is well known to be a cause of HTN [46]. Via activation of the AT-I receptor, angiotensin II induces aldosterone synthesis in the adrenal cortex and also stimulates antidiuretic hormone release which in turn acts to increase renal absorption of sodium. Angiotensin II also directly causes vasoconstriction and strengthens the activity of the sympathetic nervous system [47].

The role of inflammatory cytokines merits to be commented on since it plays a part in the pathogenesis of endothelial dysfunction and HTN. In a study including children with T1DM, hyperglycemia was related to an elevation in the proinflammatory cytokines IL-1alfa, IL-4, and IL-6 [48].

In the presence of diabetes, the kidney progressively deteriorates not only at the glomerular level but also in the tubule-interstitial structures that finally reduce the renal blood flow and the glomerular filtration rate as it progresses to chronic kidney disease and finally to end-stage renal disease [49, 50].

2.3 Type 2 Diabetes Mellitus

2.3.1 Introduction

In the past few decades, the incidence of youth-onset T2DM has progressively increased, likely due to the rising rates of childhood obesity, representing a substantial clinical and public health burden. Before the mid-1990s, only few children with DM (1%–2%) were classified as having T2DM. However, as obesity has increased in recent years, the incidence of T2DM has increased to 25%–45% of all youth diagnosed with DM [51, 52]. In order to better recognize the current and potential burden of diabetes, it is important to know its incidence and the trends over the years. In 2002–2003, the incidence of youth-onset T2DM in the USA was 9.0 cases/100,000 youths per year increasing to 12.5 cases/100,000 youths per year in 2011–2012 [10]. This trend has been observed in other parts of the world [51], and conventionally considered a disease of the middle and older age, it is increasingly diagnosed at a younger age with an average age onset at 13 years [53].

Pediatric T2DM is an aggressive disease with a greater risk of end-organ damage and comorbidities than pediatric T1DM or adult-onset T2DM [54–56]. The long-term prognosis of youth with T2DM is not currently known, but it is estimated that these youths may have a loss of up to 15 years of life expectancy and increased risk of serious health complications by the time they reach their fourth decade, depending on their level of glycemic control and CV risk factors. Within organ damage, the kidneys are notable early targets of T2DM representing the main microvascular diabetic complication and associated with the highest rates of excess mortality observed in youth with T2DM, despite a shorter disease duration than T1DM and comparable glycemic control [57, 58]. Taking all of these into consideration, early and sustained interventions to delay T2DM onset and improve blood glucose control and CV risk profiles are essential to reduce morbidity and mortality.

2.3.2 Prevalence of Hypertension and Risk Factors

Research has demonstrated that many youths with T2DM already have early signs of microvascular and macrovascular complications, HTN, dyslipidemia, and fatty liver [59, 60]. According to the Treatment Options for Type 2 Diabetes in Adolescents and Youth, the TODAY trial, with 704 youths with T2DM with less than 2 years of follow-up, 26% had systolic HTN, 80% had low HDL cholesterol levels, 10% had high triglyceride levels, and most were obese [61].

The prevalence of HTN and albuminuria as a marker of incipient renal damage is not well known in patients with T2DM. Recently, a systematic review and meta-analysis focused on the prevalence of HTN and albuminuria in these patients has been published [62]. Thirty-one studies including 4363 patients with T2DM reported the prevalence of HTN. The pooled prevalence was 25% with a high heterogeneity across the studies due to the different definitions of HTN. When assessing the prevalence of HTN in different racial groups, Indigenous and Pacific Islander youth have the highest rates of HTN when compared to other groups. Likewise, there were high levels of heterogeneity in terms of the prevalence of albuminuria. The review also demonstrated that between one and four pediatric patients with T2DM had albuminuria. However, very few studies report the persistence of albuminuria despite being a key criterion for albuminuria diagnosis [18, 63, 64]. These data have several important implications; early renal damage in T2DM exerts a much higher burden than that seen in children with T1DM [58, 65].

Recently interesting data have been published from the TODAY clinical trial [66] in which participants were 10–17 years of age and had a duration of T2DM of less than 2 years. Participants were followed for an average of 3.9 years and the mean time since the diagnosis of T2DM was 13 ± 1.8 years. The prevalence of HTN at the time of enrollment was 19.2%, and the cumulative incidence at 15 years was 67.5%. Dyslipidemia was present in 20.8% of patients at baseline and the cumulative incidence at 15 years was 51.65%. In this cohort, the accumulation of complications was tightly associated with hyperglycemia, insulin resistance, HTN, and dyslipidemia [66].

2.3.3 Pathophysiology

The pathogenesis of the long-term vascular complications associated with early-onset T2DM is not well characterized, although the mechanisms for the development of complications may be similar to T2DM in adults. Recent evidence suggests an accelerated course in people with early-onset T2DM [55]. Proposed for more aggressive evolution included a longer lifetime exposure to the adverse diabetic milieu and/or early-onset T2DM representing an inherently more aggressive metabolic phenotype with rapid onset of beta cell failure and insulin resistance compared with late-onset disease [67].

Several are the mechanisms implicated in the progression of micro- and macrovascular disease in youth with T2DM. Insulin resistance is independently associated with a higher risk of HTN in the general population [68, 69]. The link between insulin resistance and HTN can be partially explained by the fact that this condition can induce renal sodium retention [70] and overactivity of the RAAS [71, 72] and sympathetic nervous system [73]. These elements stimulate peripheral and renal vascular resistance as well as an increment in intravascular volume [73, 74].

Adipose tissue plays an important role in the increment of risk. A misbalance of substances derived from the visceral adipose tissue contributes to the development of both high BP levels and insulin resistance. The imbalance is reflected by an increment in the secretion of leptin, advanced glycation end products (AGEs), plasminogen activator inhibition (PAI I), and other inflammatory cytokines; on the other hand, a reduction in adiponectin is present. In addition, a partial resistance of leptin and the decreased secretion of adiponectin produce vasoconstriction and insulin resistance. Concurrently, an increase in angiotensin II and PAI-I produces vasoconstriction and a procoagulant state. Moreover, cytokines produce vascular inflammation and insulin resistance in the liver and in the muscle [75].

Finally, it is worthy to comment about the implication of the kidney in the development of abnormalities associated with T2DM. The pathophysiology of a diabetic kidney disease is multifactorial and is characterized by progression to chronic kidney disease and end-stage kidney disease. When renal damage develops, micro- and macrovascular diseases progress rapidly. The mechanisms implicated are similar to those describe in T1DM [49, 50].

2.4 Management

Considering the impact of T1DM and T2DM on the early development of CVD, pediatricians and staff involved in the diagnosis and management of patients with DM need to be more aware of the modifiable risk factors and devastating consequences.

2.4.1 Lifestyle Approach

In patients with T1DM, lifestyle interventions include dietary modification and increased exercise, if appropriate, aimed at weight control. Lifestyle modification is recommended in all children and adolescents with T2DM. Concerning lifestyle habits, exercise can improve other risk factors such as HTN, dyslipidemia, and insulin resistance [1]. Moderate to vigorous exercise is recommended, even though some youth with T2DM may have impaired exercise capacity and may need a personalized approach [76]. Unfortunately, these recommendations are often difficult to attain, especially in adolescents, when newfound freedoms from parental oversight and other social pressures often have negative effects on diet or other health behaviors [77]. In order to meet these recommendations, the goals need to be established realistically, tailored to individual and family characteristics, involving the family as partners in the behavioral change process, providing educational support and materials [1, 2]. Motivational interviewing approaches have been shown to be effective in reducing weight in the clinical trial setting [78, 79] and should be considered when treating diabetic children and adolescents with overweight or obesity. Those subjects treated with lifestyle measures should be followed up regularly to monitor the effect of treatment and to encourage continued adherence.

2.4.2 Optimal Treatment

Targeting euglycemia and minimizing CV risk factors remain the cornerstones in the management of T1DM and T2DM. Poor glycemic control is the primary modifiable risk factor for CVD in youth with T1DM. Subsequently, the primary focus of management is to improve glycemic control by intensifying insulin therapy [80]. Despite advances in insulin treatment, over 75% of adolescents do not reach recommended targets for HbA1c [81]. Metformin deserves special attention; although there is no strong evidence in terms of glycemic control, its use has been shown to lead to small reductions in total daily insulin dose and weight [82]. Prospective studies are required to provide additional evidence before metformin could be recommended as an adjunct therapy in T1DM.

The optimal treatment in youth with T2DM includes both medical and lifestyle interventions [83]. For glycemic control, the TODAY trial is the largest randomized controlled trial available to examine treatment of T2DM in youth [84]. In this national multisite study, 669 participants from 10 to 17 years of age with recently diagnosed T2DM (mean 7.8 months) were randomized to either monotherapy with metformin, metformin plus rosiglitazone, or metformin plus a family lifestyle intervention program focused on weight loss through modification of eating habits and physical activity. Over a mean follow-up of 3.9 years, metformin monotherapy provided durable glycemic control in only half the participants. Interestingly, the addition of rosiglitazone was superior to metformin alone in maintaining glycemic control. Whether the effect shown in the study is specific for rosiglitazone, a more general effect of thiazolidinediones, or a feature of combination therapy, is unclear. This issue is of particular interest due to the fact that rosiglitazone has a restricted status for use in pediatric patients in both the USA and Europe and is not yet considered a medication option for youth with T2DM. The addition of an intensive lifestyle intervention was not more effective than metformin alone [84]. This study reinforced the idea of premature and rapid deterioration of beta cell function in T2DM.

In childhood and adolescence, there is a need for aggressive prevention and eventual combination treatment or insulin therapy early after diagnoses, frequently within a few years [51]. Insulin therapy is recommended when children and adolescents present with ketosis or ketoacidosis, or when random blood glucose levels are ≥250 mg/dL or HbA1C levels >9% at diagnosis. In youth, insulin is also added to metformin therapy when glycemic goals are not maintained by metformin alone. Glucagon-like peptide (GLP-1) is part of the family of incretin hormones, and in 2019, the FDA approved liraglutide for the management of T2DM in children older than 10 years of age. Metformin, insulin, and GLP1 receptor agonists are the only medications approved for diabetes treatment in youth [84, 85].

2.4.3 Therapeutic Approach for HTN

Blood pressure treatment includes defining the BP goal, how achievement of this goal will be checked, and which class of antihypertensive drug will be more appropriate. The BP goal for diabetic patients is a relevant and controversial issue in children. Because of some evidence that youths with T1DM or T2DM develop early atherosclerotic lesions before the age of 30 years [86], the American Heart Association suggests the BP goal to be lower than the 90th percentile for age, sex, and height [87]. A post hoc analysis of a trial on T1DM suggests that a lower BP target may be beneficial in reducing urinary albumin excretion (UAE) and the risk of developing proteinuria [88]. The goals recommended by the European Society of HTN Guidelines in Children and Adolescents are shown in Table 2.3. The goal below the 90th percentile (or below 130/80 mmHg at age 16 years and above) may be achieved in both children and adolescents, if provided treatment is well tolerated [1].

At the time of selecting the antihypertensive drugs, two key issues should be considered; the most relevant is to achieve the BP goal over 24 h and the necessity to reduce salt intake due to the sodium-dependent component of HTN in diabetes [89]. Lifestyle interventions are important because they can delay the need for drug treatment or complement the BP-lowering effect of antihypertensive treatment. Nevertheless, if the lifestyle changes do not achieve an appropriate control within 3–6 months of initiation, pharmacologic treatment should be considered [90] usually with an angiotensin-converting enzyme inhibitor (ACE) or angiotensin receptor blocker (ARB) due to their associated effects of reduced microalbuminuria and reduced cardiovascular and renal outcomes [1, 90]. The introduction of these drugs needs to be accompanied with reproductive counseling due to the potential teratogenicity of both drug classes.

Monotherapy with long-acting drugs that can be dosed once daily is preferred, but additional agents may be needed to reach optimal BP levels. Antihypertensive drugs in children and adolescents are generally prescribed in a stepped-care manner. The child is initially started on the lowest recommended dose, and then the dose is

Table 2.3 Antihypertensive medications for use in children and adolescents

Class of drug	Drug	Recommended starting dose (per day)	Maximal dose (per day)	Dosing interval
ACE inhibitors	Benazepril	0.2 mg/kg up to 10 mg	0.6 mg/kg up to 40 mg	Daily
	Captopril	0.3–0.5 mg/kg	6 mg/kg	Twice/three times daily
	Enalapril	0.08–0.6 mg/kg		Daily
	Fosinopril	0.1–0.6 mg/kg	40 mg	Daily
	Lisinopril	0.08–0.6 mg/kg	0.6 mg/kg up to 40 mg	Daily
	Ramipril	2.5–6 mg		Daily
ARBs	Candesartan	0.16–0.5 mg/kg		Daily
	Irbesartan	75–150 mg	300 mg	Daily
	Losartan	0.7 mg/kg up to 50 mg	1.4 mg/kg up to 100 mg	Daily
	Valsartan	0.4 mg/kg	40–80 mg	Daily
Calcium channel blockers	Amlodipine	0.06–0.3 mg/kg	5–10 mg	Daily
	Felodipine	2.5 mg	10 mg	Daily
	Nifedipine (extended release form)	0.25–0.5 mg/kg	3 mg/kg up to 120 mg	Daily to twice daily
Diuretics	Furosemide	0.5–2 mg/kg	6 mg/kg	Daily to twice daily

Adapted from the European Society of Hypertension Guidelines in Children and Adolescents [1]

increased until the highest recommended dose is reached at which point a second drug from a different class should be added, and so on, until the desired BP goal is reached [1, 2]. Dihydropyridine calcium channel blockers are suitable for the combination [1, 2, 91]. Henle loop diuretics should be used if a reduction in glomerular filtration rate exists [1, 2, 91]. The antihypertensive medications for use in children and adolescents are shown in Table 2.3.

Finally, treated children require periodic laboratory monitoring to assess for electrolyte disturbances and other medication-related toxicities. Once medication treatment has been initiated, it is important to ensure that BP goals are accomplished and maintained. An ACE inhibitor or an ARB is also recommended for those patients with persistently elevated urinary albumin to creatinine ratio >30 mg/g [90].

Once started on antihypertensive medications, patients should be seen frequently at first, perhaps every 6–8 weeks, so that drugs can be titrated, and then less often once a stable regimen is established and the BP goal is attained. Home BP monitoring is a useful tool to help determine response to medication treatment. Repeated ABPM may also be used and is mandatory in children and adolescents with HTN [1, 2]. The BP goals for office, ABPM, and home BP are shown in Table 2.4.

Only one study has been performed reporting the impact of ACE inhibitors and statins in T1DM, the AdDIT study. This is the first large randomized clinical trial evaluating the use of ACE inhibitors and statins during adolescence to protect

Table 2.4 Blood pressure goal in hypertensive children and adolescents (for office, home, and 24-h ambulatory blood pressure measurements)

General hypertensive population[a]	
Blood pressure goal	<95th pct is recommended <90th pct should be considered
Diabetes type 1 and type 2[b]	
Blood pressure goal	<90th pct is recommended <75th pct is recommended in children with nonproteinuric CKD <50th pct is recommended in children with proteinuric CKD
Children with CKD[c]	
Blood pressure goal	<75th pct is recommended in children with nonproteinuric CKD <50th pct is recommended in children with proteinuric CKD

Adapted from the ESH Guidelines on Hypertension in Children and Adolescents [1]
[a]In subjects aged 16 years or older, the adult cutoff values are used, 140/90 mmHg
[b]In subjects aged 16 years or older, the adult cutoff values are used, 130/80 mmHg or 125/75 mmHg with proteinuric CKD
[c]In subjects aged 16 years or older, the adult cutoff values are used, 130/80 mmHg or 125/75 mmHg with proteinuric CKD

against T1DM vascular complications [92]. The trial showed that statins can reduce exposure to high lipid levels and ACE inhibitors can reduce new cases of microalbuminuria. These changes could potentially lead to protection against future complications [92]. In addition, a post hoc analysis of a subgroup of the trial population showed that ACE inhibitors improved endothelial function (assessed by flow-mediated vasodilation) in high-risk adolescents transitioning through puberty and may therefore offer long-term cardiorenal benefits during this potentially critical time period for the development of CVD [93].

2.5 Conclusions

During the last decades, the prevalence of diabetes (T1DM and T2DM) in youth has increased, representing a substantial clinical and public health burden considering the fact that there are many challenges in disease management as well as risks of acute and chronic complications.

Diabetes in children and adolescents is associated with long-term complications that result in increased morbidity and mortality. In addition to issues with glycemic control, it is important to screen and meet targets for BP, obesity, dyslipidemia, and smoking. Even though during the past decades there have been improvements regarding the management of diabetes, wide gaps still exist in the ability to standardize clinical care and decrease disease-associated complications and burdens. To improve CVD outcomes and related mortality, a whole life approach starting from childhood is mandatory.

Hypertension, being one of the main risk factors for developing CVD over the life span, needs to be taken into careful consideration in terms of early diagnosis and management. Hypertension in children with diabetes is probably more prevalent than previously realized and can be associated with subtle patterns that would only become apparent on a 24-h ABPM.

References

1. Lurbe E, Agabiti-Rosei E, Cruickshank JK, Dominiczak A, Erdine S, Hirth A, et al. 2016 European Society of Hypertension guidelines for the management of high blood pressure in children and adolescents. J Hypertens. 2016;34:1887–920.
2. Flynn JT, Kaelber DC, Baker-Smith CM, Blowey D, Carroll AE, Daniels SR, et al. Subcommittee on Screening and Management of High Blood Pressure in Children. Clinical practice guideline for screening and management of high blood pressure in children and adolescents. Pediatrics. 2017;140:e20171904.
3. Falkner B, Lurbe E. The USPSTF call to inaction on blood pressure screening in children and adolescents. Pediatr Nephrol. 2021;36:1327–9.
4. Falkner B, Lurbe E. Primary hypertension beginning in childhood and risk for future cardiovascular disease. J Pediatr. 2021;238:16–25.
5. Rabi DM, McBrien KA, Sapir-Pichhadze R, Nakhla M, Ahmed SB, Dumanski SM, et al. Hypertension Canada's 2020 comprehensive guidelines for the prevention, diagnosis, risk assessment, and treatment of hypertension in adults and children. Can J Cardiol. 2020;36:596–624.
6. Lurbe A, Redón J, Pascual JM, Tacons J, Alvarez V, Batlle DC. Altered blood pressure during sleep in normotensive subjects with type I diabetes. Hypertension. 1993;21:227–35.
7. Wühl E, Witte K, Soergel M, Mehls O, Schaefer F, German Working Group on Pediatric Hypertension. Distribution of 24-h ambulatory blood pressure in children: normalized reference values and role of body dimensions. J Hypertens. 2002;20:1995–2007. Erratum in: J Hypertens. 2003; 21:2205–6.
8. Stergiou GS, Palatini P, Parati G, O'Brien E, Januszewicz A, Lurbe E, et al. European Society of Hypertension Council and the European Society of Hypertension Working Group on Blood Pressure Monitoring and Cardiovascular Variability. 2021 European Society of Hypertension practice guidelines for office and out-of-office blood pressure measurement. J Hypertens. 2021;39:1293–302.
9. Lurbe E, Redon J, Kesani A, Pascual JM, Tacons J, Alvarez V, et al. Increase in nocturnal blood pressure and progression to microalbuminuria in type 1 diabetes. N Engl J Med. 2002;347:797–805.
10. Mayer-Davis EJ, Lawrence JM, Dabelea D, Divers J, Isom S, Dolan L, et al. SEARCH for Diabetes in Youth Study. Incidence trends of type 1 and type 2 diabetes among youths, 2002-2012. N Engl J Med. 2017;376:1419–29.
11. Patterson CC, Harjutsalo V, Rosenbauer J, Neu A, Cinek O, Skrivarhaug T, et al. Trends and cyclical variation in the incidence of childhood type 1 diabetes in 26 European centres in the 25 year period 1989-2013: a multicentre prospective registration study. Diabetologia. 2019;62:408–17.
12. IDF Diabetes Atlas 9th edition 2019. Available online at: https://diabetesatlas.org/atlas/ninth-edition/. Accessed 9 Dec 2021.
13. Lind M, Svensson A, Kosiborod M, Gudbjörnsdottir S, Pivodic A, Wedel H, et al. Glycemic control and excess mortality in type 1 diabetes. N Engl J Med. 2014;371:1972–82.
14. Epidemiology of Diabetes Interventions and Complications (EDIC). Design, implementation, and preliminary results of a long-term follow-up of the Diabetes Control and Complications Trial cohort. Diabetes Care. 1999;22:99–111.

15. Soedamah-Muthu SS, Chaturvedi N, Witte D, Stevens LK, Porta M, Fuller JH, For the EURODIAB Prospective Complications Study Group. Relationship between risk factors and mortality in type 1 diabetic patients in Europe: the EURODIAB Prospective Complications Study (PCS). Diabetes Care. 2008;31:1360–6.
16. Livingstone SJ, Levin D, Looker HC, Lindsay RS, Wild SH, Joss N, et al. Scottish Diabetes Research Network Epidemiology Group; Scottish Renal Registry. Estimated life expectancy in a Scottish cohort with type 1 diabetes, 2008-2010. JAMA. 2015;313:37–44.
17. Nambam B, DuBose SN, Nathan BM, Beck RW, Maahs DM, Wadwa RP, et al. T1D Exchange Clinic Network. Therapeutic inertia: underdiagnosed and undertreated hypertension in children participating in the T1D Exchange Clinic Registry. Pediatr Diabetes. 2016;17:15–20.
18. American Diabetes Association. 13. Children and adolescents: standards of medical care in diabetes-2019. Diabetes Care. 2019;42(Suppl 1):S148–64.
19. National High Blood Pressure Education Program Working Group on High Blood Pressure in Children and Adolescents. The fourth report on the diagnosis, evaluation, and treatment of high blood pressure in children and adolescents. Pediatrics. 2004;114:555–76.
20. Neuhauser HK, Thamm M, Ellert U, Hense HW, Rosario AS. Blood pressure percentiles by age and height from nonoverweight children and adolescents in Germany. Pediatrics. 2011;127:e978–88.
21. Dost A, Bechtold S, Fink K, Bonfig W, Wiemann D, Kapellen TM, et al. Initiative DPV-Science and the German Diabetes Research Center. 2017 American Academy of Pediatrics Clinical Practice Guideline: impact on prevalence of arterial hypertension in children and adolescents with type 1 diabetes. Diabetes Care. 2020;43:1311–8.
22. Rodriguez BL, Dabelea D, Liese AD, Fujimoto W, Waitzfelder B, Liu L, et al. SEARCH Study Group. Prevalence and correlates of elevated blood pressure in youth with diabetes mellitus: the SEARCH for diabetes in youth study. J Pediatr. 2010;157:245–51.
23. Margeirsdottir HD, Larsen JR, Brunborg C, Overby NC, Dahl-Jørgensen K. Norwegian Study Group for Childhood Diabetes. High prevalence of cardiovascular risk factors in children and adolescents with type 1 diabetes: a population-based study. Diabetologia. 2008;51:554–61.
24. Schwab KO, Doerfer J, Hecker W, Grulich-Henn J, Wiemann D, Kordonouri O, et al. DPV Initiative of the German Working Group for Pediatric Diabetology. Spectrum and prevalence of atherogenic risk factors in 27,358 children, adolescents, and young adults with type 1 diabetes: cross-sectional data from the German diabetes documentation and quality management system (DPV). Diabetes Care. 2006;29:218–25.
25. Eppens MC, Craig ME, Cusumano J, Hing S, Chan AK, Howard NJ, et al. Prevalence of diabetes complications in adolescents with type 2 compared with type 1 diabetes. Diabetes Care. 2006;29:1300–6.
26. De Ferranti SD, De Boer IH, Fonseca V, Fox CS, Golden SH, Lavie CJ, et al. Type 1 diabetes mellitus and cardiovascular disease: a scientific statement from the American Heart Association and American Diabetes Association. Diabetes Care. 2014;37:2843–63.
27. Katsimardou A, Imprialos K, Stavropoulos K, Sachinidis A, Doumas M, Athyros VG. Treatment strategies for hypertension in patients with type 1 diabetes. Expert Opin Pharmacother. 2020;21:1241–52.
28. Dabelea D, Talton JW, D'Agostino R Jr, Wadwa RP, Urbina EM, Dolan LM, et al. Cardiovascular risk factors are associated with increased arterial stiffness in youth with type 1 diabetes: the SEARCH CVD study. Diabetes Care. 2013;36:3938–43.
29. Urbina EM, Dabelea D, D'Agostino RB Jr, Shah AS, Dolan LM, Hamman RF, et al. Effect of type 1 diabetes on carotid structure and function in adolescents and young adults. Diabetes Care. 2013;36:2597–9.
30. Atabek ME, Akyürek N, Eklioglu BS, Alp H. Impaired systolic blood dipping and nocturnal hypertension: an independent predictor of carotid intima–media thickness in type 1 diabetic patients. J Diabetes Complicat. 2014;28:51–5.
31. Ahmadizar F, Souverein P, de Boer A, Maitland-van der Zee AH. Undertreatment of hypertension and hypercholesterolaemia in children and adolescents with type 1 diabetes: long-term

follow-up on time trends in the occurrence of cardiovascular disease, risk factors and medications use. Br J Clin Pharmacol. 2018;84:776–85.
32. Urbina EM, Isom S, Bell RA, Bowlby DA, D'Agostino R Jr, Daniels SR, et al. SEARCH for Diabetes in Youth Study Group. Burden of cardiovascular risk factors over time and arterial stiffness in youth with type 1 diabetes mellitus: the SEARCH for Diabetes in Youth Study. J Am Heart Assoc. 2019;8:e010150.
33. Stankute I, Dobrovolskiene R, Danyte E, Razanskaite-Virbickiene D, Jasinskiene E, Mockeviciene G, et al. Factors affecting cardiovascular risk in children, adolescents, and young adults with type 1 diabetes. J Diabetes Res. 2019;2019:9134280.
34. Krepel Volsky S, Shalitin S, Fridman E, Yackobovitch-Gavan M, Lazar L, Bello R, et al. Dyslipidemia and cardiovascular disease risk factors in patients with type 1 diabetes: a single-center experience. World J Diabetes. 2021;12:56–68.
35. Tommerdahl KL, Baumgartner K, Schäfer M, Bjornstad P, Melena I, Hegemann S, et al. Impact of obesity on measures of cardiovascular and kidney health in youth with type 1 diabetes as compared with youth with type 2 diabetes. Diabetes Care. 2021;44:795–803.
36. Koebnick C, Imperatore G, Jensen ET, Stafford JM, Shah AS, Mottl AK, et al. Progression to hypertension in youth and young adults with type 1 or type 2 diabetes: the SEARCH for Diabetes in Youth Study. J Clin Hypertens. 2020;22:888–96.
37. Prevalence of Obesity. World Obesity Federation: https://www.worldobesity.org/about/about-obesity/prevalence-of-obesity. Last visited 15 Nov 2021.
38. DuBose SN, Hermann JM, Tamborlane WV, Beck RW, Dost A, DiMeglio LA, et al. Obesity in youth with type 1 diabetes in Germany, Austria, and the United States. J Pediatr. 2015;167:627–32.e4.
39. Redondo MJ, Foster NC, Libman IM, Mehta SN, Hathway JM, Bethin KE, et al. Prevalence of cardiovascular risk factors in youth with type 1 diabetes and elevated body mass index. Acta Diabetol. 2015;53:271–7.
40. Phelan H, Clapin H, Bruns L, Cameron FJ, Cotterill AM, Couper JJ, et al. The Australasian Diabetes Data Network: first national audit of children and adolescents with type 1 diabetes. Med J. 2017;206:121–5.
41. Purnell JQ, Hokanson JE, Marcovina SM, Steffes MW, Cleary PA, Brunzell JD. Effect of excessive weight gain with intensive therapy of type 1 diabetes on lipid levels and blood pressure: results from the DCCT. Diabetes Control and Complications Trial. JAMA. 1998;280:140–6. Erratum in: JAMA. 1998;280:1484.
42. Marlow AL, Rowe CW, Anderson D, Wynne K, King BR, Howley P, et al. Young children, adolescent girls and women with type 1 diabetes are more overweight and obese than reference populations, and this is associated with increased cardiovascular risk factors. Diabet Med. 2019;36:1487–93.
43. Downie ML, Ulrich EH, Noone DG. An update on hypertension in children with type 1 diabetes. Can J Diabetes. 2018;42:199–204.
44. Roberts AC, Porter KE. Cellular and molecular mechanisms of endothelial dysfunction in diabetes. Diab Vasc Dis Res. 2013;10:472–82.
45. Son SM. Reactive oxygen and nitrogen species in pathogenesis of vascular complications of diabetes. Diabetes Metab J. 2012;36:190–8.
46. Te Riet L, van Esch JH, Roks AJ, van den Meiracker AH, Danser AH. Hypertension: renin-angiotensin-aldosterone system alterations. Circ Res. 2015;116:960–75.
47. Di Marzio D, Mohn A, Mokini ZH, Giannini C, Chiarelli F. Macroangiopathy in adults and children with diabetes: from molecular mechanisms to vascular damage (part 1). Horm Metab Res. 2006;38:691–705.
48. Rosa JS, Flores RL, Oliver SR, Pontello AM, Zaldivar FP, Galassetti PR. Sustained IL-1alpha, IL-4, and IL-6 elevations following correction of hyperglycemia in children with type 1 diabetes mellitus. Pediatr Diabetes. 2008;9:9–16.
49. Anders HJ, Huber TB, Isermann B, Schiffer M. CKD in diabetes: diabetic kidney disease versus nondiabetic kidney disease. Nat Rev Nephrol. 2018;14:361–77.

50. Gilbert RE. Proximal tubulopathy: prime mover and key therapeutic target in diabetic kidney disease. Diabetes. 2017;66:791–800.
51. Pulgaron ER, Delamater AM. Obesity and type 2 diabetes in children: epidemiology and treatment. Curr Diab Rep. 2014;14:508.
52. Kaufman F. Type 2 diabetes in youth: rates, antecedents, treatment, problems and prevention. Pediatr Diabetes. 2007;8:4–6.
53. Rosenbloom AL, Silverstein JH, Amemiya S, Zeitler P, Klingensmith G. ISPAD clinical practice consensus guidelines 2006-2007. Type 2 diabetes mellitus in the child and adolescent. Pediatr Diabetes. 2009;9:512–26.
54. Nanayakkara N, Curtis AJ, Heritier S, Gadowski AM, Pavkov ME, Kenealy T, et al. Impact of age at type 2 diabetes mellitus diagnosis on mortality and vascular complications: systematic review and meta-analyses. Diabetologia. 2021;64:275–87.
55. Song SH, Hardisty CA. Early-onset type 2 diabetes mellitus: an increasing phenomenon of elevated cardiovascular risk. Expert Rev Cardiovasc Ther. 2008;6:315–22.
56. Sullivan MD, Anderson RT, Aron D, Atkinson HH, Bastien A, Chen GJ, et al. ACCORD Study Group. Health-related quality of life and cost-effectiveness components of the Action to Control Cardiovascular Risk in Diabetes (ACCORD) trial: rationale and design. Am J Cardiol. 2007;99:90i–102i.
57. Afkarian M. Diabetic kidney disease in children and adolescents. Pediatr Nephrol. 2015;30:65–74.
58. Constantino MI, Molyneaux L, Limacher-Gisler F, Al-Saeed A, Luo C, Wu T, et al. Long-term complications and mortality in young-onset diabetes: type 2 diabetes is more hazardous and lethal than type 1 diabetes. Diabetes Care. 2013;36:3863–9.
59. Dean HJ, Sellers EA. Comorbidities and microvascular complications of type 2 diabetes in children and adolescents. Pediatr Diabetes. 2007;8(Suppl 9):35–41.
60. Pinhas-Hamiel O, Zeitler P. Acute and chronic complications of type 2 diabetes mellitus in children and adolescents. Lancet. 2007;369:1823–31.
61. Copeland KC, Zeitler P, Geffner M, Guandalini C, Higgins J, Hirst K, et al. for the TODAY Study Group. Characteristics of adolescents and youth with recent-onset type 2 diabetes: The TODAY cohort at baseline. J Clin Endocrinol Metab. 2011;96:159–67.
62. Cioana M, Deng J, Hou M, Nadarajah A, Qiu Y, Chen SSJ, et al. Prevalence of hypertension and albuminuria in pediatric type 2 diabetes: a systematic review and meta-analysis. JAMA Netw Open. 2021;4:e216069.
63. Dart AB, Sellers EA, Martens PJ, Rigatto C, Brownell MD, Dean HJ. High burden of kidney disease in youth-onset type 2 diabetes. Diabetes Care. 2012;35:1265–71.
64. Panagiotopoulos C, Hadjiyannakis S, Henderson M. Diabetes Canada Clinical Practice Guidelines Expert Committee. Type 2 diabetes in children and adolescents. Can J Diabetes. 2018;42(suppl 1):S247–54.
65. Maahs DM, Snively BM, Bell RA, Dolan L, Hirsch I, Imperatore G, et al. Higher prevalence of elevated albumin excretion in youth with type 2 than type 1 diabetes: the SEARCH for Diabetes in Youth study. Diabetes Care. 2007;30:2593–8.
66. TODAY Study Group, Bjornstad P, Drews KL, Caprio S, Gubitosi-Klug R, Nathan DM, Tesfaldet B, et al. Long-term complications in youth-onset type 2 diabetes. N Engl J Med. 2021;385:416–26.
67. Gungor N, Hannon T, Libman I, Bacha F, Arslanian S. Type 2 diabetes mellitus in youth: the complete picture to date. Pediatr Clin North Am. 2005;52:1579–609.
68. Amatruda M, Gembillo G, Giuffrida AE, Santoro D, Conti G. The aggressive diabetic kidney disease in youth-onset type 2 diabetes: pathogenetic mechanisms and potential therapies. Medicina (Kaunas). 2021;57:868.
69. Wang F, Han L, Hu D. Fasting insulin, insulin resistance and risk of hypertension in the general population: a meta-analysis. Clin Chim Acta. 2017;464:57–63.
70. DeFronzo RA. The effect of insulin on renal sodium metabolism. A review with clinical implications. Diabetologia. 1981;21:165–71.

71. Nickenig G, Röling J, Strehlow K, Schnabel P, Böhm M. Insulin induces upregulation of vascular AT1 receptor gene expression by posttranscriptional mechanisms. Circulation. 1998;98:2453–60.
72. Fonseca VA. Insulin resistance, diabetes, hypertension, and renin-angiotensin system inhibition: Reducing risk for CV disease. J Clin Hypertens. 2006;8:713–20.
73. Anderson EA, Hoffman RP, Balon TW, Sinkey CA, Mark AL. Hyperinsulinemia produces both sympathetic neural activation and vasodilation in normal humans. J Clin Investig. 1991;87:2246–52.
74. Busija DW, Miller AW, Katakam P, Erdös B. Insulin resistance and associated dysfunction of resistance vessels and arterial hypertension. Minerva Med. 2005;96:223–32.
75. Chait A, den Hartigh LJ. Adipose tissue distribution, inflammation and its metabolic consequences, including diabetes and cardiovascular disease. Front Cardiovasc Med. 2020;7:22.
76. Narasimhan S, Weinstock RS. Youth-onset type 2 diabetes mellitus: lessons learned from the TODAY study. Mayo Clin Proc. 2014;89:806–16.
77. Cameron FJ, Garvey K, Hood KK, Acerini CL, Codner E. ISPAD clinical practice consensus guidelines 2018: diabetes in adolescence. Pediatr Diabetes. 2018;19:250–61.
78. Davoli AM, Broccoli S, Bonvicini L, Fabbri A, Ferrari E, D'Angelo S, et al. Pediatrician-led motivational interviewing to treat overweight children: an RCT. Pediatrics. 2013;132:e1236–46.
79. Broccoli S, Davoli AM, Bonvicini L, Fabbri A, Ferrari E, Montagna G, et al. Motivational interviewing to treat overweight children: 24-month follow-up of a randomized controlled trial. Pediatrics. 2016;137(1):e20151979.
80. Donaghue KC, Marcovecchio ML, Wadwa RP, Chew EY, Wong TY, Calliari LE, et al. ISPAD Clinical Practice Consensus Guidelines 2018: microvascular and macrovascular complications in children and adolescents. Pediatr Diabetes. 2018;19:262–74.
81. Foster NC, Beck RW, Miller KM, Clements MA, Rickels MR, DiMeglio LA, et al. State of type 1 diabetes management and outcomes from the T1D exchange in 2016–2018. Diabetes Technol Ther. 2019;21:66–72.
82. Al Khalifah RA, Alnhdi A, Alghar H, Alanazi M, Florez ID. The effect of adding metformin to insulin therapy for type 1 diabetes mellitus children: a systematic review and meta-analysis. Pediatr Diabetes. 2017;18:664–7.
83. George MM, Copeland KC. Current treatment options for type 2 diabetes mellitus in youth: today's realities and lessons from the TODAY study. Curr Diab Rep. 2013;13:72–80.
84. The TODAY Study Group. A clinical trial to maintain glycemic control in youth with type 2 diabetes. N Engl J Med. 2012;366:2247–56.
85. Piani F, Reinicke T, Borghi C, Tommerdahl KL, Cara-Fuentes G, Johnson RJ, et al. Acute kidney injury in pediatric diabetic kidney disease. Front Pediatr. 2021;9:668033.
86. Expert Panel on Integrated Guidelines for Cardiovascular Health and Risk Reduction in Children and Adolescents. National Heart, Lung, and Blood Institute. Expert panel on integrated guidelines for cardiovascular health and risk reduction in children and adolescents: summary report. Pediatrics. 2011;128:S213–56.
87. Maahs DM, Daniels SR, de Ferranti SD, Dichek HL, Flynn J, Goldstein BI, et al. American Heart Association Atherosclerosis, Hypertension and Obesity in Youth Committee of the Council on Cardiovascular Disease in the Young, Council on Clinical Cardiology, Council on Cardiovascular and Stroke Nursing, Council for High Blood Pressure Research, and Council on Lifestyle and Cardiometabolic Health. Cardiovascular disease risk factors in youth with diabetes mellitus: a scientific statement from the American Heart Association. Circulation. 2014;130:1532–58.
88. de Boer IH, Rue TC, Cleary PA, Lachin JM, Molitch ME, Steffes MW, et al. Diabetes Control and Complications Trial/Epidemiology of Diabetes Interventions and Complications Study Research Group. Long-term renal outcomes of patients with type 1 diabetes mellitus and microalbuminuria: an analysis of the Diabetes Control and Complications Trial/Epidemiology of Diabetes Interventions and Complications cohort. Arch Intern Med. 2011;171:412–20.
89. Giunti S, Barit D, Cooper ME. Diabetic nephropathy: from mechanisms to rational therapies. Minerva Med. 2006;97:241–62.

90. American Diabetes Association. 13. Children and adolescents: standards of medical care in diabetes-2021. Diabetes Care. 2021;44(Suppl 1):S180–99.
91. Williams B, Mancia G, Spiering W, Agabiti Rosei E, Azizi M, Burnier M, et al; List of authors/ Task force members. 2018 practice guidelines for the management of arterial hypertension of the European Society of Hypertension and the European Society of Cardiology: ESH/ESC Task Force for the Management of Arterial Hypertension. J Hypertens. 2018;36:2284–309.
92. Marcovecchio ML, Chiesa ST, Bond S, Daneman D, Dawson S, Donaghue KC, et al. AdDIT Study Group. ACE inhibitors and statins in adolescents with type 1 diabetes. N Engl J Med. 2017;377:1733–45.
93. Chiesa ST, Marcovecchio ML, Benitez-Aguirre P, Cameron FJ, Craig ME, Couper JJ, et al. Adolescent Type 1 Diabetes Cardio-Renal Intervention Trial (AdDIT) Study Group. Vascular effects of ACE (Angiotensin-Converting Enzyme) inhibitors and statins in adolescents with type 1 diabetes. Hypertension. 2020;76:1734–43.

Hypertension and Type 2 Diabetes

3

Josep Redon and Fernando Martinez

3.1 Introduction

Type 2 diabetes mellitus (T2DM), defined by the criteria of hyperglycemia, increased glycosylated hemoglobin (HbA1c) levels, or both, is a common multifactorial disease with an elevated prevalence. It is characterized by dysregulation of carbohydrate, lipid, and protein metabolism, as a consequence of insulin resistance, impaired insulin secretion, or a combination of both. Diabetes mellitus (DM) affects over 350 million people worldwide and it is expected that the prevalence will increase by 60% by the year 2035 [1], with another one billion people being prediabetic who may eventually end up with full-blown diabetes [2]. The disorder is rapidly increasing in both developed and developing countries associated with a modern lifestyle. T2DM is seen all over the world; however, large differences in prevalence exist among ethnic populations. Specifically, the Western Pacific, Southeast Asia, Middle East, and Europe have a higher prevalence. T2DM conveys many adverse consequences, and it is estimated that having T2DM reduces life expectancy by up to 10 years, the main cause of mortality being cardiovascular disease [3].

The relationship of T2DM with hypertension (HTN) has been recognized as having common causal links and relevant bidirectional consequences [4]. The

J. Redon (✉)
Cardiovascular and Renal Research Group, INCLIVA Research Institute, University of Valencia, Valencia, Spain

CIBERObn Carlos III Institute, Madrid, Spain
e-mail: josep.redon@uv.es

F. Martinez
Cardiovascular and Renal Research Group, INCLIVA Research Institute, University of Valencia, Valencia, Spain

Internal Medicine Hospital Clínico de Valencia, Valencia, Spain

A. E. Berbari, G. Mancia (eds.), *Blood Pressure Disorders in Diabetes Mellitus*, Updates in Hypertension and Cardiovascular Protection,
https://doi.org/10.1007/978-3-031-13009-0_3

relationship between HTN and diabetes is complex since both of them share causal factors, obesity being the most common link between them. Furthermore, in the last decades, pharmacological treatments initially used to reduce blood pressure (BP) or blood glucose have demonstrated to be beneficial in the treatment of both HTN and T2DM [5, 6].

In the present chapter, an overview of the epidemiology, mechanisms, consequences, and therapeutic approaches is presented.

3.2 Epidemiology of Hypertension in T2DM

Prevalence rates of HTN in T2DM are high throughout the world. T2DM increases with age and is normally a disease of the adult and elderly population; however, the prevalence in people below 40 years of age is already increasing due to the obesity epidemic. At the time of diagnosis of T2DM, at least 30–40% of patients are hypertensive, and the prevalence increases progressively to 75% in diabetics with more than 15 years of living with the disease [7]. An example of the prevalence of HTN in diabetes across age can be seen with data from the Mediterranean Region [8], as shown in Fig. 3.1. Relevance of the association is also observed when considering that around 30% of diabetics are among patients with HTN attended to at a hypertension clinic (Fig. 3.2).

Hypertension is also becoming relevant in adolescents with T2DM as it is associated with obesity. In this young population, the TODAY study identified that HTN was present in up to 11% of subjects at the beginning of the study and progressively increased to 33.8% in early adult life [9].

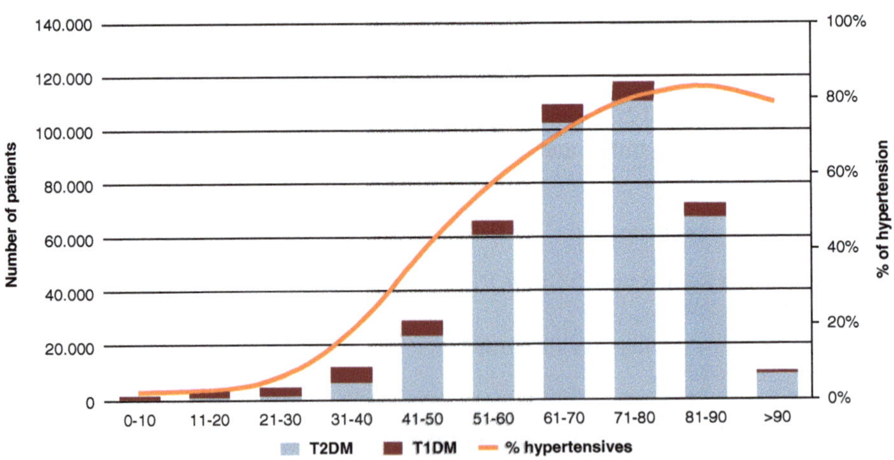

Fig. 3.1 Prevalence of HTN in diabetic subjects ($N = 422949$)

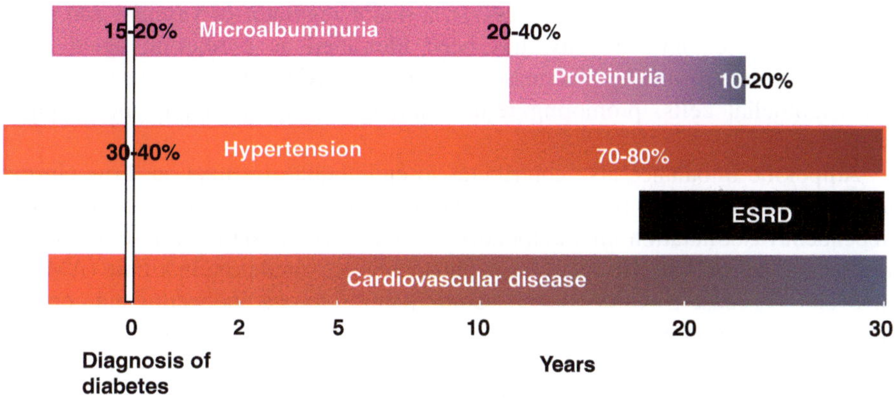

Fig. 3.2 Natural history of HTN in T2DM

3.3 Mechanisms of BP Elevation in T2DM

Many mechanisms have been proposed to explain why hypertension and T2DM coexist in the same individuals. While many of the mechanisms underlying the development of T2DM are the same that produce HTN, others are the result of organic alterations produced by the micro- and macrovascular impact of T2DM [10]. The main driving mechanisms are maladaptive endothelial dysfunction, RAAS and sympathetic overactivity, abnormal sodium handling, renal dysfunction, and vascular stiffness [11]. These mechanisms initiate and develop due to the interaction of hyperglycemia, insulin resistance, angiotensin II, aldosterone, adipokine, oxidative stress, low-grade inflammation, dietary sodium and potassium intake, excessive caloric intake, a sedentary lifestyle, and innate and adaptive immunity among others [12].

3.3.1 Endothelial Dysfunction

Hyperglycemia and insulin resistance result in a decrease in sensitivity or responsiveness to the metabolic actions of insulin and decreased normal vascular actions of insulin, in turn promoting vasoconstriction and reducing vasodilatory capacity. Both elevated blood glucose and insulin resistance increment the burden of reactive oxygen species (ROS), reducing nitric oxide (NO) and uncoupling endothelial nitric oxide synthase (eNOS) which produce superoxide, increasing endothelin (ET-1) and NADPH oxidase [13]. Vasoconstriction reduces the lumen of vessels which increments peripheral resistance. Likewise, enhanced remodeling and vascular wall stiffness further contribute to the increment of peripheral resistance. Recently, the role of glucocorticoid kinase 1 (SGK-1), a major regulator of vascular and renal sodium (Na^+) channel activity, has been identified as a relevant agent [14]. Aldosterone and insulin both increase the activity of SGK-1 that upturns Na^+ flux in the endothelial cells, promoting remodeling of the cytoskeleton and vascular stiffening.

Adipokine imbalance also contributes to endothelial dysfunction. Low plasma adiponectin levels have been shown to be associated with impaired endothelium-dependent vasodilatation since adiponectin increases NO by a PI-3 kinase-dependent mechanism as well as activity of monophosphate-activated protein kinase (AMPK) or cyclooxygenase-2 (COX-2) [15]. Consequently, hypoadiponectinemia contributes to the development of obesity-related hypertension via a direct effect on the vasculature. In contrast, leptin elevation stimulates oxidative stress, inflammation, thrombosis, and arterial stiffness [16].

Other physiological mechanisms of endothelial function in the resistant arteries are also affected such as flow-mediated vasodilatation and myogenic reactivity to blood pressure increment [17].

3.3.2 RAAS Overactivity

The RAAS, exerts actions not only through an endocrine and systemic manner, but also paracrine and autocrine, at tissular levels [18]. The sequential inappropriate increment of RAAS is considered the leading mechanism of HTN in T2DM. An increment in renin secretion, which activates the RAAS, is produced by a reduction of sodium arriving at the juxtaglomerular apparatus, an increment in reabsorption in the proximal tubule, and afferent sympathetic activity. In turn, RAAS overactivity increases the sympathetic neuronal traffic with a systemic and renal effect on the autonomic nervous system. Angiotensin II-induced vasoconstriction, increment of blood volume, and aldosterone secretions elevate BP which contributes to the deterioration of the renal structures [19]. The relevance of these mechanisms is strongly supported since drugs that reduce the activity of the RAAS and/or aldosterone reduce the impact of HTN on T2DM.

3.3.3 Sympathetic Overactivity

Dysregulation of the autonomic system is present in T2DM due to the coexistence of central obesity, insulin resistance, sleep apnea syndrome, and RAAS overactivity. Sympathetic overactivity produces not only an increment in the heart rate and vasoconstriction of the arterioles, but it also increases renin production in the juxtaglomerular apparatus of the kidney. In addition, efferent activity of the sympathetic traffic in the kidney also increases tubular reabsorption of water and sodium and renal vascular resistance and reduces glomerular filtration [20].

3.3.4 Abnormal Sodium Handling

High salt intake-induced HTN is associated with increased sympathetic traffic activity and intrarenal angiotensin II production and enhanced oxidative stress and inflammatory cytokines. All of the above result not only in an increment in vasoconstriction and peripheral resistance but they also increase intravascular volume [21].

3.3.5 Renal Dysfunction

In the presence of diabetes, the kidneys progressively deteriorate not only at the glomerular level but also in the tubulointerstitial structures where there is a reduction in the renal blood flow and the glomerular filtration rate, progressing to chronic kidney disease (CKD) and finally to end-stage renal disease (ESRD) [22].

Hemodynamic and metabolic effects induce cellular and tissue remodeling. Although initially the alterations are functional, they progress and result in permanent damage. At the tubular level, the presence of glucose results in hyper-reabsorption stress with an increment in oxygen consumption, hypertrophy, and finally atrophy of the tubular cells. In the endothelial cells, diabetes produces a loss of the glycocalyx with loss of fenestration and microvascular rarefaction. In podocytes, hyperfiltration stress initially induces podocyte hypertrophy with an increment in detachment and glomerulosclerosis. Moreover, low-level inflammation, scarring, and tubulointerstitial fibrosis contribute to the progression of renal damage [23, 24]. As a consequence, abnormal sodium handling increases the intravascular volume and activates the RAAS and the afferent sympathetic traffic, thereby elevating BP.

3.3.6 Vascular Stiffness

Hyperglycemia causes accelerated arterial stiffening, which contributes to the elevated risk for cardiovascular disease in T2DM [25]. Production of advanced glycation end products (AGEs) and decreased NO bioavailability lead to a faster increment in PWV over the years and as a result systolic BP increases, predominantly producing a wide pulse pressure [26].

3.3.7 Genetic Association

Genetic studies to identify the locus associated with the risk of T2DM [27] or HTN [28] have concluded that both diseases are polygenic. One study tried to identify whether certain gene expressions in T2DM could predict the incidence of developing HTN [29]. Six genes, *RTP4*, *FXYD6*, *GDF11*, *IFNAR1*, *NOX3*, and *HLA-DQ2*, seem to be related to the dynamics of future hypertension incidence in T2DM. Of these, two have previously been associated with the mechanisms of HTN.

3.4 Characteristics of High BP in T2DM

As a result of the interaction between the mechanisms leading to BP elevation and the impact induced by T2DM in the vessels and the kidneys, HTN in T2DM has a characteristic phenotype. Among the most frequent characteristics are systolic BP elevations with wide pulse pressure, high variability, non-dipping pattern, salt sensitivity, and refractory hypertension together with a trend of hyperkalemia.

3.4.1 Isolated Systolic Hypertension

In T2DM a high prevalence of isolated systolic hypertension (ISH), a systolic BP equal or superior to 140 mmHg, and diastolic blood pressure less than 90 mmHg are observed due to the stiffness of large arteries. In normal conditions, a progressive increment in arterial stiffness is observed with aging, but in the presence of diabetes, the process is accelerated which explains the higher prevalence of ISH in diabetics. The increment of pulse wave velocity and wide pulse pressure are part of the consequence of arterial stiffness [30]. PWV has been considered a marker of hypertension-induced organ damage by the ESC/ESH guidelines with a prognostic value for CV morbidity and mortality. However, the prognostic value of changes over time is not totally demonstrated [31]. A wide pulse pressure with low diastolic values introduces the question if excessive DBP reduction can increase CV risk and could be a limitation at the time of HTN treatment [32].

3.4.2 High Variability

Blood pressure variability, greater fluctuations at given mean pressures, both short-term and intrinsic variability [33, 34], and between-visit [35] variability are characteristics of T2DM that have been considered to be risk factors for CV events. While intrinsic variability is produced by autonomic neuropathy, the between-visit variability indicated a lack of stable BP control. In the first case, intrinsic variability, reduction of variability is not an easy task [36], while in the second, between-visit variability, efforts should be done for better BP control with drugs that cover 24 h.

3.4.3 Non-Dipping Pattern

Blunted physiological nocturnal reduction of BP, the so-called non-dipping pattern, is frequently observed in T2DM and produces persistently elevated BP values during the resting period [37]. The principal mechanisms implicated in this phenomenon are cardiovascular autonomic neuropathy and endothelial dysfunction, although salt sensitivity, early renal microvascular damage, and diminished baroreceptor sensitivity can also contribute to the blunted circadian variability. Persistence of elevated BP at night is an indirect marker of organ damage with frequent albuminuria and a prognostic factor for CV disease and the development of diabetic nephropathy. This BP pattern requires monitoring during follow-up using 24-h ambulatory blood pressure monitoring, reduction of nocturnal BP being the target rather than reversing the non-dipping pattern.

3.4.4 Salt Sensitivity

The pressure-natriuresis curve is a mechanism where BP elevation increases diuresis and natriuresis in order to restore equilibrium in the body [38]. In normal conditions, salt intake in excess is rapidly eliminated by the kidney; however, when the capacity is reduced or there is an overload, it increases the intravascular volume. The reduced capacity to control salt intake, salt sensitivity, is a situation frequent in T2DM [39]. This is the consequence of reduced flow-mediated vasodilatation due to a reduced capacity to modulate the autonomic nervous system and the increment of asymmetric dimethylarginine (ADMA), an endogenous nitric oxide synthase inhibitor that reduces nitric oxide activity [39]. Consequently, salt intake reduction needs to be a key therapeutic recommendation in these patients.

3.4.5 Toward Hyperkalemia

Hyperkalemia, defined as plasma potassium level >5.5 mmol/L, is a potentially life-threatening condition produced by many causes; however, in T2DM, the most frequent are hyporeninemic hypoaldosteronism [40] or secondary to the pharmacological blockade of angiotensin II or the use of potassium-sparing diuretics, nonsteroidal anti-inflammatory drugs, or calcineurin inhibitors. Hyporeninemic hypoaldosteronism (HH) occurs more frequently in patients around 60 years of age with diabetic nephropathy with mild or moderate CKD [41]. The presence of HH, which usually is asymptomatic and consequently not diagnosed, introduces more complexity at the time of treating BP elevation in T2DM since renin-angiotensin blockers precipitate severe hyperkalemia.

3.4.6 Resistant Hypertension

Frequently, T2DM requires more than three antihypertensive drugs to achieve a recommended BP goal in order to reduce cardiovascular and renal risk; this is called a state of resistant HTN. This is a very-high-risk condition which requires actions to be taken without delay [42]. The main causes for this resistant state are volume overload, peripheral resistance, vascular stiffness, and sympathetic overactivity. In T2DM, usually there is not just one factor present and it is necessary to exclude secondary hypertension, primary hyperaldosteronism, or renal artery stenosis, optimize diuretic treatment, and add a fourth antihypertensive drug [43]. If the patient is obese, action should be taken to reduce weight. If the triple combination of RAS blockers, calcium channel blockers, and diuretic is not sufficient for BP control, the most used drugs to introduce are spironolactone, eplerenone, doxazosin, and beta-blockers. Valsartan-sacubitril [44] and other new drugs such as aprocitentan [45] and Firibastat [46] and nonpharmacological treatments with renal denervation [47, 48] will soon be introduced on the market and open new perspectives for the future.

3.5 Impact of HTN on the Organ Damage in T2DM Patients

Hypertension and diabetes are well-known risk factors for the development of cardiovascular disease [49–52]. As hypertension and diabetes interact, risks might be different when these conditions coexist. Macrovascular and microvascular lesions of T2DM, mainly arteriosclerosis and renal damage, largely increase as a consequence of the interaction of both T2DM and HTN. Although the typical lesion associated with diabetes is renal, the main cause of mortality is cardiovascular atherosclerosis-driven such as acute myocardial infarction, stroke, and heart failure.

T2DM increases the risk of CKD and progression to end-stage kidney disease (ESKD), diabetes being the first cause of ESKD in developed and developing countries. Decline of renal function is faster in the coexistence of HTN and occurs with or without an increment of albuminuria/proteinuria. In fact, 25% of diabetics which progressed to CKD did not develop albuminuria [53]. In a large population of 156363 T2DM patients, 66 years old on average, the prevalence of renal status classified by the KDIGO risk chart was 66%, 22%, 8%, and 5% in stages 1–4, respectively [54].

The impact of HTN on T2DM is observed in Figs. 3.3 and 3.4, which include real-world data from 345083 diabetics from our community. These figures represent the increment of risk in developing different CV events in the presence of HTN as compared with T2DM without HTN. The increased risk for heart failure, atrial fibrillation, peripheral vascular disease, acute myocardial infarction, and stroke is plotted in both sexes by age group. The impact of HTN on risk is higher in the youngest patients, with the difference decreasing as the patients become older due to the impact of other comorbidities on T2DM and the reduced survival of those with much more risk [54].

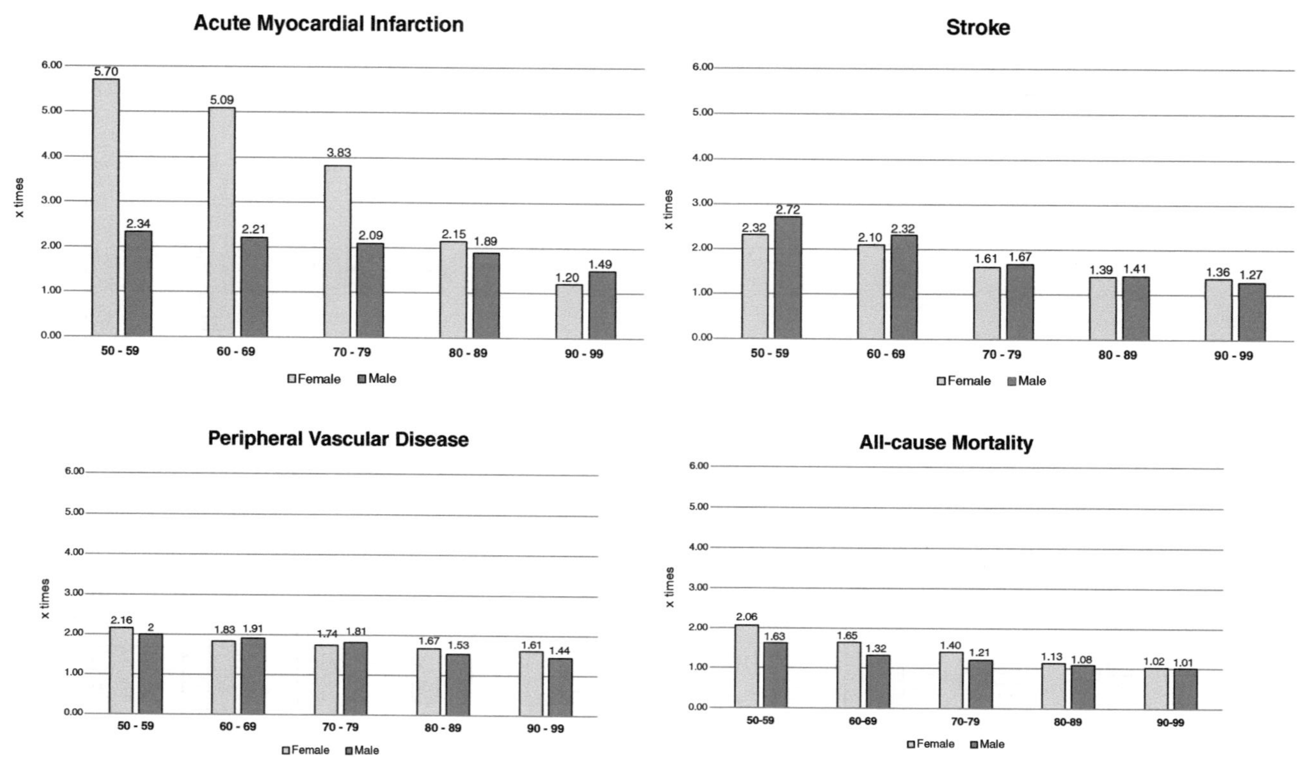

Fig. 3.3 Increment of risk to develop CV events and all-cause mortality in the presence of HTN as compared with T2DM without HTN (345083 T2DM)

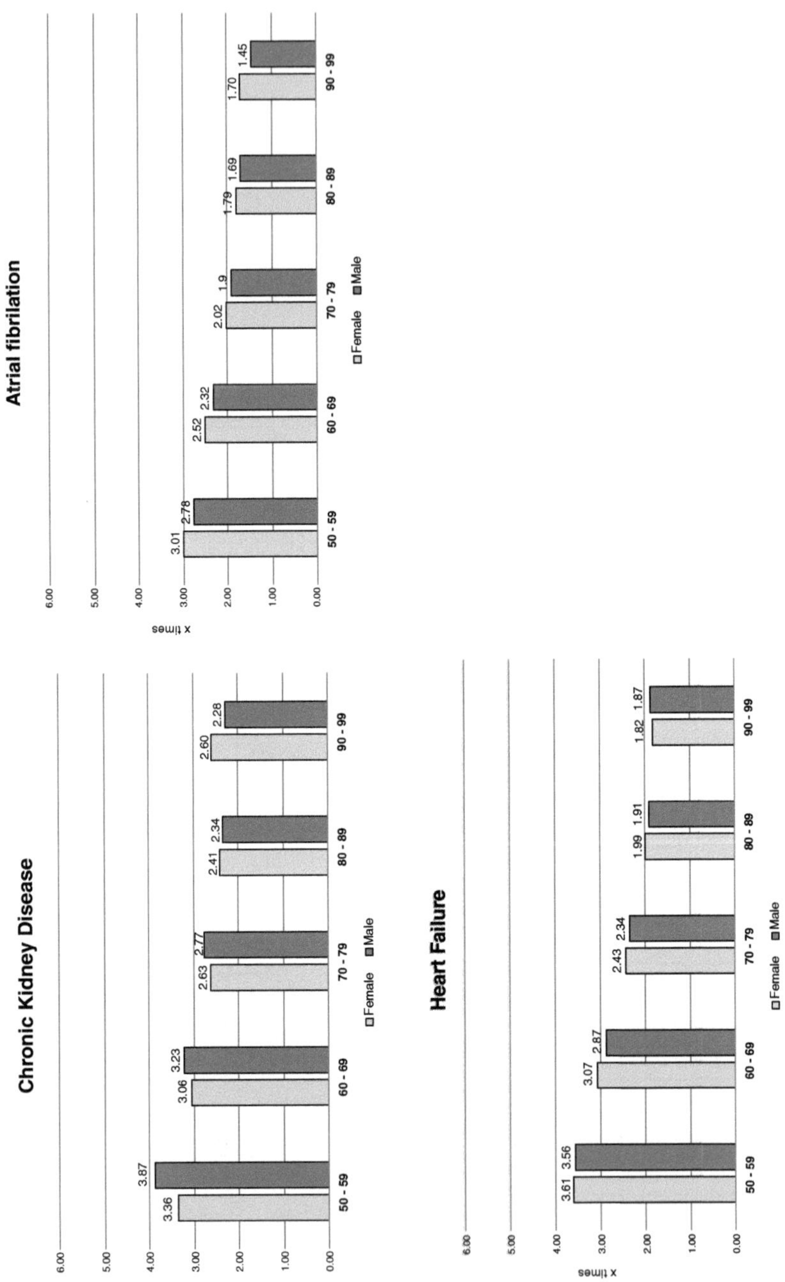

Fig. 3.4 Increment of risk to develop renal and cardiac dysfunction in the presence of HTN as compared with T2DM without HTN (345083 T2DM)

3.6 Treatment Strategies to Reduce CV Risk

Type 2 diabetes requires treatment from the moment of diagnosis. In addition, treatment should be started in prediabetes (fasting baseline blood glucose level of 100–125 mg/dL or HbA1c level 5.7%–6.4%) due to the high risk of T2D and CVD. In this situation, especially with baseline blood glucose level between 110 and 125 mg/dL or HbA1c level 6.1%–6.4%, where the risk of CVD and T2D is increased, benefits of treatment with lifestyle changes have been established [55]. The ADA recommends treatment with metformin in subjects with prediabetes, especially in those with BMI >35, age >60 years, and in women with a history of gestational diabetes [56]. At the time of starting glycemic control, HTN and dyslipidemia as well as weight control should be targeted to reduce the present CV risk and to avoid and/or delay progression.

3.7 BP Treatment in T2DM

Guidelines of the ESC/ESH published in 2018 [57] recommend starting pharmacological treatment with BP equal or higher than 140/90 mmHg, to achieve a goal of 130 mmHg or lower if tolerated, but not to reduce the value below 120 mmHg. However, in the same guidelines, it is recommended that in patients with CKD, which is a condition usually present in T2DM, BP should not be reduced to less than 130 mmHg. Publications of guidelines have raised debates about what is the best strategy to reduce CV and renal risk in the hypertensive T2DM patient.

Discrepancies are not unexpected since the concept of diabetes included different clinical conditions. It is not the same case between patients with more than 15 years of diabetes who are at very high risk and possibly with a previous CV event and those with short-term diabetes in the absence of relevant organ damage. Likewise, it is important to consider that the necessary holistic treatment should consider how glucose metabolism control is faced, intensive or not, and what kind of glucose-lowering drugs (GLDs) should be used. There are also five main issues relevant to discuss: class of antihypertensive drugs, the role of new glucose-lowering drugs (GLDs), if it is better to apply an intensive BP-lowering treatment or a standard one, what to do when renal damage is present, and the utility of 24-h ambulatory BP monitoring (ABPM).

3.7.1 Class of Antihypertensive Drugs

Pharmacological treatment of HTN in T2DM patients requires following ESC/ESH guidelines in terms of using drugs that block the RAS in combination with calcium channel blockers, dihydropyridines, and/or diuretics, dependent on the initial BP level [58]. The use of antialdosterone drugs, spironolactone, eplerenone, or finerenone, in the case of resistant HTN, needs to be administered under strict control of potassium levels [59].

3.7.2 New GLDs, When and for Whom?

In the last few years in the armamentarium to control diabetes, two new classes of GLDs have been introduced: sodium glucose cotransporter 2 inhibitors (SGLT2i) [60] and the glucagon-like peptide 1 (GLP-1) [61]. Both classes of drugs, besides glucose control, have demonstrated additional protection: SGLT2i cardiovascular and renal and GLP-1 cardiovascular and inducing weight loss [62–65]. The introduction of these drugs has been recommended by the ESC/EASD guidelines for the first step in patients with a previous CV event, target organ damage, or multiple risk factors [66]. Obese subjects may obtain benefits with GLP-1 and those with albuminuria or CKD3a with SGLT2i. It is worthy to comment that SGLT2i produces additional BP reduction combined with or without renin-angiotensin blockers [67].

3.7.3 Intensive vs Standard Antihypertensive Treatment

The controversy to use an intensive antihypertensive treatment to achieve BP around 120 mmHg SBP and 70 mmHg DBP or to maintain a treatment that achieves BP goals in the range of those recommended in the ESC/ESH guidelines still exists.

Several studies (ONTARGET [68] and ACCORD [69]) and meta-analyses (Bangalore 2011 [70], Ettehad 2015 [71], Brüstrom 2015 [72], Tomopoulos 2018 [73]) support the use of standard treatment. Overall, starting treatment at systolic BP levels in the 130–140 mmHg range reduces the risk of stroke. However, antihypertensive treatment should be implemented with caution because of the possibility of untoward cardiac effects that could counterbalance the beneficial consequences of aggressive BP reduction for stroke. The ONTARGET trial concluded that the recommendation of not excessively reducing BP should also be applied to diastolic BP values of 67 mmHg or less [31].

The design and results of the ACCORD trial in T2DM permitted the assessment of the impact of interaction of two parallel strategies of intensive treatment, for BP reduction and for glucose control. The main results of the trial were "patients with type 2 diabetes at high risk for cardiovascular events, targeting a systolic blood pressure of less than 120 mmHg, intensive treatment, as compared with less than 140 mmHg, standard treatment, did not reduce the rate of a composite outcome of fatal and nonfatal major cardiovascular events with the exception of stroke that was reduced." The post hoc analyses provided information that can be used as a hypotheses generated for future studies. The first of these post hoc analyses splits the results in two groups of glucose control: intensive and standard. In the intensive glucose control group, intensive antihypertensive treatment resulted in an increment in CV outcomes and mortality. On the contrary, in the standard glucose treatment group, intensive antihypertensive treatment reduced CV events and mortality [74]. A second post hoc analysis was performed splitting the study population into those with or without criteria similar to the SPRINT trial. The patients with SPRINT eligible criteria obtained more benefits with intensive antihypertensive treatment [75].

In these post hoc analyses, the impact of treatment in events was also analyzed in the scope of DBP. The impact of intensive BP lowering is independent of the baseline DBP in patients with glucose-lowering standard treatment. The authors concluded that low baseline DBP is not an impediment to intensive antihypertensive treatment [76].

3.7.4 Diabetic Nephropathy: What About Goals for Diabetic CKD

The impact of lowering BP on renal outcomes is a matter of concern. Overall, a greater BP reduction significantly decreases the incidence of albuminuria or the values (if they are present); however, no beneficial impact is observed in reducing the risk of progressing toward ESKD [77]. In the ACCORD trial and ACCORDION [78], a long-term follow-up of patients of the trial observed that intensive BP control may increase the risk for adverse renal events reflected in doubling serum creatinine levels. By measuring markers of tubular damage in the ACCORD patients, it was tested whether or not this increment in serum creatinine level was the consequence of real renal damage or if it was a functional reduction due to the RAS blockade. While creatinine increased, a reduction in albuminuria as well as in KIM-1, IL-18, MCP-1, and YKL-40 was observed, favoring the hypothesis of a functional impact more than a structural one [79]. Recently, KDIGO released recommendations for BP control in patients with CKD without renal replacement therapy. The recommendation is to reduce SBP <120 mmHg; however, there is no evidence available in patients with diabetes [80]. Until more ground data will be available, if intensive antihypertensive treatment is introduced, strict monitoring of creatinine and potassium levels should be recommended.

3.7.5 Use of 24-h ABPM

Considering the frequent blunted decline of BP during resting periods in T2DM, the use of 24-h ABPM is recommended in order to assess if antihypertensive treatment is effective in controlling nocturnal BP due to its relevance in CV and renal risk [81]. Although today there is a lack of ground data to establish the BP goal to achieve during 24 h and at night, 24-h ABPM results are useful in the clinical management of T2DM.

3.8 Future Trends

The increment of T2DM prevalence worldwide driven by the obesity pandemic is a real threat to health care systems due to the impact on CV and renal disease as well as other microvascular complications. Treatment and control of HTN is one of the key instruments in reducing the impact. Research on new strategies to prevent the development of T2DM and on the development of new therapeutic approaches for both T2DM and HTN is essential.

References

1. International Diabetes Federation. IDF Diabetes Atlas 6th Edition. IDF [online]; 2013. http://www.idf.org/sites/default/files/EN_6E_Atlas_Full_0.pdf
2. Lotfy M, Adeghate J, Kalasz H, Singh J, Adeghate E. Chronic complications of diabetes mellitus: a mini review. Curr Diabetes Rev. 2017;13:3–10. https://doi.org/10.2174/1573399812666151016101622.
3. DeFronzo RA, Ferrannini E, Groop L, Henry RR, Herman WH, Holst JJ, et al. Type 2 diabetes mellitus. Nat Rev Dis Primers. 2015;1:15019. https://doi.org/10.1038/nrdp.2015.19.
4. Pavlou DI, Paschou SA, Anagnostis P, Spartalis M, Spartalis E, Vryonidou A, et al. Hypertension in patients with type 2 diabetes mellitus: targets and management. Maturitas. 2018;112:71–7. https://doi.org/10.1016/j.maturitas.2018.03.013.
5. Marso SP, Daniels GH, Brown-Frandsen K, Kristensen P, Mann JF, Nauck MA, et al. LEADER Steering Committee; LEADER Trial Investigators. Liraglutide and cardiovascular outcomes in type 2 diabetes. N Engl J Med. 2016;375:311–22. https://doi.org/10.1056/NEJMoa1603827.
6. Wanner C, Inzucchi SE, Lachin JM, Fitchett D, von Eynatten M, Mattheus M, et al. EMPA-REG OUTCOME Investigators. Empagliflozin and progression of kidney disease in type 2 diabetes. N Engl J Med. 2016;375:323–34. https://doi.org/10.1056/NEJMoa1515920.
7. Colosia AD, Palencia R, Khan S. Prevalence of hypertension and obesity in patients with type 2 diabetes mellitus in observational studies: a systematic literature review. Diabetes Metab Syndr Obes. 2013;6:327–38. https://doi.org/10.2147/DMSO.S51325.
8. Sauri I, Uso R, Trillo JL, Fernandez A, Holgado JL, Lopez C, et al. Impact of hypertension in the morbidity and mortality in diabetes mellitus: a real world data. J Hypertens. 2021;39(e23)
9. Tryggestad JB, Willi SM. Complications and comorbidities of T2DM in adolescents: findings from the TODAY clinical trial. J Diabetes Complications. 2015;29:307–12. https://doi.org/10.1016/j.jdiacomp.2014.10.009.
10. Castro Torres Y, Katholi RE. Novel treatment approaches in hypertensive type 2 diabetic patients. World J Diabetes. 2014;5:536–45. https://doi.org/10.4239/wjd.v5.i4.536.
11. Yerram P, Whaley-Connell A. Novel role for the incretins in blood pressure regulation. Curr Opin Nephrol Hypertens. 2012;21:463–8. https://doi.org/10.1097/MNH.0b013e328356bccd.
12. van der Zijl NJ, Moors CC, Goossens GH, Blaak EE, Diamant M. Does interference with the renin-angiotensin system protect against diabetes? Evidence and mechanisms. Diabetes Obes Metab. 2012;14:586–95. https://doi.org/10.1111/j.1463-1326.2012.01559.x.
13. Rizvi S, Raza ST, Rahman Q, Eba A, Zaidi ZH, Mahdi F. Association of endothelial nitric oxide synthase (eNOS) and norepinephrine transporter (NET) genes polymorphism with type 2 diabetes mellitus. Mol Biol Rep. 2019;46:5433–41. https://doi.org/10.1007/s11033-019-04998-y.
14. Ferrelli F, Pastore D, Capuani B, Lombardo MF, Blot-Chabaud M, Coppola A, et al. Serum glucocorticoid inducible kinase (SGK)-1 protects endothelial cells against oxidative stress and apoptosis induced by hyperglycaemia. Acta Diabetol. 2015;52:55–64. https://doi.org/10.1007/s00592-014-0600-4.
15. Rojas E, Rodríguez-Molina D, Bolli P, Israili ZH, Faría J, Fidilio E, et al. The role of adiponectin in endothelial dysfunction and hypertension. Curr Hypertens Rep. 2014;16:463–75. https://doi.org/10.1007/s11906-014-0463-7.
16. Katsiki N, Mikhailidis DP, Banach M. Leptin, cardiovascular diseases and type 2 diabetes mellitus. Acta Pharmacol Sin. 2018;39:1176–88. https://doi.org/10.1038/aps.2018.40.
17. Hill MA, Yang Y, Zhang L, Sun Z, Jia G, Parrish AR, Sowers JR. Insulin resistance, cardiovascular stiffening and cardiovascular disease. Metabolism. 2021;119:154766. https://doi.org/10.1016/j.metabol.2021.154766.
18. Vargas Vargas RA, Varela Millán JM, Fajardo Bonilla E. Renin-angiotensin system: basic and clinical aspects—a general perspective. Endocrinol Diabetes Nutr. 2022;69:52–62.
19. Hussain M, Awan FR. Hypertension regulating angiotensin peptides in the pathobiology of cardiovascular disease. Clin Exp Hypertens. 2018;40:344–52.
20. Lips MA, de Groot GH, De Kam M, Berends FJ, Wiezer R, Van Wagensveld BA, et al. Autonomic nervous system activity in diabetic and healthy obese female subjects and the effect

of distinct weight loss strategies. Eur J Endocrinol. 2013;169:383–90. https://doi.org/10.1530/EJE-13-0506.
21. Libianto R, Batu D, MacIsaac RJ, Cooper ME, Ekinci EI. Pathophysiological links between diabetes and blood pressure. Can J Cardiol. 2018;34:585–94. https://doi.org/10.1016/j.cjca.2018.01.010.
22. Gupta R, Woo K, Yi JA. Epidemiology of end-stage kidney disease. Semin Vasc Surg. 2021;34:71–8. https://doi.org/10.1053/j.semvascsurg.2021.02.010.
23. Anders HJ, Huber TB, Isermann B, Schiffer M. CKD in diabetes: diabetic kidney disease versus nondiabetic kidney disease. Nat Rev Nephrol. 2018;14:361–77. https://doi.org/10.1038/s41581-018-0001-y.
24. Gilbert RE. Proximal tubulopathy: prime mover and key therapeutic target in diabetic kidney disease. Diabetes. 2017;66:791–800. https://doi.org/10.2337/db16-0796.
25. Wijkman M, Länne T, Östgren CJ, Nystrom FH. Aortic pulse wave velocity predicts incident cardiovascular events in patients with type 2 diabetes treated in primary care. J Diabetes Complications. 2016;30:1223–8. https://doi.org/10.1016/j.jdiacomp.2016.06.008.
26. Stehouwer CD, Henry RM, Ferreira I. Arterial stiffness in diabetes and the metabolic syndrome: a pathway to cardiovascular disease. Diabetologia. 2008;51:527–39. https://doi.org/10.1007/s00125-007-0918-3.
27. Venkatachalapathy P, Padhilahouse S, Sellappan M, Subramanian T, Kurian SJ, Miraj SS, et al. Pharmacogenomics and personalized medicine in type 2 diabetes mellitus: potential implications for clinical practice. Pharmgenomics Pers Med. 2021;14:1441–55. https://doi.org/10.2147/PGPM.S329787.
28. Padmanabhan S, Dominiczak AF. Genomics of hypertension: the road to precision medicine. Nat Rev Cardiol. 2021;18:235–50. https://doi.org/10.1038/s41569-020-00466-4.
29. Radkowski P, Wątor G, Skupien J, Bogdali A, Wołkow P. Analysis of gene expression to predict dynamics of future hypertension incidence in type 2 diabetic patients. BMC Proc. 2016;10(Suppl 7):113–7. https://doi.org/10.1186/s12919-016-0015-z.
30. Battistoni A, Michielon A, Marino G, Savoia C. Vascular aging and central aortic blood pressure: from pathophysiology to treatment. High Blood Press Cardiovasc Prev. 2020;27:299–308. https://doi.org/10.1007/s40292-020-00395-w.
31. Laurent S, Chatellier G, Azizi M, Calvet D, Choukroun G, Danchin N, et al. SPARTE Investigators. SPARTE Study: Normalization of arterial stiffness and cardiovascular events in patients with hypertension at medium to very high risk. Hypertension. 2021;78:983–95.
32. Redon J, Mancia G, Sleight P, Schumacher H, Gao P, Pogue J, et al. ONTARGET Investigators. Safety and efficacy of low blood pressures among patients with diabetes: subgroup analyses from the ONTARGET (ONgoing Telmisartan Alone and in combination with Ramipril Global Endpoint Trial). J Am Coll Cardiol. 2012;59:74–83. https://doi.org/10.1016/j.jacc.2011.09.040.
33. Ozawa M, Tamura K, Iwatsubo K, Matsushita K, Sakai M, Tsurumi- Ikeya Y, et al. Ambulatory blood pressure variability is increased in diabetic hypertensives. Clin Exp Hypertens. 2008;30:213–24.
34. Palatini P, Reboldi G, Beilin LJ, Casiglia E, Eguchi K, Imai Y, et al. Added predictive value of night-time blood pressure variability for cardiovascular events and mortality: the Ambulatory Blood Pressure-International Study. Hypertension. 2014;64:487–93.
35. Rothwell PM, Howard SC, Dolan E, O'Brien E, Dobson JE, Dahlof B, et al. Prognostic significance of visit-to-visit variability, maximum systolic blood pressure, and episodic hypertension. Lancet. 2010;375:895–905.
36. Zhou TL, Kroon AA, Reesink KD, Schram MT, Koster A, Schaper NC, et al. Blood pressure variability in individuals with and without (pre)diabetes: the Maastricht study. J Hypertens. 2018;36:259–67. https://doi.org/10.1097/HJH.0000000000001543.
37. Kim YS, Davis SCAT, Stok WJ, van Ittersum FJ, van Lieshout JJ. Impaired nocturnal blood pressure dipping in patients with type 2 diabetes mellitus. Hypertens Res. 2019;42:59–66. https://doi.org/10.1038/s41440-018-0130-5.
38. O'Connor PM, Cowley AW Jr. Modulation of pressure-natriuresis by renal medullary reactive oxygen species and nitric oxide. Curr Hypertens Rep. 2010;12:86–92.

39. Päivä H, Laakso J, Kähönen M, Turjanmaa V, Kööbi T, Majahalme S, et al. Asymmetric dimethylarginine and hemodynamic regulation in middle-aged men. Metabolism. 2006;55:771–7.
40. Sousa AG, Cabral JV, El-Feghaly WB, de Sousa LS, Nunes AB. Hyporeninemic hypoaldosteronism and diabetes mellitus: pathophysiology assumptions, clinical aspects and implications for management. World J Diabetes. 2016;7:101–11. https://doi.org/10.4239/wjd.v7.i5.101.
41. Rodríguez Soriano J. Renal tubular acidosis: the clinical entity. J Am Soc Nephrol. 2002;13:2160–70.
42. Redon J. Improving knowledge of arterial resistant hypertension: what is relevant? Rev Esp Cardiol (Engl Ed). 2014;67:251–3. https://doi.org/10.1016/j.rec.2013.11.015.
43. Aronow WS. Approaches for the management of resistant hypertension in 2020. Curr Hypertens Rep. 2020;22:3–15. https://doi.org/10.1007/s11906-019-1013-0.
44. Crea F, The ESC. Guidelines on heart failure, sacubitril-valsartan in resistant hypertension, and new therapeutic targets in myocardial hypertrophy. Eur Heart J. 2021;42:3581–5. https://doi.org/10.1093/eurheartj/ehab627.
45. McCoy EK, Lisenby KM. Aprocitentan (a dual endothelin-receptor antagonist) for treatment-resistant hypertension. J Cardiovasc Pharmacol. 2021;77:699–706. https://doi.org/10.1097/FJC.0000000000001023.
46. Alomar SA, Alghabban SA, Alharbi HA, Almoqati MF, Alduraibi Y, Abu-Zaid A. Firibastat, the first-in-class brain aminopeptidase a inhibitor, in the management of hypertension: a review of clinical trials. Avicenna J Med. 2021;11:1–7. https://doi.org/10.4103/ajm.ajm_117_20.
47. Pisano A, Iannone LF, Leo A, Russo E, Coppolino G, Bolignano D. Renal denervation for resistant hypertension. Cochrane Database Syst Rev. 2021;11(11):CD011499. https://doi.org/10.1002/14651858.CD011499.pub3.
48. Schmieder RE, Mahfoud F, Mancia G, Azizi M, Böhm M, Dimitriadis K, et al. Members of the ESH Working Group on Device-Based Treatment of Hypertension. European Society of Hypertension position paper on renal denervation 2021. J Hypertens. 2021;39:1733–41. https://doi.org/10.1097/HJH.0000000000002933.
49. Ferrannini E, Cushman WC. Diabetes and hypertension: the bad companions. Lancet. 2012;380:601–10.
50. Perreault L, Pan Q, Aroda VR, Barrett-Connor E, Dabelea D, Dagogo-Jack S, et al. Diabetes Prevention Program Research Group. Exploring residual risk for diabetes and microvascular disease in the Diabetes Prevention Program Outcomes Study (DPPOS). Diabet Med. 2017;34:1747–55.
51. Wei GS, Coady SA, Goff DC Jr, Brancati FL, Levy D, Selvin E, Vasan RS, Fox CS. Blood pressure and the risk of developing diabetes in African Americans and whites: ARIC, CARDIA, and the Framingham heart study. Diabetes Care. 2011;34:873–9.
52. Aroda VR, Knowler WC, Crandall JP, Perreault L, Edelstein SL, Jeffries SL, et al. Diabetes Prevention Program Research Group. Metformin for diabetes prevention: insights gained from the Diabetes Prevention Program/Diabetes Prevention Program Outcomes Study. Diabetologia. 2017;60:1601–11.
53. de Boer IH, Rue TC, Hall YN, Heagerty PJ, Weiss NS, Himmelfarb J. Temporal trends in the prevalence of diabetic kidney disease in the United States. JAMA. 2011;305(24):2532–9. https://doi.org/10.1001/jama.2011.861.
54. Ruiz A, Fernandez A, Holgado JL, Lopez C, Vela S, Bea C, et al. BP values and control rates in a general population: Impact of the ESC-ESH and ACC-AHA guidelines. J Hypertens. 2021;39(Suppl 1):e234.
55. Grams J, Garvey WT. Weight loss and the prevention and treatment of type 2 diabetes using lifestyle therapy, pharmacotherapy, and bariatric surgery: mechanisms of action. Curr Obes Rep. 2015;4:287–302. https://doi.org/10.1007/s13679-015-0155-x.
56. Lende M, Rijhsinghani A. Gestational diabetes: overview with emphasis on medical management. Int J Environ Res Public Health. 2020;17:9573. https://doi.org/10.3390/ijerph17249573.
57. Williams B, Mancia G, Spiering W, Agabiti Rosei E, Azizi M, Burnier M, et al. Authors/Task Force Members. 2018 ESC/ESH Guidelines for the management of arterial hypertension: the Task Force for the management of arterial hypertension of the European Society

of Cardiology and the European Society of Hypertension. J Hypertens. 2018;36:1953–2041. https://doi.org/10.1097/HJH.0000000000001940.
58. Ott C, Schmieder RE. Diagnosis and treatment of arterial hypertension 2021. Kidney Int. 2022;101:36–46. https://doi.org/10.1016/j.kint.2021.09.026.
59. Lamirault G, Artifoni M, Daniel M, Barber-Chamoux N. Nantes University Hospital Working Group on Hypertension. Resistant hypertension: novel insights. Curr Hypertens Rev. 2020;16:61–72. https://doi.org/10.2174/1573402115666191011111402.
60. Li J, Fagbote CO, Zhuo M, Hawley CE, Paik JM. Sodium-glucose cotransporter 2 inhibitors for diabetic kidney disease: a primer for deprescribing. Clin Kidney J. 2019;12:620–8. https://doi.org/10.1093/ckj/sfz100.
61. Verma S, McGuire DK, Bain SC, Bhatt DL, Leiter LA, Mazer CD, et al. Effects of glucagon-like peptide-1 receptor agonists liraglutide and semaglutide on cardiovascular and renal outcomes across body mass index categories in type 2 diabetes: Results of the LEADER and SUSTAIN 6 trials. Diabetes Obes Metab. 2020;22:2487–92. https://doi.org/10.1111/dom.14160.
62. Reifsnider OS, Kansal AR, Wanner C, Pfarr E, Koitka-Weber A, Brand SB, et al. Cost-effectiveness of empagliflozin in patients with diabetic kidney disease in the united states: findings based on the EMPA-REG OUTCOME Trial. Am J Kidney Dis. 2022:796-806. https://doi.org/10.1053/j.ajkd.2021.09.014.
63. Furtado RHM, Bonaca MP, Raz I, Zelniker TA, Mosenzon O, Cahn A, et al. Dapagliflozin and cardiovascular outcomes in patients with type 2 diabetes mellitus and previous myocardial infarction. Circulation. 2019;139:2516–27. https://doi.org/10.1161/CIRCULATIONAHA.119.039996.
64. Neal B, Perkovic V, Mahaffey KW, de Zeeuw D, Fulcher G, Erondu N, et al. CANVAS Program Collaborative Group. Canagliflozin and cardiovascular and renal events in type 2 diabetes. N Engl J Med. 2017;377:644–57. https://doi.org/10.1056/NEJMoa1611925.
65. Perkovic V, Jardine MJ, Neal B, Bompoint S, Heerspink HJL, Charytan DM, et al. CREDENCE Trial Investigators. Canagliflozin and renal outcomes in type 2 diabetes and nephropathy. N Engl J Med. 2019;380:2295-306. https://doi.org/10.1056/NEJMoa1811744.
66. Cosentino F, Grant PJ, Aboyans V, Bailey CJ, Ceriello A, Delgado V, et al. ESC Scientific Document Group. 2019 ESC guidelines on diabetes, pre-diabetes, and cardiovascular diseases developed in collaboration with the EASD. Eur Heart J. 2020;41:255–323. https://doi.org/10.1093/eurheartj/ehz486.
67. Mancia G, Cannon CP, Tikkanen I, Zeller C, Ley L, Woerle HJ, et al. Impact of empagliflozin on blood pressure in patients with type 2 diabetes mellitus and hypertension by background antihypertensive medication. Hypertension. 2016;68:1355–64. https://doi.org/10.1161/HYPERTENSIONAHA.116.07703.
68. ONTARGET Investigators, Yusuf S, Teo KK, Pogue J, Dyal L, Copland I, Schumacher H, et al. Telmisartan, ramipril, or both in patients at high risk for vascular events. N Engl J Med. 2008;358:1547–59. https://doi.org/10.1056/NEJMoa0801317.
69. ACCORD Study Group, Cushman WC, Evans GW, Byington RP, Goff DC Jr, Grimm RH Jr, Cutler JA, et al. Effects of intensive blood-pressure control in type 2 diabetes mellitus. N Engl J Med. 2010;362:1575–85. https://doi.org/10.1056/NEJMoa1001286.
70. Bangalore S, Kumar S, Lobach I, Messerli FH. Blood pressure targets in subjects with type 2 diabetes mellitus/impaired fasting glucose: observations from traditional and bayesian random-effects meta-analyses of randomized trials. Circulation. 2011;123:2799–810. https://doi.org/10.1161/CIRCULATIONAHA.110.016337.
71. Ettehad D, Emdin CA, Kiran A, Anderson SG, Callender T, Emberson J, et al. Blood pressure lowering for prevention of cardiovascular disease and death: a systematic review and meta-analysis. Lancet. 2016;387:957–67. https://doi.org/10.1016/S0140-6736(15)01225-8.
72. Brunström M, Carlberg B. Association of blood pressure lowering with mortality and cardiovascular disease across blood pressure levels: a systematic review and meta-analysis. JAMA Intern Med. 2018;178:28–36. https://doi.org/10.1001/jamainternmed.2017.6015.
73. Thomopoulos C, Parati G, Zanchetti A. Effects of blood pressure-lowering treatment on cardiovascular outcomes and mortality: 13—benefits and adverse events in older and younger

patients with hypertension: overview, meta-analyses and meta-regression analyses of randomized trials. J Hypertens. 2018;36:1622–36. https://doi.org/10.1097/HJH.0000000000001787.
74. Beddhu S, Chertow GM, Greene T, Whelton PK, Ambrosius WT, Cheung AK, et al. Effects of intensive systolic blood pressure lowering on cardiovascular events and mortality in patients with type 2 diabetes mellitus on standard glycemic control and in those without diabetes mellitus: reconciling results from ACCORD BP and SPRINT. J Am Heart Assoc. 2018;7:e009326. https://doi.org/10.1161/JAHA.118.009326.
75. Buckley LF, Dixon DL, Wohlford GF 4th, Wijesinghe DS, Baker WL, Van Tassell BW. Intensive versus standard blood pressure control in SPRINT-eligible participants of ACCORD-BP. Diabetes Care. 2017;40:1733–8. https://doi.org/10.2337/dc17-1366.
76. Ilkun OL, Greene T, Cheung AK, Whelton PK, Wei G, Boucher RE, et al. The influence of baseline diastolic blood pressure on the effects of intensive blood pressure lowering on cardiovascular outcomes and all-cause mortality in type 2 diabetes. Diabetes Care. 2020;43:1878–84. https://doi.org/10.2337/dc19-2047.
77. Böhm M, Schumacher H, Teo KK, Lonn EM, Mahfoud F, Emrich I, et al. Renal outcomes and blood pressure patterns in diabetic and nondiabetic individuals at high cardiovascular risk. J Hypertens. 2021;39:766–74. https://doi.org/10.1097/HJH.0000000000002697.
78. Beddhu S, Greene T, Boucher R, Cushman WC, Wei G, Stoddard G, et al. Intensive systolic blood pressure control and incident chronic kidney disease in people with and without diabetes mellitus: secondary analyses of two randomised controlled trials. Lancet Diabetes Endocrinol. 2018;6:555–63. https://doi.org/10.1016/S2213-8587(18)30099-8.
79. Nadkarni GN, Chauhan K, Rao V, Ix JH, Shlipak MG, Parikh CR, et al. Effect of intensive blood pressure lowering on kidney tubule injury: findings from the ACCORD trial study participants. Am J Kidney Dis. 2019;73:31–8. https://doi.org/10.1053/j.ajkd.2018.07.016.
80. Tomson CRV, Cheung AK, Mann JFE, Chang TI, Cushman WC, Furth SL, et al. Management of blood pressure in patients with chronic kidney disease not receiving dialysis: synopsis of the 2021 KDIGO clinical practice guideline. Ann Intern Med. 2021;174:1270–81. https://doi.org/10.7326/M21-0834.
81. Minutolo R, Gabbai FB, Agarwal R, Chiodini P, Borrelli S, Bellizzi V, et al. Assessment of achieved clinic and ambulatory blood pressure recordings and outcomes during treatment in hypertensive patients with CKD: a multicenter prospective cohort study. Am J Kidney Dis. 2014;64:744–52. https://doi.org/10.1053/j.ajkd.2014.06.014.

Diabetes Complicating Pregnancy and Hypertension

4

Nicholas Baranco, Robert K. Silverman, John T. Nosovitch Jr, Robert Eden, and D. S. Mastrogiannis

4.1 Introduction

Diabetes complicating pregnancy and hypertensive disorders in pregnancy are common complications and are significant causes of maternal and fetal morbidity and mortality. In this chapter, we will discuss the definitions of gestational diabetes, hypertensive disorders in pregnancy, common etiologic and pathophysiologic factors, and the management of the pregnant diabetic with hypertension.

4.2 Diabetes Mellitus in Pregnancy

Diabetes mellitus is a common medical condition which precedes or develops during pregnancy.

Gestational diabetes is defined as diabetes that is first recognized during pregnancy (ACOG) [1].

Specifically in the United States, about 1–2% of pregnancies are complicated with pregestational diabetes (diabetes that precedes pregnancy) and another 6–18% develop diabetes during the gestation according to criteria used for the diagnosis.

It has been observed that the incidence of diabetic pregnancies is increasing. Gestational diabetes increased by 56% from 2000 to 2010, while type I or type 2 diabetes increased by 37% in the same period.

This increase parallels the increase in obesity rates in the United States. Obesity is significantly associated with the development of type II or gestational diabetes.

N. Baranco · R. K. Silverman · J. T. Nosovitch Jr · R. Eden · D. S. Mastrogiannis (✉)
Division of Maternal Fetal Medicine, Department of OB Gyn, SUNY, Upstate Medical University, Syracuse, NY, USA
e-mail: barancon@upstate.edu; silvermr@upstate.edu; nosovitj@upstate.edu; edenr@upstate.edu; mastrogd@upstate.edu

A. E. Berbari, G. Mancia (eds.), *Blood Pressure Disorders in Diabetes Mellitus*, Updates in Hypertension and Cardiovascular Protection,
https://doi.org/10.1007/978-3-031-13009-0_4

Diabetes in pregnancy significantly increases the risk of various maternal and fetal complications. It is associated with significantly higher risk of pregnancy-related hypertension, preterm delivery (iatrogenic or spontaneous), and increased rates of cesarean section and its fetal effects include birth defects, macrosomia, and birth injury.

4.3 Hypertensive Disorders of Pregnancy

Hypertensive disorders of pregnancy include preexisting chronic hypertension and hypertension that develops during pregnancy such as gestational hypertension, preeclampsia, and chronic hypertension with superimposed preeclampsia[2].

Chronic hypertension complicates 1.5% of pregnant women. A significant number of pregnancies associated with chronic hypertension may develop superimposed preeclampsia (20%–50%).

Preeclampsia is a syndrome defined by hypertension and proteinuria; the exact pathogenesis of preeclampsia remains unclear but involves vasoconstriction and endothelial damage. It can cause damage to almost any maternal organ along with fetal growth restriction, placental abruption, intrauterine fetal demise (IUFD), and iatrogenic preterm birth[3]. GDM has been consistently linked to an increased risk of preeclampsia, and management of GDM with lifestyle modification and pharmacologic treatment can decrease this risk [4, 5].

Hypertensive disorders complicated 8–10% of all pregnancies.

Hypertensive disorders in pregnancy are a very significant risk factor for pregnancy complications including risks for the mother and fetus.

Hypertension in pregnancy accounts for 14% of maternal deaths worldwide and 12.9% of deaths in the developed world. While this percentage has decreased over time, it remains the second most common cause of obstetric maternal mortality[6]. These disorders include chronic hypertension, gestational hypertension, preeclampsia, preeclampsia with severe features, and chronic hypertension with superimposed preeclampsia[2]. The rates of hypertensive disorders in pregnancy have increased over time[7]. The severity of hypertension in pregnancy can vary widely from mild and asymptomatic to severe and life-threatening with intractable symptoms and acute end-organ failure, but all hypertensive disorders in pregnancy increase the risk of maternal and fetal morbidity and mortality[2].

4.4 Classification of Hypertension

In pregnancy, hypertension is commonly defined as a systolic blood pressure of 140 mmHg or higher or a diastolic blood pressure of 90 mmHg or higher. Recent changes to cardiology guidelines in the United States [8] may change the definition and management of chronic hypertension in pregnancy to include blood pressure elevations of 130–139 mmHg systolic and/or 80–89 mmHg diastolic over time; these slight elevations are associated with increased risks in pregnancy[9], but 140 mmHg systolic and 90 mmHg diastolic continue to define gestational hypertension and preeclampsia. Chronic hypertension in pregnancy is hypertension identified before pregnancy or before 20 weeks of gestation during pregnancy.

Gestational hypertension is defined as systolic blood pressure of 140 mmHg or greater and/or diastolic blood pressure of 90 mmHg or greater on two measurements at least 4 h apart after 20 weeks of gestation in the absence of new-onset proteinuria [2]. Gestational hypertension with severely elevated blood pressure (systolic 160 mmHg or greater and/or diastolic 110 mmHg or greater) should be considered preeclampsia with severe features.

Preeclampsia without severe features is gestational hypertension with new-onset proteinuria (either 300 mg or more on 24-h urine collection, 0.3 or higher on urine total protein to creatinine ratio, or less reliably on 2+ urine dipstick if quantitative testing is not available.) The word "mild" is no longer used to describe preeclampsia because it remains a serious condition even without "severe" features.

Preeclampsia with severe features is preeclampsia or gestational hypertension with severely elevated blood pressures (systolic more or equal 160 mmHg and diastolic more or equal to 110 mmHg measured 15–20 min apart) or new-onset hypertension with or without proteinuria along with one or more of a varied list of severe features, the diversity of which emphasizes the systemic nature of preeclampsia and its consequences. These features include laboratory abnormalities (transaminases greater than twice the upper limit of normal, creatinine of 1.1 mg/dL or higher, doubling of baseline creatinine, platelet count less than 100×10^9/L), persistent symptoms (headache, vision changes, right upper quadrant pain), and pulmonary edema. Severe proteinuria, oliguria, and intrauterine growth restriction which were previously part of the definition of preeclampsia with severe features (severe preeclampsia) are no longer considered indicators of severe features.

Superimposed preeclampsia is preeclampsia on top of preexisting chronic hypertension. It can be diagnosed by an increase in blood pressure, new-onset proteinuria, worsening of preexisting proteinuria, or the development of severe features of preeclampsia. Superimposed preeclampsia is challenging to diagnose and requires a careful evaluation including laboratory testing, quantitative assessment of proteinuria, and serial measurements of blood pressure.

Hemolysis, elevated liver enzymes, low platelet (HELLP) syndrome, and eclampsia are uncommon, highly morbid conditions related to preeclampsia and gestational hypertension. Eclampsia is new-onset seizure activity without another clear cause such as epilepsy. The HELLP syndrome is often defined as lactate dehydrogenase level of 600 IU/L or greater, transaminases greater than twice the upper limit of normal, and platelet count less than 100×10^9/L. Both conditions are more common in the context of preeclampsia but can occur without elevated blood pressure and/or without proteinuria.

4.5 Treatment of Hypertension in Pregnancy

The treatment of hypertension in pregnancy is primarily indicated to prevent acute complications such as maternal hemorrhagic or ischemic stroke, heart failure, acute kidney injury, and myocardial ischemia[2]. In one case series of maternal stroke, systolic blood pressure of 160 mmHg or more was present in over 95% of cases immediately before the stroke event[10]. Severely elevated blood pressure confirmed on two measurements at least 15 minutes apart should be promptly treated (as soon as reasonably possible within 30–60 min) with a goal of reducing the systolic blood pressure to 140–150 mmHg and the diastolic blood pressure to 90–100 mmHg. This should be considered a hypertensive emergency during pregnancy, labor, or the postpartum period with or without symptoms. It is important to note the lower blood pressure thresholds and shorter timeframe to lower blood pressure compared to asymptomatic, nonpregnant adults due to an association with maternal stroke[10, 11].

There are limited data to guide the choice of antihypertensive medication to treat severe hypertension in pregnancy; a systematic review and meta-analysis did not find significant differences between intravenous (IV) labetalol, IV hydralazine, and oral nifedipine capsules (not sublingual) [12], and these agents have been recommended in national guidelines [2]. A more recent randomized trial showed that oral nifedipine controls blood pressure faster and is more likely to achieve target blood pressure than IV labetalol. Magnesium sulfate should not be used as an antihypertensive but is frequently indicated for seizure prophylaxis during the treatment of severe hypertension in pregnancy [12]. The choice of agent and protocol for treatment should be standardized to improve patient outcomes [13] (Table 4.1).

The benefit of treating mildly elevated blood pressure in pregnancy is less clearly defined. An early randomized trial failed to show any decrease in complications with treatment of preeclampsia without severe features in an inpatient setting compared to inpatient observation alone, but antihypertensive treatment did increase the risk of small-for-gestational-age infants [14]. A meta-analysis of further trials showed that antihypertensive treatment halved the risk of developing severely elevated blood pressure but did not find a significant difference in maternal or fetal complications and did not find an increase in small-for-gestational-age infants [15]. Some experts initiate antihypertensive medication once blood pressure is severely elevated but do not treat lesser elevations in the absence of a clear decrease in complications in randomized trials. Given the rare but catastrophic nature of maternal stroke, we strongly consider initiation of antihypertensive medication when systolic blood pressure is 150 mmHg or more and diastolic pressure is 100 mmHg or more

Table 4.1 Medications for the treatment of chronic hypertension

Drug	Starting dose	Maximum dose
Labetalol	100–200 mg BID	2400 mg/daily
Hydralazine	10 mg QID	25–50 mg QID
Nifedipine	30 mg extended-release (XL) daily	120 mg XL daily

to prevent a delay in treatment of severely elevated blood pressure. Randomized trials are unlikely to ever have the power to show a decrease in such rare complications, but unrecognized severe hypertension is likely an important contributor to maternal mortality [11], and treatment of mildly elevated blood pressure does not appear to cause harm [15]. We are careful to remember that treatment of hypertension does not cure preeclampsia and should not change the overall management.

Labetalol and nifedipine are common first-line choices for the treatment of mildly elevated blood pressure or after severely elevated blood pressure has been resolved. Other options include oral hydralazine, oral or transdermal clonidine, and methyldopa. **Angiotensin-converting enzyme inhibitors and angiotensin receptor blockers should not be used in pregnancy.**

In the context of diabetes complicating pregnancy, nifedipine might be preferable as a first-choice agent.

The definitions and treatment of preeclampsia and gestational hypertension have changed over time. Recent guidelines from the American College of Obstetrics and Gynecology recommend treating preeclampsia and gestational hypertension as essentially the same disorder. These guidelines also included severe gestational hypertension as a form of preeclampsia with severe features. Varying definitions make it difficult to specifically define associations and effects of treatment. Hypertensive disorders of pregnancy have also been a secondary outcome in randomized trials on the treatment of GDM [1, 2]

4.6 Insulin Resistance and Diabetes in Pregnancy

Insulin resistance appears to be a common culprit for the development of hypertensive disorders of pregnancy and gestational diabetes [16]. Normal pregnancy induces significant insulin resistance in all women by decreasing the concentration of IRS-1 in skeletal muscle [17]. This results in decreased uptake of glucose by skeletal muscle. In women with GDM, phosphorylation of insulin receptor substrate-1 (IRS-1) is also decreased which further decreases glucose uptake and decreases attenuation of hepatic glucose production by insulin [18]. The placenta is the likely cause of these changes as it produces multiple hormones including human placental lactogen, estrogen, and progesterone, and it has wide-ranging effects on maternal physiology. The placenta also induces increased maternal adipose mass. Human placental lactogen, estrogen, progesterone, tumor necrosis factor-α, free fatty acids, and many other cytokines and substances have been studied as mechanisms of insulin resistance, and the mechanism is almost certainly a combination of multiple factors [19]. Glucose is the primary nutrient for the fetus and is transported from the maternal blood to the placenta and then to the fetal circulation by several glucose transporters via facilitated diffusion. The efficiency of this transport is so high that the transfer of glucose is almost directly proportional to placental perfusion and maternal blood glucose concentration [20]. Increased maternal hepatic glucose synthesis and increased postprandial glucose in normal pregnancy are an adaptive change to facilitate fetal growth.

Insulin resistance increases similarly in glucose-tolerant pregnancy and pregnancy complicated by GDM. As such, the risk factors for GDM are nearly identical to the risk factors for type 2 diabetes mellitus (T2DM). Insulin and insulin resistance increase in the third trimester. In women with preexisting insulin resistance without glucose intolerance, this can lead to GDM. Glucose challenge testing after pregnancy is normal for most women with GDM [21], but the lifetime risk of T2DM is extremely high [1].

4.7 Increased Risk for Hypertension with Gestational Diabetes

GDM, increased insulin resistance, and increased maternal insulin levels are all associated with preeclampsia and gestational hypertension. The odds ratio (OR) for preeclampsia in women diagnosed with GDM compared to women with normal glucose tolerance in one large cohort was 1.50 (confidence interval [CI] 1.28–1.76) [22]. In a cohort of women with GDM, the OR for preeclampsia was 1.81 (CI 1.3–2.51) when fasting plasma glucose (FPG) was greater than 105 mg/dL at the time of glucose challenge testing. The risk of preeclampsia is also increased with calculated insulin resistance greater than the 75th percentile for a low-risk cohort of women with normal glucose tolerance both in the second trimester (OR 2.57, CI 2.04–3.24) and third trimester (OR 2.63, CI 2.07–3.34) [23]. The HAPO trial was a large, blinded cohort study that followed over 20,000 women through pregnancy. Women with overt diabetes were excluded, and the remaining patients were stratified into groups by glucose ranges. Preeclampsia was a secondary outcome of the initial study, and OR for preeclampsia was 1.21 (CI 1.13–1.37) for each 6.9 mg/dL increase in FPG. This showed a nearly linear increase in risk with increasing FPG from less than 70 mg/dL to 105 mg/dL [24]. The HAPO data was reanalyzed with preeclampsia as a primary outcome to assess the roles of maternal insulin (C-peptide used as a proxy marker) and glucose and to control for obesity, and the OR for increasing FPG decreased to 1.08 (CI 1.0–1.16) for both maternal insulin (OR 1.28, CI 1.20–1.36) and obesity (OR 1.6, CI 1.51–1.70) for each standard deviation increase in fasting C-peptide and body mass index (BMI) [25]. These data strongly suggest that the association of hyperglycemia with preeclampsia in GDM is largely caused by increased maternal insulin level which tends to increase with glucose in GDM. The strong association with obesity after controlling for maternal insulin and glucose in the HAPO cohort demonstrates the importance of shared risk factors for GDM and preeclampsia that are independent of the actual GDM disease process.

4.8 Treatment of Gestational Diabetes Decreases the Risk of Hypertension

Treatment of GDM decreased the risk of preeclampsia in two large, randomized trials compared to routine obstetric care. In one trial, women with a fasting plasma glucose less than 140 mg/dL but abnormal glucose tolerance on a 75 -g, 2-h glucose challenge test were randomized to diet and lifestyle modifications plus insulin if needed to maintain fasting capillary glucose less than 99 mg/dL and 2-h postprandial less than 126 mg/dL. Twenty percent of women in the intervention group were treated with insulin[4]. Women in the intervention group had a relative risk for preeclampsia of 0.7 (confidence interval [CI] 0.51–0.95). The second trial evaluated women with glucose intolerance but without overt hyperglycemia[5]. Women with plasma glucose between 135 and 200 mg/dL after a 50-g, 1-h glucose challenge followed by an abnormal 100-g, 3-h glucose challenge but also a fasting plasma glucose of less than 95 mg/dL were randomized. The intervention group was treated with dietary modification and insulin if needed to maintain fasting capillary glucose less than 95 mg/dL and 2-h postprandial less than 120 mg/dL. Eight percent of women in the intervention group received insulin. The relative risk for preeclampsia in the intervention group was 0.46 (CI 0.22–0.97). These trials provided high-quality evidence that treating GDM decreases the risk of preeclampsia and that this benefit extends to GDM without overt hyperglycemia and can be achieved with diet modification alone in most women.

The role of metformin in the treatment of GDM has been explored in recent studies. A randomized trial established the short-term safety of metformin versus insulin to treat gestational diabetes; it also showed a nonsignificant decrease in the risk of gestational hypertension in the metformin group[21]. Further trials have also shown a nonsignificant trend, and a meta-analysis showed a relative risk of gestational hypertension of 0.55 (CI 0.37–0.85) but did not show a significant decrease in preeclampsia [26]. Another meta-analysis specifically focused on the risk of gestational hypertension and preeclampsia with metformin versus other treatments for GDM [27] found a 92.7% chance that metformin decreased the risk of preeclampsia, a 92.8% chance that it decreased the risk of pregnancy-induced hypertension, and a 99.2% chance that it decreased the risk of all hypertensive disorders of pregnancy.

Trials comparing metformin to other treatments for GDM have generally initiated treatment in the third trimester [27]. Metformin decreases gestational weight gain [21], which is a plausible mechanism for decreasing late-onset PIH. Early-onset preeclampsia is associated with specific biochemical markers including soluble fms-like tyrosine kinase (s-Flt-1) [28]. In vitro research has demonstrated that metformin significantly decreases s-Flt-1 in human cells and that it overall promotes vasodilation and inhibits endothelial dysfunction suggesting that it may be able to prevent or treat early-onset preeclampsia [29]. There is currently no clear evidence to support the clinical use of metformin to prevent preeclampsia before the diagnosis of GDM.

4.9 The Role of Aspirin in Prevention of Hypertension

Aspirin has also been shown to decrease the risk of preeclampsia [30, 31]. It preferentially inhibits thromboxane A_2 at low doses [32] which is associated with early-onset preeclampsia. Aspirin is most frequently used for patients with risk factors for preeclampsia including obesity, advanced maternal age, chronic hypertension, and multifetal gestation. These risk factors are shared between GDM and hypertensive disorders of pregnancy [1, 2] and likely also indicate a risk of increased insulin levels. Aspirin treatment initiated in the first trimester based on risk for preeclampsia is also likely to treat many women who will be subsequently diagnosed with GDM and therefore have a further increase in preeclampsia risk.

One meta-analysis showed a much stronger protective effect when aspirin was initiated before 16 weeks gestational age [30], before most patients are screened for GDM from 24 to 28 weeks gestation, and current guidelines only recommend aspirin be initiated before 28 weeks gestation [1]. Another meta-analysis used individual participant data investigating groups with randomization at multiple gestational ages; it found a similar reduction in preeclampsia risk for patients randomized to aspirin or placebo from 24 to 27 weeks gestation and greater than 28 weeks gestation compared to lower gestational age at randomization [31]. This suggests that patients diagnosed with GDM in the third trimester who did not already qualify for aspirin treatment may also benefit from aspirin for preeclampsia prevention.

4.10 The Effect of Hypertensive Treatment on Diabetes

Once GDM and a hypertensive disorder of pregnancy have been diagnosed, treatment of hypertension is not expected to influence glycemic control. Some beta blockers and thiazide diuretics can worsen glycemic control, but standard treatments of hypertension in pregnancy including labetalol, nifedipine, and hydralazine are not expected to increase glucose levels [15]. Hydrochlorothiazide may increase glucose if it is continued during pregnancy by decreasing intracellular potassium and directly inhibiting insulin secretion. Treatment of hypertension in pregnancy should not be altered by the presence of gestational diabetes.

4.11 Weight Loss to Reduce Risk

As previously noted, obesity is a strong risk factor for both GDM and hypertensive disorders of pregnancy. No randomized trials on weight loss surgery and pregnancy have been performed. A review of cohort studies compared pregnancy outcome in women who underwent restrictive or malabsorptive surgery to women without weight loss surgery with BMI matched to the treatment group before the weight loss surgery; it found a strong reduction in GDM (OR 0.21, CI 0.12–0.36) [33]. There was also a strong reduction in all hypertensive disorders (OR 0.38, CI 0.27–0.53) but not a significant reduction in preeclampsia (OR 0.59, CI 0.32–1.09) indicating the primary reduction was likely chronic hypertension.

4.12 Hypertensive Disorders Complicating Diabetes Worsen the Maternal Fetal Outcome

In a study done in 2012, our group showed that coexistence of hypertension and diabetes increased with advancing maternal age as expected. A combination of hypertension and diabetes in pregnancy increased the risk of preterm deliveries, neonatal intensive care unit admissions, neonatal seizures, low Apgar scores, and longer NICU stays compared to the presence of diabetes or hypertension alone [34].

4.13 Management of Diabetic Patient with Chronic Hypertension

The principles of management of diabetic patients with chronic hypertension is management of a diabetic patient with gestational hypertension and preeclampsia including preconceptual and early pregnancy evaluations to assess the severity of diabetes and hypertension, optimize medication (angiotensin receptor antagonist and ARBs should not be used in pregnancy; they should be replaced by antihypertensives friendly to pregnancy; see Table 4.1), and evaluate the patient for end-organ damage. During pregnancy, the principles of management include maintenance of appropriate blood pressures with medications or not, maintenance of good diabetic control, evaluation and follow-up of the fetus, and surveillance of the patient for the development of superimposed preeclampsia. Specific management issues are addressed in Table 4.2.

Table 4.2 Management of the diabetic patient with chronic hypertension

Periconceptual period
Baseline workup to assess hypertension, document severity.
Evaluation for end-organ damage (heart, kidney, thyroid gastroparesis, neuropathy, etc.).
Obtain prior obstetrical history.
Discontinuation of antihypertensive medications incompatible with pregnancy because of fetal concerns such as angiotensin-converting enzyme inhibitors, or angiotensin receptor blockers, and replacement with medications commonly used in pregnancy such as labetalol, nifedipine, and hydralazine.
Weight control.
Optimization of hemoglobin A1c to less than or equal to 7.
Gestational period
Maintain blood pressures below or equal to 140–150 mmHg systolic BP over 70–90 mmHg diastolic BP.
Adjust medications to achieve goal.
First trimester ultrasound to assess viability and establish dating (of note, uncontrolled diabetes is associated with increased risk of miscarriages).
First trimester genetic testing.

(continued)

Table 4.2 (continued)

Periconceptual period
Baseline laboratories to assess renal function (24-h urine for protein and creatinine clearance or urine protein to creatinine ratio, serum creatinine), liver enzymes (AST, ALT), thyroid function, hemoglobin A1c, CBC with platelets.
Optimize glucose control as early as possible, due to increased risk of congenital abnormalities in the periconceptional period in uncontrolled diabetes.
Target glucose values are fasting less than or equal to 95 mg/dL and 2-h postprandials less than or equal to 120 mg/dL (if 1-h postprandial is used, the target is less than or equal to 140 mg/dL).
Second trimester anatomic ultrasound/consider fetal echocardiogram to rule out congenital abnormalities.
Follow-up fetal growth.
Continue maintaining appropriate glucose control with target values as above.
Continue maintaining blood pressure control as above.
Start fetal well-being testing (with nonstress test/BPP/AFI as needed) between 28 and 32 weeks as indicated based on severity of hypertension and diabetes and fetal findings.
Fetal kick counts.
Follow-up the patient for development of superimposed preeclampsia.
In the absence of superimposed preeclampsia or severe hypertension with blood pressures over or equal to 160 mmHg systolic or more that 110 mmHg diastolic, the patient can be delivered at 37–39 weeks based on glycemic control, fetal growth abnormalities, severity of hypertension, fetal well-being tests, and other obstetrical parameters (earlier delivery might be indicated based on standard obstetrical indications).
If the patient develops signs or symptoms of superimposed preeclampsia, manage as preeclamptic.

4.14 Management of Diabetic Patient with Preeclampsia

The principles of management of the diabetic patient with preeclampsia is to assess the type of preeclampsia, with or without severe features, based on blood pressure readings, additional symptomatology, or abnormal laboratories [2]. Initial hospitalization should be considered. Patients with preeclampsia without severe features can be managed expectantly with serial maternal and fetal evaluations and to be delivered at 37 weeks (Table 4.3).

Patients with preeclampsia with severe features need to be managed as inpatients with emergent control of blood pressure (see Table 4.4) with careful and frequent follow-ups to assess for contraindication of expectant management. Delivery at 34 weeks is recommended unless the patient develops additional severe features or has nonreassuring fetal testing (Table 4.5).

Table 4.3 Management of diabetic patient with preeclampsia without severe features

Management of diabetic patient with preeclampsia
(Elevated blood pressure over or equal to 140/90 mmHg 4 h apart and proteinuria over or equal to 300 mg of protein per 24 h over or equal to 0.3 protein to creatinine ratio on random urine sample)
Gestational age 23–37 weeks
Management of preeclampsia without severe features
Blood pressure less than 160/110 mmHg plus proteinuria
Consider hospitalization for initial workup
Preeclamptic laboratory workup (CBC, LFTs, serum creatinine, uric acid, LDH, 24-h urine for protein and creatinine clearance for protein to creatinine ratio and random sample)
Steroids for pulmonary maturity (betamethasone 2 mg intramuscularly every 24 h for two doses or alternative)
Adjust or add insulin because betamethasone will decompensate glucose control, to maintain target values as indicated
Fetal evaluation with ultrasound (estimated fetal weight, BPP, AFI, Doppler ultrasound if intrauterine growth restriction)
Daily maternal evaluations to rule out severe features
Daily fetal evaluation to assess fetal well-being
After initial hospitalization, evaluate the patient for discharge and outpatient management
Outpatient management of preeclampsia without severe features
Instruct the patient regarding preeclamptic constitutional symptomatology
Twice-weekly fetal testing in the office (NST/BPP/AFI as needed) and maternal evaluation
Weekly maternal preeclamptic laboratories
Fetal kick counts
In the absence of preeclampsia with severe features, deliver patient at 37 weeks (or earlier if clinically indicated due to standard obstetrical conditions)
If induction of labor is visible, maintain blood glucoses less than or equal to 120 mg/dL for optimal neonatal outcome. Consider insulin pump versus intermittent blood glucose monitoring and insulin administration

Table 4.4 Medications to manage and treat hypertensive emergencies

Drug	Dose	Timing to re-dose if unresolved	Maximum daily dose	Next medication if unresolved
Labetalol	20–80 mg IV	10 min	300 mg IV	Hydralazine
Hydralazine	5–10 mg IV	20 min	20 mg IV	Labetalol
Nifedipine	10–20 mg oral capsule	20 min	180 mg	Labetalol

Table 4.5 Management of diabetic patient with preeclampsia with severe features

Blood pressures more than or equal to 160 mmHg systolic or 110 mmHg diastolic 15–20 min apart, constitutional symptomatology, severe features.
Upon diagnosis, hospitalization is indicated.
Admission to labor and delivery.
Emergency management of blood pressure to maintain blood pressures below 160/110 mmHg.
Preeclamptic laboratories.
Fetal evaluation with ultrasound, BPP, AFI, and Doppler ultrasound if IUGR.
Consider continuous fetal monitoring.

(continued)

Table 4.5 (continued)

Pulmonary maturation therapy with betamethasone 12 mg intramuscularly every 24 h for two doses.
Adjust or add insulin to maintain blood glucose targets.
Magnesium sulfate administration for 24 h and then reevaluate (discontinue magnesium sulfate after 24 h if the patient is stable).
Daily maternal evaluations.
Consider lab trending because disease can progress acutely.
Daily fetal evaluations with nonstress test and backup biophysical evaluation as needed.
Continue hospitalization until 34 weeks if patient is stable.
Delivery at 34 weeks is indicated in the patient with preeclampsia with severe features.
Delivery before 34 weeks needs to be considered in cases of:
Persistent constitutional symptomatology (headaches, epigastric pain, blurred vision)
Pulmonary edema
Uncontrolled severe blood pressures despite maximal antihypertensive therapy
Fetal growth restriction with reversed end-diastolic flow less than or equal to 32 weeks based on additional testing
Evidence of HELLP syndrome
Eclampsia
DIC
Elevated laboratories (LFTs equal to or twice normal)
Thrombocytopenia less than or equal to 100,000 platelets
Elevated serum creatinine to more than 1.1 mg/dL
Nonreassuring fetal testing
Evidence of placental abruption
Less than 23 weeks or in case of fetal anomalies or IUFD
If induction of labor is visible, maintain optimal blood glucoses during labor with blood glucose less than or equal to 120 mg/dL using insulin pump or intermittent boluses.

4.15 Conclusion

Gestational diabetes and hypertensive disorders of pregnancy are important contributors to both maternal and fetal morbidity and mortality in pregnancy. After diagnosis, the medical and obstetric management of diabetes and hypertension in pregnancy is largely unchanged. The primary interactions of the two conditions are measures to prevent the development of hypertension once diabetes in pregnancy is diagnosed, including optimal control of diabetes, consideration of metformin for diabetes control, and initiation of low-dose aspirin to prevent preeclampsia. Gestational diabetes and hypertensive disorders in pregnancy should be managed by providers experienced in these conditions, the potential complications, and the decision-making around the timing of delivery with both hypertension and diabetes. While the obstetric management and timing of delivery may be difficult, ideal control of both blood pressure and blood glucose helps to optimize maternal and fetal outcomes.

References

1. ACOG Practice Bulletin No. 190: gestational diabetes mellitus. Obstet Gynecol. 2018;131(2):e49–64.
2. ACOG Practice Bulletin No. 202: gestational hypertension and preeclampsia. Obstet Gynecol. 2019;133(1):e1–25.

3. Steegers EA, Cluver CA, Kingdom J, Tong S. Pre-eclampsia. Lancet. 2010;376(9741):631–44.
4. Crowther CA, Hiller JE, Moss JR, McPhee AJ, Jeffries WS, Robinson JS. Effect of treatment of gestational diabetes mellitus on pregnancy outcomes. N Engl J Med. 2005;352(24):2477–86.
5. Landon MB, Spong CY, Thom E, Carpenter MW, Ramin SM, Casey B, et al. A multicenter, randomized trial of treatment for mild gestational diabetes. N Engl J Med. 2009;361(14):1339–48.
6. Say L, Chou D, Gemmill A, Tunçalp O, Moller A, Daniels J, et al. Global causes of maternal death: a WHO systematic analysis. Lancet Glob Health. 2014;2(6):e323–33.
7. Ananth CV, Keyes KM, Wapner RJ. Pre-eclampsia rates in the United States, 1980-2010: age-period-cohort analysis. BMJ. 2013;347:f6564.
8. Whelton PK, Carey RM, Aronow WS, Casey DE Jr, Collins KJ, Himmelfarb CD et al. 2017 ACC/AHA/AAPA/ABC/ACPM/AGS/APhA/ASH/ASPC/NMA/PCNA guideline for the prevention, detection, evaluation, and management of high blood pressure in adults: a report of the American College of Cardiology/American Heart Association Task Force on clinical practice guidelines. Hypertension. 2018;71(6):e13–115.
9. Hauspurg A, Sutton EF, Catov JM, Caritis SN. Aspirin effect on adverse pregnancy outcomes associated with stage 1 hypertension in a high-risk cohort. Hypertension. 2018;72(1):202–7.
10. Martin JN Jr, Thigpen BD, Moore RC, Rose CH, Cushman J, May W. Stroke and severe preeclampsia and eclampsia: a paradigm shift focusing on systolic blood pressure. Obstet Gynecol. 2005;105(2):246–54.
11. Judy AE, McCain CL, Lawton ES, Morton CH, Main EK, Druzin ML. Systolic hypertension, preeclampsia-related mortality, and stroke in California. Obstet Gynecol. 2019;133(6):1151–9.
12. Duley L, Meher S, Jones L. Drugs for treatment of very high blood pressure during pregnancy. Cochrane Database Syst Rev. 2013;2013(7):CD001449.
13. ACOG Committee Opinion No. 767: Emergent therapy for acute-onset, severe hypertension during pregnancy and the postpartum period. Obstet Gynecol. 2019;133(2):e174–80.
14. Sibai BM, Gonzalez AR, Mabie WC, Moretti M. A comparison of labetalol plus hospitalization versus hospitalization alone in the management of preeclampsia remote from term. Obstet Gynecol. 1987;70(3 Pt 1):323–7.
15. Abalos E, Duley L, Steyn DW, Henderson-Smart DJ. Antihypertensive drug therapy for mild to moderate hypertension during pregnancy. Cochrane Database Syst Rev. 2018;10(10):CD002252.
16. Mastrogiannis DS, Spiliopoulos M, Mulla W, Homko CJ. Insulin resistance: the possible link between gestational diabetes mellitus and hypertensive disorders of pregnancy. Curr Diab Rep. 2009;9(4):296–302.
17. Ryan EA, Enns L. Role of gestational hormones in the induction of insulin resistance. J Clin Endocrinol Metab. 1988;67(2):341–7.
18. Friedman JE, Ishizuka T, Shao J, Huston L, Highman T, Catalano P. Impaired glucose transport and insulin receptor tyrosine phosphorylation in skeletal muscle from obese women with gestational diabetes. Diabetes. 1999;48(9):1807–14.
19. Resnik R, Lockwood C, Moore TR, Greene MF, Copel JA, Silver RM. Creasy and Resnik's Maternal-fetal medicine: principles and practice. 8th ed. Philadephia: Elsevier; 2019.
20. Illsley NP, Baumann MU. Human placental glucose transport in fetoplacental growth and metabolism. Biochim Biophys Acta Mol Basis Dis. 2020;1866(2):165359.
21. Rowan JA, Hague WM, Gao W, Battin MR, Moore MP, MiG Trial Investigators. Metformin versus insulin for the treatment of gestational diabetes. N Engl J Med. 2008;358(19):2003–15.
22. Bryson CL, Ioannou GN, Rulyak SJ, Critchlow C. Association between gestational diabetes and pregnancy-induced hypertension. Am J Epidemiol. 2003;158(12):1148–53.
23. Parretti E, Lapolla A, Dalfrà M, Pacini G, Mari A, Cioni R, et al. Preeclampsia in lean normotensive normotolerant pregnant women can be predicted by simple insulin sensitivity indexes. Hypertension. 2006;47(3):449–53.
24. Metzger BE, Lowe LP, Dyer AR, Trimble ER, Chaovarindr U, Coustan DR, et al. Hyperglycemia and adverse pregnancy outcomes. N Engl J Med. 2008;358(19):1991–2002.
25. Yogev Y, Chen R, Hod M, Coustan D, Oats JJN, McIntyre HD, et al. Hyperglycemia and adverse pregnancy outcome (HAPO) study cooperative research group. Hyperglycemia and adverse pregnancy outcome (HAPO) study: preeclampsia. Am J Obstet Gynecol. 2010;202(3):255.e1–7.

26. Butalia S, Gutierrez L, Lodha A, Aitken E, Zakariasen A, Donovan L. Short- and long-term outcomes of metformin compared with insulin alone in pregnancy: a systematic review and meta-analysis. Diabet Med. 2017;34(1):27–36.
27. Kalafat E, Sukur YE, Abdi A, Thilaganathan B, Khalil A. Metformin for prevention of hypertensive disorders of pregnancy in women with gestational diabetes or obesity: systematic review and meta-analysis of randomized trials. Ultrasound Obstet Gynecol. 2018;52(6):706–14.
28. Zeisler H, Llurba E, Chantraine F, Vatish M, Staff AC, Sennström M, et al. Predictive value of the sFlt-1:PlGF ratio in women with suspected preeclampsia. N Engl J Med. 2016;374(1):13–22.
29. Brownfoot FC, Hastie R, Hannan NJ, Cannon P, Tuohey L, Parry LJ, et al. Metformin as a prevention and treatment for preeclampsia: effects on soluble fms-like tyrosine kinase 1 and soluble endoglin secretion and endothelial dysfunction. Am J Obstet Gynecol. 2016;214(3):356.e1–356.e15.
30. Roberge S, Nicolaides K, Demers S, Hyett J, Chaillet N, Bujold E. The role of aspirin dose on the prevention of preeclampsia and fetal growth restriction: systematic review and meta-analysis. Am J Obstet Gynecol. 2017;216(2):110–20.
31. Meher S, Duley L, Hunter K, Askie L. Antiplatelet therapy before or after 16 weeks' gestation for preventing preeclampsia: an individual participant data meta-analysis. Am J Obstet Gynecol. 2017;216(2):121–8.
32. Benigni A, Gregorini G, Frusca T, Chiabrando C, Ballerini S, Valcamonico A, et al. Effect of low-dose aspirin on fetal and maternal generation of thromboxane by platelets in women at risk for pregnancy-induced hypertension. N Engl J Med. 1989;321(6):357–62.
33. Kwong W, Tomlinson G, Feig DS. Maternal and neonatal outcomes after bariatric surgery; a systematic review and meta-analysis: do the benefits outweigh the risks? Am J Obstet Gynecol. 2018;218(6):573–80.
34. Potti S, Jain NJ, Mastrogiannis DS, Dandolu V. Obstetric outcomes in pregnant women with diabetes versus hypertensive disorders versus both. J Matern Fetal Neonatal Med. 2012;25(4):385–8.

Part III

Screening and Diagnostic Approaches in Diabetic Hypertensive Patients

Office/Out-of-Office Blood Pressure Measurements

5

Paolo Verdecchia, Gianpaolo Reboldi, and Fabio Angeli

5.1 Introduction

Several studies have been conducted over the past 30 years to investigate whether the superiority of out-of-office blood pressure (BP) over office BP for improving cardiovascular risk stratification, initially obtained from mixed cohorts of diabetic and nondiabetic subjects [1–4], is suitably extendible to fully diabetic cohorts. Dealing with diabetes, these studies mostly focused on diabetic microvascular complications at the renal, retinal, and neural level, in addition to macrovascular complications and mortality.

Extensive reviews and commentaries have been published on this issue [5–7]. Here, we will provide a clinically oriented overview of clinical studies, which investigated the impact of office versus out-of-office BP, either at home or during 24-h ambulatory BP monitoring, on target organ damage and major cardiovascular events in diabetic subjects. Table 5.1 summarizes the main areas of interest.

P. Verdecchia (✉)
Fondazione Umbra Cuore e Ipertensione-ONLUS and Division of Cardiology, Hospital S. Maria della Misericordia, Perugia, Italy

G. Reboldi
Department of Medicine, and Centro di Ricerca Clinica e Traslazionale (CERICLET), University of Perugia, Perugia, Italy

F. Angeli
Department of Medicine and Surgery, University of Insubria, Varese, Italy

Department of Medicine and Cardiopulmonary Rehabilitation, Maugeri Care and Research Institute, IRCCS Tradate, Tradate, Italy

A. E. Berbari, G. Mancia (eds.), *Blood Pressure Disorders in Diabetes Mellitus*, Updates in Hypertension and Cardiovascular Protection,
https://doi.org/10.1007/978-3-031-13009-0_5

Table 5.1 Out-of-office blood pressure in subjects with diabetes: main areas of interest

Masked hypertension
White-coat hypertension
24-h BP and day-night BP changes
Self-measured home BP
BP variability
Therapeutic implications

5.2 Masked Hypertension

Initially coined by Pickering in year 2002 [8], the term "masked hypertension" (MH) is defined as untreated subjects with normal BP during the clinical visit associated with abnormally elevated BP out of the clinical setting (i.e., self-measured at home or during 24-h ambulatory BP monitoring). Such definition has been subsequently extended to treated subjects apparently controlled by treatment, using the term "uncontrolled masked hypertension" [9].

The prevalence of MH is generally elevated in diabetic subjects. In the IDACO (*International Database on Ambulatory Blood Pressure in Relation to Cardiovascular Outcomes*) study, the prevalence of MH, defined by 24-h ambulatory BP monitoring in untreated subjects, was 29%, versus 19% among nondiabetics [10]. When the analysis was restricted to treated subjects, the prevalence of MH was 42% among diabetics and 30% among nondiabetics [10]. In other studies conducted with 24-h ambulatory BP monitoring, the prevalence of MH among diabetics was 30% [11] and 47% [12]. In a study from Japan with MH detected using self-measured home BP in diabetic patients, the prevalence of MH was 41% (112 subjects over 270 with normal home BP) [13]. In a recent study, the prevalence of MH was 29% in offspring of patients with diabetes, versus only 3% in offspring of nondiabetic subjects [14].

Which are the predictors of MH? As shown in Table 5.2, several factors including diabetes have been associated with a higher probability of MH.

5.2.1 Masked Hypertension and Organ Damage

Diabetic subjects with MH generally present greater organ damage when compared with diabetic controls with normal out-of-office blood pressure. In studies from independent laboratories, diabetic subjects with MH showed an increased left ventricular mass at echocardiography [22, 23] and a reduction of active diastolic relaxation [23] when compared with diabetic normotensive controls. A meta-analysis of published studies showed a nonsignificant trend towards a higher left ventricular mass in diabetic subjects with MH [24]. Urinary albumin excretion rate (UAER) has been found increased in diabetic subjects with MH [22] and the progression from microalbuminuria to macroproteinuria was eightfold more frequent in diabetic subjects with MH [13].

Table 5.2 Predictors of masked hypertension

Prehypertension [15]
High physical or mental stress at work/home [16]
Diabetes [10]
Smoking [17]
Metabolic syndrome [18]
Chronic kidney disease [19]
Obstructive sleep apnea [20]
Elderly subjects, with office BP taken after a large meal [21]

Eguchi et al. found an excess risk of silent cerebral infarctions in diabetic subjects with MH [12]. In a study from Sweden, diabetic subjects with MH defined by a normal office BP associated with an isolated raise in nighttime BP (30 out of 100 subjects) showed an increased pulse wave velocity and central blood pressure, reflecting increased large artery stiffness [25].

5.2.2 Masked Hypertension and Outcome

MH is associated with a markedly increased risk of major cardiovascular events. In a meta-analysis from our group, the risk of major CV events was higher in subjects with MH than in the normotensive subjects regardless of whether MH was defined according to self-measured BP at home (hazard ratio [HR] 2.13; 95% confidence interval [CI], 1.35–3.35; $P = 0.001$) or 24-h ambulatory BP (HR 2.00; 95% CI: 1.54–2.60; $P < 0.001$) [26].

The IDACO study specifically investigated the prognostic impact of MH among diabetic subjects. Overall, 229 diabetic and 5486 nondiabetic subjects who underwent 24-h ambulatory BP monitoring were followed for a median of 11 years [10]. After adjustment for potential confounders, the excess risk of total cardiovascular events (Fig. 5.1) in untreated subjects with diabetes and MH tended to be higher than that in diabetic normotensive subjects (HR 1.96; 95% CI 0.97–3.97; $P = 0.059$), not dissimilar from subjects with stage 1 hypertension (HR, 1.07; 95% CI 0.58–1.98; $P = 0.82$) and definitely lower than in subjects with stage 2 hypertension (HR 0.53; CI 0.29–0.99; $P = 0.048$) [10]. The prognostic impact of MH tended to disappear in treated subjects: in this subgroup, the risk of cardiovascular events did not differ between those with MH and the normotensive group (HR 1.13; 95% CI 0.54–2.35; $P = 0.75$), as well as with the group with stage 1 hypertension (HR, 0.91; 95% CI 0.49–1.69; $P = 0.76$) and stage 2 hypertension (HR 0.65; 95% CI, 0.35–1.20; $P = 0.17$) [10].

In addition to 24-h ambulatory BP, self-measured home BP may be useful to identify diabetic subjects with MH and increased cardiovascular risk. In the HONEST (*Home BP measurement with Olmesartan Naive patients to Establish Standard Target blood pressure*) study, which included treated diabetic patients, the incidence of major cardiovascular events was 13.2/1.000 patients/year in the group with masked uncontrolled hypertension, versus 6.1/1.000 patients/year (HR 2.77) in the normotensive subgroup [27].

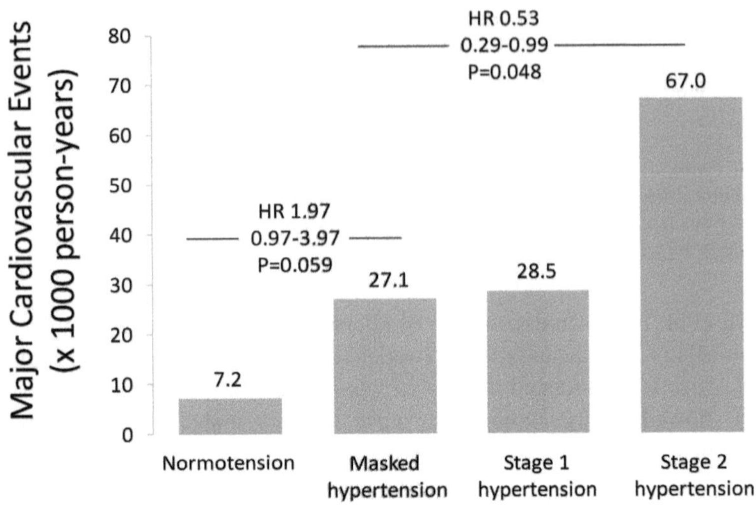

Fig. 5.1 Incidence of major cardiovascular events in diabetic subjects with normotension, masked hypertension, stage 1 hypertension, and stage 2 hypertension. From Franklin et al. [10], modified

An interesting finding noted in the PAMELA (*Pressioni Arteriose Monitorate E Loro Associazioni*) study was the increased risk to develop diabetes in the long term among initially nondiabetic subjects with MH [28]. This finding may be accounted for by the unfavorable metabolic profile of these subjects even in a prediabetic phase [28].

The recent European Hypertension Guidelines provided some important recommendations on the management of subjects with MH [29] and there is no reason why these recommendations should not be extended to diabetic subjects [29]. First, "In masked hypertension, lifestyle changes are recommended to reduce cardiovascular risk, with regular follow-up, including periodic out-of-office BP monitoring" (I C recommendation) [29]. Second, "antihypertensive drug treatment should be considered in masked hypertension to normalize the out-of-office BP, based on the prognostic importance of out-of-office BP elevation" (IIa C recommendation) [29] Third, "antihypertensive drug up-titration should be considered in treated patients whose outof-office BP is not controlled (i.e. masked uncontrolled hypertension), because of the high CV risk of these patients" (IIa C recommendation) [29].

Taken together, these findings strongly suggest the usefulness of 24-h ambulatory BP monitoring in diabetic subjects with normal office BP, particularly in those who are still untreated, with the aim to identify the high-risk subgroup with MH. These subjects should be treated with the aim to normalize out-of-office blood pressure.

Notwithstanding the utility of regular self-measurements of BP at home in the long term, 24-hour ABPM remains strongly recommended at least in the initial diagnostic phase because self-measured BP at home may miss about 25% of subjects with MH [30]. Thus, 24-h ABP monitoring may be particularly recommended when one or more predictors for MH (Table 5.2) in addition to diabetes coexist in the same individual.

5.3 White-Coat Hypertension

White-coat hypertension (WCH) is defined by an elevated office BP combined with normal BP at home or during 24-h ambulatory BP monitoring [31]. Such definition relies on the belief that WCH is mostly accounted for by the alerting reaction and the transient rise in BP which commonly occur during the clinical visit [32]. WCH mostly applies to untreated subjects because drug treatment could induce a different drop in BP as captured by office and out-of-office BP measurement [1]. Subsequently, the term "white-coat uncontrolled hypertension" has been introduced to define, in treated subjects, a condition with elevated office BP and normal home or 24-hour ABP as opposed to a condition of "sustained uncontrolled hypertension" with elevation of both office and out-of-office BP [29].

The prognostic impact of WCH hypertension has been extensively debated [1, 29]. It is generally believed that such condition should be considered at intermediate cardiovascular risk between normotension (i.e., office plus out-of-office normotension) and sustained hypertension (i.e., elevation in both office and out-of-office BP) [1, 29].

In patients with type 2 diabetes, the prevalence of WCH was around 18% [33]. Some studies addressed the issue of target organ damage in diabetic patients with WCH, but results are limited by the generally low sample sizes of these studies. For example, WCH was not associated with diabetic nephropathy or left ventricular hypertrophy in some studies [34, 35], while other studies found a greater organ damage in diabetic patients with WCH, which included increased arterial stiffness [36], silent cerebral infarcts [37], and diabetic retinopathy and nephropathy [38].

Evidence from a long-term outcome study is limited. In a longitudinal study of 262 patients with type 2 diabetes followed for about 4 years, the incidence of major cardiovascular events was significantly lower among patients with WCH than in those with sustained hypertension [33]. Unfortunately, such study did not include clinically normotensive individuals [33]. As a consequence of such uncertainty, the medical literature hosted some hot debates over the past few years about whether clinically hypertensive patients with diabetes and WCH should receive drug treatment [39] or not [40].

More recently, an important contribution on this topic came from a longitudinal analysis of the IDACO (International Database on Ambulatory Blood Pressure Monitoring) study, in which 653 untreated subjects with WCH and 653 normotensive controls were followed for a median of 10.8 years [41]. Notably, the subjects with WCH were divided into "low" and "high" cardiovascular risk on the basis of established risk factors (diabetes, male sex, smoking, obesity, dyslipidemia). Of course, the prevalence of diabetes was 0% in the subgroup at "low" risk versus 19%–23% in the subgroup at "high" risk [41]. During follow-up, the incidence of new cardiovascular events was significantly higher in the WCH group than in the age-matched normotensive group (HR 2.06, 95% CI 1.10–3.84, $P = 0.023$) [41]. However, the higher risk in WCH was restricted to the high-risk subjects aged 60 years or more (HR 2.19, 95% CI 1.09–4.37) not to the low-risk subgroup (HR 0.88, 95% CI 0.51–1.53, $P = 0.66$). The P-value for interaction between the two groups was statistically significant ($P = 0.04$) [41].

Taken together, all these findings suggest that WCH may not be an innocent phenotype in patients with diabetes, differently from other clinical lower-risk phenotypes.

5.4 24-Hour Day-Night BP Changes

The superiority of ambulatory BP over office BP for cardiovascular risk stratification in mixed populations of diabetic and nondiabetic subjects is well established [2, 29, 42]. In 1994, we provided the first longitudinal evidence that WCH and a non-dipping pattern were independent predictors of major cardiovascular events after adjustment for several potential confounders including diabetes [3].

Over the subsequent years, a growing number of studies investigated the prognostic impact of 24-hour ambulatory BP in cohorts of diabetic subjects.

5.4.1 Relationship with Organ Damage

A blunted fall in BP from day to night has been associated with increased urinary albumin excretion in patients with diabetes [43–46], but it was not clear whether the major determinant of albuminuria was the blunted day-night BP drop or the increased nighttime BP in itself. In a study, a blunted decline in BP from day to night antedated the progressive worsening of renal function in diabetic subjects [47]. The percent decline in glomerular filtration rate (GFR) over a follow-up period of 3.6 years was 21.8% among diabetics, versus 6.6% among nondiabetics ($P < 0.001$), and it was greater in non-dippers (−15.9%) than in dippers (+1.3%) [47]. Notably, a mean 24-h systolic BP >136 mmHg was an additional independent predictor of GFR decline even after adjustment for non-dipping ($P = 0.04$) [47].

Ambulatory BP also showed a closer association with echocardiographic left ventricular mass [48–50] and carotid atherosclerosis [48] when compared with office BP in diabetic patients. Some authors have also found that a blunted day-night BP fall is associated with diabetic neuropathy independently from pain-related sleep disorders and obstructive sleep apnea [51].

Subjects with diabetes are more prone to develop cognitive decline and dementia and hypertension is believed to increase the likelihood of neurological deficits. However, both low and high 24-h BP values are associated with impaired global cognitive functioning, consistent with a U-curve phenomenon [52].

5.4.2 Relationship with Outcome

Knudsen et al. first noted that diabetic subjects with a history of macrovascular events had an increased BP at night [53]. The first longitudinal evidence that ambulatory BP predicts outcome in diabetic subjects dates back to year 2000, when Sturrock et al. published a small study of 75 diabetic subjects followed for 4 years

[54]. In that study, a non-dipping pattern was associated with an increased risk of mortality [54]. In 2004, a larger study from Japan conducted in initially hospitalized diabetic subjects followed up for about 7 years found that the mean 24-h pulse pressure and mean nighttime systolic BP were independent predictors of major cardiovascular events, independent of the day-night BP changes [55]. These findings have been subsequently confirmed from longitudinal studies conducted in Italy [56] and Japan [57]. In 2009, a longitudinal study of 1178 diabetic patients found that a blunted day-night rhythm of heart rate, in addition to the ambulatory arterial stiffness index (a measure of the dynamic relationship between systolic and diastolic BP reflecting arterial stiffness), were independent predictors of mortality [58].

An important longitudinal study in this area, the *Rio de Janeiro type 2 Diabetes Cohort Study* (RIO-T2D), was published in 2013 by Salles et al. [59]. In brief, 565 subjects with type 2 diabetes were followed for 5.75 years and 24-h ambulatory BP monitoring was performed at baseline and during follow-up [59]. After controlling other cardiovascular risk factors, 24-h systolic BP and 24-h pulse pressure were stronger predictors of major cardiovascular events than office BP. Notably, achieved BP was more potent than baseline BP on risk stratification [59]. The multivariate spline analysis showed that the risk of events in these subjects increased when 24-h ambulatory BP levels exceeded 120/75 mmHg, which corresponds to 130/80 mmHg for daytime BP and 110/65 mmHg for nighttime BP [59]. Although not being a randomized trial between more intensive and less intensive ambulatory BP targets, the study by Salles generates the hypothesis that lower ambulatory BP goals may be beneficial in the management of patients with diabetes.

5.4.3 Impact on Chronotherapy

In a prospective, randomized study in 448 hypertensive patients with type 2 diabetes followed for 5.4 years, Hermida et al. found that administration of at least one antihypertensive drug at bedtime was associated with a significant reduction of a composite outcome of major cardiovascular events (Fig. 5.2) as compared with administration of all antihypertensive drugs in the morning [60]. Whereas daytime BP at follow-up did not differ between the two groups (127/71 mmHg in both), asleep BP was lower in the group with at least one antihypertensive drug at bedtime (115/60 vs 122/64 mmHg) [60]. In a commentary, Friedman and Banrji noted that these results partly disagree with the *Action to Control Cardiovascular Risk in Diabetes* (ACCORD) study, which did not find a different incidence of major cardiovascular events between the groups randomized to a more intensive (<120 mmHg) or less intensive systolic BP goals (<140 mmHg) [61]. In a subsequent study conducted in a smaller diabetic cohort, bedtime administration of antihypertensive drugs was associated with lower nighttime and 24-h BP, increased natriuresis, and lower levels of C-reactive protein, the latter suggesting a reduction in low-grade inflammation [62].

Taken together, these data suggest the potential usefulness of bedtime administration of antihypertensive drugs in diabetic patients, particularly in those with

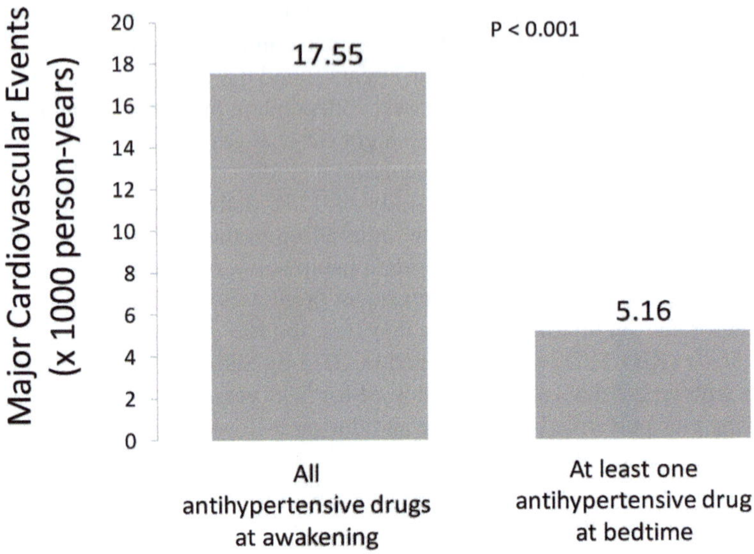

Fig. 5.2 Incidence of major cardiovascular events in hypertensive subjects randomized to receive all antihypertensive drugs at awakening, or at least one drug at bedtime. From Hermida et al. [60], modified

elevated nighttime BP values. A caveat to consider is that the sleep disturbances possibly caused by cuff inflations during nocturnal BP monitoring could trigger a monitoring-related raise in nighttime BP, which might invalidate its prognostic impact [63]. Further, randomized studies are urgently needed to provide a definite answer to this question.

5.5 Self-Measured Home Blood Pressure

Several longitudinal studies conducted in mixed cohorts of diabetic and nondiabetic subjects clearly demonstrated that BP self-measured by patients at home (home BP) is superior to office BP for the prediction of major cardiovascular events and mortality [64–68].

Some cross-sectional and longitudinal studies investigated the applicability of these findings to diabetic subjects. Cross-sectional studies found an association of home BP with diabetic nephropathy, retinopathy, and history of major cardiovascular complications [69, 70]. In a longitudinal study, the progression of diabetic nephropathy from normo-albuminuria to micro- and macroproteinuria was more frequent among subjects with home BP in the range of 120–129 mmHg than among those with home BP <120 mmHg (OR 2.72, $P = 0.035$) even after adjustment for other potential determinants of proteinuria. Of note, the risk of coronary events did not increase (i.e., there was no “J-curve”) among the subjects with home BP <120 mmHg [71].

In the *Hypertension Objective Treatment Based on Measurement by Electrical Devices of Blood Pressure* (HOMED-BP) trial, 979 patients with impaired fasting glucose (IFG) or type 2 diabetes were followed for a median of 5.45 years. At entry, home systolic BP was a significant predictor of major cardiovascular events in the total population of subjects with IFG or diabetes (HR 1.68, 95% CI 1.26–2.26, $P = 0.0005$] [72]. Home BP recorded during follow-up was a significant predictor of cardiovascular events even after adjustment for clinic BP, which did not achieve significance in the multivariate analysis. Since only 26 events occurred in the diabetic subgroup, this study could not assess the prognostic impact of home BP in these subjects. Notably, home BP values <125/75 mmHg were associated with a 47% (systolic BP) and 55% (diastolic BP) lower risk of cardiovascular events when compared with subjects with higher home BP [72].

The *Japan Morning Surge Home Blood Pressure* (J-HOP) study provided important data on the prognostic value of home BP in diabetic subjects [73]. In that study, 1057 subjects with diabetes and 3251 without diabetes were followed for a median of 4.0 years. After adjustment for confounders, home systolic BP ≥135 mmHg was associated with increased risk of cardiovascular events both in the diabetic (HR 2.45, $P = 0.017$) and nondiabetic (HR 1.79, $P = 0.024$) cohorts. Conversely, home systolic BP ≥125 mmHg predicted an increased risk of cardiovascular events only in the diabetic cohort (HR 4.35, $P = 0.045$), not in the other cohort [73]. Again, although it was not a randomized study between different treatment goals, the J-HOP study generates the hypothesis that home systolic BP should be kept below 125 mmHg for an optimal protection from major cardiovascular events.

As discussed above, home BP may be useful to identify diabetic subjects with white-coat or masked hypertension, as shown in the HONEST study [27]. An interesting point to be kept present when interpreting the data is represented by the seasonal variations in home BP. A study from Japan conducted in patients with type 2 diabetes showed that home BP is considerably lower in August (about 126/70 mmHg) than in January (about 140/77 mmHg) [74].

Diabetic patients should be instructed to share the results of home BP measurements with their doctors. A study specifically conducted in 566 subjects with diabetes clearly showed that the patient-clinician communication of results of home BP monitoring is an independent factor associated with a better BP control [75].

5.6 Blood Pressure Variability

BP variability is a complex phenomenon which results from the interaction between extrinsic (physical activity, psychological stress, temperature, etc.) and intrinsic (neural and humoral mechanisms) factors [7]. BP variability can be detected beat-by-beat using intra-arterial BP recoding, or over longer time windows using 24-h noninvasive BP monitoring (BP variability during the day, night, or over 24 h) or home BP measurements (day-to-day and seasonal variability). When using 24-h ambulatory BP monitoring, BP variability can be estimated through the standard deviation of daytime, nighttime, or 24-h BP, the latter being more properly an expression of the day-night dipping pattern (see above). Unfortunately, the standard deviation of daytime and nighttime BP may not be sensitive enough to short or very short changes in BP that may occur during day or night.

BP variability during the day, night, and over 24 h tends to be increased in hypertensive subjects with diabetes as compared with subjects without diabetes [76, 77]. In subjects at risk of diabetes due to overweight or obesity, a visit-to-visit variability of systolic BP of at least 10 mmHg predicted an increased likelihood to develop diabetes over time [78]. A study in diabetic subjects showed that day-to-day home BP variability is more closely associated with daytime variability than with nighttime variability from 24-h ambulatory BP monitoring [79].

Several factors including increased arterial stiffness, autonomic dysfunction, and elevated adrenergic activity could explain the increased BP variability in subjects with diabetes [76, 80, 81]. An elevated variability of systolic BP during the night and 24-hour BP has also been linked with coronary artery disease [82].

The prognostic impact of blunted day-night BP variability has been discussed above. Coming to the day-to-day BP variability, there is large evidence that such variability is associated with a greater organ damage and a higher risk of major cardiovascular events [7]. Increased home BP variability predicted a higher risk of development and progression of diabetic nephropathy [83, 84]. In subjects with type 1 diabetes, the year-to-year BP variability was linked with a higher risk of subsequent diabetic nephropathy, but not retinopathy [85]. In a study from Japan conducted in subjects with type 2 diabetes, the standard deviation and the coefficient of variation of home BP measured in the morning were significantly associated with the risk of progression from micro- to macroalbuminuria over 2 years even after adjustment for important confounders including sex, duration of diabetes, obesity, glycosylated hemoglobin, serum creatinine, and antihypertensive treatment [86]. These data have been confirmed in a large study from the United States [87]. In another longitudinal study, day-to-day variability was associated with greater arterial stiffness, reflected by pulse wave velocity and urinary albumin excretion, in a large cohort of subjects with type 2 diabetes [88].

The *Action in Diabetes and Vascular Disease: Preterax and Diamicron Modified Release Controlled Evaluation* (ADVANCE) study, conducted in 8811 subjects with diabetes and no previous cardiovascular events, strongly supported the prognostic value of visit-to-visit BP variability [89]. In this study, the association between systolic BP variability and macrovascular and microvascular events was continuous even after adjustment for mean systolic BP and other confounding factors. The HRs in the upper tenth versus the lowest tenth were 1.54 (0.99–2.39) for macrovascular events and 1.84 (1.19–2.84) for microvascular events [89].

5.7 Blood Pressure Targets

The 2018 ESC/ESH Guidelines [29] and the 2019 ESC Guidelines on diabetes, prediabetes, and cardiovascular diseases [90] recommended that in subjects with diabetes:

(a) Antihypertensive treatment is needed when office BP is ≥140/90 mmHg (I A recommendation).
(b) Systolic BP should be targeted to 130 mmHg and <130 mmHg if tolerated, but not <120 mmHg (I A recommendation).
(c) In people aged ≥65 years, systolic BP should be targeted to 130–139 mmHg (I A recommendation).
(d) Diastolic BP should be targeted to <80 mmHg, but not <70 mmHg (I C recommendation) [29, 90].

Conversely, the 2017 Guidelines issued by the American College of Cardiology, the American Heart Association, and other scientific societies recommend starting antihypertensive drug treatment when office BP is 130/80 mmHg or higher, with the aim to reduce it to <130/80 mmHg [91].

The *Standards of Medical Care in Diabetes-2019* issued by the American Diabetes Association suggest that BP should be targeted <130/80 mmHg in diabetic hypertensive subjects at high cardiovascular risk (history of cardiovascular disease, or 10-year atherosclerotic cardiovascular disease risk >15%) and to <140/90 mmHg in those at lower risk (no history of cardiovascular disease, or 10-year atherosclerotic cardiovascular disease risk <15%) [92].

While office BP targets in subjects with diabetes appear to be well established, out-of-office BP targets remain undefined. Home BP should be kept below 125/75 mmHg according to the HOMED-BP study [72]. Also the J-HOP study [73] and the HONEST study [27] suggested that home systolic BP <125 mmHg is an appropriate target. Thus, a home BP target <125/75 mmHg sounds like a reasonable proposal.

As for ambulatory BP monitoring, the RIO-T2D study concluded that achieved 24-h systolic BP values <120/75 mmHg are associated with significant cardiovascular protection [59].

Despite the reported association between a blunted day-night BP decline and organ damage (see above), uncertainty remains whether the higher nocturnal BP in itself or the blunted day-night BP drop is the main determinant of outcome [47, 55]. Similar caveats may apply to long-term (i.e., visit-to-visit) BP variability, although the ADVANCE study provided clear evidence that the relation between visit-to-visit systolic BP variability and outcome is continuous and independent from the mean BP [89].

5.8 Conclusions

The above data strongly suggest that, owing to the continuous rise in the incidence of diabetes worldwide, the deleterious impact of elevated BP in these subjects, and the superiority of out-of-office versus office BP for cardiovascular risk stratification in diabetic subjects, further studies with home BP and 24-h ambulatory BP in diabetes are urgently needed. In the meantime, the use of both techniques of out-of-office BP measurements should be encouraged in the clinical practice. This review provides some out-of-office BP goals based on available outcome-based studies.

Acknowledgment This study was supported in part by the nonprofit Fondazione Umbra Cuore e Ipertensione-ONLUS, Perugia, Italy.

References

1. Mancia G, Verdecchia P. Clinical value of ambulatory blood pressure: evidence and limits. Circ Res. 2015;116:1034–45.
2. Verdecchia P. Prognostic value of ambulatory blood pressure : current evidence and clinical implications. Hypertension. 2000;35:844–51.
3. Verdecchia P, Porcellati C, Schillaci G, Borgioni C, Ciucci A, Battistelli M, et al. Ambulatory blood pressure. An independent predictor of prognosis in essential hypertension. Hypertension. 1994;24(6):793–801.
4. Boggia J, Li Y, Thijs L, Hansen TW, Kikuya M, Bjorklund-Bodegard K, et al. Prognostic accuracy of day versus night ambulatory blood pressure: a cohort study. Lancet. 2007;370:1219–29.
5. Bursztyn M, Ben-Dov IZ. Diabetes mellitus and 24-hour ambulatory blood pressure monitoring. Hypertension. 2009;53:110–1.
6. Parati G, Bilo G. Should 24-h ambulatory blood pressure monitoring be done in every patient with diabetes? Diabetes Care. 2009;32(Suppl 2):S298–304.
7. Parati G, Ochoa JE, Salvi P, Lombardi C, Bilo G. Prognostic value of blood pressure variability and average blood pressure levels in patients with hypertension and diabetes. Diabetes Care. 2013;36(Suppl 2):S312–24.
8. Pickering TG, Davidson K, Gerin W, Schwartz JE. Masked hypertension. Hypertension. 2002;40(6):795–6.
9. Franklin SS, O'Brien E, Staessen JA. Masked hypertension: understanding its complexity. Eur Heart J. 2017;38:1112–8.
10. Franklin SS, Thijs L, Li Y, Hansen TW, Boggia J, Liu Y, et al. Masked hypertension in diabetes mellitus: treatment implications for clinical practice. Hypertension. 2013;61(5):964–71.
11. Leitao CB, Canani LH, Kramer CK, Moehlecke M, Pinto LC, Ricardo ED, et al. Blood pressure means rather than nocturnal dipping pattern are related to complications in Type 2 diabetic patients. Diabet Med. 2008;25(3):308–13.
12. Eguchi K, Ishikawa J, Hoshide S, Pickering TG, Shimada K, Kario K. Masked hypertension in diabetes mellitus: a potential risk. J Clin Hypertens (Greenwich). 2007;9(8):601–7.
13. Ushigome E, Oyabu C, Tanaka T, Hasegawa G, Ohnishi M, Tsunoda S, et al. Impact of masked hypertension on diabetic nephropathy in patients with type II diabetes: a KAMOGAWA-HBP study. J Am Soc Hypertens. 2018;12(5):364–71.
14. Mahfouz RA, Gouda M, Alawady W. Determinants and impact of masked hypertension in offspring of patients with diabetes: relation with coronary flow and cardiac function. Blood Press. 2019;28(1):57–63.
15. Diaz KM, Veerabhadrappa P, Brown MD, Whited MC, Dubbert PM, Hickson DA. Prevalence, determinants, and clinical significance of masked hypertension in a population-based sample of African Americans: the Jackson heart study. Am J Hypertens. 2015;28(7):900–8.
16. Trudel X, Brisson C, Milot A. Job strain and masked hypertension. Psychosom Med. 2010;72(8):786–93.
17. Seki M, Inoue R, Ohkubo T, Kikuya M, Hara A, Metoki H, et al. Association of environmental tobacco smoke exposure with elevated home blood pressure in Japanese women: the Ohasama study. J Hypertens. 2010;28(9):1814–20.
18. Hanninen MR, Niiranen TJ, Puukka PJ, Jula AM. Metabolic risk factors and masked hypertension in the general population: the Finn-Home study. J Hum Hypertens. 2014;28(7):421–6.
19. Bangash F, Agarwal R. Masked hypertension and white-coat hypertension in chronic kidney disease: a meta-analysis. Clin J Am Soc Nephrol. 2009;4(3):656–64.
20. Hermida RC, Ayala DE, Mojon A, Fernandez JR. Sleep-time blood pressure and the prognostic value of isolated-office and masked hypertension. Am J Hypertens. 2012;25(3):297–305.

21. Tabara Y, Okada Y, Uetani E, Nagai T, Igase M, Kido T, et al. Postprandial hypotension as a risk marker for asymptomatic lacunar infarction. J Hypertens. 2014;32(5):1084–90; discussion 90.
22. Leitao CB, Canani LH, Kramer CK, Boza JC, Pinotti AF, Gross JL. Masked hypertension, urinary albumin excretion rate, and echocardiographic parameters in putatively normotensive type 2 diabetic patients. Diabetes Care. 2007;30(5):1255–60.
23. Marchesi C, Maresca AM, Solbiati F, Franzetti I, Laurita E, Nicolini E, et al. Masked hypertension in type 2 diabetes mellitus. Relationship with left-ventricular structure and function. Am J Hypertens. 2007;20(10):1079–84.
24. Pierdomenico SD, Cuccurullo F. Ambulatory blood pressure monitoring in type 2 diabetes and metabolic syndrome: a review. Blood Press Monit. 2010;15(1):1–7.
25. Wijkman M, Lanne T, Engvall J, Lindstrom T, Ostgren CJ, Nystrom FH. Masked nocturnal hypertension–a novel marker of risk in type 2 diabetes. Diabetologia. 2009;52(7):1258–64.
26. Angeli F, Reboldi G, Verdecchia P. Masked hypertension: evaluation, prognosis, and treatment. Am J Hypertens. 2010;23(9):941–8.
27. Kushiro T, Kario K, Saito I, Teramukai S, Sato Y, Okuda Y, et al. Increased cardiovascular risk of treated white coat and masked hypertension in patients with diabetes and chronic kidney disease: the HONEST Study. Hypertens Res. 2017;40(1):87–95.
28. Mancia G, Bombelli M, Facchetti R, Madotto F, Quarti-Trevano F, Grassi G, et al. Increased long-term risk of new-onset diabetes mellitus in white-coat and masked hypertension. J Hypertens. 2009;27(8):1672–8.
29. Williams B, Mancia G, Spiering W, Agabiti Rosei E, Azizi M, Burnier M, et al. 2018 ESC/ESH Guidelines for the management of arterial hypertension. Eur Heart J. 2018;39(33):3021–104.
30. Zhang L, Li Y, Wei FF, Thijs L, Kang YY, Wang S, et al. Strategies for classifying patients based on office, home, and ambulatory blood pressure measurement. Hypertension. 2015;65(6):1258–65.
31. Pickering TG, James GD, Boddie C, Harshfield GA, Blank S, Laragh JH. How common is white coat hypertension? JAMA. 1988;259(2):225–8.
32. Mancia G, Bertinieri G, Grassi G, Parati G, Pomidossi G, Ferrari A, et al. Effects of blood-pressure measurement by the doctor on patient's blood pressure and heart rate. Lancet. 1983;2(8352):695–8.
33. Eguchi K, Hoshide S, Ishikawa J, Ishikawa S, Pickering TG, Gerin W, et al. Cardiovascular prognosis of sustained and white-coat hypertension in patients with type 2 diabetes mellitus. Blood Press Monit. 2008;13(1):15–20.
34. Nielsen FS, Gaede P, Vedel P, Pedersen O, Parving HH. White coat hypertension in NIDDM patients with and without incipient and overt diabetic nephropathy. Diabetes Care. 1997;20(5):859–63.
35. Ng CM, Yiu SF, Choi KL, Choi CH, Ng YW, Tiu SC. Prevalence and significance of white-coat hypertension and masked hypertension in type 2 diabetics. Hong Kong Med J. 2008;14(6):437–43.
36. Ribeiro L, Gama G, Santos A, Asmar R, Martins L, Polonia J. Arterial distensibility in subjects with white-coat hypertension with and without diabetes or dyslipidaemia: comparison with normotensives and sustained hypertensives. Blood Press Monit. 2000;5(1):11–7.
37. Eguchi K, Kario K, Shimada K. Greater impact of coexistence of hypertension and diabetes on silent cerebral infarcts. Stroke. 2003;34(10):2471–4.
38. Kramer CK, Leitao CB, Canani LH, Gross JL. Impact of white-coat hypertension on microvascular complications in type 2 diabetes. Diabetes Care. 2008;31(12):2233–7.
39. Mancia G, Sega R, Bombelli M, Quarti-Trevano F, Facchetti R, Grassi G. Should white-coat hypertension in diabetes be treated? Pro. Diabetes Care. 2009;32(Suppl 2):S305–9.
40. Bursztyn M, Ben-Dov IZ. White-coat hypertension should not be treated in subjects with diabetes. Diabetes Care. 2009;32(suppl_2):S310–3.
41. Franklin SS, Thijs L, Asayama K, Li Y, Hansen TW, Boggia J, et al. The cardiovascular risk of white-coat hypertension. J Am Coll Cardiol. 2016;68(19):2033–43.

42. Parati G, Stergiou G, O'Brien E, Asmar R, Beilin L, Bilo G, et al. European Society of Hypertension practice guidelines for ambulatory blood pressure monitoring. J Hypertens. 2014;32(7):1359–66.
43. Fogari R, Zoppi A, Malamani GD, Lazzari P, Albonico B, Corradi L. Urinary albumin excretion and nocturnal blood pressure in hypertensive patients with type II diabetes mellitus. Am J Hypertens. 1994;7(9 Pt 1):808–13.
44. Pinkney JH, Denver AE, Mohamed-Ali V, Foster C, Yudkin JS. Insulin resistance in non-insulin-dependent diabetes mellitus is associated with microalbuminuria independently of ambulatory blood pressure. J Diabetes Complications. 1995;9(4):230–3.
45. Equiluz-Bruck S, Schnack C, Kopp HP, Schernthaner G. Nondipping of nocturnal blood pressure is related to urinary albumin excretion rate in patients with type 2 diabetes mellitus. Am J Hypertens. 1996;9(11):1139–43.
46. Mitchell TH, Nolan B, Henry M, Cronin C, Baker H, Greely G. Microalbuminuria in patients with non-insulin-dependent diabetes mellitus relates to nocturnal systolic blood pressure. Am J Med. 1997;102(6):531–5.
47. Davidson MB, Hix JK, Vidt DG, Brotman DJ. Association of impaired diurnal blood pressure variation with a subsequent decline in glomerular filtration rate. Arch Intern Med. 2006;166(8):846–52.
48. Li S, Wang X, Zhao L, Chen M, Long J, Cheng W, et al. The characteristics of 24-hour ambulatory blood pressure monitoring and its relationship with cardiovascular target organ damage in Chinese Han patients with concomitant type 2 diabetes and hypertension. Blood Press Monit. 2019;24(4):167–73.
49. Devereux RB, Roman MJ, Paranicas M, O'Grady MJ, Lee ET, Welty TK, et al. Impact of diabetes on cardiac structure and function: the strong heart study. Circulation. 2000;101(19):2271–6.
50. Palmieri V, Bella JN, Arnett DK, Liu JE, Oberman A, Schuck MY, et al. Effect of type 2 diabetes mellitus on left ventricular geometry and systolic function in hypertensive subjects: Hypertension Genetic Epidemiology Network (HyperGEN) study. Circulation. 2001;103(1):102–7.
51. D'Amato C, Morganti R, Di Gennaro F, Greco C, Marfia GA, Spallone V. A novel association between nondipping and painful diabetic polyneuropathy. Diabetes Care. 2014;37(9):2640–2.
52. Spauwen PJ, van Boxtel MP, Verhey FR, Kohler S, Sep SJ, Koster A, et al. Both low and high 24-hour diastolic blood pressure are associated with worse cognitive performance in type 2 diabetes: the Maastricht study. Diabetes Care. 2015;38(8):1473–80.
53. Knudsen ST, Poulsen PL, Hansen KW, Ebbehoj E, Bek T, Mogensen CE. Pulse pressure and diurnal blood pressure variation: association with micro- and macrovascular complications in type 2 diabetes. Am J Hypertens. 2002;15(3):244–50.
54. Sturrock ND, George E, Pound N, Stevenson J, Peck GM, Sowter H. Non-dipping circadian blood pressure and renal impairment are associated with increased mortality in diabetes mellitus. Diabet Med. 2000;17(5):360–4.
55. Nakano S, Ito T, Furuya K, Tsuda S, Konishi K, Nishizawa M, et al. Ambulatory blood pressure level rather than dipper/nondipper status predicts vascular events in type 2 diabetic subjects. Hypertens Res. 2004;27(9):647–56.
56. Mannucci E, Lambertucci L, Monami M, Fedeli A, Chiasserini V, Marchionni N, et al. Pulse pressure and mortality in hypertensive type 2 diabetic patients. A cohort study. Diabetes Metab Res Rev. 2006;22(3):172–5.
57. Eguchi K, Pickering TG, Hoshide S, Ishikawa J, Ishikawa S, Schwartz JE, et al. Ambulatory blood pressure is a better marker than clinic blood pressure in predicting cardiovascular events in patients with/without type 2 diabetes. Am J Hypertens. 2008;21(4):443–50.
58. Palmas W, Pickering TG, Teresi J, Schwartz JE, Moran A, Weinstock RS, et al. Ambulatory blood pressure monitoring and all-cause mortality in elderly people with diabetes mellitus. Hypertension. 2009;53(2):120–7.
59. Salles GF, Leite NC, Pereira BB, Nascimento EM, Cardoso CR. Prognostic impact of clinic and ambulatory blood pressure components in high-risk type 2 diabetic patients: the Rio de Janeiro Type 2 Diabetes Cohort Study. J Hypertens. 2013;31(11):2176–86.

60. Hermida RC, Ayala DE, Mojon A, Fernandez JR. Sleep-time blood pressure as a therapeutic target for cardiovascular risk reduction in type 2 diabetes. Am J Hypertens. 2012;25(3):325–34.
61. Friedman EA, Banerji MA. Chronobiology impacts response to antihypertensive drug regimen in type 2 diabetes. Diabetes Care. 2011;34(6):1438–9.
62. Rossen NB, Knudsen ST, Fleischer J, Hvas AM, Ebbehoj E, Poulsen PL, et al. Targeting nocturnal hypertension in type 2 diabetes mellitus. Hypertension. 2014;64(5):1080–7.
63. Verdecchia P, Angeli F, Borgioni C, Gattobigio R, Reboldi G. Ambulatory blood pressure and cardiovascular outcome in relation to perceived sleep deprivation. Hypertension. 2007;49(4):777–83.
64. Bobrie G, Chatellier G, Genes N, Clerson P, Vaur L, Vaisse B, et al. Cardiovascular prognosis of "masked hypertension" detected by blood pressure self-measurement in elderly treated hypertensive patients. JAMA. 2004;291(11):1342–9.
65. Kario K, Saito I, Kushiro T, Teramukai S, Tomono Y, Okuda Y, et al. Morning home blood pressure is a strong predictor of coronary artery disease: the HONEST study. J Am Coll Cardiol. 2016;67(13):1519–27.
66. Ohkubo T, Imai Y, Tsuji I, Nagai K, Kato J, Kikuchi N, et al. Home blood pressure measurement has a stronger predictive power for mortality than does screening blood pressure measurement: a population-based observation in Ohasama, Japan. J Hypertens. 1998;16(7):971–5.
67. Sega R, Facchetti R, Bombelli M, Cesana G, Corrao G, Grassi G, et al. Prognostic value of ambulatory and home blood pressures compared with office blood pressure in the general population: follow-up results from the Pressioni Arteriose Monitorate e Loro Associazioni (PAMELA) study. Circulation. 2005;111(14):1777–83.
68. Yasui D, Asayama K, Ohkubo T, Kikuya M, Kanno A, Hara A, et al. Stroke risk in treated hypertension based on home blood pressure: the Ohasama study. Am J Hypertens. 2010;23(5):508–14.
69. Kamoi K, Miyakoshi M, Soda S, Kaneko S, Nakagawa O. Usefulness of home blood pressure measurement in the morning in type 2 diabetic patients. Diabetes Care. 2002;25(12):2218–23.
70. Kamoi K, Tanaka M, Ikarashi T, Miyakoshi M. Effect of the 2004 Mid-Niigata Prefecture earthquake on home blood pressure measurement in the morning in type 2 diabetic patients. Clin Exp Hypertens. 2006;28(8):719–29.
71. Ushigome E, Hamaguchi M, Matsumoto S, Oyabu C, Omoto A, Tanaka T, et al. Optimal home SBP targets for preventing the progression of diabetic nephropathy in patients with type 2 diabetes mellitus. J Hypertens. 2015;33(9):1853–9; discussion 9.
72. Noguchi Y, Asayama K, Staessen JA, Inaba M, Ohkubo T, Hosaka M, et al. Predictive power of home blood pressure and clinic blood pressure in hypertensive patients with impaired glucose metabolism and diabetes. J Hypertens. 2013;31(8):1593–602.
73. Eguchi K, Hoshide S, Kario K. Target home morning SBP be below 125mmHg in type 2 diabetes patients. J Hypertens. 2018;36(6):1284–90.
74. Ushigome E, Kitagawa N, Kitae A, Kimura T, Iwai K, Oyabu C, et al. Seasonal variation in home blood pressure and its relationship with room temperature in patients with type 2 diabetes. Diab Vasc Dis Res. 2020;17(1):1479164119883986.
75. Naik AD, Kallen MA, Walder A, Street RL Jr. Improving hypertension control in diabetes mellitus: the effects of collaborative and proactive health communication. Circulation. 2008;117(11):1361–8.
76. Ozawa M, Tamura K, Iwatsubo K, Matsushita K, Sakai M, Tsurumi-Ikeya Y, et al. Ambulatory blood pressure variability is increased in diabetic hypertensives. Clin Exp Hypertens. 2008;30(3):213–24.
77. Zhou TL, Kroon AA, Reesink KD, Schram MT, Koster A, Schaper NC, et al. Blood pressure variability in individuals with and without (pre)diabetes: The Maastricht Study. J Hypertens. 2018;36(2):259–67.
78. Joshipura KJ, Munoz-Torres FJ, Campos M, Rivera-Diaz AD, Zevallos JC. Association between within-visit systolic blood pressure variability and development of pre-diabetes and diabetes among overweight/obese individuals. J Hum Hypertens. 2017;32(1):26–33.

79. Iuchi H, Sakamoto M, Matsutani D, Suzuki H, Kayama Y, Takeda N, et al. Association between day-by-day and ambulatory blood pressure variability in type 2 diabetes patients. Blood Press Monit. 2017;22(6):351–4.
80. Frattola A, Parati G, Gamba P, Paleari F, Mauri G, Di Rienzo M, et al. Time and frequency domain estimates of spontaneous baroreflex sensitivity provide early detection of autonomic dysfunction in diabetes mellitus. Diabetologia. 1997;40(12):1470–5.
81. Ruiz J, Monbaron D, Parati G, Perret S, Haesler E, Danzeisen C, et al. Diabetic neuropathy is a more important determinant of baroreflex sensitivity than carotid elasticity in type 2 diabetes. Hypertension. 2005;46(1):162–7.
82. Tamura K, Tsurumi Y, Sakai M, Tanaka Y, Okano Y, Yamauchi J, et al. A possible relationship of nocturnal blood pressure variability with coronary artery disease in diabetic nephropathy. Clin Exp Hypertens. 2007;29(1):31–42.
83. Tamura K, Azushima K, Umemura S. Day-by-day home-measured blood pressure variability: another important factor in hypertension with diabetic nephropathy? Hypertens Res. 2011;34(12):1249–50.
84. Ushigome E, Fukui M, Hamaguchi M, Senmaru T, Sakabe K, Tanaka M, et al. The coefficient variation of home blood pressure is a novel factor associated with macroalbuminuria in type 2 diabetes mellitus. Hypertens Res. 2011;34(12):1271–5.
85. Kilpatrick ES, Rigby AS, Atkin SL. The role of blood pressure variability in the development of nephropathy in type 1 diabetes. Diabetes Care. 2010;33(11):2442–7.
86. Ushigome E, Matsumoto S, Oyabu C, Kitagawa N, Tanaka T, Hasegawa G, et al. Prognostic significance of day-by-day variability of home blood pressure on progression to macroalbuminuria in patients with diabetes. J Hypertens. 2018;36(5):1068–75.
87. Sohn MW, Epstein N, Huang ES, Huo Z, Emanuele N, Stukenborg G, et al. Visit-to-visit systolic blood pressure variability and microvascular complications among patients with diabetes. J Diabetes Complications. 2017;31(1):195–201.
88. Okada H, Fukui M, Tanaka M, Inada S, Mineoka Y, Nakanishi N, et al. Visit-to-visit variability in systolic blood pressure is correlated with diabetic nephropathy and atherosclerosis in patients with type 2 diabetes. Atherosclerosis. 2012;220(1):155–9.
89. Hata J, Arima H, Rothwell PM, Woodward M, Zoungas S, Anderson C, et al. Effects of visit-to-visit variability in systolic blood pressure on macrovascular and microvascular complications in patients with type 2 diabetes mellitus: the ADVANCE trial. Circulation. 2013;128(12):1325–34.
90. Wheeler DC, Valensi P, Sousa-Uva M, Seferović PM, Sattar N, Roffi M, et al. 2019 ESC Guidelines on diabetes, pre-diabetes, and cardiovascular diseases developed in collaboration with the EASD. Eur Heart J. 2020;41(2):255–323.
91. Whelton PK, Carey RM, Aronow WS, Casey DE, Collins KJ, Dennison Himmelfarb C, et al. 2017 ACC/AHA/AAPA/ABC/ACPM/AGS/APhA/ASH/ASPC/NMA/PCNA Guideline for the Prevention, Detection, Evaluation, and Management of High Blood Pressure in Adults: A Report of the American College of Cardiology/American Heart Association Task Force on Clinical Practice Guidelines. Hypertension. 2018;71(6):e13–e115.
92. American Diabetes Association. 10. Cardiovascular disease and risk management: standards of medical care in diabetes-2019. Diabetes Care. 2019;42(Suppl 1):S103–23.

Laboratory Indices/Bioimaging

6

Maria Lorenza Muiesan, Claudia Agabiti-Rosei, Carolina De Ciuceis, Massimo Salvetti, and Anna Paini

6.1 Laboratory Indices

As suggested by ESC guidelines [1], the diagnosis of diabetes should include both fasting glucose measurements and hemoglobin A1c, and in case of inconclusive results, an oral glucose tolerance test should be performed to identify impaired glucose intolerance or fasting hyperglycemia.

Routine assessment of microalbuminuria is mandatory in patients at risk of developing or already presenting with high or very high risk of developing renal dysfunction and/or CVD. The gold standard for the measurement of albuminuria is 24-h urine collection (albuminuria normal values are less than 30 mg/day, microalbuminuria is 30–300 mg/day, and macroalbuminuria is >300 mg/day). Although 24-h urine collection is the gold standard for the detection of albuminuria, it has been suggested that screening can be carried out more simply and albuminuria can be tested from the first morning urine sample. In recent years, the albumin-to-creatinine ratio (UACR) from spot urine, preferably the first voided in the morning, may be considered equivalent to the values during a 24-h urine collection. When albumin concentration is between 30 and 300 mg/day in a 24-h urine collection or 30–300 mg/g of creatinine in a first morning sample, the term microalbuminuria is used; when albuminuria is more than 300 mg/day or UACR is greater than 300 mg/g, it is considered macroalbuminuria.

In diabetic patients, UACR values identify two stages of diabetic nephropathy—micro- and macroalbuminuria. In addition to the risk of developing diabetic

M. L. Muiesan (✉) · C. Agabiti-Rosei · C. De Ciuceis · M. Salvetti · A. Paini
Clinica Medica, Department of Clinical and Experimental Sciences, University of Brescia, Brescia, Italy
e-mail: marialorenza.muiesan@unibs.it; claudia.agabitirosei@unibs.it; carolina.deciuceis@unibs.it; massimo.salvetti@unibs.it

A. E. Berbari, G. Mancia (eds.), *Blood Pressure Disorders in Diabetes Mellitus*, Updates in Hypertension and Cardiovascular Protection,
https://doi.org/10.1007/978-3-031-13009-0_6

nephropathy, CV diseases starts when UACR values are still within the normoalbuminuric range [2, 3]

Microalbuminuria may progress to macroalbuminuria, although not in all patients and may even regress to normoalbuminuria. Available prospective studies in type 1 and type 2 diabetic patients have shown that the progression from normoalbuminuria or microalbuminuria to macroalbuminuria is influenced by higher baseline levels of blood pressure (BP) and glycated hemoglobin (HbA1c).

In normoalbuminuric type 1 diabetic patients, the progression to microalbuminuria or proteinuria is related to hypertension, worse baseline glomerular lesions, and lower glomerular filtration rate.

Insulin resistance seems to play a central role in causing renal injury with functional as well as structural nephron loss and contribute to elevated BP, which in turn may further damage renal function, in addition to other suboptimal control of hemodynamic and metabolic abnormalities [4].

Recently it has been observed that patients with type 2 DM and chronic kidney disease (CKD) with normoalbuminuria had a less unfavorable clinical course, as compared with those with micro- and macroalbuminuria; concomitant treatment with renin–angiotensin–aldosterone system blockade and ongoing medical care could have played a role in the progression to end-stage renal disease [5].

Renal function should be also measured by the estimation of glomerular filtration rate, calculated by the 2009 CKD-Epidemiology Collaboration formula, since albuminuria and kidney function may both have a predictive role for CV and renal outcomes [6].

According to the 2018 ESH/ESC Guidelines, the assessment of serum creatinine and the calculation of estimated glomerular filtration rate (eGFR) is recommended to assess renal excretory function [7] and urinary albumin excretion is considered a biomarker of early renal damage. Both measurements are low cost and easy to perform. In the presence of CKD, albuminuria and eGFR evaluation should be repeated annually [7].

Novel methods for evaluating early mediators of renal injury in the assessment of diabetic/hypertensive nephropathy development and progression have been proposed, including serum uric acid, insulin sensitivity, vasopressin, and sodium–glucose cotransport-2 inhibition, transforming growth factor-β, and bone morphogenic growth factor-7 in serum and urine. The routine assessment of novel biomarkers is not recommended for CV risk stratification, although the precise role of these laboratory parameters will be investigated by future studies.

6.2 Other Circulating Biomarkers

In patients with DM and without known CVD, the measurement of some inflammatory markers (C-reactive protein or fibrinogen) did not provide a significant improvement in risk assessment [8].

Recent evidence suggests that high-sensitivity cardiac troponin T (hsTnT) and troponin I (hsTnI) may be considered markers of CV disease and mortality risk, reflecting the cumulative impact of diabetes and hypertension, in addition to other comorbidities, on cardiac damage, especially in individuals of older age.

In individuals with DM type 2, hsTNT was associated with all-cause and CV mortality [9], and more recently in older type 2 DM patients (age 67–89 years) enrolled into the ARIC (Atherosclerosis Risk in Communities) study, both hsTNT and hsTNI improved the prediction of CV events independently of associated comorbidities, including hypertension [10].

In the SAVOR-TIMI 53 study (Saxagliptin Assessment of Vascular Outcomes Recorded in patients with diabetes mellitus—Thrombolysis in Myocardial Infarction 53 trial), enrolling patients with type 2 DM and elevated CV risk, increased levels of hs-TNT, indicating subclinical myocardial injury, were associated with lower values of diastolic BP (<80 mmHg) possibly causing insufficient coronary perfusion [11].

In diabetic patients with type 1 DM, elevated hsTnT was an independent predictor of renal decline and CV events [12].

N-terminal pro-B-type natriuretic peptide (NT-proBNP), another marker of cardiac damage, may be measured in hypertensive patients with DM [13]. In an unselected cohort of individuals with DM, it was shown that low levels of NT-proBNP were associated with a benign short-term prognosis [14–16].

In diabetic patients, however, the concomitant presence of obesity and hyperinsulinemia may influence the levels of natriuretic peptides. In the PARADIGM-HF trial, patients with diabetes had lower NT-proBNP than those without diabetes [17]. In patients with obesity and heart failure, measuring plasma levels of proBNP is more precise than measuring the plasma levels of either NT-proBNP or BNP.

The measurement of NT-proBNP has been proposed for the detection of left ventricular hypertrophy (LVH) and it was observed that NT-proBNP was superior to ECG, although it remained unsuitable for detecting echocardiographic LVH [18].

Gamella-Pozuelo et al. [19] have measured cardiotrophin-1 and found that hypertensive or diabetic patients have higher plasma cardiotrophin-1 than control patients; a positive correlation was found between cardiotrophin-1 and basal glycaemia, systolic and diastolic BP and pulse pressure (PP), the presence of cardiac (LVH), arterial damage (increased intima-media thickness [IMT] and decreased ankle–brachial index [ABI]), and renal damage (microalbuminuria and elevated UACR). The relationship between cardiotrophin-1 and cardiac and vascular damage remained significant at multivariate analysis, suggesting that increased plasma levels of cardiotrophin-1 are strongly related to the degree of subclinical target organ damage in hypertensive and diabetic patients.

6.3 Bioimaging

The ESH/ESC societies [1, 7] recommend a resting electrocardiogram (ECG) in patients with DM and hypertension, and/or if CV disease is suspected.

Other tests, such as transthoracic echocardiography, coronary artery calcium (CAC) score, ABI, and IMT may be considered to test for structural heart and vascular disease or as risk modifiers in those at moderate or high risk of CV disease.

6.3.1 Electrocardiography

ECG abnormalities may be present in patients with diabetes in the absence of coronary artery disease. Some ECG alterations have been advocated as a specific pattern of diabetes: abnormal repolarization, increase of QRS duration [20], and "strain" pattern [21].

When DM is associated with hypertension, an increased Cornell voltage–duration product [22], a prolonged QTc interval [23], and impaired heart rate variability [24] have been described. Another ECG finding, suggesting a worse prognosis, is T-wave axis deviation; in a general population study, ECG-LVH was more prevalent in patients with DM and hypertension and was associated with a higher prevalence of T-wave axis deviation [25].

In patients with diabetes and hypertension, ECG-LVH may be observed using criteria on the basis of the Cornell product and the Sokolow–Lyon voltage combination. It should be underlined that the concomitant presence of obesity might influence the detection of LVH according to the used criterion and the Cornell product should be preferred over the Sokolow–Lyon voltage [26].

In the LIFE study, the reduction or the absence of ECG LVH predicted a reduced incidence of DM in a large group of hypertensive patients [27], whereas in the same study regression of LVH was impaired in diabetic patients as compared to nondiabetics [28].

In the ACCORD study, including hypertensive diabetic patients, an intensive BP control has been associated with more regression of baseline LVH and lower rate of developing new LVH, compared to standard BP lowering [29].

A previous silent myocardial infarction may be detected by a resting ECG in 4% of patients with DM [30]. This finding has been associated with increased risks of all-cause mortality (hazard ratio 1.50, 95% confidence interval 1.30–1.73), CV mortality (2.33, 1.66–3.27), and major adverse cardiac events (1.61, 1.38–1.89) compared with the absence of myocardial infarction, as demonstrated by a recent meta-analysis [31].

In both type 1 and type 2 DM, an increase in heart rate detected at resting ECG is associated with the risk of CV disease, while a low heart rate variability (a marker of diabetic CV autonomic neuropathy) has been associated with an increased risk of fatal and nonfatal coronary artery disease (CAD).

6.4 Imaging Techniques

6.4.1 Echocardiography

Echocardiography is the first choice to evaluate structural and functional abnormalities associated with DM and hypertension. Two-dimensional transthoracic echocardiography provides information about left ventricular geometry, left atrial volume, aortic root dimensions, left ventricular systolic and diastolic function, pump performance, and output impedance [7] (Table 6.1). Increased left ventricular (LV) mass,

Table 6.1 Echocardiographic cutoff values for the definition of left ventricular hypertrophy, concentric geometry, left ventricular chamber size, and left atrial dilatation

Parameter measure	Abnormality threshold
LVH	
Left ventricular mass/height2.7 (g/m2.7)	>50 (men) >47 (women)
Left ventricular mass/BSA (g/m^2)	>115 (men) >95 (women)
Left ventricular concentric geometry RWT	≥0.43
Left ventricular and atrial chamber size	
Left ventricular end-diastolic diameter/height (cm/m)	>3.4 (men) >3.3 (women)
Left atrial volume/height^2 (mL/m^2)	>18.5 (men) >16.5 (women)

concentric geometry, diastolic dysfunction, and impaired LV deformation have been reported in asymptomatic patients with both hypertension and DM and are more severe than in patients with either hypertension or diabetes [32–36].

In patients with DM, associated with obesity and hypertension, a higher severity of diastolic function (lower e' velocities and higher filling pressures determined by the E/e' ratio) was observed, as compared with patients with DM alone [37]. In this study, a greater susceptibility of women with diastolic dysfunction to CV impact of type 2 DM was identified [37].

6.4.2 Cardiac Magnetic Resonance

Cardiac magnetic resonance is the gold standard for cardiac anatomical and functional quantification [38]. Tissue characterization techniques have shown that patients with DM have diffuse myocardial fibrosis as the mechanism of LV systolic and diastolic dysfunction, even in the absence of coronary artery disease [39]. LV deformation, diastolic dysfunction, and myocardial perfusion detected by CMR are further impaired by the presence of DM in hypertensive patients [40].

The prognostic value of these advanced imaging techniques in routine practice has not yet been extensively demonstrated.

6.4.3 Coronary Calcium Score

Multislice computed tomography allows the detection of coronary artery calcium (CAC), in order to identify subclinical coronary atherosclerosis, mainly stable coronary plaques containing calcium.

CAC scores range from 0 to >1000, with a score ≥100 being significant and ≥400 being at high risk.

The prevalence and severity of coronary calcium are higher in hypertensive patients compared with normotensive subjects [41, 42] and in diabetics, as compared to nondiabetic individuals [42]. Valenti et al. [43] have shown that in asymptomatic patients with type 2 DM and with a CAC score of 0, the prognosis is favorable, while each increment in CAC score (from 1–99 to 100–399 and >400) is associated with a 25%–33% higher relative risk of mortality.

Diabetes, in addition to BP increase and hypertension duration, could promote the development of atherosclerotic plaques with calcium accumulation in coronary and lower limbs vascular beds. In a cross-sectional study of patients free of coronary heart disease with type 2 DM, CAC score was independently associated with systolic BP and waist to hip ratio in a multivariate analysis [44].

A meta-analysis of seven studies, examining 12,682 individuals, has shown that the main predictors of CAC presence in order of importance were hypertension (OR = 1.71, $p < 0.00001$), male sex (OR = 1.47, $p = 0.02$), diabetes (OR = 1.34, $p = 0.03$), and age (OR = 1.07, $p = 0.04$) [45].

The CAC score by computed tomography may noninvasively estimate the atherosclerotic burden and computed tomography coronary angiography may identify stenotic atherosclerotic plaques.

It should be underlined, however, that the identification of CAC does not correspond to the presence of ischemia, and stress echocardiography or myocardial perfusion imaging should be performed, because of the contribution of coronary microcirculation impairment to ischemia, in addition to epicardial coronary vessel disease [46]. Positron emission tomography (PET) can assess myocardial blood flow and helps in the estimation of coronary flow reserve. The disadvantage of PET scan that sets back its utility in clinical practice is its prohibitive cost.

An extensive routine screening of silent ischemia and CAD in asymptomatic DM is still controversial [47]. However, in asymptomatic hypertensive or diabetic individuals at moderate risk, the presence of an increased CAC score could modify the risk from moderate to high; in addition stress testing or CT coronary angiography may be indicated in very-high-risk asymptomatic individuals, i.e., those with peripheral arterial disease, a high CAC score, proteinuria, or renal failure [47].

Exercise ECG has a moderate sensitivity (45%–61%) and better specificity (70%–90%) for the detection of silent ischemia in asymptomatic diabetic patients. The presence of repolarization abnormalities at baseline ECG and patients' incapacity to exercise may limit the use of this widely available and low-cost test [47].

6.4.4 Carotid Intima-Media Thickness

Carotid intima-media thickness (IMT) is an ultrasound biomarker of atherosclerosis, considered as a marker of subclinical organ damage [48, 49]. A greater carotid IMT was observed in diabetic patients, as compared with those without diabetes; carotid IMT seems to increase progressively from individuals without diabetes to those with impaired glucose tolerance, newly diagnosed diabetes, and established diabetes [50–52]. A relationship between albuminuria and carotid IMT was observed in patients with DM type 2 [53, 54]. However, European guidelines [1, 7] do not recommend routine carotid imaging and IMT measurements for CV risk re-stratification.

Carotid ultrasound may be clinically indicated in patients with a carotid bruit, previous cerebrovascular disease, or extensive peripheral vascular disease, in order to identify the presence of a carotid plaque (i.e., an IMT at least 1.5 mm, or by a focal increase in thickness of 0.5 mm or 50% of the surrounding carotid IMT value) [55].

The detection of a carotid plaque has shown incremental value over carotid intima-media thickness to detect coronary artery disease in asymptomatic DM [56]. The ultrasound evidence of an echolucent plaque and an increased plaque thickness are independent predictors of CV morbidity and mortality [57].

6.4.5 Aortic Stiffness

Increased arterial stiffness involving the aorta and femoral, carotid, and brachial arteries has been consistently documented in asymptomatic patients with T2D compared to healthy subjects. Concomitant hypertension and DM associated with vessel aging may accelerate the vascular stiffening process.

The measurement of aortic (carotid–femoral) pulse wave velocity (cfPWV) is a well-established technique for the assessment of arterial stiffness and a widely used methodology to study the relationship between arterial stiffness and disease outcomes. By arterial tonometry, aortic PWV may be measured and the threshold of 10 m/s indicates the presence of increased large artery stiffening [7].

DM is a contributory factor to the increased cfPWV values in hypertensive patients at different ages [58–60]. The increase in arterial stiffness in individuals with DM and arterial hypertension was greater than in those without diabetes and with hypertension [59, 61]. Moreover, it has been shown that in hypertensive patients with diabetes mellitus, exercise induces a greater increase in aortic stiffness in those with type 2 diabetes as compared to those without [62].

A recent study has assessed baseline cfPWV and its 3-year change in patients with type 2 diabetes and has shown that the risk of CKD progression was associated with aortic stiffness at baseline and 3-year changes. In this study the reclassification of the risk of progressive CKD was improved by including cfPWV, above and beyond traditional risk factors [63], supporting the hypothesis that arterial stiffness should be considered in the management of individuals with type 2 diabetes and hypertension [64]. In the presence of diabetes and hypertension, the kidney may be more susceptible to loss of the protective autoregulation on blood flow which results in exacerbation of the pulsatile energy transmission, damage of glomerular vasculature, and progressive loss of kidney function.

6.4.6 Ankle–Brachial Index (ABI)

In a healthy subject, systolic BP is greater in the lower than in the upper limbs, because reflection and amplification of pulse wave and vascular walls changes induced by hydrostatic pressure; the ratio between systolic BP measured at ankle and brachial levels may quantify this difference [65]. A reduction of ABI to <0.9 is due to atherosclerotic stenosis of lower limb vasculature and is widely accepted for the diagnosis of peripheral artery diseases. An ABI >1.4 indicated medial calcinosis and is associated with lower limb arterial disease in 50% of cases.

A low ABI (<0.9) is associated with several CV risk factors, including hypertension, diabetes, dyslipidemia, smoking, and others more recently identified (inflammatory markers and CKD) [65, 66].

CV risk stratification may be improved by ABI assessment [67] and ABI is associated with an increased risk of all-cause and CV mortality in DM and non-DM patients [68]. Two recent retrospective analyses of the Catalan Primary Care (SIDIAP) database have shown that different levels of ABI are independently associated with diabetes complications in type 2 DM patients (70% prevalence of hypertension) [69] and that in hypertensive patients a high ABI (>1.3) is associated with a mortality risk similar to the group with an ABI of at least 0.9 [70].

Repeated evaluation of ABI during follow-up may imply a clinical advantage, as shown by Criqui et al. [71].

6.5 Conclusions

The majority of patients with both diabetes mellitus and hypertension are at high or very high risk of CV disease and CKD [72]. Routine laboratory examination, including albuminuria and eGFR, may identify the degree of hypertensive/diabetic nephropathy. The evaluation of cardiac and vascular subclinical organ damage may integrate laboratory tests (cardiac troponin and NT-proBNP), ECG, and echocardiography. The prognostic value of advanced imaging techniques, such as strain imaging or CV magnetic resonance with tissue characterization, will be validated in the future in prospective cohorts. Asymptomatic patients with a high risk of coronary artery disease (carotid plaque, peripheral artery disease, proteinuria) may undergo CAC score assessment and may be referred for functional imaging or CTCA in the presence of high CAC (if CAC score >400).

References

1. Cosentino F, Grant PJ, Aboyans V, Bailey CJ, Ceriello A, Delgado V, et al. 2019 ESC Guidelines on diabetes, pre-diabetes, and cardiovascular diseases developed in collaboration with the EASD. Eur Heart J. 2020;41(2):255–323. https://doi.org/10.1093/eurheartj/ehz486.
2. de Zeeuw D, Remuzzi G, Parving HH, Keane WF, Zhang Z, Shahinfar S, et al. Proteinuria, a target for renoprotection in patients with type 2 diabetic nephropathy: lessons from RENAAL. Kidney Int. 2004;65(6):2309–20.
3. Wachtell K, Ibsen H, Olsen MH, Borch-Johnsen K, Lindholm LH, Mogensen CE, et al. Albuminuria and cardiovascular risk in hypertensive patients with left ventricular hypertrophy: the LIFE study. Ann Intern Med. 2003;139(11):901–6. https://doi.org/10.7326/0003-4819-139-11-200312020-00008.

4. Mancusi C, Izzo R, di Gioia G, Losi MA, Barbato E, Morisco C. Insulin resistance the hinge between hypertension and type 2 diabetes. High Blood Press Cardiovasc Prev. 2020;27(6):515–26. https://doi.org/10.1007/s40292-020-00408-8.
5. Koye DN, Magliano DJ, Reid CM, Keane WF, Zhang Z, Shahinfar S, et al. Risk of progression of nonalbuminuric CKD to end-stage kidney disease in people with diabetes: the CRIC (Chronic Renal Insufficiency Cohort) Study. Am J Kidney Dis. 2018;72(5):653–61.
6. Ninomiya T, Perkovic V, de Galan BE, Zoungas S, Pillai A, Jardine M, et al. ADVANCE Collaborative Group. Albuminuria and kidney function independently predict cardiovascular and renal outcomes in diabetes. J Am Soc Nephrol. 2009;20:1813–21.
7. Williams B, Mancia G, Spiering W, Agabiti Rosei E, Azizi M, Burnier M, et al. Authors/Task Force Members. 2018 ESC/ESH Guidelines for the management of arterial hypertension: the task force for the management of arterial hypertension of the European Society of Cardiology and the European Society of Hypertension: The Task Force for the management of arterial hypertension of the European Society of Cardiology and the European Society of Hypertension. J Hypertens. 2018;36(10):1953–2041.
8. Emerging Risk Factors Collaboration, Kaptoge S, Di Angelantonio E, Pennells L, Wood AM, White IR, Gao P, et al. Creactive protein, fibrinogen, and cardiovascular disease prediction. N Engl J Med. 2012;367:1310–20.
9. Hendriks SH, van Dijk PR, van Hateren KJ, van Pelt JL, Groenier KH, Bilo HJ, et al. High-sensitive troponin T is associated with all-cause and cardiovascular mortality in stable outpatients with type 2 diabetes (ZODIAC-37). Am Heart J. 2016;174:43–50.
10. Tang O, Daya N, Matsushita K, Coresh J, Sharrett AR, Hoogeveen R, et al. Performance of high-sensitivity cardiac troponin assays to reflect comorbidity burden and improve mortality risk stratification in older adults with diabetes. Diabetes Care. 2020;43(6):1200–8. https://doi.org/10.2337/dc19-2043.
11. Bergmark BA, Scirica BM, Steg PG, Fanola CL, Gurmu Y, Mosenzon O, et al. SAVOR-TIMI 53 Investigators.Blood pressure and cardiovascular outcomes in patients with diabetes and high cardiovascular risk. Eur Heart J. 2018;39(24):2255–62. https://doi.org/10.1093/eurheartj/ehx809.
12. Galsgaard J, Persson F, Hansen TW, Jorsal A, Tarnow L, Parving HH, Rossing P. Plasma high-sensitivity troponin T predicts end-stage renal disease and cardiovascular and all-cause mortality in patients with type 1 diabetes and diabetic nephropathy. Kidney Int. 2017;92:1242–8.
13. Hildebrandt P, Richards MA. Amino-terminal pro-B-type natriuretic peptide testing in patients with diabetes mellitus and with systemic hypertension. Am J Cardiol. 2008;101(3A):21–4. https://doi.org/10.1016/j.amjcard.2007.11.015.
14. Tarnow L, Hildebrandt P, Hansen BV, Borch-Johnsen K, Parving HH. Plasma N-terminal pro-brain natriuretic peptide as an independent predictor of mortality in diabetic nephropathy. Diabetologia. 2005;48:149–55.
15. Gaede P, Hildebrandt P, Hess G, Parving HH, Pedersen O. Plasma N-terminal pro-brain natriuretic peptide as a major risk marker for cardiovascular disease in patients with type 2 diabetes and microalbuminuria. Diabetologia. 2005;48:156–63.
16. Huelsmann M, Neuhold S, Strunk G, Moertl D, Berger R, Prager R, et al. NT-proBNP has a high negative predictive value to rule-out short-term cardiovascular events in patients with diabetes mellitus. Eur Heart J. 2008;29:2259–64.
17. Rorth R, Jhund P, Kristensen S, Desai A, Køber L, Rouleau J, et al. The prognostic value of troponin T and N-terminal pro B-type natriuretic peptide, alone and in combination, in heart failure patients with and without diabetes. Eur J Heart Fail. 2019;21:40–9.
18. Somaratne JB, Whalley GA, Poppe KK, ter Bals MM, Wadams G, Pearl A, et al. Screening for left ventricular hypertrophy in patients with type 2 diabetes mellitus in the community. Cardiovasc Diabetol. 2011;10:29. https://doi.org/10.1186/1475-2840-10-29.
19. Gamella-Pozuelo L, Fuentes-Calvo I, Gómez-Marcos MA, Recio-Rodriguez JI, Agudo-Conde C, Fernández-Martín JL, et al. Plasma cardiotrophin-1 as a marker of hypertension

and diabetes-induced target organ damage and cardiovascular risk. Medicine (Baltimore). 2015;94(30):e1218. https://doi.org/10.1097/MD.0000000000001218.

20. Bacharova L, Krivosikova Z, Wsolova L, Gajdos M. Alterations in the QRS complex in the offspring of patients with metabolic syndrome and diabetes mellitus: early evidence of cardiovascular pathology. J Electrocardiol. 2012;45:244–51.
21. Flugelman MY, Kanter Y, Abinader EG, Lewis BS, Barzilai D. Electrocardiographic patterns in diabetics without clinical ischemic heart disease. Isr J Med Sci. 1983;19:252–5.
22. Okin PM, Devereux RB, Nieminen MS, Jern S, Oikarinen L, Viitasalo M, et al. Electrocardiographic strain pattern and prediction of new-onset congestive heart failure in hypertensive patients. The Losartan Intervention for Endpoint Reduction in Hypertension (LIFE) Study. Circulation. 2006;113:67–73.
23. Li X, Ren H, Xu Z, Liu Y, Yang X, Liu J. Prevalence and risk factors of prolonged QTc Interval among Chinese patients with type 2 diabetes. Exp Diabetes Res. 2012;2012:234084. https://doi.org/10.1155/2012/234084.
24. Cerutti F, Rabbia F, Rabbonei I, Bobbio A, Ignaccolo MG, Greco G, et al. Impairment of cardiovascular autonomic pattern in obese adolescents with type 2 diabetes mellitus. J Endocrinol Investig. 2010;33:539–43.
25. Assanelli D, Di Castelnuovo A, Rago L, Badilini F, Vinetti G, Gianfagna F, et al. Moli-sani Project Investigators. T-wave axis deviation and left ventricular hypertrophy interaction in diabetes and hypertension. J Electrocardiol. 2013;46(6):487–91. https://doi.org/10.1016/j.jelectrocard.2013.08.002.
26. Muiesan ML, Salvetti M, Di Castelnuovo A, Paini A, Assanelli D, Costanzo S, et al. Moli-sani Study Investigators. Obesity and ECG left ventricular hypertrophy. J Hypertens. 2017;35(1):162–9. https://doi.org/10.1097/HJH.0000000000001121.
27. Okin PM, Devereux RB, Harris KE, Jern S, Kjeldsen SE, Lindholm LH, et al. LIFE Study Investigators. In-treatment resolution or absence of electrocardiographic left ventricular hypertrophy is associated with decreased incidence of new-onset diabetes mellitus in hypertensive patients: the Losartan Intervention for Endpoint reduction in hypertension (LIFE) Study. Hypertension. 2007;50:984–90.
28. Okin PM, Devereux RB, Gerdts E, Snapinn SM, Harris KE, Jern S, et al. LIFE Study Investigators. Impact of diabetes mellitus on regression of electrocardiographic left ventricular hypertrophy and the prediction of outcome during antihypertensive therapy: the Losartan Intervention For Endpoint (LIFE) Reduction in Hypertension Study. Circulation. 2006;113(12):1588–96.
29. Soliman E, Byington R, Bigger T, Evans G, Okin P, Goff D, et al. Effect of intensive blood pressure lowering on left ventricular hypertrophy in patients with diabetes mellitus: action to control cardiovascular risk in Diabetes Blood Pressure Trial. Hypertension. 2015;66(6):1123–9. https://doi.org/10.1161/HYPERTENSIONAHA.115.06236.
30. Hadaegh F, Ehteshami-Afshar S, Hajebrahimi MA, Hajsheikholeslami F, Azizi F. Silent coronary artery disease and incidence of cardiovascular and mortality events at different levels of glucose regulation; results of greater than a decade follow-up. Int J Cardiol. 2015;182:334–9.
31. Yang Y, Li W, Zhu H, Pan XF, Hu Y, Arnott C, et al. Prognosis of unrecognised myocardial infarction determined by electrocardiography or cardiac magnetic resonance imaging: systematic review and meta-analysis. BMJ. 2020;369:m1184. https://doi.org/10.1136/bmj.m1184.
32. Devereux RB, Roman MJ, Paranicas M, O'Grady MJ, Lee ET, Welty TK, et al. Impact of diabetes on cardiac structure and function: the strong heart study. Circulation. 2000;101(19):2271–6. https://doi.org/10.1161/01.CIR.101.19.2271.
33. Cioffi G, Faggiano P, Lucci D, Di LA, Mureddu GF, Tarantini L, et al. Inappropriately high left ventricular mass in patients with type 2 diabetes mellitus and no overt cardiac disease. The DYDA Study. J Hypertens. 2011;29(10):1994–2003. https://doi.org/10.1097/HJH.0b013e32834acc6d.
34. Palmieri V, Bella JN, Arnett DR, Liu JE, Oberman A, Schuck M-Y, et al. Effect of type 2 diabetes mellitus on left ventricular geometry and systolic function in hypertensive subjects: Hypertension Genetic Epidemiology Network (HyperGEN) Study. Circulation. 2001;103:102–7.

35. Bella JN, Devereux RB, Roman MJ, Palmieri V, Liu JE, Paranicas M, et al. Separate and joint effects of systemic hypertension and diabetes mellitus on left ventricular structure and function in American Indians (the Strong Heart Study). Am J Cardiol. 2001;87:1260–5.
36. Ernande L, Audureau E, Jellis CL, Bergerot C, Henegar C, Sawaki D, et al. Clinical implications of echocardiographic phenotypes of patients with diabetes mellitus. J Am Coll Cardiol. 2017;70:1704–16.
37. Gerdts E, Okin PM, Omvik P, Wachtell K, Dahlöf B, Hildebrandt P, et al. Impact of diabetes on treatment-induced changes in left ventricular structure and function in hypertensive patients with left ventricular hypertrophy. The LIFE study. Nutr Metab Cardiovasc Dis. 2009;19(5):306–12.
38. Perrone-Filardi P, Coca A, Galderisi M, Paolillo S, Alpendurada F, de Simone G, et al. Noninvasive cardiovascular imaging for evaluating subclinical target organ damage in hypertensive patients: a consensus article from the European Association of Cardiovascular Imaging, the European Society of Cardiology Council on Hypertension and the European Society of Hypertension. J Hypertens. 2017;35(9):1727–41.
39. Tadic M, Cuspidi C, Calicchio F, Grassi G, Mancia G. Diabetic cardiomyopathy: how can cardiac magnetic resonance help? Acta Diabetol. 2020;57(9):1027–34.
40. Li XM, Jiang L, Guo YK, Ren Y, Han P, Peng L, et al. The additive effects of type 2 diabetes mellitus on left ventricular deformation and myocardial perfusion in essential hypertension: a 3.0 T cardiac magnetic resonance study. Cardiovasc Diabetol. 2020;19(1):161.
41. Valenti V, Hartaigh O, Heo R, Schulman-Marcus J, Cho I, Kalra DK, et al. Long-term prognosis for individuals with hypertension undergoing coronary artery calcium scoring. Int J Cardiol. 2015;187:534–40.
42. Uddin SMI, Mirbolouk M, Kianoush S, Orimoloye OA, Dardari Z, Whelton SP, et al. Role of coronary artery calcium for stratifying cardiovascular risk in adults with hypertension. Hypertension. 2019;73:983–9.
43. Valenti V, Hartaigh BO, Cho I, Schulman-Marcus J, Gransar H, Heo R, et al. Absence of coronary artery calcium identifies asymptomatic diabetic individuals at low near-term but not long-term risk of mortality: a 15-year follow-up study of 9715 patients. Circ Cardiovasc Imaging. 2016;9:e003528.
44. Elkeles RS, Feher MD, Flather MD, Godsland IF, Nugara F, Richmond W, et al. The association of coronary calcium score and conventional cardiovascular risk factors in Type 2 diabetic subjects asymptomatic for coronary heart disease (The PREDICT Study). Diabet Med. 2004;21(10):1129–34.
45. Nicoll R, Zhao Y, Ibrahimi P, Olivecrona G, Henein M. Diabetes and hypertension consistently predict the presence and extent of coronary artery calcification in symptomatic patients: a systematic review and meta-analysis. Int J Mol Sci. 2016;17(9):1481. https://doi.org/10.3390/ijms17091481.
46. Murtaza G, Virk HUH, Khalid M, Lavie CJ, Ventura H, Mukherjee D, et al. Diabetic cardiomyopathy a comprehensive updated review. Prog Cardiovasc Dis. 2019;62(4):315–26.
47. Makrilakis K, Liatis S. Cardiovascular screening for the asymptomatic patient with diabetes: more cons than pros. J Diabetes Res. 2017;2017:8927473.
48. O'Leary DH, Polak JF, Kronmal RA, Manolio TA, Burke GL, Wolfson SK Jr. Carotid artery intima-media thickness as a risk factor for myocardial infarction and stroke in older adults. N Engl J Med. 1999;340:14–22.
49. Lorenz MW, Price JF, Robertson C, Bots ML, Polak JF, Poppert H, et al. Carotid intima-media thickness progression and risk of vascular events in people with diabetes: results from the PROG-IMT Collaboration. Diabetes Care. 2015;38(10):1921–9. https://doi.org/10.2337/dc14-2732.
50. Wagenknecht LE, D'Agostino RB Jr, Haffner SM, Savage PJ, Rewers M. Impaired glucose tolerance, type 2 diabetes, and carotid wall thickness: the Insulin Resistance Atherosclerosis Study. Diabetes Care. 1998;21:1812–8.
51. Temelkova-Kurktschiev TS, Koehler C, Leonhardt W, Schaper F, Henkel E, Siegert G, et al. Increased intimal-medial thickness in newly detected type 2 diabetes: risk factors. Diabetes Care. 1999;22:333–8.

52. Brohall G, Odén A, Fagerberg B. Carotid artery intima-media thickness in patients with type 2 diabetes mellitus and impaired glucose tolerance: a systematic review. Diabet Med. 2006;23:609–16.
53. Mykkanen L, Zaccaro D, O'Leary D, Howard G, Robbins D, Haffner S. Microalbuminuria and carotid artery intima-media thickness in nondiabetic and NIDDM subjects: the Insulin Resistance Atherosclerosis Study (IRAS). Stroke. 1997;28:1710–6.
54. Agewall S, Wikstrand J, Ljungman S, Fagerberg B. Urinary albumin excretion is associated with the intima-media thickness of the carotid artery in hypertensive males with non-insulin-dependent diabetes mellitus. J Hypertens. 1995;13:463–9.
55. Touboul PJ, Hennerici MG, Meairs S, Adams H, Amarenco P, Desvarieux M, et al. Advisory Board of the 3rd Watching the Risk Symposium 2004, 13th European Stroke Conference. Mannheim intima-media thickness consensus. Cerebrovasc Dis. 2004;18:346–9.
56. Akazawa S, Tojikubo M, Nakano Y, Nakamura S, Tamai H, Yonemoto K, et al. Usefulness of carotid plaque (sum and maximum of plaque thickness) in combination with intima-media thickness for the detection of coronary artery disease in asymptomatic patients with diabetes. J Diabetes Investig. 2016;7:396–403.
57. Irie Y, Katakami N, Kaneto H, Takahara M, Nishio M, Kasami R, et al. The utility of ultrasonic tissue characterization of carotid plaque in the prediction of cardiovascular events in diabetic patients. Atherosclerosis. 2013;230:399–405.
58. Tedesco MA, Natale F, Di Salvo G, Caputo S, Capasso M, Calabro R. Effects of coexisting hypertension and type II diabetes mellitus on arterial stiffness. J Hum Hypertens. 2004;18(7):469–73. https://doi.org/10.1038/sj.jhh.1001690.
59. Bruno RM, Penno G, Daniele G, Pucci L, Lucchesi D, Stea F, et al. Type 2 diabetes mellitus worsens arterial stiffness in hypertensive patients through endothelial dysfunction. Diabetologia. 2012;55(6):1847–55. https://doi.org/10.1007/s00125-012-2517-1.
60. Galvão RDV, Pereira CS, Freitas EGB, Lima DRART, Santos WAM, Souza DF, et al. Association between diabetes mellitus and central arterial stiffness in elderly patients with systemic arterial hypertension. Clin Exp Hypertens. 2020;42(8):728–32.
61. Yeboah K, Antwi DA, Gyan B, Govoni V, Mills CE, Cruickshank JK, et al. Arterial stiffness in hypertensive and type 2 diabetes patients in Ghana: comparison of the cardio-ankle vascular index and central aortic techniques. BMC Endocr Disord. 2016;16(1):53.
62. Cooke AB, Dasgupta K, Spronck B, Sharman JE, Daskalopoulou SS. Adults with type 2 diabetes mellitus exhibit a greater exercise-induced increase in arterial stiffness and vessel hemodynamics. Hypertension. 2020;75(6):1565–73.
63. Liu JJ, Liu S, Lee J, Gurung RL, Yiamunaa M, Ang K, et al. Aortic pulse wave velocity, central pulse pressure, augmentation index and chronic kidney disease progression in individuals with type 2 diabetes: a 3-year prospective study. BMC Nephrol. 2020;21(1):359.
64. Vlachopoulos C, Aznaouridis K, O'Rourke MF, Safar ME, Baou K, Stefanadis C. Prediction of cardiovascular events and all-cause mortality with central haemodynamics: a systematic review and meta-analysis. Eur Heart J. 2010;31:1865–71.
65. Aboyans V, Criqui MH, Abraham P, Allison MA, Creager MA, Diehm C, et al. American Heart Association Council on Peripheral Vascular Disease; Council on Epidemiology and Prevention; Council on Clinical Cardiology; Council on Cardiovascular Nursing; Council on Cardiovascular Radiology and Intervention, and Council on Cardiovascular Surgery and Anesthesia. Measurement and interpretation of the ankle-brachial index: a scientific statement from the American Heart Association. Circulation. 2012;126(24):2890–909.
66. Criqui MH, Langer RD, Fronek A, Feigelson HS, Klauber MR, McCann TJ, et al. Mortality over a period of 10 years in patients with peripheral arterial disease. N Engl J Med. 1992;326(6):381–6.
67. Ankle Brachial Index Collaboration, Fowkes FG, Murray GD, Butcher I, Heald CL, Lee RJ, Chambless LE, et al. Ankle brachial index combined with Framingham Risk Score to predict cardiovascular events and mortality: a meta-analysis. JAMA. 2008;300(2):197–208.
68. Hanssen NM, Huijberts MS, Schalkwijk CG, Nijpels G, Dekker JM, Stehouwer CD. Associations between the ankle-brachial index and cardiovascular and all cause mortality

are similar in individuals without and with type 2 diabetes: nineteen-year follow-up of a population-based cohort study. Diabetes Care. 2012;35:1731–5.

69. Alves-Cabratosa L, Comas-Cufí M, Ponjoan A, Garcia-Gil M, Martí-Lluch R, Blanch J, et al. Levels of ankle-brachial index and the risk of diabetes mellitus complications. BMJ Open Diabetes Res Care. 2020;8(1):e000977. https://doi.org/10.1136/bmjdrc-2019-000977.
70. Alves-Cabratosa L, Elosua-Bayes M, García-Gil M, Comas-Cufí M, Martí-Lluch R, Ponjoan A. Hypertension and high ankle brachial index: the overlooked combination. J Hypertens. 2019;37(1):92–8.
71. Criqui MH, Ninomiya JK, Wingard DL, Ji M, Fronek A. Progression of peripheral arterial disease predicts cardiovascular disease morbidity and mortality. J Am Coll Cardiol. 2008;52(21):1736–42.
72. Piepoli MF, Hoes AW, Agewall S, Albus C, Brotons C, Catapano AL, et al. 2016 European Guidelines on cardiovascular disease prevention in clinical practice: The Sixth Joint Task Force of the European Society of Cardiology and Other Societies on Cardiovascular Disease Prevention in Clinical Practice (constituted by representatives of 10 societies and by invited experts) Developed with the special contribution of the European Association for Cardiovascular Prevention & Rehabilitation (EACPR). Eur Heart J. 2016;37:2315–81.

Part IV

Pathophysiological Mechanisms

Molecular Mechanisms Underlying Vascular Disease in Diabetes

7

Rhian M. Touyz, Omotayo Eluwole, Livia L. Camargo, Francisco J. Rios, Rheure Alves-Lopes, Karla B. Neves, Muzi J. Maseko, Tomasz Guzik, John Petrie, and Augusto C. Montezano

7.1 Introduction

Diabetes mellitus is the heterogeneous derangement of metabolism characterized primarily by chronic hyperglycaemia and insulin resistance [1]. This is due to impaired insulin secretion and/or impaired insulin action [2]. Among all types of diabetes, type 2 diabetes, which was formally referred to as noninsulin-dependent diabetes or adult-onset diabetes, accounts for 90%–95% of all diabetes. Hypertension and type 2 diabetes are common comorbidities that are inextricably linked [3–5]. The former is twice as frequent in patients with diabetes compared with those who do not have diabetes. Patients with hypertension often exhibit insulin resistance and are at greater risk of developing diabetes than normotensive individuals [6]. As comorbidities, hypertension and diabetes correlate with worse outcomes and more

R. M. Touyz (✉)
Institute of Cardiovascular and Medical Sciences, BHF Glasgow Cardiovascular Research Centre, University of Glasgow, Glasgow, UK

Research Institute of McGill University Health Centre, McGill University, Montreal, Canada
e-mail: Rhian.touyz@mcgill.ca

O. Eluwole
Department of Physiology, University of Witwatersrand, Johannesburg, South Africa

Obafemi Awolowo University, Ile-Ife, Osun State, Nigeria

L. L. Camargo · F. J. Rios · R. Alves-Lopes · K. B. Neves · T. Guzik · J. Petrie · A. C. Montezano
Institute of Cardiovascular and Medical Sciences, BHF Glasgow Cardiovascular Research Centre, University of Glasgow, Glasgow, UK

M. J. Maseko
Department of Physiology, University of Witwatersrand, Johannesburg, South Africa

A. E. Berbari, G. Mancia (eds.), *Blood Pressure Disorders in Diabetes Mellitus*, Updates in Hypertension and Cardiovascular Protection,
https://doi.org/10.1007/978-3-031-13009-0_7

disability than in patients with only diabetes or hypertension [7]. Type 2 diabetes typically occurs in the setting of abdominal obesity, hypertension, hyperlipidaemia and increased coagulability, features that are also common in metabolic syndrome.

Many of the complications of diabetes are linked to vascular injury [8]. Vascular changes typically involve inflammation and prothrombotic processes that manifest as capillary basement membrane thickening, vascular fibrosis, microvascular calcification and endothelial dysfunction [4, 8]. These vascular changes are amplified in obesity and changes in the gut microbiome may be a trigger for metabolic inflammation in obesity and diabetes [9]. Molecular processes underlying these events include oxidative stress, immune responses, activation of the renin-angiotensin system and formation of advanced glycation end products (AGEs) [4, 10]. Recent data indicate an important role for microRNAs in the vasculopathy of diabetes [11]. Hypertension and obesity are important risk factors for diabetes-associated vascular complications, because these conditions are also associated with vascular dysfunction and injury.

This chapter provides a comprehensive update on vascular complications of diabetes and the molecular mechanisms that underlie the vasculopathy of diabetes. In particular, the role of advanced glycation end products (AGEs), oxidative stress and inflammation are highlighted.

7.2 Macrovascular and Microvascular Disease in Diabetes

Diabetes is associated with both macrovascular (large arteries) and microvascular disease (small arteries and capillaries). Macrovascular disease leads to myocardial infarction, stroke and peripheral artery disease, primarily due to atherosclerosis. The process of atherosclerosis is accelerated in diabetes [12–14]. Patients with type 2 diabetes have poorer cardiovascular outcomes than patients without diabetes [15]. Diabetes is a frequent and strong risk factor for large artery disease and coronary artery calcification [16]. Individuals with diabetes consistently have higher levels of calcification than do those without diabetes [16]. Vascular calcification and atherosclerosis in diabetes contribute to increased risk of myocardial infarction. Type 2 diabetes acts as an independent risk factor for the development of ischaemic disease. Major modifiable risk factors for macrovascular disease in diabetes are hypertension, dyslipidaemia, obesity and cigarette smoking [17, 18]. Increased risk of cardiovascular disease starts during prediabetes in association with insulin resistance and impaired glucose tolerance [19].

Microvascular disease leads to retinopathy, nephropathy and neuropathy with target organ damage. These are the major causes of morbidity and mortality in patients with diabetes [20–22]. Microvascular dysfunction seems to precede structural vascular changes. During the early phases of diabetes and/or cardiometabolic disease, each can cause reversible microvascular damage with associated dysfunction. With time these changes may become irreversible leading to target organ damage and consequent vision loss, renal insufficiency and neuropathy [23]. Microvascular disease in diabetes can also cause heart failure, sarcopenia, cognitive decline and worsening of metabolic dysfunction [24]. Processes underlying microvascular injury include increased endothelial permeability, inflammation and oxidative stress [10, 23]. Diabetic retinopathy is the most common microvascular complication of diabetes often leading to blindness [4]. Diabetic nephropathy, characterized by microalbuminuria, is the leading cause of end-stage renal disease worldwide [25]. Microalbuminuria commonly coexists with hypertension and may reflect endothelial dysfunction in both conditions. Although the underlying cause of microalbuminuria is controversial, it is thought to be a renal manifestation of generalized vascular endothelial dysfunction and is strongly linked to increased cardiovascular risk [26]. Moreover, systemic inflammation precedes microalbuminuria in diabetes, suggesting that by the time microalbuminuria is detected, there is already evidence of vascular injury [26]. Accordingly, screening for microalbuminuria is important for the intervention and prevention of further complications such as end-stage renal disease and cardiovascular disease.

7.3 Pathophysiology of Vascular Disease in Diabetes

7.3.1 Insulin Resistance

Physiologically, insulin maintains glucose homeostasis by integrated actions on carbohydrate, protein and lipid metabolism [27]. These actions occur mainly in the liver, skeletal muscle and adipose tissue. Glucose can alter insulin sensitivity in muscle and fat, as well as decrease insulin secretion from β-cells of the pancreatic tissue. In pathological conditions, hyperglycaemia promotes loss of sensitivity to insulin in insulin-sensitive tissue resulting in insulin resistance, which is associated with type 2 diabetes, obesity, hypertension and other cardiometabolic diseases [28, 29]. Many factors play a role in insulin resistance including AGEs, which inhibit insulin signalling by increasing Ser-307 phosphorylation of IRS-1 and forming methylglyoxal-IRS-1. In addition, in the context of obesity, adipocytes undergo hypertrophy and assume a pro-inflammatory phenotype, which contribute to vascular injury in diabetes [30, 31]. These changes have been shown to coincide with the onset of insulin resistance and provide a pathophysiological link between metabolic and vascular disease.

Activation of the renin-angiotensin system plays an important role in vascular inflammation and injury in diabetes and hypertension [32, 33]. Ang II opposes the actions of insulin to enhance glucose uptake in skeletal muscle and may lead to insulin resistance in the vasculature [34]. Important cross-talk between insulin and Ang II signalling has been demonstrated in VSMCs, where Ang II opposes the effects of insulin [35].

7.3.2 Endothelial Dysfunction

Endothelial dysfunction is a key feature in vascular disease and is typically observed in hypertension, diabetes and obesity [36, 37]. Impaired endothelial function is associated with reduced vasorelaxation, inflammation, prothrombotic state, increased permeability and increased production of vasoactive and mitogenic factors [38, 39]. Abnormal endothelium-dependent vasodilatation may also contribute to or exacerbate insulin resistance by reducing the delivery of glucose to target tissues [40].

7.3.3 Vascular Remodeling

The vasculopathy of diabetes is associated not only with functional alterations, but with structural changes of small and large vessels [41]. Vascular smooth muscle cells (VSMCs) undergo dedifferentiation from a contractile phenotype to a pro-migratory and proliferative form [42]. In addition, they produce pro-inflammatory mediators and pro-fibrotic factors that contribute to chronic low-grade inflammation, vascular fibrosis and increased stiffness, which resemble processes that occur with 'vascular ageing' [43–45]. The vasculopathy of diabetes has been considered as a condition of 'premature' vascular ageing, similar to what has been described in hypertension, since the vascular changes observed in diabetes in young individuals is similar to that observed in non-diabetic elderly people [46].

7.4 Molecular Mechanisms of Vascular Dysfunction and Damage During Diabetes

7.4.1 Advanced Glycation End Products (AGEs) and Activation of the AGE-Receptor AGE (RAGE) System

AGEs are a diverse group of macromolecules formed via the process of non-enzymatic glycation of proteins and lipids [47]. This process is accelerated during hyperglycaemia, oxidative stress, ageing, advanced renal disease and inflammation [48]. AGEs accumulate in the extracellular matrix of vessels and contribute to vascular damage in diabetes [49]. AGEs interact with two main types of cell surface receptors: scavenger receptors, which remove and degrade AGEs, and receptors for AGEs (RAGE), which trigger specific cellular signalling responses on AGE binding [50]. AGEs stimulate the production of reactive oxygen species (ROS), which reversibly enhance AGE formation [51, 52]. AGEs are antigenic and induce immune and inflammatory responses [53]. RAGE is a receptor and member of the immunoglobulin family and binds many ligands besides AGEs. AGE-RAGE signals through transforming growth factor (TGF)-b, NFκB, mitogen-activated protein kinases (MAPK; ERK1/2, p38MAPK) and nicotinamide adenine dinucleotide phosphate (NADPH) oxidases (Nox) and induces expression of vascular adhesion molecule 1, E-selectin, vascular endothelial growth factor and pro-inflammatory cytokines (IL-1b, IL-6, TNF-a) [54].

In diabetes, activation of AGE-RAGE signalling pathways is increased in VSMCs leading to inflammation, pro-thrombotic effects, fibrosis and calcification, which underlie diabetic nephropathy, retinopathy, neuropathy and atherosclerotic cardiovascular disease [55]. In the presence of hypertension these processes are amplified leading to accelerated vasculopathy in diabetes [56]. Patients with diabetes have increased tissue and circulating concentrations of AGEs and soluble RAGE, which predict cardiovascular events [57]. Accordingly urinary and plasma AGE levels and soluble RAGE have been considered as putative biomarkers for vascular disease in diabetes [58] (Fig. 7.1).

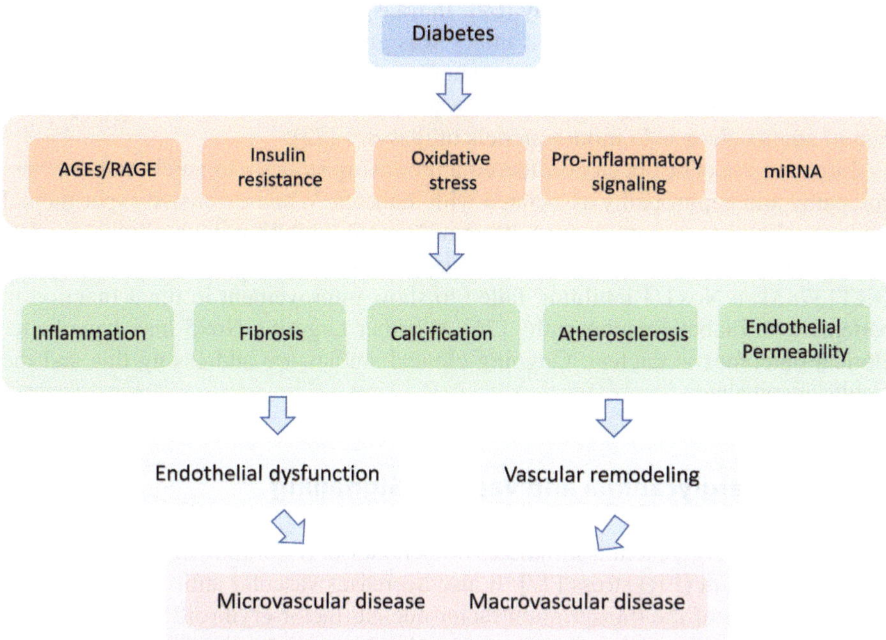

Fig. 7.1 Schematic demonstrating vascular processes whereby diabetes predisposes to microvascular and macrovascular disease, which leads to cardiovascular disease. Activation of AGE/RAGE signaling, oxidative stress, pro-inflammatory signaling and miRNAs lead to vascular injury and dysfunction that manifest as microvascular and macrovascular disease. *AGEs* Advanced glycation end products, *RAGE* Receptor AGE

7.4.2 Oxidative Stress and Vascular Injury in Diabetes

Oxidative stress (increased bioavailability of ROS) is a key mechanism of glucotoxicity in diabetes, as evidenced by increased vascular ROS generation in response to hyperglycaemia and accumulation of oxidation by-products of lipids, proteins and nucleic acids [59, 60]. NADPH oxidases (Nox) and dysfunctional eNOS are principal sources of increased vascular ROS in diabetes [61, 62]. Diabetes-/hypertension-associated oxidative stress is caused by multiple processes that increase and decrease pro-oxidant and antioxidants, respectively [63]. Increased vascular oxidative stress in diabetes and hypertension promotes posttranslational oxidative modification of proteins, causing cellular damage, endothelial dysfunction and vascular inflammation and injury. Oxidative stress and activation of Noxs are increased in patients with diabetes and in preclinical models of diabetes and obesity [62, 64].

Of the seven Nox isoforms (Nox1–5, Duox1, Duox2), Nox1, Nox2, Nox4 and Nox5 have been implicated in cardiovascular and renal oxidative stress in diabetes [65–68]. Nox1 and Nox4 are important in renal injury and atherosclerosis in mouse models of diabetes [66–68]. Nox5 may also be important in diabetes-associated vascular injury and nephropathy [69, 70]. Renal Nox5 expression is increased in patients with diabetic nephropathy [69]. In transgenic mice with podocyte-specific expression of human Nox5, renal injury was amplified by diabetes [71]. Similar findings were observed in mice expressing human Nox5 in a VSMC-specific manner [72]. Vascular/mesangial cell Nox5 overexpression is associated with amplification of atherosclerosis in mouse models of diabetes [73].

Targeting Noxs has been considered a promising strategy to ameliorate the vasculopathy and nephropathy associated with diabetes. While extensive experimental evidence showed a renoprotective effect of Nox1/4 inhibition in preclinical models of diabetes, clinical studies have been less positive [74, 75]. A clinical trial using GKT137831, a Nox1/4 inhibitor, failed to show improvement in renal function in patients with diabetic nephropathy [76]. Whether targeting Nox5 may have better clinical outcomes is unclear. Ongoing clinical studies are addressing this and the results are awaited.

7.4.3 Hyperglycaemia and Vascular Signalling

In diabetes, hyperglycaemia stimulates mitochondrial respiration and induces endoplasmic reticulum (ER) stress [77]. It also decreases vascular antioxidant capacity, reduces activity of the transcription factor nuclear factor-erythroid 2-related factor (Nrf-2) and promotes activation of vascular Nox isoforms leading to oxidative stress in diabetes [63, 68]. Oxidative stress is also associated with reduced bioavailability of the vasodilator nitric oxide (NO) and increased production of injurious peroxynitrite, causing endothelial dysfunction and inflammation [78]. At the molecular level hyperglycaemia induces activation of redox-sensitive protein kinase C (PKC), MAPKs, calcium channels, pro-inflammatory genes and polyol and hexosamine pathways, further contributing to mitochondrial dysfunction, oxidative stress, ER stress and consequent vascular inflammation and damage [62, 79].

7.4.4 Inflammation and Vascular Injury in Diabetes

It is well established that inflammatory polarization of immune cells occurs in many tissues, including adipose tissue, heart, kidney, skeletal muscle, liver, gut and vessels [80]. Subclinical inflammation contributes to obesity-linked metabolic dysfunctions, leading to insulin resistance and type 2 diabetes mellitus. Obesity triggers metabolically activated immune cells thereby contributing to the adverse regulation of adipocyte metabolism and adipose tissue remodelling [81]. These processes involve activation of many signalling pathways including upregulation of transcription factors such as hypoxia-inducible factor (HIF1α) [82]. Activation of HIF1α induces adipocyte expression of chemokines such as MCP-1, which contributes to adipocyte inflammation through pathways involving the JAK1/JAK2/STAT1 pathway [83]. Circulating and locally produced effector cytokines such as TNF-α, interferon-gamma (IFN-γ), IL-1β and IL-12 [84, 85] may influence the insulin sensitivity of peripheral tissues and, in the pancreatic islets, can modulate insulin release [86, 87]. Increased glucotoxicity and lipotoxicity have been associated with immune cell infiltration of target tissues, thereby affecting diabetes-associated target organ damage and cardiovascular complications [87–89].

Epigenetics is another mechanism that may influence inflammation and immunometabolism in diabetes [90]. Histone deacetylase (HDAC) inhibitors cause NFκB inhibition through acetylation of the p65 subunit. ITF2357, an orally active HDAC inhibitor, has been shown to prevent the development of diabetes [91]. Similarly, activation of sirtuin1 (Sirt1), involved in inflammation, metabolism and ageing, has been shown to have anti-inflammatory properties in diabetes [92].

Extensive experimental evidence has shown a close association between vascular inflammation, diabetes and cardiovascular morbidity [90, 93]. This is already evident in prediabetes [94]. Clinical studies also support the role of inflammation in cardiovascular complications of diabetes. Patients with type 2 diabetes have increased total leukocyte counts, particularly neutrophils and lymphocytes, that correlate with insulin sensitivity [58], and inflammatory changes of adipose tissue [95–97]. The link between inflammation, insulin resistance and type 2 diabetes is further supported by genetic studies and clinical trials showing the protective effects of immune-targeted therapies and anti-inflammatory actions of classical anti-diabetic drugs [98].

To further support the notion that inflammation and activation of the immune system are involved in the pathophysiology of diabetes and its vascular complications, studies integrating metabochip approaches with GWAS have shown that classical immunometabolic genes including JNK signalling pathways, NFκB regulators (MACROD1), inflammasome activators (NRF3) and interferon gamma receptor genes associate with type 2 diabetes [99, 100]. This also corresponds to results of GWAS that identified genes related to macrophage function and antigen presentation. Inflammation and oxidative stress are thus key elements underlying vascular disease and cardiovascular complications in diabetes [101].

7.5 MicroRNAs, Diabetes and Vascular Complications

MicroRNAs (miRNAs) are a group of small, single-stranded, 22–25-nucleotide-long, non-coding RNAs that are multifunctional [102]. They normally bind to the 3′ untranslated region of their target mRNA, leading to translational inhibition and/or mRNA degradation. miRNAs regulate over 90% of all protein-encoding mRNAs and their biological events [103]. They are detected in blood serum/plasma as well as in urine, saliva, tears and breast milk. Over 1000 miRNAs discovered in the human genome have been recognized to be useful diagnostic indicators. They fine-tune gene expression and have been implicated in various pathological processes including diabetes, insulin resistance and cardiovascular disease.

Normally, miRNAs are essential in maintaining physiological homeostasis, metabolism and energy balance. With respect to insulin biology, they control β-cell genesis, β-cell death (miR-21), insulin production (miR-30d, miR-204, and miR-124a) and α/β-cell mass balance (miR-375) [104, 105]. miRNAs are crucial in regulating adipogenesis (formation of adipocytes), metabolic homeostasis and endocrine functions of adipocytes [106]. Many miRNAs have been identified to be differentially regulated during adipogenesis, including let-7c, miR-143, miR-210, miR-221, miR-27 and miR-30a-e [106, 107]. In obesity, the expression of miR-132 is downregulated and its expression level is related to the activation of NFκB signalling and transcription of MCP-1 and IL-8. Expressions of miR-132 and miR-155 are also associated with macrophage infiltration in adipose tissue [106, 107].

In pathological conditions such as diabetes mellitus and cardiovascular disorders, miRs are differentially expressed [108]. Pancreatic β-cell-specific miRNAs, including miR-375, miR-124a, miR-96, miR-7a, miR7a2, miR-30d, miR-9, miR-200, miR-184 and let-7 are dysregulated in diabetes [109]. Differential miRNA signatures have been identified in prediabetic individuals, diabetic patients and patients with diabetes and vascular complications, suggesting that miRNAs may be novel biomarkers [110]. Diabetic cardiovascular complications are associated with increased levels of miR-223, miR-320, miR-501, miR504 and miR1 and decreased levels of miR-16, miR-133, miR-492 and miR-373 [110, 111]. Detection of deregulated miRNA profile in circulating peripheral blood cells or vascular cells may potentially be associated with diabetes-associated vascular disease.

7.6 Conclusions

Diabetes is associated with an increased risk of cardiovascular disease, which is exaggerated with coexistent hypertension and obesity. Many of the underlying molecular mechanisms, including oxidative stress, inflammation and fibrosis, causing microvascular and macrovascular complications in diabetes, also cause vascular remodelling and dysfunction in hypertension. Preventing vascular injury and inflammation in diabetes may protect against the devastating complications associated with retinopathy, nephropathy and neuropathy. Some of the newer anti-diabetic drugs seem to have vasoprotective effects.

Acknowledgements This work was supported by grants from the British Heart Foundation (BHF) (RG/13/7/30099, RE/13/5/30177).

Conflict of Interest There are no conflicts to declare.

References

1. Pearson ER. Type 2 diabetes: a multifaceted disease. Diabetologia. 2019;62(7):1107–12.
2. Rachdaoui N. Insulin: the friend and the foe in the development of type 2 diabetes mellitus. Int J Mol Sci. 2020;21(5):1770.
3. Tsimihodimos V, Gonzalez-Villalpando C, Meigs JB, Ferrannini E. Hypertension and diabetes mellitus: coprediction and time trajectories. Hypertension. 2018;71(3):422–8.

4. Petrie JR, Guzik TJ, Touyz RM. Diabetes, hypertension, and cardiovascular disease: clinical insights and vascular mechanisms. Can J Cardiol. 2018;34(5):575–84.
5. Ohishi M. Hypertension with diabetes mellitus: physiology and pathology. Hypertens Res. 2018;41(6):389–93.
6. D'Elia L, Strazzullo P. Excess body weight, insulin resistance and isolated systolic hypertension: potential pathophysiological links. High Blood Press Cardiovasc Prev. 2018;25(1):17–23.
7. Koenen M, Hill MA, Cohen P, Sowers JR. Obesity, adipose tissue and vascular dysfunction. Circ Res. 2021;128(7):951–68.
8. Manrique C, Lastra G, Sowers JR. New insights into insulin action and resistance in the vasculature. Ann N Y Acad Sci. 2014;1311(1):138–50.
9. Scheithauer TPM, Rampanelli E, Nieuwdorp M, Vallance BA, Verchere CB, van Raalte DH, et al. Gut microbiota as a trigger for metabolic inflammation in obesity and type 2 diabetes. Front Immunol. 2020;11:571731.
10. Brownlee M. The pathobiology of diabetic complications: a unifying mechanism. Diabetes. 2005;54(6):1615–25.
11. Zhang Y, Sun X, Icli B, Feinberg MW. Emerging roles for microRNAs in diabetic microvascular disease: novel targets for therapy. Endocr Rev. 2017;38(2):145–68.
12. Kattoor AJ, Pothineni NVK, Palagiri D, Mehta JL. Oxidative stress in atherosclerosis. Curr Atheroscler Rep. 2017;19(11):42–60.
13. Juutilainen A, Lehto S, Rönnemaa T, Pyörälä K, Laakso M. Type 2 diabetes as a "coronary heart disease equivalent": an 18-year prospective population-based study in Finnish subjects. Diabetes Care. 2005;28(12):2901–7.
14. Haffner SM, Lehto S, Ronnemaa T, Pyorala K, Laakso M. Mortality from coronary heart disease in subjects with type 2 diabetes and in nondiabetic subjects with and without prior myocardial infarction. N Engl J Med. 1998;339:229–34.
15. Abbott RD, Donahue RP, Kannel WB, Wilson PW. The impact of diabetes on survival following myocardial infarction in men vs women. The Framingham Study. JAMA. 1988;260(23):3456–60.
16. Snell-Bergeon JK, Budoff MJ, Hokanson JE. Vascular calcification in diabetes: mechanisms and implications. Curr Diab Rep. 2013;13(3):391–402.
17. Viigimaa M, Sachinidis A, Toumpourleka M, Koutsampasopoulos K, Alliksoo S, Titma T. Macrovascular complications of type 2 diabetes mellitus. Curr Vasc Pharmacol. 2020;18(2):110–6.
18. Gæde P, Oellgaard J, Carstensen B, Rossing P, Lund-Andersen H, Parving HH, et al. Years of life gained by multifactorial intervention in patients with type 2 diabetes mellitus and microalbuminuria: 21 years follow-up on the Steno-2 randomised trial. Diabetologia. 2016;59(11):2298–307.
19. Balkau B, Eschwège E, Papoz L, Richard JL, Claude JR, Warnet JM, et al. Risk factors for early death in non-insulin dependent diabetes and men with known glucose tolerance status. BMJ. 1993;307(6899):295–9.
20. Fong DS, Aiello LP, Ferris FL 3rd, Klein R. Diabetic retinopathy. Diabetes Care. 2004;27(10):2540–53.
21. Ruta LM, Magliano DJ, Lemesurier R, Taylor HR, Zimmet PZ, Shaw JE. Prevalence of diabetic retinopathy in Type 2 diabetes in developing and developed countries. Diabet Med. 2013;30(4):387–98.
22. Barrett EJ, Liu Z, Khamaisi M, King GL, Klein R, Klein BEK, et al. Diabetic microvascular disease: an endocrine society scientific statement. J Clin Endocrinol Metab. 2017;102(12):4343–410.
23. Horton WB, Barrett EJ. Microvascular dysfunction in diabetes mellitus and cardiometabolic disease. Endocr Rev. 2021;42(1):29–55.
24. Zhang X, Saaddine JB, Chou CF, Cotch MF, Cheng YJ, Geiss LS, et al. Prevalence of diabetic retinopathy in the United States, 2005-2008. JAMA. 2010;304(6):649–56.

25. Faselis C, Katsimardou A, Imprialos K, Deligkaris P, Kallistratos M, Dimitriadis K. Microvascular complications of type 2 diabetes mellitus. Curr Vasc Pharmacol. 2020;18(2):117–24.
26. Scurt FG, Menne J, Brandt S, Bernhardt A, Mertens PR, Haller H, et al. ROADMAP Steering Committee. Systemic inflammation precedes microalbuminuria in diabetes. Kidney Int Rep. 2019;4(10):1373–86.
27. da Silva Rosa SC, Nayak N, Caymo AM, Gordon J. Mechanisms of muscle insulin resistance and the cross-talk with liver and adipose tissue. Physiol Rep. 2020;8(19):e14607.
28. Ferrannini E, Buzzigoli G, Bonadonna R, Giorico MA, Oleggini M, Graziadei L, et al. Insulin resistance in essential hypertension. N Engl J Med. 1987;317(6):350–7.
29. Giordano A, Murano I, Mondini E, Perugini J, Smorlesi A, Severi I, et al. Obese adipocytes show ultrastructural features of stressed cells and die of pyroptosis. J Lipid Res. 2013;54(9):2423–36.
30. Antoniades C. 'Dysfunctional' adipose tissue in cardiovascular disease: a reprogrammable target or an innocent bystander? Cardiovasc Res. 2017;113:997–8.
31. Camastra S, Vitali A, Anselmino M, Gastaldelli A, Bellini R, Berta R, et al. Muscle and adipose tissue morphology, insulin sensitivity and beta-cell function in diabetic and nondiabetic obese patients: effects of bariatric surgery. Sci Rep. 2017;7(1):9007.
32. Das S, Zhang E, Senapati P, Amaram V, Reddy MA, Stapleton K, et al. A novel angiotensin II-induced long noncoding RNA giver regulates oxidative stress, inflammation, and proliferation in vascular smooth muscle cells. Circ Res. 2018;123(12):1298–312.
33. Touyz RM, Savoia C, He Y, Endemann D, Pu Q, Ko EA, et al. Increased inflammatory biomarkers in hypertensive type 2 diabetic patients: improvement after angiotensin II type 1 receptor blockade. J Am Soc Hypertens. 2007;1(3):189–99.
34. Touyz RM, Tolloczko B, Schiffrin EL. Blunted attenuation of angiotensin II-mediated Ca2+ transients by insulin in cultured unpassaged vascular smooth muscle cells from spontaneously hypertensive rats. Am J Hypertens. 1995;8(2):104–12.
35. Muniyappa R, Yavuz S. Metabolic actions of angiotensin II and insulin: a microvascular endothelial balancing act. Mol Cell Endocrinol. 2013;378(1–2):59–69.
36. Su Y, Liu XM, Sun YM, Wang YY, Luan Y, Wu Y. Endothelial dysfunction in impaired fasting glycemia, impaired glucose tolerance, and type 2 diabetes mellitus. Am J Cardiol. 2008;102(4):497–8.
37. Scuteri A, Tesauro M, Rizza S, Iantorno M, Federici M, Lauro D, et al. Endothelial function and arterial stiffness in normotensive normoglycemic first-degree relatives of diabetic patients are independent of the metabolic syndrome. Nutr Metab Cardiovasc Dis. 2008;18:349–56.
38. Creager MA, Lüscher TF, Cosentino F, Beckman JA. Diabetes and vascular disease: pathophysiology, clinical consequences, and medical therapy: Part I. Circulation. 2003;108(12):1527–32.
39. Weiss N, Keller C, Hoffmann U, Loscalzo J. Endothelial dysfunction and atherothrombosis in mild hyperhomocysteinemia. Vasc Med. 2002;7:227–39.
40. Meijer RI, De Boer MP, Groen MR, Eringa EC, Rattigan S, Barrett EJ, et al. Insulin-induced microvascular recruitment in skin and muscle are related and both are associated with whole-body glucose uptake. Microcirculation. 2012;19(6):494–500.
41. Kannenkeril D, Bosch A, Harazny J, Karg M, Jung S, Ott C, et al. Early vascular parameters in the micro- and macrocirculation in type 2 diabetes. Cardiovasc Diabetol. 2018;17(1):128.
42. Savoia C, Sada L, Zezza L, Pucci L, Lauri FM, Befani A, et al. Vascular inflammation and endothelial dysfunction in experimental hypertension. Int J Hypertens. 2011;2011:281240.
43. Harvey A, Montezano AC, Touyz RM. Vascular biology of ageing—implications in hypertension. J Mol Cell Cardiol. 2015;83:112–21.
44. Guzik TJ, Touyz RM. Oxidative stress, inflammation, and vascular aging in hypertension. Hypertension. 2017;70(4):660–7.
45. Zieman SJ, Melenovsky V, Kass DA. Mechanisms, pathophysiology, and therapy of arterial stiffness. Arterioscler Thromb Vasc Biol. 2005;25(5):932–43.

46. Aberdeen H, Battles K, Taylor A, Garner-Donald J, Davis-Wilson A, Rogers BT, et al. The aging vasculature: glucose tolerance, hypoglycemia and the role of the serum response factor. J Cardiovasc Dev Dis. 2021;8(5):58.
47. Perrone A, Giovino A, Benny J, Martinelli F. Advanced glycation end products (AGEs): biochemistry, signaling, analytical methods, and epigenetic effects. Oxid Med Cell Longev. 2020;2020:3818196.
48. Moldogazieva NT, Mokhosoev IM, Mel'nikova TI, Porozov YB, Terentiev AA. Oxidative stress and advanced lipoxidation and glycation end products (ALEs and AGEs) in aging and age-related diseases. Oxid Med Cell Longev. 2019;2019:3085756.
49. Strieder-Barboza C, Baker NA, Flesher CG, Karmakar M, Neeley CK, Polsinelli D, et al. Advanced glycation end-products regulate extracellular matrix-adipocyte metabolic crosstalk in diabetes. Sci Rep. 2019;9(1):19748.
50. Taneja S, Vetter SW, Leclerc E. Hypoxia and the receptor for advanced glycation end products (RAGE) signaling in cancer. Int J Mol Sci. 2021;22(15):8153.
51. Yamagishi S, Maeda S, Matsui T, Ueda S, Fukami K, Okuda S. Role of advanced glycation end products (AGEs) and oxidative stress in vascular complications in diabetes. Biochim Biophys Acta. 2012;1820(5):663–71.
52. Nigro C, Leone A, Raciti GA, Longo M, Mirra P, Formisano P, et al. Methylglyoxal-glyoxalase 1 balance: the root of vascular damage. Int J Mol Sci. 2017;18(1):188–202.
53. Leung SS, Forbes JM, Borg DJ. Receptor for advanced glycation end products (RAGE) in type 1 diabetes pathogenesis. Curr Diab Rep. 2016;16(10):100.
54. Manigrasso MB, Juranek J, Ramasamy R, Schmidt AM. Unlocking the biology of RAGE in diabetic microvascular complications. Trends Endocrinol Metab. 2014;25(1):15–22.
55. Koulis C, Watson AM, Gray SP, Jandeleit-Dahm KA. Linking RAGE and Nox in diabetic micro- and macrovascular complications. Diabetes Metab. 2015;41(4):272–81.
56. Frimat M, Daroux M, Litke R, Nevière R, Tessier FJ, Boulanger E. Kidney, heart and brain: three organs targeted by ageing and glycation. Clin Sci (Lond). 2017;131(11):1069–92.
57. Reyaz A, Alam S, Chandra K, Kohli S, Agarwal S. Methylglyoxal and soluble RAGE in type 2 diabetes mellitus: association with oxidative stress. J Diabetes Metab Disord. 2020;19(1):515–21.
58. Schmidt AM. 2016 ATVB plenary lecture: receptor for advanced glycation endproducts and implications for the pathogenesis and treatment of cardiometabolic disorders: spotlight on the macrophage. Arterioscler Thromb Vasc Biol. 2017;37(4):613–21.
59. Yaribeygi H, Atkin SL, Sahebkar A. A review of the molecular mechanisms of hyperglycemia-induced free radical generation leading to oxidative stress. J Cell Physiol. 2019;234(2):1300–12.
60. Van der Zwan LP, Scheffer PG, Dekker JM, Stehouwer CD, Heine RJ, Teerlink T. Hyperglycemia and oxidative stress strengthen the association between myeloperoxidase and blood pressure. Hypertension. 2010;55(6):1366–72.
61. Adeshara KA, Diwan AG, Tupe RS. Diabetes and complications: cellular signaling pathways, current understanding and targeted therapies. Curr Drug Targets. 2016;17(11):1309–28.
62. Sedeek M, Montezano AC, Hebert RL, Gray SP, Di Marco E, Jha JC, et al. Oxidative stress, Nox isoforms and complications of diabetes-potential targets for novel therapies. J Cardiovasc Transl Res. 2012;5(4):509–18.
63. Newsholme P, Cruzat VF, Keane KN, Carlessi R, de Bittencourt PI Jr. Molecular mechanisms of ROS production and oxidative stress in diabetes. Biochem J. 2016;473(24):4527–50.
64. Zhang Y, Murugesan P, Huang K, Cai H. NADPH oxidases and oxidase crosstalk in cardiovascular diseases: novel therapeutic targets. Nat Rev Cardiol. 2020;17(3):170–94.
65. Gray SP, Di Marco E, Okabe J, Szyndralewiez C, Heitz F, Montezano AC, et al. NADPH oxidase 1 plays a key role in diabetes mellitus accelerated atherosclerosis. Circulation. 2013;127:1888–902.
66. Gray SP, Di Marco E, Kennedy K, Chew P, Okabe J, El-Osta A, et al. Reactive oxygen species can provide atheroprotection via NOX4-dependent inhibition of inflammation and vascular remodeling. Arterioscler Thromb Vasc Biol. 2016;36(2):295–307.

67. Jha JC, Gray SP, Barit D, Okabe J, El-Osta A, Namikoshi T, et al. Genetic targeting or pharmacologic inhibition of NADPH oxidase nox4 provides renoprotection in long-term diabetic nephropathy. J Am Soc Nephrol. 2014;25(6):1237–54.
68. Sedeek M, Gutsol A, Montezano AC, Burger D, Nguyen Dinh Cat A, Kennedy CR, et al. Renoprotective effects of a novel Nox1/4 inhibitor in a mouse model of Type 2 diabetes. Clin Sci (Lond). 2013;124(3):191–202.
69. Touyz RM, Anagnostopoulou A, Rios F, Montezano AC, Camargo LL. NOX5: Molecular biology and pathophysiology. Exp Physiol. 2019;104(5):605–16.
70. Camargo LL, Montezano AC, Hussain M, Wang Y, Zou Z, Rios FJ, et al. Central role of c-Src in NOX5- mediated redox signaling in vascular smooth muscle cells in human hypertension. Cardiovasc Res. 2022;118(5):1359–73.
71. Holterman CE, Thibodeau JF, Towaij C, Gutsol A, Montezano AC, Parks RJ, et al. Nephropathy and elevated BP in mice with podocyte-specific NADPH oxidase 5 expression. J Am Soc Nephrol. 2014;25(4):784–97.
72. Jha JC, Banal C, Okabe J, Gray SP, Hettige T, Chow BSM, et al. NADPH oxidase Nox5 accelerates renal injury in diabetic nephropathy. Diabetes. 2017;66(10):2691–703.
73. Petheő GL, Kerekes A, Mihálffy M, Donkó Á, Bodrogi L, Skoda G, et al. Disruption of the NOX5 gene aggravates atherosclerosis in rabbits. Circ Res. 2021;128(9):1320–2.
74. Yang Q, Wu FR, Wang JN, Gao L, Jiang L, Li HD, et al. Nox4 in renal diseases: an update. Free Radic Biol Med. 2018;124:466–72.
75. Pavlov TS, Palygin O, Isaeva E, Levchenko V, Khedr S, Blass G, et al. NOX4-dependent regulation of ENaC in hypertension and diabetic kidney disease. FASEB J. 2020;34(10):13396–408.
76. Mooradian AD. Targeting select cellular stress pathways to prevent hyperglycemia-related complications: shifting the paradigm. Drugs. 2016;76(11):1081–91.
77. De Livera AM, Reutens A, Cooper M, Thomas M, Jandeleit-Dahm K, Shaw JE, et al. Evaluating the efficacy and safety of GKT137831 in adults with type 1 diabetes and persistently elevated urinary albumin excretion: a statistical analysis plan. Trials. 2020;21(1):459.
78. Förstermann U, Xia N, Li H. Roles of vascular oxidative stress and nitric oxide in the pathogenesis of atherosclerosis. Circ Res. 2017;120(4):713–35.
79. Stefano GB, Challenger S, Kream RM. Hyperglycemia-associated alterations in cellular signaling and dysregulated mitochondrial bioenergetics in human metabolic disorders. Eur J Nutr. 2016;55(8):2339–45.
80. Domingueti CP, Dusse LM, Carvalho M, de Sousa LP, Gomes KB, Fernandes AP. Diabetes mellitus: the linkage between oxidative stress, inflammation, hypercoagulability and vascular complications. J Diabetes Complications. 2016;30(4):738–45.
81. Saxton SN, Clark BJ, Withers SB, Eringa EC, Heagerty AM. Mechanistic links between obesity, diabetes, and blood pressure: role of perivascular adipose tissue. Physiol Rev. 2019;99(4):1701–63.
82. Packer M. Mechanisms leading to differential hypoxia-inducible factor signaling in the diabetic kidney: modulation by SGLT2 inhibitors and hypoxia mimetics. Am J Kidney Dis. 2021;77(2):280–6.
83. Belmokhtar K, Bourguignon T, Worou ME, Khamis G, Bonnet P, Domenech J, et al. Regeneration of three layers vascular wall by using BMP2-treated MSC involving HIF-1alpha and Id1 expressions through JAK/STAT pathways. Stem Cell Rev Rep. 2011;7(4):847–59.
84. Banerjee M, Saxena M. Interleukin-1 (IL-1) family of cytokines: role in type 2 diabetes. Clin Chim Acta. 2012;413:1163–70.
85. Mishra M, Kumar H, Bajpai S, Singh RK, Tripathi K. Level of serum IL-12 and its correlation with endothelial dysfunction, insulin resistance, proinflammatory cytokines and lipid profile in newly diagnosed type 2 diabetes. Diabetes Res Clin Pract. 2011;94:255–61.
86. Gao D, Madi M, Ding C, Fok M, Steele T, Ford C, et al. Interleukin-1beta mediates macrophage-induced impairment of insulin signaling in human primary adipocytes. Am J Physiol Endocrinol Metab. 2014;307(3):E289–304.
87. Donath MY, Dinarello CA, Mandrup-Poulsen T. Targeting innate immune mediators in type 1 and type 2 diabetes. Nat Rev Immunol. 2019;19(12):734–46.

88. Zatterale F, Longo M, Naderi J, Raciti GA, Desiderio A, Miele C, et al. Chronic adipose tissue inflammation linking obesity to insulin resistance and type 2 diabetes. Front Physiol. 2020;10:1607.
89. Ieronymaki E, Daskalaki MG, Lyroni K, Tsatsanis C. Insulin signaling and insulin resistance facilitate trained immunity in macrophages through metabolic and epigenetic changes. Front Immunol. 2019;10:1330.
90. Guzik TJ, Cosentino F. Epigenetics and immunometabolism in diabetes and aging. Antiox Redox Sig. 2018;29(3):257–74.
91. Besancon A, Goncalves T, Valette F, Dahllöf MS, Mandrup-Poulsen T, Chatenoud L, et al. Oral histone deacetylase inhibitor synergises with T cell targeted immunotherapy to preserve beta cell metabolic function and induce stable remission of new-onset autoimmune diabetes in NOD mice. Diabetologia. 2018;61(2):389–98.
92. Gillum MP, Kotas ME, Erion DM, Kursawe R, Chatterjee P, Nead KT, et al. SirT1 regulates adipose tissue inflammation. Diabetes. 2011;60:3235–45.
93. Bessueille L, Magne D. Inflammation: a culprit for vascular calcification in atherosclerosis and diabetes. Cell Mol Life Sci. 2015;72(13):2475–89.
94. Wasserman DH, Wang TJ, Brown NJ. The vasculature in prediabetes. Circ Res. 2018;122(8):1135–50.
95. Lorenzo C, Hanley AJ, Haffner SM. Differential white cell count and incident type 2 diabetes: the Insulin Resistance Atherosclerosis Study. Diabetologia. 2014;57:83–92.
96. Vacca M, Di Eusanio M, Cariello M, Graziano G, D'Amore S, Petridis FD, et al. Integrative miRNA and whole-genome analyses of epicardial adipose tissue in patients with coronary atherosclerosis. Cardiovasc Res. 2016;109:228–39.
97. Passacquale G, Di Giosia P, Ferro A. The role of inflammatory biomarkers in developing targeted cardiovascular therapies: lessons from the cardiovascular inflammation reduction trials. Cardiovasc Res. 2016;109:9–23.
98. Donath MY. Targeting inflammation in the treatment of type 2 diabetes: time to start. Nat Rev Drug Discov. 2014;13:465–76.
99. Hotamisligil GS. Inflammation, metaflammation and immunometabolic disorders. Nature. 2017;542:177–85.
100. Strawbridge RJ, Laumen H, Hamsten A, Breier M, Grallert H, Hauner H, Arner P, et al. Effects of genetic loci associated with central obesity on adipocyte lipolysis. PloS One. 2016;11:e0153990.
101. Guzik TJ, Mussa S, Gastaldi D, Sadowski J, Ratnatunga C, Pillai R, et al. Mechanisms of increased vascular superoxide production in human diabetes mellitus: role of NAD(P)H oxidase and endothelial nitric oxide synthase. Circulation. 2002;105:1656–62.
102. Guzik TJ, Skiba D, Touyz RM, Harrison DG. The role of infiltrating immune cells in dysfunctional adipose tissue. Cardiovasc Res. 2017;113:1009–23.
103. Zhang Y, Bai R, Liu C, Ma C, Chen X, Yang J, et al. MicroRNA single-nucleotide polymorphisms and diabetes mellitus: a comprehensive review. Clin Genet. 2019;95(4): 451–61.
104. Zampetaki A, Kiechl S, Drozdov I, Willeit P, Mayr U, Prokopi M, et al. Plasma microRNA profiling reveals loss of endothelial miR-126 and other microRNAs in type 2 diabetes. Circ Res. 2010;107(6):810–7.
105. Januszewski AS, Cho YH, Joglekar MV, Farr RJ, Scott ES, Wong WKM, et al. Insulin microsecretion in Type 1 diabetes and related microRNA profiles. Sci Rep. 2021;11(1):11727.
106. Hathaway QA, Pinti MV, Durr AJ, Waris S, Shepherd DL, Hollander JM. Regulating microRNA expression: at the heart of diabetes mellitus and the mitochondrion. Am J Physiol Heart Circ Physiol. 2018;314(2):H293–310.
107. Zeinali F, Aghaei Zarch SM, Jahan-Mihan A, Kalantar SM, Vahidi Mehrjardi MY, Fallahzadeh H, et al. Circulating microRNA-122, microRNA-126-3p and microRNA-146a are associated with inflammation in patients with pre-diabetes and type 2 diabetes mellitus: a case control study. PLoS One. 2021;16(6):e0251697.

108. Banerjee J, Nema V, Dhas Y, Mishra N. Role of microRNAs in type 2 diabetes and associated vascular complications. Biochimie. 2017;139:9–19.
109. LaPierre MP, Stoffel M. MicroRNAs as stress regulators in pancreatic beta cells and diabetes. Mol Metab. 2017;6(9):1010–23.
110. Sidorkiewicz I, Niemira M, Maliszewska K, Erol A, Bielska A, Szalkowska A, et al. Circulating miRNAs as a predicticve biomarker of the progression from prediabetes to diabetes: outcomes of a 5-year prospective observational study. J Clin Med. 2020;9(7):2184–204.
111. Shantikumar S, Caporali A, Emanueli C. Role of microRNAs in diabetes and its cardiovascular complications. Cardiovasc Res. 2012;93(4):583–93.

Insulin and Blood Pressure Relationships

8

Peter M. Nilsson and Andrea Natali

8.1 Observational Studies: Epidemiology

Already in 1987 a first report indicated that insulin sensitivity is impaired in subjects with essential hypertension and that hyperinsulinaemia is a consequence of this phenomenon [1], as later summarized [2]. In 1988, Gerald Reaven stated in his Banting Lecture that insulin resistance could be a unifying factor for impaired glucose metabolism, dyslipidaemia and elevated blood pressure [3], often considered together as representing the so-called metabolic syndrome and linked to (abdominal) obesity as the 'deadly quartet' [4]. Numerous studies later on reported that hyperinsulinaemia, as a marker of insulin resistance, in subjects with elevated blood pressure or hypertension [5–7] is a phenomenon that could also be influenced by the drugs used for the reduction of blood pressure. Some antihypertensive drugs seem to be beneficial for insulin sensitivity (RAS blockers, moxonidine, alpha-receptor blockers), others are mostly neutral (calcium antagonists), but some may even be detrimental, especially when used at higher dosages (thiazide diuretics, beta-receptor blockers) [8–10]. However, among beta-receptor blockers there exist also vasodilating drugs with less negative impact on glucose metabolism. The weight increase of a mean 2–4 kg induced by more traditional beta-receptor blockers could be a contributing factor for the concomitant decrease in insulin sensitivity (increased insulin resistance).

When epidemiological correlations have been studied between insulin and blood pressure, it was noted that such correlations are stronger when more

P. M. Nilsson (✉)
Department of Clinical Sciences, Lund University, Skane University Hospital, Malmö, Sweden
e-mail: Peter.Nilsson@med.lu.se

A. Natali
Department of Clinical and Experimental Medicine, Università di Pisa (UNIPI), Pisa, Italy

A. E. Berbari, G. Mancia (eds.), *Blood Pressure Disorders in Diabetes Mellitus*, Updates in Hypertension and Cardiovascular Protection,
https://doi.org/10.1007/978-3-031-13009-0_8

sophisticated measures are used for reflecting glucose metabolism and blood pressure control than more simple methods. One example was then oral glucose tolerance testing (OGTT), and hyperinsulinaemic and euglycaemic clamp data for insulin sensitivity were used together with 24-h ambulatory blood pressure monitoring (ABPM), showing stronger correlations, in contrast to using only fasting insulin and office blood pressure correlations [11]. The study concluded that the apparent association between blood pressure and insulin resistance not only is obscured by measurement error, but is also affected by the particular measures of insulin resistance and blood pressure used. The study thus provided further evidence that a relationship exists between blood pressure levels and hyperinsulinaemia or insulin resistance [11]. Similar findings were also obtained from a cohort of patients with type 2 diabetes [12] and one cohort consisting only of middle-aged women [13].

The importance of sex differences for these associations have been discussed in two other studies as men are more prone to abdominal obesity and insulin resistance than women, at least before menopause [14, 15].

The problem of proving a causal link between insulin metabolism and blood pressure regulation can be addressed by applying genetic analyses via Mendelian randomization (causal inference) methodology. In a recent publication applying genetic methods, several biomarkers were found to be causally related to blood pressure, among them insulin-like growth factor binding protein 3 (IGF-BP3), but not the biomarker insulin itself [16]. However, insulin sensitivity is not a single biomarker like that, but more complex, and if impaired insulin sensitivity (insulin resistance) is causally related to blood pressure regulation, it might be a better choice to go for intervention studies directed towards insulin resistance and then follow the effects on blood pressure.

It could also be the other way around, i.e. that pathophysiological changes associated with hypertension increases the risk of insulin resistance. One study supported the hypothesis that genes in the blood pressure pathway may play a role in insulin resistance in Mexican-Americans, a population with a high prevalence of abdominal obesity and the metabolic syndrome [17].

Finally, it should be noted that patients with insulinoma do not in general have elevated blood pressure in spite of hyperinsulinaemia [18], indicating that it may be insulin resistance per se that after all is more important for blood pressure regulation than hyperinsulinaemia itself.

8.2 Mechanistic Studies Linking Insulin, Insulin Resistance and Blood Pressure Regulation

The precise mechanism linking insulin resistance to blood pressure is still unknown probably simply because there is not just one, but many, each not efficient enough either in terms of potency or prevalence, but all together they do justify the observed epidemiologic association. Classically these mechanisms can be divided in *three groups* according to the type of cause-effect relationship.

8.2.1 Insulin Resistance Facilitates Elevated Blood Pressure

Insulin resistance, observed at the whole-body level, is caused by a reduced liver, adipose and skeletal muscle tissues response to insulin, while it neither affects the kidney nor the sympathetic nervous system (SNS), which in insulin-resistant individuals respond normally to insulin. Therefore, the resulting compensatory day-long relative hyperinsulinemia—faced by insulin-resistant subjects—will produce an overstimulation of these two tissues with possible consequences on blood pressure control. Indeed, insulin directly acts on the kidney at the tubular level by promoting sodium reabsorption similarly in healthy subjects and in patients with essential hypertension and insulin resistance [19], while it increases the SNS tone similarly in lean and obese insulin-resistant subjects [20]. These effects, modest in quantitative terms and transient during the day (fed > fasting), are unlikely to be responsible of large blood pressure changes, but might become effective synergizing with others of similar nature, like environmental stress and a high-salt diet [21].

On the other hand, insulin also acts on the endothelium by facilitating nitric oxide release [22], but the endothelium in insulin-resistant individuals is also less responsive [23, 24]; therefore, this 'hypotensive' effect is lost. The direct link between insulin sensitivity and endothelial function has been shown also in an intervention study in which in subjects with type 2 diabetes the glucose control was improved with either metformin or rosiglitazone, but only the latter treatment was able to improve both mechanisms and to a similar extent [25].

8.2.2 Elevated Blood Pressure Facilitates Insulin Resistance

Essential hypertension and obesity are associated with variable degrees of endothelial dysfunction and microvascular rarefaction [26]. Insulin, in order to exert its full metabolic effect (glucose uptake), requires an optimal skeletal muscle perfusion, which in turn requires a normal endothelial function [27] and a normal microvascular recruitment [28]. It is thus possible to hypothesize that in the hypertensive subjects in whom either component is affected, there is also a blunted insulin function. In a series of experiments, a research group in Pisa, Italy, tried to verify this elegant hypothesis by first improving skeletal muscle capillary recruitment with adenosine [29] and subsequently by improving overall tissue perfusion with sodium nitroprusside (a nitric oxide donor) [30] in subjects with established essential hypertension, but neither intervention was associated with improvement in skeletal muscle insulin resistance. Possibly, the vasodilation induced through drugs does not reproduce the capillary recruitment of the nutritive network, as it occurs with insulin, or the network is structurally compromised due to capillary rarefaction [31]. Endothelial dysfunction per se probably is not effective on metabolism unless it is associated with other chronic metabolic stress. Indeed, in genetically manipulated mice the selective partial deletion of endothelial nitric oxide produced insulin resistance and hypertension only when the animals were submitted to a chronic high-fat diet [32].

A second mechanism through which hypertension might facilitate insulin resistance is through the negative effect on insulin action of some antihypertensive drugs and it will be addressed in the next paragraph. Nevertheless, this would only explain in part the observed epidemiologic association and does not shed light on the mechanism since insulin resistance has been demonstrated also in untreated lean subjects with essential hypertension [1].

8.2.3 Factors Able to Induce Simultaneously Insulin Resistance and Elevated Blood Pressure

At least four major factors are involved through distinct mechanisms in the simultaneous regulation of blood pressure and insulin action.

Stress hormones (catecholamines and glucocorticoids) induce insulin resistance and elevates blood rather effectively. This is clearly seen in conditions of abnormal secretion of either hormone or when glucocorticoids are given for therapeutic purposes or when voluptuary substances increasing the SNS adrenergic tone are consumed. A series of elegant studies in monkeys [33] has clearly demonstrated that social stress induces abdominal obesity, elevated blood pressure and insulin resistance, as well as coronary atherosclerosis. Whether also in humans the physiologic response to stress, when protracted, is able to achieve the hormone levels that are effective both on metabolism and on blood pressure in humans is uncertain. In an elegant nested case-control study, subjects with metabolic syndrome showed an enhanced cortisol and catecholamine 24-h urinary secretion when compared to healthy controls [34]. A peculiar condition of intermittent but rather persistent stress response activation is represented by obstructive sleep apnoea (OSA) and indeed this affection is known to be associated with both hypertension [35] and insulin resistance [36]. The treatment of OSA is beneficial for both conditions [37, 38].

Lack of physical activity is able to produce biochemical changes in the skeletal muscle cells that makes them less responsive to insulin [39] and is also able to modify the vascular network so as to reduce peripheral resistances [40]. Training programmes are indeed almost invariably associated with improvements in both insulin sensitivity [41] and reduced blood pressure [42].

Elevated free fatty acids (FFA) are able to induce impaired endothelial function and skeletal muscle insulin resistance when their concentration is raised through experimental manipulations [43]. Whether the mild FFA elevations observed in obese individuals and in stress conditions (beta adrenergic-induced lipolysis) are effective in this regards is uncertain and still to be demonstrated.

Low-grade inflammation induces insulin resistance [44], impairs endothelial function [45] and promotes arterial stiffness [46]. Plasma C reactive protein predicts both hypertension [47] and diabetes [48], and in a cohort of subjects with type 2 diabetes, we observed a clustering of inflammation, insulin resistance and endothelial dysfunction [49]. A poor diet, a poor hygiene, environmental pollution and smoking are all conditions of low-grade inflammation as well as factors predisposing to both type 2 diabetes and hypertension [50].

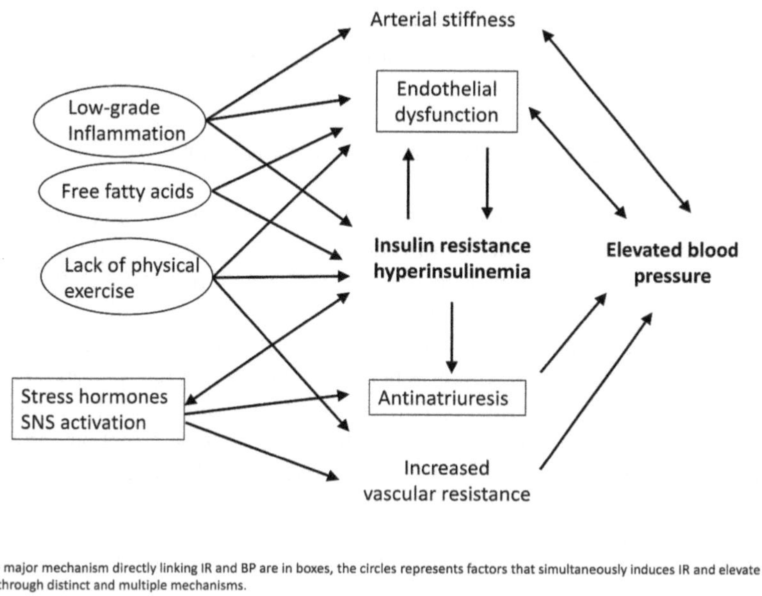

Fig. 8.1 The major mechanism directly linking IR and BP are in boxes, the circles represents factors that simultaneously induces IR and elevate BP through distinct and multiple mechanisms

In summary the mechanism directly linking blood pressure to insulin resistance are depicted in Fig. 8.1. These are based essentially on endothelial dysfunction, anti-natriuresis and the activity of stress hormones, as well as increased SNS activity [51]. Then there are a number of factors, mostly related to the environment that acts on one or more of these mechanism and reinforce the link.

8.3 Intervention Studies

8.3.1 Lifestyle Intervention: Weight Loss and Physical Exercise

There are different ways to reduce insulin resistance and hyperinsulinaemia in order to evaluate the effects on blood pressure regulation and levels.

First of all, different lifestyle modifications (diet, physical exercise) have been shown to be of special benefit to people with hyperinsulinaemia, as shown in a 1-year randomized, controlled study from Sweden when also office blood pressure was lowered [52]. As there were several metabolic effects induced by this multimodality lifestyle intervention, keeping a constant drug usage over the study period, it could be problematic to disentangle if the beneficial effect was due to weight loss, improved physical activity and muscle activation, or a more direct effect on insulin resistance causing hyperinsulinaemia by stress reduction, or unknown mechanisms linked to improved lifestyle [52].

Even calorie restriction alone, without the physical exercise component, may impact on insulin resistance and lower blood pressure [53].

8.3.2 Drug Effects on Insulin and Blood Pressure

As already mentioned, the various antihypertensive drugs commonly used may have shifting effects on body weight, insulin sensitivity, insulin levels and blood pressure regulation [8–10, 54]. Some of these drugs are of special relevance as they improve insulin sensitivity and reduce blood pressure levels at the same time, both measured as office blood pressure and 24-h ambulatory blood pressure. One of the drugs, moxonidine, seems to work via central nervous inhibition of the SNS via its interaction with imidazolidine receptors [10]. However, it is not enough to show these favourable metabolic and haemodynamic effects, but also the effect on cardiovascular endpoints must be evaluated. For example, even if alpha-receptor blockers have been shown to improve insulin sensitivity and lower blood pressure, the selective alpha-blocker doxazosin did not show special clinical benefits in the ALLHAT study when compared with the ACE-inhibitor lisinopril and the diuretic chlorthalidone; in fact congestive heart failure increased in the doxazosin arm [55].

Finally, also some anti-diabetic drugs have documented benefits for reducing insulin resistance and at the same time lower blood pressure levels. One such drug is rosiglitazone (a thiazolidinedione) with favourable metabolic and haemodynamic effects [56–58]. On the other hand, there was a tendency for volume retention and peripheral oedema that could increase the risk of congestive heart failure in susceptible patients with type 2 diabetes. In a randomized trial (RECORD), the risk of cardiovascular events in general was, however, not different between rosiglitazone treatment and other per-oral anti-diabetes drugs [59]. The lesson from this is that in the end it is the cardiovascular preventive effect of a specific drug that matters, not the different ways (mechanisms) this is achieved. Even drugs that may increase body weight and worsen insulin sensitivity (but lower peripheral blood pressure) may show protective effects on the risk of re-infarction, for example, selective beta-receptor blockers in secondary prevention post-myocardial infarction.

Finally, also metformin has been investigated for blood pressure-lowering properties but with conflicting results even if this drug may increase hepatic insulin sensitivity and stabilize glucose metabolism [60]. The newer anti-diabetes drugs (SGLT-2 inhibitors, GLP-1 receptor agonists, RA) may reduce body weight and blood pressure [61], but the effect on hyperinsulinaemia and insulin resistance is less clear. In fact, incretin-active drugs such as DPP-4 inhibitors and GLP-1 RA may in fact increase insulin secretion, but blood pressure is at least not elevated by this influence. Experimental studies have indicated a role of GLP-1 receptor signalling for blood pressure regulation. In one study in rodents, endogenous GLP-1R signalling exerted a physiologically relevant effect on BP control, which may be attributable, in part, to its tonic actions on the proximal tubule NHE3-mediated sodium reabsorption, intrarenal renin-angiotensin system and insulin sensitivity [62].

8.4 Summary

There are many observational studies to show associations between insulin levels, or insulin sensitivity, with blood pressure levels, and with more sophisticated methods stronger associations can be shown as compared to the use of more simple methods. Several mechanisms have been described to mediate these effects of insulin regulation on blood pressure levels, most importantly involving the endothelium [63], sodium retention, SNS activation and vascular remodelling. It is possible to favourably reduce hyperinsulinaemia and insulin resistance, either by lifestyle alone (weight loss, physical exercise, smoking cessation) or by some antihypertensive and anti-diabetic drugs.

Future studies may shed more light on these associations, including determination of causality by genetic methods [16, 17], and newer drugs may be designed to better target insulin resistance without side effects. Blood pressure and central haemodynamics should then be evaluated by more sophisticated methods such as 24-h ABPM and measurement of central blood pressure, as well as aortic stiffness by use of pulse wave velocity and pulse wave analyses.

Acknowledgements This review was supported by the Research Council of Sweden and the Heart and Lung Foundation of Sweden to PMN.

References

1. Ferrannini E, Buzzigoli G, Bonadonna R, Giorico MA, Oleggini M, Graziadei L, et al. Insulin resistance in essential hypertension. N Engl J Med. 1987;317(6):350–7.
2. Ferrannini E, Natali A, Capaldo B, Lehtovirta M, Jacob S, Yki-Järvinen H. Insulin resistance, hyperinsulinemia, and blood pressure: role of age and obesity. European Group for the Study of Insulin Resistance (EGIR). Hypertension. 1997;30(5):1144–9.
3. Reaven GM. Banting lecture 1988. Role of insulin resistance in human disease. Diabetes. 1988;37(12):1595–607.
4. Kaplan NM. The deadly quartet. Upper-body obesity, glucose intolerance, hypertriglyceridemia, and hypertension. Arch Intern Med. 1989;149(7):1514–20.
5. Nilsson P, Lindholm L, Schersté́n B. Hyperinsulinaemia and other metabolic disturbances in well-controlled hypertensive men and women: an epidemiological study of the Dalby population. J Hypertens. 1990;8(10):953–9.
6. Bonora E, Capaldo B, Perin PC, Del Prato S, De Mattia G, Frittitta L, et al. Group of Italian Scientists of Insulin Resistance (GISIR). Hyperinsulinemia and insulin resistance are independently associated with plasma lipids, uric acid and blood pressure in non-diabetic subjects. The GISIR database. Nutr Metab Cardiovasc Dis. 2008;18(9):624–31.
7. Wang F, Han L, Hu D. Fasting insulin, insulin resistance and risk of hypertension in the general population: a meta-analysis. Clin Chim Acta. 2017;464:57–63.
8. Lithell HO, Andersson PE. Antihypertensive treatment in insulin resistant patients. Hypertens Res. 1996;19(Suppl 1):S75–9.
9. Quiñones-Galvan A, Pucciarelli A, Ciociaro D, Masoni A, Franzoni F, Natali A, et al. Metabolic effects of combined antihypertensive treatment in patients with essential hypertension. J Cardiovasc Pharmacol. 2002;40(6):916–21.
10. Haenni A, Lithell H. Moxonidine improves insulin sensitivity in insulin-resistant hypertensives. J Hypertens Suppl. 1999;17(3):S29–35.

11. Nilsson PM, Lind L, Andersson PE, Hänni A, Berne C, Baron J, Lithell HO. On the use of ambulatory blood pressure recordings and insulin sensitivity measurements in support of the insulin-hypertension hypothesis. J Hypertens. 1994;12(8):965–9.
12. Pinkney JH, Mohamed-Ali V, Denver AE, Foster C, Sampson MJ, Yudkin JS. Insulin resistance, insulin, proinsulin, and ambulatory blood pressure in type II diabetes. Hypertension. 1994;24(3):362–7.
13. Nilsson P, Schwan A. Independent association between fasting plasma insulin and ambulatory blood pressure in 50-year-old women. Blood Press. 1995;4(5):283–6.
14. Nilsson PM, Lind L, Pollare T, Berne C, Lithell H. Differences in insulin sensitivity and risk markers due to gender and age in hypertensives. J Hum Hypertens. 2000;14(1):51–6.
15. Petrie JR, Malik MO, Balkau B, Perry CG, Højlund K, Pataky Z, et al. RISC Investigators. Euglycemic clamp insulin sensitivity and longitudinal systolic blood pressure: role of sex. Hypertension. 2013;62(2):404–9.
16. Thériault S, Sjaarda J, Chong M, Hess S, Gerstein H, Paré G. Identification of circulating proteins associated with blood pressure using mendelian randomization. Circ Genom Precis Med. 2020;13(1):e002605.
17. Guo X, Cheng S, Taylor KD, Cui J, Hughes R, Quiñones MJ, et al. Hypertension genes are genetic markers for insulin sensitivity and resistance. Hypertension. 2005;45(4):799–803.
18. O'Brien T, Young WF Jr, Palumbo PJ, O'Brien PC, Service FJ. Hypertension and dyslipidemia in patients with insulinoma. Mayo Clin Proc. 1993;68(2):141–6.
19. Muscelli E, Natali A, Bianchi S, Bigazzi X, Galvan AQ, Sironi AN, et al. Effect of insulin on renal sodium and uric acid handling in essential hypertension. Am J Hypertens. 1996;9(8):746–52.
20. Muscelli E, Emdin M, Natali A, Pratali L, Camastra S, Gastaldelli A, et al. Autonomic and hemodynamic responses to insulin in lean and obese humans. J Clin Endocrinol Metab. 1998;83(6):2084–90.
21. Facchini FS, DoNascimento C, Reaven GM, Yip JW, Ni XP, Humphreys MH. Blood pressure, sodium intake, insulin resistance, and urinary nitrate excretion. Hypertension. 1999;33(4):1008–12.
22. Scherrer U, Randin D, Vollenweider P, Vollenweider L, Nicod P. Nitric-oxide release accounts for insulins vascular effects in humans. J Clin Invest. 1994;94(6):2511–5.
23. Taddei S, Virdis A, Mattei P, Natali A, Ferrannini E, Salvetti A. Effect of insulin on acetylcholine-induced vasodilation in normotensive subjects and patients with essential-hypertension. Circulation. 1995;92(10):2911–8.
24. Vollenweider P, Randin D, Tappy L, Jequier E, Nicod P, Scherrer U. Impaired insulin-induced sympathetic neural activation and vasodilation in skeletal-muscle in obese humans. J Clin Invest. 1994;93(6):2365–71.
25. Natali A, Baldeweg S, Toschi E, Capaldo B, Barbaro D, Gastaldelli A, et al. Vascular effects of improving metabolic control with metformin or rosiglitazone in type 2 diabetes. Diabetes Care. 2004;27(6):1349–57.
26. de Jongh RT, Serne EH, Ijzerman RG, de Vries G, Stehouwer CDA. Impaired microvascular function in obesity: implications for obesity-associated microangiopathy, hypertension, and insulin resistance. Circulation. 2004;109(21):2529–35.
27. Baron AD, Steinberg HO, Chaker H, Leaming R, Johnson A, Brechtel G. Insulin-mediated skeletal-muscle vasodilation contributes to both insulin sensitivity and responsiveness in lean humans. J Clin Invest. 1995;96(2):786–92.
28. Vincent MA, Clerk LH, Lindner JR, Klibanov AL, Clark MG, Rattigan S, et al. Microvascular recruitment is an early insulin effect that regulates skeletal muscle glucose uptake in vivo. Diabetes. 2004;53(6):1418–23.
29. Natali A, Bonadonna R, Santoro D, Galvan AQ, Baldi S, Frascerra S, et al. Insulin resistance and vasodilation in essential hypertension. Studies with adenosine. J Clin Invest. 1994;94(4):1570–6.
30. Natali A, Galvan AQ, Pecori N, Sanna G, Toschi E, Ferrannini E. Vasodilation with sodium nitroprusside does not improve insulin action in essential hypertension. Hypertension. 1998;31(2):632–6.

31. Clark MG, Wallis MG, Barrett EJ, Vincent MA, Richards SM, Clerk LH, et al. Blood flow and muscle metabolism: a focus on insulin action. Am J Physiol Endocrinol Metab. 2003;284(2):E241–58.
32. Cook S, Hugli O, Egli M, Ménard B, Thalmann S, Sartori C, et al. Partial gene deletion of endothelial nitric oxide synthase predisposes to exaggerated high-fat diet-induced insulin resistance and arterial hypertension. Diabetes. 2004;53(8):2067–72.
33. Shively CA, Register TC, Clarkson TB. Social stress, visceral obesity, and coronary artery atherosclerosis: product of a primate adaptation. Am J Primatol. 2009;71(9):742–51.
34. Brunner EJ, Hemingway H, Walker BR, Page M, Clarke P, Juneja M, et al. Adrenocortical, autonomic, and inflammatory causes of the metabolic syndrome: nested case-control study. Circulation. 2002;106(21):2659–65.
35. Peppard PE, Young T, Palta M, Skatrud J. Prospective study of the association between sleep-disordered breathing and hypertension. N Engl J Med. 2000;342(19):1378–84.
36. Ip MSM, Lam B, Ng MMT, Lam WK, Tsang KWT, Lam KSL. Obstructive sleep apnea is independently associated with insulin resistance. Am J Resp Crit Care Med. 2002;165(5):670–6.
37. Harsch IA, Schahin SP, Radespiel-Troger M, Weintz O, Jahreiss H, Fuchs FS, et al. Continuous positive airway pressure treatment rapidly improves insulin sensitivity in patients with obstructive sleep apnea syndrome. Am J Resp Crit Care Med. 2004;169(2):156–62.
38. Norman D, Loredo JS, Nelesen RA, Ancoli-Israel S, Mills PJ, Ziegler MG, et al. Effects of continuous positive airway pressure versus supplemental oxygen on 24-hour ambulatory blood pressure. Hypertension. 2006;47(5):840–5.
39. Alibegovic AC, Sonne MP, Hojbjerre L, Bork-Jensen J, Jacobsen S, Nilsson E, et al. Insulin resistance induced by physical inactivity is associated with multiple transcriptional changes in skeletal muscle in young men. Am J Physiol Endocrinol Metab. 2010;299(5):E752–63.
40. Thijssen DHJ, Maiorana AJ, O'Driscoll G, Cable NT, Hopman MTE, Green DJ. Impact of inactivity and exercise on the vasculature in humans. Eur J Appl Physiol. 2010;108(5):845–75.
41. Henriksen EJ. Invited review: effects of acute exercise and exercise training on insulin resistance. J Applied Physiol. 2002;93(2):788–96.
42. Cornelissen VA, Buys R, Smart NA. Endurance exercise beneficially affects ambulatory blood pressure: a systematic review and meta-analysis. J Hypertens. 2013;31(4):639–48.
43. Steinberg HO, Tarshoby M, Monestel R, Hook G, Cronin J, Johnson A, et al. Elevated circulating free fatty acid levels impair endothelium-dependent vasodilation. J Clin Invest. 1997;100(5):1230–9.
44. Romeo GR, Lee J, Shoelson SE. Metabolic syndrome, insulin resistance, and roles of inflammation—mechanisms and therapeutic targets. Art Thromb Vasc Biol. 2012;32(8):1771–6.
45. Hingorani AD, Cross J, Kharbanda RK, Mullen MJ, Bhagat K, Taylor M, et al. Acute systemic inflammation impairs endothelium-dependent dilatation in humans. Circulation 2000; 102(9):994-9.
46. van Bussel BC, Schouten F, Henry RM, Schalkwijk CG, de Boer MR, Ferreira I, et al. Endothelial dysfunction and low-grade inflammation are associated with greater arterial stiffness over a 6-year period. Hypertension. 2011;58(4):588–95.
47. Sesso HD, Buring JE, Rifai N, Blake GJ, Gaziano JM, Ridker PM. C-reactive protein and the risk of developing hypertension. JAMA. 2003;290(22):2945–51.
48. Thorand B, Lowel H, Schneider A, Kolb H, Meisinger C, Frohlich M, et al. C-reactive protein as a predictor for incident diabetes mellitus among middle-aged men: results from the MONICA Augsburg Cohort Study, 1984–1998. Arch Internal Med. 2003;163(1):93–9.
49. Natali A, Toschi E, Baldeweg S, Ciociaro D, Favilla S, Sacca L, et al. Clustering of insulin resistance with vascular dysfunction and low-grade inflammation in type 2 diabetes. Diabetes. 2006;55(4):1133–40.
50. Furman D, Campisi J, Verdin E, Carrera-Bastos P, Targ S, Franceschi C, et al. Chronic inflammation in the etiology of disease across the life span. Nature Med. 2019;25(12):1822–32.
51. Reaven GM, Lithell H, Landsberg L. Hypertension and associated metabolic abnormalities—the role of insulin resistance and the sympathoadrenal system. N Engl J Med. 1996;334(6):374–81.

52. Nilsson PM, Lindholm LH, Scherstén BF. Life style changes improve insulin resistance in hyperinsulinaemic subjects: a one-year intervention study of hypertensives and normotensives in Dalby. J Hypertens. 1992;10(9):1071–8.
53. Nicoll R, Henein MY. Caloric restriction and its effect on blood pressure, heart rate variability and arterial stiffness and dilatation: a review of the evidence. Int J Mol Sci. 2018;19(3):751.
54. Lithell HO, Pollare T, Berne C. Insulin sensitivity in newly detected hypertensive patients—influence of Captopril and other antihypertensive agents on insulin sensitivity and related biological parameters. J Cardiovasc Pharmacol. 1990;15:S46–52.
55. ALLHAT Collaborative Research Group. Major cardiovascular events in hypertensive patients randomized to doxazosin vs chlorthalidone: the antihypertensive and lipid-lowering treatment to prevent heart attack trial (ALLHAT). JAMA. 2000;283(15):1967–75. Erratum in: JAMA 2002; 288(23):2976.
56. Sarafidis PA, Lasaridis AN, Nilsson PM, Pagkalos EM, Hitoglou-Makedou AD, Pliakos CI, et al. Ambulatory blood pressure reduction after rosiglitazone treatment in patients with type 2 diabetes and hypertension correlates with insulin sensitivity increase. J Hypertens. 2004;22(9):1769–77.
57. Sarafidis PA, Nilsson PM. The effects of thiazolidinediones on blood pressure levels—a systematic review. Blood Press. 2006;15(3):135–50.
58. Nilsson PM, Hedblad B, Donaldson J, Berglund G. Rosiglitazone reduces office and diastolic ambulatory blood pressure following 1-year treatment in non-diabetic subjects with insulin resistance. Blood Press. 2007;16(2):95–100.
59. Mahaffey KW, Hafley G, Dickerson S, Burns S, Tourt-Uhlig S, White J, et al. Results of a reevaluation of cardiovascular outcomes in the RECORD trial. Am Heart J. 2013;166(2):240–9.e1.
60. Thomopoulos C, Katsimagklis G, Makris T. Metformin and blood pressure lowering: a questioned association. J Hypertens. 2017;35(1):27–8.
61. Berra C, Manfrini R, Regazzoli D, Radaelli MG, Disoteo O, Sommese C, et al. Blood pressure control in type 2 diabetes mellitus with arterial hypertension. The important ancillary role of SGLT2-inhibitors and GLP1-receptor agonists. Pharmacol Res. 2020;160:105052.
62. Martins FL, Bailey MA, Girardi ACC. Endogenous activation of glucagon-like peptide-1 receptor contributes to blood pressure control: role of proximal tubule Na+/H+ exchanger isoform 3, renal angiotensin II, and insulin sensitivity. Hypertension. 2020;76(3):839–48.
63. Morgantini C, Stea F, Boldrini B, Duranti E, Ghiadoni L, Natali A. Effect of mild hyperisulinemia on conduit vessel endothelial function: role of noradrenergic activation. J Hypertens. 2012;30(4):720–4.

Mechanisms of Diabetic Nephropathy in Humans and Experimental Animals

9

Charbel C. Khoury, Sheldon Chen, and Fuad N. Ziyadeh

9.1 Introduction

Diabetic kidney disease (DKD) remains one of the main causes of end-stage kidney disease (ESKD) in the industrialized world and many developing countries and is likely to continue increasing given the pandemic of diabetes and obesity. While still considered a microvascular complication of diabetes, nephropathy involves more than just kidney capillaries, extending its damage across the various kidney cells and associated extracellular structures. This chapter will provide a comprehensive review of our current understanding of the pathophysiology of DKD especially focusing on lessons learned from experimental animal models.

9.2 Pathology

Histopathological changes of DKD in humans and in experimental animals involve all compartments of the kidney and correlate with functional and clinical manifestations of the disease. One of the earliest quantifiable changes in DKD is thickening of the glomerular basement membrane (GBM), a predictor of renal survival in patients with DKD [1]. Increased synthesis of extracellular matrix (ECM) components such as type IV collagen, laminins, and nidogen/entactin and decreased ECM degradation result in a near doubling of the GBM size [2]. More dramatic changes

C. C. Khoury
Washington University, St. Louis, MO, USA

S. Chen
MD Anderson Cancer Center, Houston, TX, USA

F. N. Ziyadeh (✉)
Faculty of Medicine, American University of Beirut, Beirut, Lebanon
e-mail: fz05@aub.edu.lb

A. E. Berbari, G. Mancia (eds.), *Blood Pressure Disorders in Diabetes Mellitus*, Updates in Hypertension and Cardiovascular Protection,
https://doi.org/10.1007/978-3-031-13009-0_9

to the GBM are noted by ultrastructural studies, including denudation, abnormal folding, and the presence of shallow craterlike cavities and tunnels in fragmented segments of the GBM. Concurrently, there is a change in the composition of the GBM due to increased synthesis of the α1 chain of collagen IV and of perlecan by endothelial cells usually seen during embryonic development, along with overproduction of the mature GBM components (α3 and α5 chains of collagen IV and agrin) by podocytes [3, 4]. This transition, along with changes in nonenzymatic glycosylation, redistribution of GBM components, and nonspecific trapping of serum protein, likely affects the quality of the GBM and could explain, at least in part, the correlation of GBM thickness with its functional properties such as "leakiness" of serum macromolecules or the magnitude of proteinuria [5].

Aside from the altered GBM structure and function, the cellular components of the glomerular filtration barrier, namely, the podocytes and the endothelial cells, are both compromised in diabetes. The podocytes undergo cytoskeletal rearrangement, dedifferentiation, and autophagy manifested by effacement of their foot processes and decrease in slit diaphragm length with downregulation of its core components, such as nephrin [6]. Importantly, reduction in podocyte density secondary to detachment and dropout of the cells or apoptosis might be a useful predictor of DKD and its progression [7, 8]. On the other side of the GBM, the glomerular endothelium is a highly specialized, fenestrated layer coated by a negatively charged endothelial surface layer (ESL) with two components: the glycocalyx, which refers to membrane-bound proteoglycans (PG), and the endothelial cell coat that contains secreted PGs, negatively charged glycosaminoglycans (GAG), glycoproteins, and soluble proteins. Alteration of the composition and amount of PGs in the ESL leads to a reduced thickness of the ESL and decreased negative charge, but may also lead to disturbances in local signaling events [9, 10].

Another histopathologic hallmark of DKD is expansion of the mesangium. This is mostly due to increased deposition of extracellular mesangial matrix components and only minimally to mesangial cell hypertrophy and/or proliferation [11, 12]. Recent evidence suggests that mesangial expansion may also be due to, at least in part, overproduced GBM material that spreads into the mesangium. In general, mesangial expansion in DKD is diffusely uniform within the glomerulus [4]. As collagen deposition progresses with advanced nephropathy, diffuse diabetic glomerulosclerosis ensues and eventually leads to scarring of the glomeruli. Nodular glomerulosclerosis or the so-called Kimmelstiel–Wilson lesions may also be present in up to 50% of diabetic patients. Kimmelstiel–Wilson lesions are usually focal, segmental, and only occasionally diffuse. These develop due to continued local expansion of the mesangial matrix, or more likely as a result of mesangiolysis, with separation of the glomerular capillary from the mesangium and the formation of capillary aneurysms. The new capillary space is subsequently filled with mesangial matrix [13].

As for the renal vasculature in diabetes, a common finding is the accumulation of periodic acid–Schiff (PAS)-positive material around both the afferent and efferent arterioles, referred to as arteriolar hyalinosis. Hyalinosis of both arterioles is typical of DKD. The deposition of similar material in the subendothelial space of the glomerular capillaries is referred to as a hyaline cap. These, together with capsular drops (hyaline material underneath the parietal epithelial cells of Bowman's capsule), constitute the exudative lesions of DKD.

Tubular basement membrane thickening develops in parallel with that of the GBM, and both correlate strongly with the degree of hyperglycemia in type 1 diabetes [6]. With progression of DKD, interstitial fibrosis and tubular atrophy develop and these changes correlate strongly with the progressive decline in kidney function as assessed by the glomerular filtration rate (GFR) [14–16]. This may be accompanied by chronic inflammatory infiltrates composed chiefly of T lymphocytes and macrophages.

To help with the staging of DKD, the Renal Pathology Society introduced a classification of the pathology of DKD, based on the degree of glomerular pathology, with a separate scoring system for tubular and vascular lesions [17] (Table 9.1). However, the classic description of DKD is mostly based on the glomerular pathology of kidneys in type 1 diabetes in humans (T1DKD). The pathognomonic glomerular changes are also identified in patients with type 2 diabetes and DKD (T2DKD) [18], but the overall pathological picture is more heterogeneous. Less than a third of T2DKD patients with microalbuminuria have the typical glomerular lesions expected in a similar stage of T1DKD [19, 20]. While there may be nuances in the pathogenesis of kidney disease in patients with type 1 compared with type 2 diabetes, these differences in pathology are more likely due to variability in the duration of DKD and the presence of comorbidities such as hypertension, obesity, and aging that have independent effects on the kidney.

Table 9.1 Glomerular classification of DKD

Class	Description	Inclusion criteria
I	Mild or nonspecific LM changes and EM-proven GBM thickening	Biopsy does not meet any of the criteria mentioned below for class II, III, or IV GBM >395 nm in female and >430 nm in male individuals 9 years of age and older (a)
IIa	Mild mesangial expansion	Biopsy does not meet criteria for class III or IV Mild mesangial expansion in >25% of the observed mesangium
IIb	Severe mesangial expansion	Biopsy does not meet criteria for class III or IV Severe mesangial expansion in >25% of the observed mesangium
III	Nodular sclerosis (Kimmelstiel–Wilson lesion)	Biopsy does not meet criteria for class IV At least one convincing Kimmelstiel–Wilson lesion
IV	Advanced diabetic glomerulosclerosis	Global glomerular sclerosis in >50% of glomeruli Lesions from classes I through III

Light microscopy (LM). (a) The basis of direct measurement of GBM width by EM, these individual cutoff levels may be considered indicative when other GBM measurements are used
From Tervaert TWC et al. [17]

9.3 Clinical Course

Tracking changes in GFR, urinary albumin excretion (UAE), and systemic arterial blood pressure, Mogensen and others classically described DKD to progress through distinct clinical stages (Fig. 9.1) [21]. In T1DKD these clinical stages correlate, in general, with the severity of renal pathology as described above. However, as with the kidney pathology, DKD in type 2 diabetes is a more heterogeneous disease, with variable degrees of glomerulosclerosis, tubulointerstitial fibrosis, and vasculopathy [22].

9.3.1 Normoalbuminuria

The initial stage of DKD is characterized by normoalbuminuria with a normal or high GFR and is overall clinically silent. However, in about a third or more of type 1 diabetes, a relatively large increase in GFR (greater than 150 mL/min/1.73 m^2) occurs and seems to be positively associated with glycemic control [23, 24]. This hyperfiltration is less common or much more attenuated in type 2 diabetic patients [25].

Hyperfiltration has been hypothesized to contribute to the initiation of nephron damage and progression of kidney disease [24]. The evidence to support that is mostly preclinical or based on observational studies. In a meta-analysis of cohort studies in type 1 diabetes, the pooled odds for the development of at least microalbuminuria was 2.71 (95% CI 1.20–6.11) in patients with hyperfiltration compared to those with normofiltration [26]. Similar findings were noted by the GFR study investigators [27]. In their longitudinal study of type 2 diabetic patients, the hazard

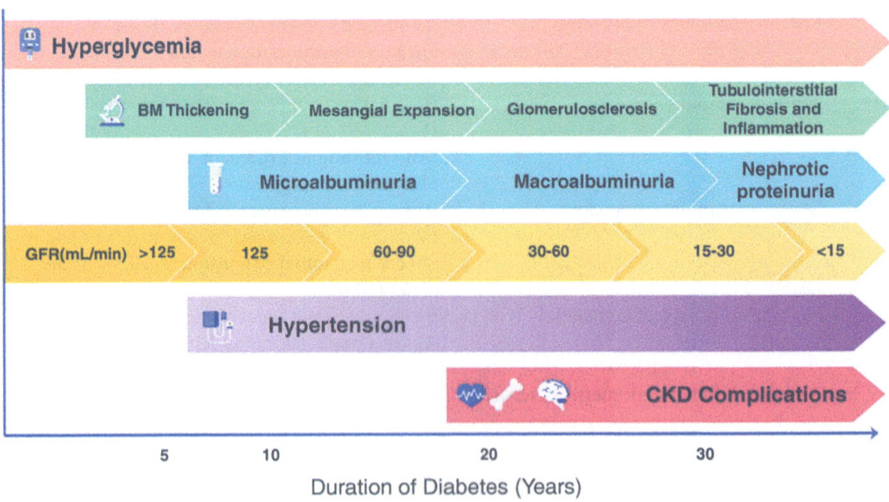

Fig. 9.1 Proposed model for clinicopathologic progression of diabetic kidney disease

ratio for progression to a minimum of microalbuminuria was 2.16 (95% CI 1.13–4.14). It was noted that 23.4% (11 of 47) of patients with persistent hyperfiltration progressed to micro- or macroalbuminuria compared to 10.6% (53 of 502) of patients who had hyperfiltration ameliorated at 6 months or who did not develop hyperfiltration since study inclusion. Dedicated prospective trials are needed to confirm whether targeting hyperfiltration improves clinically relevant end points (i.e., progressive GFR decline or incidence of ESKD). However, it remains the preferred mechanism proposed for the majority of the nephroprotective effects of drugs that intercept the renin–angiotensin–aldosterone (RAAS) system and the novel sodium–glucose cotransporter 2 inhibitors (SGLT2i).

9.3.2 Microalbuminuria

Traditionally, microalbuminuria is defined as a UAE of 30–300 mg/d or 20–200 μg/min, and it develops five years after the onset of type 1 diabetes in 20–40% of patients and can be present at the time of diagnosis of type 2 diabetes in 20–40% of patients. Hyperglycemia, hypertension, and elevated body mass index (BMI) are all independent risk factors for the development of microalbuminuria in type 1 and type 2 diabetic patients [28]. Onset of albuminuria tends to correlate pathologically with continued thickening of the glomerular and tubular basement membranes and some degree of podocyte loss. Mesangial matrix expansion and diffuse glomerulosclerosis may also be noted.

Longitudinal studies had previously suggested that approximately 80% of type 1 diabetic patients progress from microalbuminuria to proteinuria over a period of 6–14 years [29]. More recent studies suggest this could be closer to 40% [30]. While improved control of glycemia and hypertension over the years and the widespread use of RAAS blockers in microalbuminuric patients could explain these findings, it is also conceivable that microalbuminuria is not uniformly a predictor of macroalbuminuria in all diabetic patients [31]. On the other hand, UAE has been repeatedly and strongly validated as a risk factor for cardiovascular disease, peripheral vascular disease, stroke, and mortality from coronary heart disease [32–35].

Within 1 or 2 years of the onset of microalbuminuria in type 1 diabetes, patients may develop hypertension. GFR remains normal or is slightly elevated in type 1 diabetic patients with microalbuminuria [36]. On the other hand, GFR begins to normalize and then decline at rates approximating 3 to 4 mL/min/year in microalbuminuric type 2 diabetic patients [37].

9.3.3 Overt Nephropathy

With progressive podocyte loss and the onset of diffuse and/or nodular glomerulosclerosis, overt proteinuria (total urinary protein excretion exceeding 500 mg/d) or macroalbuminuria (UAE exceeding 300 mg/d) develops (Fig. 9.1). This occurs after an average of 15 years of the diabetic state in type 1 diabetes. In parallel, progressive mesangial expansion leads to a reduction in the glomerular surface area available for filtration and has been shown to inversely correlate with declining GFR [38]. Hypertension is almost always present at this stage, and its poor control starts contributing to disease progression. Proteinuria by itself is another independent risk factor for further worsening of renal damage [39].

Untreated patients may progress to nephrotic-range proteinuria, which could signal the onset of rapid decline in GFR at a mean rate of 1 mL/min/month (stage IV) until ESKD ensues (stage V). The average time from the initial diagnosis of type 1 diabetes to ESKD is around 20–25 years. However, this time course is extremely variable among individual patients.

While this proposed staging system helps align the structure and function of the kidney in diabetes, growing evidence suggests that not all patients progress in a linear manner. Regression from micro- to normoalbuminuria and direct progression to ESKD have been reported in type 1 and type 2 diabetes [31, 40]. While the more frequent use of RAAS inhibitors may contribute to this trend, some studies have failed to confirm this correlation [41].

9.4 Metabolic Dysregulation of Diabetic Nephropathy

Hyperglycemia is the main driver for the pathophysiology and progression of DKD. In fact, glycemic control can slow the advancement of nephropathy and, at times, may reverse the original pathology [42–46]. As glucose accumulates intracellularly to excess, there is increased flux through glycolysis and possibly through the tricarboxylic acid (TCA) cycle, with less efficient oxidative phosphorylation. Indeed, diabetic kidneys upregulate glucose transporters GLUT-1 and GLUT-4 in the glomeruli, as well as the glycolytic enzymes hexokinase and phosphofructokinase, thus promoting flux into anaerobic glycolysis, in a manner reminiscent of the Warburg effect [47–51]. Growing evidence has implicated mitochondria in the metabolic dysregulation of diabetes. Increased mitochondrial fission and fragmentation as well as reduced levels of peroxisome proliferator-activated receptor-γ coactivator 1α (PGC-1α) levels in the tubules, abnormalities in electron transport chain complex assembly/activity, and increased expression of uncoupling protein UCP1 have been reported [51–53]. It remains unclear whether the altered glucose metabolism is the cause or a result of diseased mitochondria in diabetic kidneys and whether the mitochondria will make a meaningful target for disease control.

Evidence is emerging that lipid metabolism may also play a role in the progression of DKD. Kimmelstiel and Wilson noted significant intratubular lipid accumulation in their seminal work on diabetic pathology [54]. Defective lipid metabolism likely contributes to lipid accumulation and may be associated with impaired mitochondrial function and the development of tubulointerstitial fibrosis [55]. Lipotoxicity can also manifest in the podocyte with intracellular accumulation of lipid droplets, abnormal glucose metabolism, inflammation, oxidative stress, endoplasmic reticulum stress, and actin cytoskeleton rearrangements [56].

The change in glucose metabolism is also manifested as an increased flux into alternative pathways: the pentose phosphate pathway, sorbitol/polyol pathway, advanced glycation end-product pathway, protein kinase C (PKC) pathway, and hexosamine pathway. These metabolic pathways had long been thought to contribute to glucotoxicity in the kidney through various mechanisms. However, research from the Joslin Medalist Study suggests that increased glycolytic flux and sorbitol/polyol pathway may protect from diabetic nephropathy by reducing the accumulation of glucose toxic metabolites and improving mitochondrial function [57, 58].

9.4.1 Advanced Glycation Reactions

Advanced glycation end products (AGEs) are proteins, lipids, or nucleic acids that are irreversibly cross-linked with reducing sugars. AGEs accumulate in both glomerular and tubular cells in experimental and human DKD [59, 60]. As renal function declines, higher concentrations of these products are retained in the plasma [61]. Experimental evidence shows that infusion of AGEs into normal rodents leads to the increased glomerular volume, accumulation of PAS-positive deposits, basement membrane widening, mesangial matrix expansion, and glomerulosclerosis [62]. Concurrently, inhibition of AGEs in experimental animal models of diabetes ameliorates albuminuria and glomerulosclerosis [63].

AGEs contribute to DKD injury by altering the function of the glycated proteins. ECM proteins, like in collagen, may become less susceptible to enzymatic hydrolysis by matrix metalloproteinases (MMPs), facilitating their accumulation in the extracellular space [64]. Glycation of sulfated proteoglycans modifies the charge-selective properties of the basement membrane and contributes to the development of microalbuminuria [65]. Concomitantly, AGEs act as signaling molecules either by acting intracellularly or by interacting with their receptor for advanced glycation end products (RAGE) that is expressed on the surfaces of podocytes and tubular epithelia. AGEs induce intracellular oxidant stress and activate NF-κB by redox-sensitive signaling pathways. They also activate PKC and regulate the expression of diverse growth factors and cytokines such as angiotensin II (Ang II) and transforming growth factor-beta1 (TGF-β1) [66, 67].

9.4.2 Protein Kinase C Signaling

As glycolytic metabolites react with glycerol phosphate, diacylglycerol (DAG), the major endogenous activator of PKC, is formed [68]. Other by-products of glucotoxicity such the polyol metabolites, AGE accumulation, RAGE activation, production of reactive oxygen species (ROS), and Ang II further activate PKC [69]. On the other hand, altered lipid metabolism and particularly the imbalance between lipid delivery and intracellular oxidation of fatty acids could lead to the accumulation of DAG [70].

PKC isoforms cooperate in the pathogenesis of DKD. While PKC-beta can lead to renal hypertrophy and glomerulosclerosis, PKC-alpha appears to contribute primarily to diabetic albuminuria by acting through vascular endothelial growth factor (VEGF) and by affecting nephrin expression [71]. Animal experiments with double knockouts of PKC-alpha and PKC-beta or the administration of an inhibitor of both PKC isoforms confirmed this hypothesis [71]. However, the PKC-beta inhibitor, ruboxistaurin, did not show a significant reduction in albumin/creatinine ratios when evaluated in a randomized clinical trial in patients [72].

9.4.3 Oxidative Stress

Oxidative stress has long been considered an integral pathogenic mechanism in the metabolic dysregulations of hyperglycemia [73]. Superoxide, hydroxyl radicals, hydrogen peroxide, and peroxynitrite, all commonly referred to as ROS, are increased in a diabetic kidney. These species, along with the oxidized proteins, lipids, nucleic acids, and the carbohydrates they produce, contribute to glomerular hypertrophy, cause injury to the podocyte, and promote fibrogenesis in the glomeruli and tubules [74, 75].

The notable sources of ROS production in the diabetic kidney are the mitochondria, the cytosolic NADPH oxidase (NOX), nitric oxide synthases, xanthine oxidase, and lipoxygenase [70, 76]. The prevailing hypothesis was that altered glucose metabolism increased mitochondrial electron transport chain activity, resulting in a high proton gradient, and high electrochemical potential differences led to the enhanced generation of mitochondrial superoxide [73]. However, measuring mitochondrial superoxide is difficult and has yielded inconsistent conclusions, with some groups finding a decrease in mitochondrial ROS [53, 70, 76, 77]. In fact, some level of mitochondrial superoxide may be beneficial and may retard organ dysfunction [76, 77]. With improved tools and real-time imaging, more sensitive spatiotemporal ROS measurements are being pursued to elucidate the role of mitochondrial ROS in DKD.

Meanwhile, NOX4, another notable source of ROS, has been consistently shown to be upregulated in animal models of diabetic kidney disease [68]. Its activity or expression appears to be influenced by various mediators of the diabetic milieu, including hyperglycemia, Ang II, TGF-β, AGEs, VEGF, endothelin, and aldosterone [74]. NOX4-mediated stimulation of PKC-alpha may contribute to many of the NOX4-dependent effects in DKD [78]. Moreover, NOX4 can inhibit fumarate hydratase, leading to the accumulation of fumarate, a TCA cycle metabolite with oncogenic properties that has been linked to the stimulation of hypoxia-inducible factor 1-alpha (HIF1α), TGF-β, and other matrix genes promoting fibrosis [79].

9.5 Glomerular Hemodynamics

As hyperfiltration is one of the earliest pathophysiologic features of DKD, it has been the target of many therapeutic interventions. Physiologically, four factors determine the GFR: (a) the glomerular plasma flow, (b) the systemic oncotic pressure, (c) the glomerular transcapillary hydraulic pressure difference, and (d) the glomerular ultrafiltration (permeability) coefficient, K_f. These factors are affected in diabetes, resulting in hyperfiltration. First, diabetic glomeruli become hypertrophied and then filtration surface area increases, leading to an increased ultrafiltration coefficient [80]. Second, and more importantly, abnormal vascular control in diabetic nephropathy leads to differential reduction in afferent glomerular arteriolar resistance and a net increase in efferent arteriolar resistance. This results in increased renal blood flow and glomerular capillary hypertension, all resulting in an elevated single-nephron GFR [81]. This change in intraglomerular hemodynamics occurs in response to an imbalance of a variety of vasoactive substances and growth factors including the RAAS, atrial natriuretic peptide, insulin-like growth factor-1, endothelin, prostanoids, eicosanoids, and the nitric oxide (NO) system secondary to endothelial dysfunction [82, 83]. The rise in glomerular capillary pressure promotes the production of various mediators of DKD [84]. Angiotensin-converting enzyme inhibitors (ACEi) and angiotensin receptor blockers (ARB) lower glomerular pressure and limit hyperfiltration by blocking the effect of Ang II on the efferent arteriole [85–88].

The impressive results from recent SGLT2i studies have shed light on the prior proposed mechanisms of glomerular hyperfiltration involving increased proximal tubular reabsorption of glucose and sodium (Na) [89]. In diabetes, hyperglycemia, tubular hypertrophy, and augmented SGLT2 expression in the proximal tubule contribute to increased Na/glucose reabsorption via SGLT2 and SGLT1, as well as increased Na reabsorption via NHE3 [90]. As a result, less sodium is delivered to the macula densa, thus attenuating tubuloglomerular feedback. This results in facilitated dilation of the afferent arteriole. Indeed, glomerular hyperfiltration is blunted in diabetic mice deficient in the adenosine receptor A1, which lack the tubuloglomerular feedback mechanism [91]. However, there have been conflicting results using this mouse model [92]. In addition, the decreased distal delivery lowers the tubular back pressure in Bowman space, which increases the effective glomerular filtration pressure and may explain a significant portion of diabetic hyperfiltration [93, 94]. Gene-targeted SGLT2 knockout and pharmacologic inhibition of SGLT2 prevent glomerular hyperfiltration in animal models of diabetes [95]. Treatment of type 1 and type 2 diabetic patients with the SGLT2i empagliflozin has been shown to attenuate renal hyperfiltration, as reflected by the estimated GFR (eGFR) [96, 97]. This effect appears to be independent of lowering blood glucose [98, 99].

After an SGLT2i was consistently observed to have excellent secondary kidney outcomes in a cardiovascular trial in patients with type 2 diabetes (as in the Empagliflozin Cardiovascular Outcome Event Trial in Type 2 Diabetes Mellitus Patients—EMPA-REG OUTCOME), other dedicated kidney outcome trials have been completed with other SGLT2i agents such as canagliflozin and dapagliflozin, all demonstrating robust benefits on primary kidney outcomes. CREDENCE (Canagliflozin and Renal Events in Diabetes with Established Nephropathy Clinical Evaluation) was a randomized, double-blind, placebo-controlled, multicenter clinical trial of patients with type 2 diabetes and albuminuric chronic kidney disease [100]. It showed that the SGLT2i was able to prevent ESKD (dialysis, transplantation, or sustained eGFR <15 mL/min/1.73m^2), doubling of serum creatinine, or death from renal causes, with a hazard ratio (HR) of 0.70 (0.59–0.82). Similarly, the DAPA-CKD (Dapagliflozin and Prevention of Adverse Outcomes in Chronic Kidney Disease) trial studied dapagliflozin in patients with chronic kidney disease, with or without type 2 diabetes. It showed significant prevention of renal outcomes (≥50% decrease in eGFR, ESKD, or death from renal or cardiovascular causes) with an HR of 0.61 (0.51–0.72). This effect appears to be additive to ACEi and ARBs. It appears that renoprotection is a consistent feature across the class of SGLT2i.

9.6 Cellular and Molecular Mechanisms of Glomerulopathy

Hyperfiltration and intraglomerular hypertension are transduced as a biomechanical stress on the endothelial cells, the mesangial cells, and the podocytes, resulting in activation of molecular signaling pathways. As such, endothelial cells have increased nitric oxide synthase (eNOS) dysfunction initiated by hyperglycemia and metabolic dysregulation [101]. Moreover, mesangial cells respond to increased mechanical stretch by upregulating GLUT-1, ECM protein accumulation, and TGF-β1 activity [102, 103].

Regarding the podocyte, complex interactions between their intricate actin-based cytoskeleton, cell–cell, and cell–matrix contact proteins allow them to maintain the glomerular filtration barrier in the face of mechanical challenges resulting from the filtration of a pulsatile blood flow [104, 105]. The morphologic and functional changes of diabetes such as glomerular hypertrophy, thickening and stiffening of the GBM, and glomerular hyperfiltration and hypertension all result in shear and tensile stresses on the podocyte that challenge the cell's attachment to the GBM [104]. Meanwhile, the metabolic dysregulation in diabetes further compromises the cytoskeletal architecture of the podocytes. Glucotoxicity, Ang II, TGF-β, VEGF, and other signaling pathways result in the downregulation of the expression of nephrin, a key protein of the slit diaphragm and of cytoskeletal function in podocytes [6]. Furthermore, hyperglycemia, AGEs, ROS, and others result in dysregulation of the Rho family of GTPases, key regulators of the actin cytoskeleton [6]. Lastly, studies have shown that podocyte integrin expression is decreased in diabetes, compromising cell–matrix interactions [6]. Altogether, these stressors result in effacement of the foot processes, detachment, and the loss of a number of podocytes and their shedding into the urinary space. Other podocytes succumb to apoptosis under the effect of hyperglycemia, ROS, and activation of the TGF-β pathway [106]. The remaining podocytes attempt to cover the newly denuded GBM by hypertrophy, with activation of the mammalian target of rapamycin (mTOR) [107]. However, once podocyte loss reaches 20%, glomerulosclerosis develops [108].

In sum, the metabolic and hemodynamic dysregulations in DKD converge and activate second messenger signaling pathways, transcription factors, and cytokines, including the RAAS, TGF-β, VEGF, and others, all of which contribute to the development of albuminuria and glomerulosclerosis, characteristic features of established diabetic nephropathy.

The RAAS is one of the most important pathways in DKD pathophysiology. Along with the systemic RAAS activation, renal cells such as mesangial cells, podocytes, and even tubular cells synthesize Ang II and express its receptors, which may contribute to the regional activation of RAAS [102, 109]. Indeed, hyperglycemia directly, and via ROS and AGEs, upregulates the expression of renin and angiotensinogen [81, 110, 111]. The RAAS drives the hemodynamic changes of DKD but also independently activates a multitude of cytokines such as TGF-β, connective tissue growth factor (CTGF), interleukin-6, monocyte chemoattractant protein-1 (MCP-1), and VEGF-A. Accordingly, high levels of Ang II can contribute to the early hyperplasia and hypertrophy of the renal cells observed in diabetes and can modulate glomerular ECM deposition in the later stages of diabetes [112]. In addition to the classical ACE/Ang II/AT1R axis, the RAAS comprises another important axis, the ACE2/Ang-(1–7)/Mas receptor, considered the counterregulatory axis of ACE/Ang II/AT1R. Indeed, an imbalance between the Ang II and Ang-(1–7) systems is associated with vascular dysfunction, inflammation, and fibrosis, making the ACE2/Ang-(1–7)/Mas receptor a potential ameliorating and therapeutic target in DKD [113].

RAAS blockers in clinical use may not be sufficient to fully arrest the activation of this system due to "aldosterone breakthrough," the increase of plasma aldosterone to basal levels after several weeks of ACEi or ARB administration. The mineralocorticoid receptor is also expressed in kidney cells outside of the aldosterone-sensitive distal nephron, such as vascular cells, podocytes, fibroblasts, and inflammatory cells. Activation of the mineralocorticoid receptor in those cells has been associated with activation of inflammatory and fibrotic pathways in the kidney, and this has deleterious effects on podocytes and mesangial cells [114]. Clinical studies show that steroidal mineralocorticoid receptor antagonists (MRAs) have an anti-albuminuric effect in diabetic kidney disease. Finerenone is a novel, nonsteroidal MRA with a better therapeutic index than the steroidal MRAs such as spironolactone and eplerenone. In the FIDELIO-DKD trial, finerenone reduced CKD progression and improved cardiovascular outcomes compared with placebo when added to an optimized regimen of renin–angiotensin–aldosterone system inhibitors. Plus, the incidence of hyperkalemia was manageably low [115].

VEGF is one of the key signaling pathways of the crosstalk between glomerular endothelium and podocytes. Healthy podocytes produce VEGF-A which helps maintain the endothelial cell's structure and function upon binding to vascular endothelial growth factor receptor 2 (VEGFR2) [116]. Targeted genetic deletion of all VEGF-A isoforms from podocytes leads to glomerular disease in healthy mice [117]. The role of VEGF signaling in diabetes was difficult to decipher initially. Some studies reported increased VEGF-A activity in diabetic glomeruli, with improvement of DKD upon inhibition of VEGF-A or VEGFR2 [118–121]. Other research showed that total glomerular VEGF-A levels decreased as diabetic nephropathy progressed and that targeted genetic deletion of all VEGF-A isoforms from podocytes accelerated nephropathy in diabetic animals [119]. More likely, the glomerular cells tightly control a state of delicate VEGF balance, and too much or too little can be pathogenic [122]. More recent evidence has also shown that the different isoforms of VEGF-A may confer additional nuances of signaling. VEGF-A_{165a} is a potent vasoactive agent, increasing vasodilation, vascular permeability, and angiogenesis [123]. Meanwhile, VEGF-A_{165b} is a protective factor in diabetic nephropathy[124]. In diabetic mice, podocyte-specific $VEGF_{165b}$ overexpression or $VEGF_{165b}$ administration maintained the glycocalyx and prevented endothelial and podocyte cell death, resulting in reduced albuminuria [124].

Other paracrine signals such as NO and angiopoietins can also feed into this crosstalk and tip the balance toward pathogenesis. New insights have revealed that endothelin-1 (ET-1), an endothelial-derived vasoconstrictor, can signal to the podocyte and then back to the endothelial cell [125]. Atrasentan, an ET-1 receptor antagonist, has been shown clinically to ameliorate early microalbuminuric diabetic kidney disease [126].

TGF-β appears to be a common pathway that leads to hypertrophic changes early on and then promotes fibrosis and sclerosis in the later stages of diabetic kidney disease [127, 128]. Under the impact of metabolic and hemodynamic forces in DKD, multiple mediators converge upon the activation of the TGF-β system. These include high glucose concentration [129], AGE-modified proteins [130], ROS [73], cyclical stretch/relaxation of mesangial cells in culture [131], PKC activation [132], and Ang II [133]. TGF-β has been shown to stimulate the synthesis of type I collagen, type IV collagen, fibronectin, and laminin. Further, TGF-β inhibits matrix metalloproteinases and can also stimulate the inhibitors of proteases, thus preventing the degradation of ECM proteins and leading to their deposition and accumulation [134]. Blocking TGF-β upstream of its receptor or downstream in the intracellular signaling cascade results in marked improvement in glomerulosclerosis, ECM deposition, GBM thickening, and other histological and molecular parameters of diabetic renal disease [82, 121, 135, 136]. This provides proof of the cytokine's central role in DKD pathophysiology.

9.7 Tubulopathy in Diabetes

Along with glomerulopathy, tubular damage plays a significant role in the pathogenesis of DKD [137]. Growing clinical and pathological data confirm that elevated baseline plasma biomarkers of tubular injury such as KIM-1 have been significantly associated with the risk of early decline of kidney function, independent of albuminuria [138]. Tubular dysfunction as well as tubulointerstitial fibrosis are known to correlate significantly with the decline in GFR and the progression of kidney disease.

Various mechanisms come into play in diabetic tubulopathy [139]. First, the increased metabolic stress in diabetes promotes a hypoxic environment for the proximal tubule. As SGLT2 and NHE3 increase their reabsorptive capacity, there is a commensurate increase in the demand for ATP to maintain the crucial activity of Na^+/K^+-ATPase to support ion transport [139]. Moreover, proximal tubular epithelial cells increase gluconeogenesis in the setting of diabetes [139]. However, because of mitochondrial injury and metabolic dysfunction, the proximal tubular cells consume more O_2 for each molecule of ATP generated. This increased demand and inefficient utilization of O_2 are met with reduced blood supply due to concomitant endothelial injury, intrinsic capillary loss within the affected tubulointerstitium, and glomerular capillary occlusion, resulting in significant hypoxia [139].

Hypoxic proximal tubular epithelial cells undergo apoptosis but also promote tubulointerstitial fibrosis via TGF-β and other mechanisms [139]. The expansion of the extracellular matrix further exacerbates hypoxia and microvascular rarefaction, starting the spiral of fibrosis and chronic kidney injury.

Several other pathomechanisms target the proximal tubule in DKD. These include the RAAS as well as the toxic effects of leaked albumin and albumin-bound fatty acids into the tubular lumen due to albuminuria, among others [139, 140].

With their advent, the new single-cell modalities such as transcriptomics, epigenetics, metabolomics, and proteomics are starting to show the effect of diabetes on various tubular segments. For instance, a recent single-nucleus RNA sequencing (snRNA-seq) on cryopreserved human diabetic kidney samples showed that the diabetic thick ascending limb, late distal convoluted tubule, and principal cells of the collecting ducts all adopt a gene expression signature consistent with increased potassium secretion, including alterations in Na^+/K^+-ATPase, WNK1, mineralocorticoid receptor, and NEDD4L expression, as well as decreased paracellular calcium and magnesium reabsorption [141].

Furthermore, there is evidence of retrograde crosstalk between the proximal tubules and the podocytes. Indeed, recent animal studies have shown that selective proximal tubular injury can lead to podocytopathy and extensive glomerular injury reminiscent of diabetes [142]. Tubular epithelial cells can protect against albuminuria in diabetes by maintaining nicotinamide mononucleotide concentrations around glomeruli and by influencing podocyte function [143].

9.8 Inflammation

Metabolic and hemodynamic abnormalities, including hyperglycemia, AGEs, ROS, Ang II, and TGF-β, have been shown to promote a proinflammatory state [144]. The immune system is involved in the pathophysiology of DKD at multiple levels [145]. First, from an innate immunity standpoint, mononuclear phagocytic cells that reside in the kidney are activated in diabetes and are joined by renal cells in the release of proinflammatory cytokines and paracrine signals [146]. Subsequently, additional monocytes and macrophages are recruited into the kidney, further amplifying cytokine and chemokine release from the kidney [147, 148]. The mast cell is another innate immune cell that infiltrates the tubulointerstitium in DKD. Its degranulation releases inflammatory mediators such as TGF-β and proteolytic enzymes, the most notable of which is chymase [145]. Mast cell chymase is 40 times more potent than ACE at converting Ang I to Ang II [149, 150].

Pattern recognition receptors (PRRs), including Toll-like receptors (TLRs) and nucleotide-binding oligomerization domain-like receptors (NOD-like receptors or NLRs) are essential to the proper function of the innate immune system. PRRs are upregulated in mononuclear phagocytic cells as well as in endothelial cells and podocytes [145]. They recognize pathogen-associated molecular patterns (PAMPs) and endogenous stress signals or damage-associated molecular patterns (DAMPs) that indicate cellular stress and injury, including uric acid, extracellular ATP, as well as glucose and ROS. Upon sensitization of PRRs, there is activation of the inflammasome and, among other effects, release of inflammatory cytokines.

Numerous interleukin cytokines have been implicated in the pathogenesis of DKD. For instance, IL-1, IL-6, and IL-18 have been linked with morphological changes of DKD, such as GBM thickening, as well as functional changes, such as albuminuria and loss of GFR [145]. Early in diabetes, both glomerular and tubular cells increase expression of TNF-α [151]. This cytokine is cytotoxic to glomerular mesangial and epithelial cells and has been demonstrated to increase vascular endothelial permeability, induce oxidative stress, and affect glomerular hemodynamics and GFR [152, 153]. Its receptors, TNFR1 and TNFR2, are candidate biomarkers of DKD. The serum level of TNFR1 was a predictor of ESKD, even after adjustment for clinical covariates in a cohort of type 1 diabetes [154].

Chemokines mediate the migration of monocytes and macrophages into kidney tissue and are also upregulated in DKD. Of particular interest is the CC chemokine ligand 2 (CCL2, also known as MCP-1). Its expression is upregulated in response to the metabolic and hemodynamic features of the diabetic milieu, including Ang II [155]. In the kidney, its receptor CCR2 is also expressed on podocytes, extending its role beyond the recruitment of macrophages to the tubulointerstitium [156]. Several studies have implicated CCR2 in the effacement of foot processes, podocytopenia, and damage to the slit diaphragm, leading to albuminuria [157]. CCR2 inhibitors are being evaluated for the management of DKD [158].

Another therapeutic target in DKD is the Janus kinase–signal transducer and activator of transcription (JAK-STAT) pathway. This pathway transduces inflammatory signals from cytokines and chemokines as well as AGEs and growth factors/hormones [159]. The JAK-STAT pathway has been shown to be upregulated in DKD, including in intrinsic renal cells. Baricitinib, an oral, reversible, selective inhibitor of JAK1 and JAK2, has shown promise as an intervention to slow the progression of DKD [159].

Overall, resident immune cells, infiltrating cells, and resident renal cells converge to activate the innate immune system in DKD. Renal cells produce cytokines and chemokines and increase the expression of adhesion molecules that facilitate adhesion of the inflammatory cells [144, 145]. Eventually, the adaptive immune system is also involved in diabetes, as T cells infiltrate the kidney in DKD, albeit not as prominently as macrophages [145]. The T helper phenotype in DKD appears to be shifted toward Th1/Th17 cells rather than regulatory T cell, Tregs [145, 160]. This promotes further macrophage-induced injury rather than repair of the kidney. There is limited evidence for the involvement of B cells in DKD.

9.9 Conclusion

The pathophysiology of DKD is complex (Fig. 9.2) and most of these pathways were the fruit of deploying various experimental animal models to elucidate mechanisms of injury at the cellular and molecular level and to inform clinical and

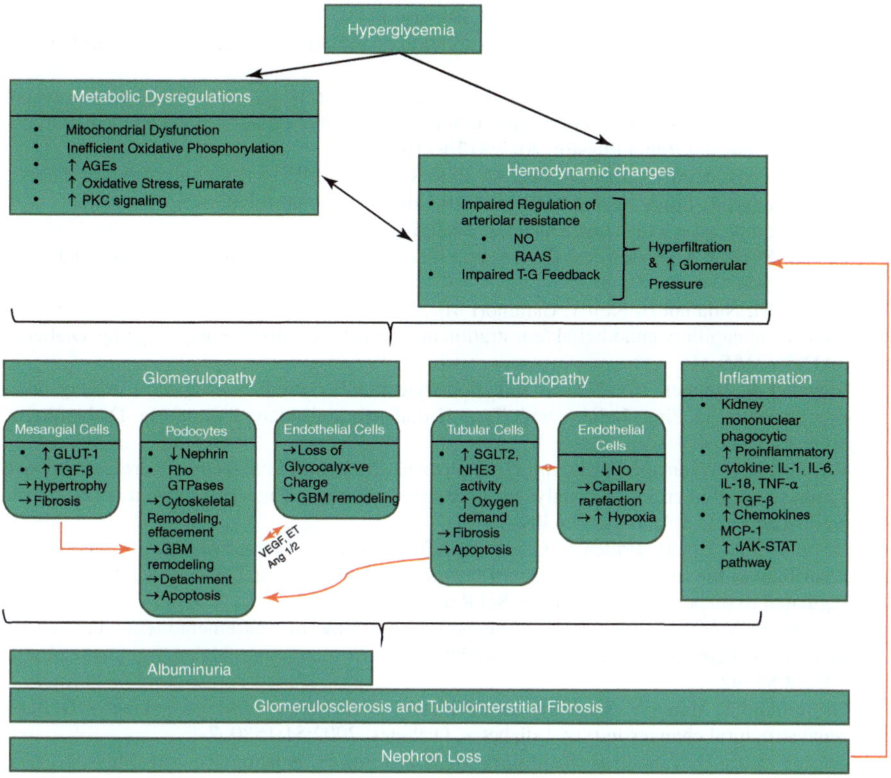

Fig. 9.2 Conceptual model of the pathogenesis of diabetic kidney disease

pathological studies in humans. Glucotoxicity and glomerular hypertension plus deleterious combinations of toxic metabolites, growth factors, and cytokines promote injury in the various compartments of the kidney, leading to albuminuria and progressive fibrosis and loss of renal function. While the treatment and prevention of DKD in clinical practice had long been dependent on ACEi and ARBs as well as the control of systemic hypertension and hyperglycemia, recent clinical studies have brought new options for the management of this disease. The SGLT2i and MRAs currently offer hope for additional nephroprotective effects. By further elucidating the pathophysiology of DKD, we expect that newer and more effective therapies will be on the horizon.

References

1. Stefan G, Stancu S, Zugravu A, Petre N, Mandache E, Mircescu G. Histologic predictors of renal outcome in diabetic nephropathy: Beyond renal pathology society classification. Medicine (Baltimore). 2019;98:e16333.
2. Fioretto P, Mauer M. Histopathology of diabetic nephropathy. Semin Nephrol. 2007;27:195–207.

3. Zhu D, Kim Y, Steffes MW, Groppoli TJ, Butkowski RJ, Mauer SM. Glomerular distribution of type IV collagen in diabetes by high resolution quantitative immunochemistry. Kidney Int. 1994;45:425–33.
4. Kriz W, Lowen J, Federico G, van den Born J, Grone E, Grone HJ. Accumulation of worn-out GBM material substantially contributes to mesangial matrix expansion in diabetic nephropathy. Am J Physiol Renal Physiol. 2017;312:F1101–11.
5. Caramori ML, Kim Y, Huang C, Fish AJ, Rich SS, Miller ME, et al. Cellular basis of diabetic nephropathy: 1. Study design and renal structural-functional relationships in patients with long-standing type 1 diabetes. Diabetes. 2002;51:506–13.
6. Lin JS, Susztak K. Podocytes: the weakest link in diabetic kidney disease? Curr Diab Rep. 2016;16:45.
7. Toyoda M, Najafian B, Kim Y, Caramori ML, Mauer M. Podocyte detachment and reduced glomerular capillary endothelial fenestration in human type 1 diabetic nephropathy. Diabetes. 2007;56:2155–60.
8. Meyer TW, Bennett PH, Nelson RG. Podocyte number predicts long-term urinary albumin excretion in Pima Indians with Type II diabetes and microalbuminuria. Diabetologia. 1999;42:1341–4.
9. Kashihara N, Watanabe Y, Makino H, Wallner EI, Kanwar YS. Selective decreased de novo synthesis of glomerular proteoglycans under the influence of reactive oxygen species. Proc Natl Acad Sci U S A. 1992;89:6309–13.
10. Khramova A, Boi R, Friden V, Granqvist AB, Nilsson U, Tenstad O, et al. Proteoglycans contribute to the functional integrity of the glomerular endothelial cell surface layer and are regulated in diabetic kidney disease. Sci Rep. 2021;11:8487.
11. Østerby R. Morphometric studies of the peripheral glomerular basement membrane in early juvenile diabetes. I. Development of initial basement membrane thickening. Diabetologia. 1972;8:84–92.
12. Drummond K, Mauer M. The early natural history of nephropathy in type 1 diabetes: II. Early renal structural changes in type 1 diabetes. Diabetes. 2002;51:1580–7.
13. Saito Y, Kida H, Takeda S, Yoshimura M, Yokoyama H, Koshino Y, et al. Mesangiolysis in diabetic glomeruli: its role in the formation of nodular lesions. Kidney Int. 1988;34:389–96.
14. Bader R, Bader H, Grund KE, Markensen-Haen S, Christ H, Bohle A. Structure and function of the kidney in diabetic glomerulosclerosis: Correlations between morphologic and functional parameters. Pathol Res Practice. 1980;167:204–16.
15. Lane PH, Steffes MW, Fioretto P, Mauer SM. Renal interstitial expansion in insulin-dependent diabetes mellitus. Kidney Int. 1993;43:661–7.
16. Ziyadeh FN, Goldfarb S. The renal tubulointerstitium in diabetes mellitus. Kidney Int. 1991;39:464–75.
17. Tervaert TW, Mooyaart AL, Amann K, Cohen AH, Cook HT, Drachenberg CB, et al. Pathologic classification of diabetic nephropathy. J Am Soc Nephrol. 2010;21:556–63.
18. Ponchiardi C, Mauer M, Najafian B. Temporal profile of diabetic nephropathy pathologic changes. Curr Diab Rep. 2013;13:592–9.
19. Fioretto P, Mauer M, Brocco E, Velussi M, Frigato F, Muollo B, et al. Patterns of renal injury in NIDDM patients with microalbuminuria. Diabetologia. 1996;39:1569–76.
20. Gambara V, Mecca G, Remuzzi G, Bertani T. Heterogeneous nature of renal lesions in type II diabetes. J Am Soc Nephrol. 1993;3:1458–66.
21. Mogensen CE, Christensen CK, Vittinghus E. The stages in diabetic renal disease. With emphasis on the stage of incipient diabetic nephropathy. Diabetes. 1983;32(Suppl 2):64–78.
22. Olivarius Nde F, Andreasen AH, Keiding N, Mogensen CE. Epidemiology of renal involvement in newly-diagnosed middle-aged and elderly diabetic patients. Cross-sectional data from the population-based study "Diabetes Care in General Practice", Denmark. Diabetologia. 1993;36:1007–16.
23. Mogensen CE, Steffes MW, Deckert T, Christiansen JS. Functional and morphological renal manifestations in diabetes mellitus. Diabetologia. 1981;21:89–93.

24. Ficociello LH, Perkins BA, Roshan B, Weinberg JM, Aschengrau A, Warram JH, et al. Renal hyperfiltration and the development of microalbuminuria in type 1 diabetes. Diabetes Care. 2009;32:889–93.
25. Myers BD, Nelson RG, Williams GW, Bennett PH, Hardy SA, Berg RL, et al. Glomerular function in Pima Indians with noninsulin-dependent diabetes mellitus of recent onset. J Clin Invest. 1991;88:524–30.
26. Magee GM, Bilous RW, Cardwell CR, Hunter SJ, Kee F, Fogarty DG. Is hyperfiltration associated with the future risk of developing diabetic nephropathy? A meta-analysis. Diabetologia. 2009;52:691–7.
27. Ruggenenti P, Porrini EL, Gaspari F, van Bommel EJ, Heerspink HJL, van Raalte DH, et al. Glomerular hyperfiltration and renal disease progression in type 2 diabetes. Diabetes Care. 2012;35:2061–8.
28. Cederholm J, Eliasson B, Nilsson PM, Weiss L, Gudbjörnsdottir S, Steering Committee of the Swedish National Diabetes Register. Microalbuminuria and risk factors in type 1 and type 2 diabetic patients. Diabetes Res Clin Pract. 2005;67:258–66.
29. Mogensen CE. Microalbuminuria predicts clinical proteinuria and early mortality in maturity-onset diabetes. N Engl J Med. 1984;310:356–60.
30. Caramori ML, Fioretto P, Mauer M. The need for early predictors of diabetic nephropathy risk: is albumin excretion rate sufficient? Diabetes. 2000;49:1399–408.
31. Perkins BA, Ficociello LH, Silva KH, Finkelstein DM, Warram JH, Krolewski AS. Regression of microalbuminuria in type 1 diabetes. New Engl J Med. 2003;348:2285–93.
32. Ninomiya T, Perkovic V, Verdon C, Barzi F, Cass A, Gallagher M, et al. Proteinuria and stroke: a meta-analysis of cohort studies. Am J Kidney Dis. 2009;53:417–25.
33. Perkovic V, Verdon C, Ninomiya T, Barzi F, Cass A, Patel A, et al. The relationship between proteinuria and coronary risk: a systematic review and meta-analysis. PLoS Med. 2008;5:1486–95.
34. Deckert T, Yokoyama H, Mathiesen E, Rønn B, Jensen T, Feldt-Rasmussen B, et al. Cohort study of predictive value of urinary albumin excretion for atherosclerotic vascular disease in patients with insulin dependent diabetes. BMJ. 1996;312:871–4.
35. Damsgaard EM, Froland A, Jorgensen OD, Mogensen CE. Microalbuminuria as predictor of increased mortality in elderly people. BMJ. 1990;300:297–300.
36. Mathiesen ER, Feldt-Rasmussen B, Hommel E, Deckert T, Parving HH. Stable glomerular filtration rate in normotensive IDDM patients with stable microalbuminuria. A 5-year prospective study. Diabetes Care. 1997;20:286–9.
37. Gaede P, Tarnow L, Vedel P, Parving H-H, Pedersen O. Remission to normoalbuminuria during multifactorial treatment preserves kidney function in patients with type 2 diabetes and microalbuminuria. Nephrol Dial Transplant. 2004;19:2784–8.
38. Mauer SM, Steffes MW, Ellis EN, Sutherland DE, Brown DM, Goetz FC. Structural-functional relationships in diabetic nephropathy. J Clin Invest. 1984;74:1143–55.
39. Remuzzi G, Bertani T. Is glomerulosclerosis a consequence of altered glomerular permeability to macromolecules? Kidney Int. 1990;38:384–94.
40. Yamada T, Komatsu M, Komiya I, Miyahara Y, Shima Y, Matsuzaki M, et al. Development, progression, and regression of microalbuminuria in Japanese patients with type 2 diabetes under tight glycemic and blood pressure control: the Kashiwa study. Diabetes Care. 2005;28:2733–8.
41. Macisaac RJ, Jerums G. Diabetic kidney disease with and without albuminuria. Curr Opin Nephrol Hypertens. 2011;20:246–57.
42. Writing Team for the Diabetes Control and Complications Trial/Epidemiology of Diabetes Interventions and Complications Research Group. Sustained effect of intensive treatment of type 1 diabetes mellitus on development and progression of diabetic nephropathy: the Epidemiology of Diabetes Interventions and Complications (EDIC) study. JAMA. 2003;290:2159–67.

43. United Kingdom Prospective Diabetes Study Group. Intensive blood-glucose control with sulphonylureas or insulin compared with conventional treatment and risk of complications in patients with type 2 diabetes (UKPDS 33). Lancet. 1998;352:837–53.
44. Fioretto P, Steffes MW, Sutherland DER, Goetz FC, Mauer M. Reversal of lesions of diabetic nephropathy after pancreas transplantation. New Engl J Med. 1998;339:69–75.
45. Barbosa J, Steffes MW, Sutherland DE, Connett JE, Rao KV, Mauer SM. Effect of glycemic control on early diabetic renal lesions. A 5-year randomized controlled clinical trial of insulin-dependent diabetic kidney transplant recipients. JAMA. 1994;272:600–6.
46. Diabetes Control and Complications Trial Research Group, Nathan DM, Genuth S, Lachin J, Cleary P, Crofford O, et al. The effect of intensive treatment of diabetes on the development and progression of long-term complications in insulin-dependent diabetes mellitus. N Engl J Med. 1993;329:977–86.
47. Heilig CW, Brosius FC, Henry DN. Glucose transporters of the glomerulus and the implications for diabetic nephropathy. Kidney Int Suppl. 1997;60:S91–9.
48. Zhang G, Darshi M, Sharma K. The Warburg effect in diabetic kidney disease. Semin Nephrol. 2018;38:111–20.
49. Tanner LB, Goglia AG, Wei MH, Sehgal T, Parsons LR, Park JO, et al. Four key steps control glycolytic flux in mammalian cells. Cell Syst. 2018;7:49–62.e8.
50. Sas KM, Kayampilly P, Byun J, Nair V, Hinder LM, Hur J, et al. Tissue-specific metabolic reprogramming drives nutrient flux in diabetic complications. JCI Insight. 2016;1:e86976.
51. Sharma K, Karl B, Mathew AV, Gangoiti JA, Wassel CL, Saito R, et al. Metabolomics reveals signature of mitochondrial dysfunction in diabetic kidney disease. J Am Soc Nephrol. 2013;24:1901–12.
52. Bhargava P, Schnellmann RG. Mitochondrial energetics in the kidney. Nat Rev Nephrol. 2017;13:629–46.
53. Galvan DL, Green NH, Danesh FR. The hallmarks of mitochondrial dysfunction in chronic kidney disease. Kidney Int. 2017;92:1051–7.
54. Kimmelstiel P, Wilson C. Intercapillary lesions in the glomeruli of the kidney. Am J Pathol. 1936;12:83–98.7.
55. Kang HM, Ahn SH, Choi P, Ko Y, Han SH, Chinga F, et al. Defective fatty acid oxidation in renal tubular epithelial cells has a key role in kidney fibrosis development. Nat Med. 2015;21:37–46.
56. Martinez-Garcia C, Izquierdo-Lahuerta A, Vivas Y, Velasco I, Yeo T, Chen S, et al. Renal lipotoxicity-associated inflammation and insulin resistance affects actin cytoskeleton organization in podocytes. PLoS One. 2015;10:e0142291.
57. Qi W, Li Q, Gordin D, King GL. Preservation of renal function in chronic diabetes by enhancing glomerular glucose metabolism. J Mol Med (Berl). 2018;96:373–81.
58. Qi W, Keenan HA, Li Q, Ishikado A, Kannt A, Sadowski T, et al. Pyruvate kinase M2 activation may protect against the progression of diabetic glomerular pathology and mitochondrial dysfunction. Nat Med. 2017;23:753–62.
59. Horie K, Miyata T, Maeda K, Miyata S, Sugiyama S, Sakai H, et al. Immunohistochemical colocalization of glycoxidation products and lipid peroxidation products in diabetic renal glomerular lesions. Implication for glycoxidative stress in the pathogenesis of diabetic nephropathy. J Clin Invest. 1997;100:2995–3004.
60. Schleicher ED, Wagner E, Nerlich AG. Increased accumulation of the glycoxidation product N(epsilon)-(carboxymethyl)lysine in human tissues in diabetes and aging. J Clin Invest. 1997;99:457–68.
61. Cooper ME. Interaction of metabolic and haemodynamic factors in mediating experimental diabetic nephropathy. Diabetologia. 2001;44:1957–72.
62. Vlassara H, Striker LJ, Teichberg S, Fuh H, Li YM, Steffes M. Advanced glycation end products induce glomerular sclerosis and albuminuria in normal rats. Proc Natl Acad Sci U S A. 1994;91:11704–8.
63. Busch M, Franke S, Rüster C, Wolf G. Advanced glycation end-products and the kidney. Eur J Clin Invest. 2010;40:742–55.

64. Catania JM, Chen G, Parrish AR. Role of matrix metalloproteinases in renal pathophysiologies. Am J Physiol Renal Physiol. 2007;292:F905–11.
65. Wautier JL, Guillausseau PJ. Advanced glycation end products, their receptors and diabetic angiopathy. Diabetes Metab. 2001;27:535–42.
66. Yamagishi S, Inagaki Y, Okamoto T, Amano S, Koga K, Takeuchi M, et al. Advanced glycation end product-induced apoptosis and overexpression of vascular endothelial growth factor and monocyte chemoattractant protein-1 in human-cultured mesangial cells. J Biol Chem. 2002;277:20309–15.
67. Fukami K, Ueda S, Yamagishi S, Kato S, Inagaki Y, Takeuchi M, et al. AGEs activate mesangial TGF-beta-Smad signaling via an angiotensin II type I receptor interaction. Kidney Int. 2004;66:2137–47.
68. Studer RK, Craven PA, DeRubertis FR. Role for protein kinase C in the mediation of increased fibronectin accumulation by mesangial cells grown in high glucose medium. Diabetes. 1993;42:118–26.
69. Thallas-Bonke V, Thorpe SR, Coughlan MT, Fukami K, Yap FY, Sourris KC, et al. Inhibition of NADPH oxidase prevents advanced glycation end product-mediated damage in diabetic nephropathy through a protein kinase C-alpha-dependent pathway. Diabetes. 2008;57:460–9.
70. Hallan S, Sharma K. The role of mitochondria in diabetic kidney disease. Curr Diab Rep. 2016;16:61.
71. Menne J, Shushakova N, Bartels J, Kiyan Y, Laudeley R, Haller H, et al. Dual inhibition of classical protein kinase C-α and protein kinase C-β isoforms protects against experimental murine diabetic nephropathy. Diabetes. 2013;62:1167–74.
72. Tuttle KR, Bakris GL, Toto RD, McGill JB, Hu K, Anderson PW. The effect of ruboxistaurin on nephropathy in type 2 diabetes. Diabetes Care. 2005;28:2686–90.
73. Brownlee M. Biochemistry and molecular cell biology of diabetic complications. Nature. 2001;414:813–20.
74. Gorin Y, Block K. Nox4 and diabetic nephropathy: with a friend like this, who needs enemies? Free Radic Biol Med. 2013;61:130–42.
75. Baynes JW. Role of oxidative stress in development of complications in diabetes. Diabetes. 1991;40:405–12.
76. Coughlan MT, Sharma K. Challenging the dogma of mitochondrial reactive oxygen species overproduction in diabetic kidney disease. Kidney Int. 2016;90:272–9.
77. Sharma K. Mitochondrial dysfunction in the diabetic kidney. In: Santulli G, editor. Mitochondrial dynamics in cardiovascular medicine. Cham: Springer International Publishing; 2017. p. 553–62.
78. Thallas-Bonke V, Jha JC, Gray SP, Barit D, Haller H, Schmidt HHHW, et al. Nox-4 deletion reduces oxidative stress and injury by PKC-α-associated mechanisms in diabetic nephropathy. Physiol Rep. 2014;2:e12192.
79. You YH, Quach T, Saito R, Pham J, Sharma K. Metabolomics reveals a key role for fumarate in mediating the effects of NADPH oxidase 4 in diabetic kidney disease. J Am Soc Nephrol. 2016;27:466–81.
80. Christiansen JS, Gammelgaard J, Frandsen M, Parving HH. Increased kidney size, glomerular filtration rate and renal plasma flow in short-term insulin-dependent diabetics. Diabetologia. 1981;20:451–6.
81. Tonneijck L, Muskiet MH, Smits MM, van Bommel EJ, Heerspink HJL, van Raalte DH, et al. Glomerular hyperfiltration in diabetes: mechanisms, clinical significance, and treatment. J Am Soc Nephrol. 2017;28:1023–39.
82. De Vriese AS, Stoenoiu MS, Elger M, Devuyst O, Vanholder R, Kriz W, et al. Diabetes-induced microvascular dysfunction in the hydronephrotic kidney: role of nitric oxide. Kidney Int. 2001;60:202–10.
83. Goligorsky MS. Endothelial cell dysfunction and nitric oxide synthase. Kidney Int. 2000;58:1360–76.
84. Hostetter TH, Rennke HG, Brenner BM. The case for intrarenal hypertension in the initiation and progression of diabetic and other gomerulopathies. Am J Med. 1982;72:375–80.

85. Anderson S, Rennke HG, Brenner BM. Therapeutic advantage of converting enzyme inhibitors in arresting progressive renal disease associated with systemic hypertension in the rat. J Clin Invest. 1986;77:1993–2000.
86. Lambers Heerspink HJ, de Borst MH, Bakker SJL, Navis GJ. Improving the efficacy of RAAS blockade in patients with chronic kidney disease. Nature Rev Nephrol. 2012;9:112–21.
87. Holtkamp FA, de Zeeuw D, Thomas MC, Cooper ME, de Graeff PA, Hillege HJL, et al. An acute fall in estimated glomerular filtration rate during treatment with losartan predicts a slower decrease in long-term renal function. Kidney Int. 2011;80:282–7.
88. Bakris GL, Weir MR. Angiotensin-converting enzyme inhibitor–associated elevations in serum creatinine: is this a cause for concern? Arch Int Med. 2000;160:685–93.
89. Vallon V, Thomson SC. Renal function in diabetic disease models: the tubular system in the pathophysiology of the diabetic kidney. Annu Rev Physiol. 2012;74:351–75.
90. Wang XX, Levi J, Luo Y, Myakala K, Herman-Edelstein M, Qiu L, et al. SGLT2 protein expression is increased in human diabetic nephropathy: SGLT2 protein inhibition decreases renal lipid accumulation, inflammation, and the development of nephropathy in diabetic mice. J Biol Chem. 2017;292:5335–48.
91. Vallon V, Schroth J, Satriano J, Blantz RC, Thomson SC, Rieg T. Adenosine A(1) receptors determine glomerular hyperfiltration and the salt paradox in early streptozotocin diabetes mellitus. Nephron Physiol. 2009;111:30–8.
92. Carmines PK. The renal vascular response to diabetes. Curr Opin Nephrol Hypértens. 2010;19:85–90.
93. Vallon V, Richter K, Blantz RC, Thomson S, Osswald H. Glomerular hyperfiltration in experimental diabetes mellitus: potential role of tubular reabsorption. J Am Soc Nephrol. 1999;10:2569–76.
94. Hallow KM, Gebremichaël Y, Helmlinger G, Vallon V. Primary proximal tubule hyperreabsorption and impaired tubular transport counterregulation determine glomerular hyperfiltration in diabetes: a modeling analysis. Am J Physiol Renal Physiol. 2017;312:F819–35.
95. Vallon V, Rose M, Gerasimova M, Satriano J, Platt KA, Koepsell H, et al. Knockout of Na-glucose transporter SGLT2 attenuates hyperglycemia and glomerular hyperfiltration but not kidney growth or injury in diabetes mellitus. Am J Physiol Renal Physiol. 2013;304:F156–67.
96. Cherney DZ, Perkins BA, Soleymanlou N, Maione M, Lai V, Lee A, et al. Renal hemodynamic effect of sodium-glucose cotransporter 2 inhibition in patients with type 1 diabetes mellitus. Circulation. 2014;129:587–97.
97. Wanner C, Inzucchi SE, Lachin JM, Fitchett D, von Eynatten M, Mattheus M, et al. Empagliflozin and progression of kidney disease in type 2 diabetes. N Engl J Med. 2016;375:323–34.
98. Thomson SC, Rieg T, Miracle C, Mansoury H, Whaley J, Vallon V, et al. Acute and chronic effects of SGLT2 blockade on glomerular and tubular function in the early diabetic rat. Am J Physiol Regul Integr Comp Physiol. 2012;302:R75–83.
99. Skrtic M, Yang GK, Perkins BA, Soleymanlou N, Lytvyn Y, von Eynatten M, et al. Characterisation of glomerular haemodynamic responses to SGLT2 inhibition in patients with type 1 diabetes and renal hyperfiltration. Diabetologia. 2014;57:2599–602.
100. Perkovic V, Jardine MJ, Neal B, Bompoint S, Heerspink HJL, Charytan DM, et al. Canagliflozin and renal outcomes in type 2 diabetes and nephropathy. N Engl J Med. 2019;380:2295–306.
101. Chade AR. Renal vascular structure and rarefaction. Compr Physiol. 2013;3:817–31.
102. Gnudi L, Thomas SM, Viberti G. Mechanical forces in diabetic kidney disease: a trigger for impaired glucose metabolism. J Am Soc Nephrol. 2007;18:2226–32.
103. Gruden G, Zonca S, Hayward A, Thomas S, Maestrini S, Gnudiet L, et al. Mechanical stretch-induced fibronectin and transforming growth factor-beta1 production in human mesangial cells is p38 mitogen-activated protein kinase-dependent. Diabetes. 2000;49:655–61.
104. Endlich K, Kliewe F, Endlich N. Stressed podocytes-mechanical forces, sensors, signaling and response. Pflugers Arch. 2017;469:937–49.

105. Kriz W, Lemley KV. A potential role for mechanical forces in the detachment of podocytes and the progression of CKD. J Am Soc Nephrol. 2015;26:258–69.
106. Schiffer M, Bitzer M, Roberts IS, Kopp JB, ten Dijke P, Mundel P, et al. Apoptosis in podocytes induced by TGF-beta and Smad7. J Clin Invest. 2001;108:807–16.
107. Inoki K, Mori H, Wang J, Suzuki T, Hong S, Yoshida S, et al. mTORC1 activation in podocytes is a critical step in the development of diabetic nephropathy in mice. J Clin Invest. 2011;121:2181–96.
108. Wharram BL, Goyal M, Wiggins JE, Sanden SK, Hussain S, Filipiak WE, et al. Podocyte depletion causes glomerulosclerosis: diphtheria toxin-induced podocyte depletion in rats expressing human diphtheria toxin receptor transgene. J Am Soc Nephrol. 2005;16:2941–52.
109. Durvasula RV, Petermann AT, Hiromura K, Blonski M, Pippin J, Mundel P, et al. Activation of a local tissue angiotensin system in podocytes by mechanical strain. Kidney Int. 2004;65:30–9.
110. Thomas MC, Tikellis C, Burns WM, Bialkowski K, Cao Z, Coughlan MT, et al. Interactions between renin angiotensin system and advanced glycation in the kidney. J Am Soc Nephrol. 2005;16:2976–84.
111. Tan ALY, Forbes JM, Cooper ME. AGE, RAGE, and ROS in diabetic nephropathy. Semin Nephrol. 2007;27:130–43.
112. Wolf G. New insights into the pathophysiology of diabetic nephropathy: from haemodynamics to molecular pathology. Eur J Clin Invest. 2004;34:785–96.
113. Zoja C, Xinaris C, Macconi D. Diabetic nephropathy: novel molecular mechanisms and therapeutic targets. Front Pharmacol. 2020;11:586892.
114. Barrera-Chimal J, Lima-Posada I, Bakris GL, Jaisser F. Mineralocorticoid receptor antagonists in diabetic kidney disease—mechanistic and therapeutic effects. Nat Rev Nephrol. 2022;18:56–70.
115. Bakris GL, Agarwal R, Anker SD, Pitt B, Ruilope LM, Rossing P, et al. Effect of finerenone on chronic kidney disease outcomes in type 2 diabetes. N Engl J Med. 2020;383:2219–29.
116. Tufro A, Veron D. VEGF and podocytes in diabetic nephropathy. Semin Nephrol. 2012;32:385–93.
117. Eremina V, Sood M, Haigh J, Nagy A, Lajoie G, Ferrara N, et al. Glomerular-specific alterations of VEGF-A expression lead to distinct congenital and acquired renal diseases. J Clin Invest. 2003;111:707–16.
118. Sung SH, Chen S, Laping NJ, Ziyadeh FN. Albuminuria is ameliorated by an inhibitor of VEGF receptors, SU5416, in diabetic db/db mice but is unaffected in Smad3-knockout mice rendered diabetic with streptozotocin. J Am Soc Nephrol. 2004:(Abstract).
119. Sivaskandarajah GA, Jeansson M, Maezawa Y, Eremina V, Baelde HJ, Quaggin SE. VEGFA protects the glomerular microvasculature in diabetes. Diabetes. 2012;61:2958–66.
120. De Vriese AS, Tilton RG, Elger M, Stephan CC, Kriz W, Lameire NH. Antibodies against vascular endothelial growth factor improve early renal dysfunction in experimental diabetes. J Am Soc Nephrol. 2001;12:993–1000.
121. Flyvbjerg A, Dagnaes-Hansen F, De Vriese AS, Schrijvers BF, Tilton RG, Rasch R. Amelioration of long-term renal changes in obese type 2 diabetic mice by a neutralizing vascular endothelial growth factor antibody. Diabetes. 2002;51:3090–4.
122. Majumder S, Advani A. VEGF and the diabetic kidney: more than too much of a good thing. J Diabetes Complications. 2017;31:273–9.
123. Bates DO. Vascular endothelial growth factors and vascular permeability. Cardiovasc Res. 2010;87:262–71.
124. Oltean S, Qiu Y, Ferguson JK, Stevens M, Neal C, Russell A, et al. Vascular endothelial growth factor-A165b is protective and restores endothelial glycocalyx in diabetic nephropathy. J Am Soc Nephrol. 2015;26:1889–904.
125. Garsen M, Lenoir O, Rops AL, Dijkman HB, Willemsen B, van Kuppevelt TH, et al. Endothelin-1 Induces proteinuria by heparanase-mediated disruption of the glomerular glycocalyx. J Am Soc Nephrol. 2016;27:3545–51.
126. de Zeeuw D, Coll B, Andress D, Brennan JJ, Tang H, Houser M, et al. The endothelin antagonist atrasentan lowers residual albuminuria in patients with type 2 diabetic nephropathy. J Am Soc Nephrol. 2014;25:1083–93.

127. Reeves WB, Andreoli TE. Transforming growth factor beta contributes to progressive diabetic nephropathy. Proc Natl Acad Sci USA. 2000;97:7667–9.
128. Ziyadeh FN. Evidence for the involvement of transforming growth factor-beta in the pathogenesis of diabetic kidney disease: are Koch's postulates fulfilled? Curr Pract Med. 1998;1:87–9.
129. Ziyadeh FN, Sharma K, Ericksen M, Wolf G. Stimulation of collagen gene expression and protein synthesis in murine mesangial cells by high glucose is mediated by autocrine activation of transforming growth factor-beta. J Clin Invest. 1994;93:536–42.
130. Yang CW, Vlassara H, Peten EP, He C-J, Striker GE, Striker LJ. Advanced glycation end products up-regulate gene expression found in diabetic glomerular disease. Proc Natl Acad Sci USA. 1994;91:9436–40.
131. Riser BL, Cortes P, Yee J, Sharba AK, Asano K, Rodriguez-Barbero A, et al. Mechanical strain- and high glucose-induced alterations in mesangial cell collagen metabolism: role of TGF-beta. J Am Soc Nephrol. 1998;9:827–36.
132. Fumo P, Kuncio GS, Ziyadeh FN. PKC and high glucose stimulate collagen alpha1(IV)transcriptional activity in a reporter mesangial cell line. Am J Physiol. 1994;267:F632–8.
133. Wolf G, Neilson EG. Angiotensin II as a hypertrophogenic cytokine for proximal tubular cells. Kidney Int Suppl. 1993;39:S100–7.
134. Sharma K, Ziyadeh FN, Alzahabi B, McGowan TA, Kapoor S, Kurnik BR, et al. Increased renal production of transforming growth factor-beta1 in patients with type II diabetes. Diabetes. 1997;46:854–9.
135. Ziyadeh FN, Hoffman BB, Han DC, Iglesias-De La Cruz MC, Hong SW, Isono M, et al. Long-term prevention of renal insufficiency, excess matrix gene expression, and glomerular mesangial matrix expansion by treatment with monoclonal anti-TGF-β antibody in db/db diabetic mice. Proc Natl Acad Sci USA. 2000:8015–20.
136. Chen S, Kasama Y, Lee JS, Jim B, Marin M, Ziyadeh FN. Podocyte-derived vascular endothelial growth factor mediates the stimulation of alpha3(IV) collagen production by transforming growth factor-beta1 in mouse podocytes. Diabetes. 2004;53:2939–49.
137. Yu SM, Bonventre JV. Acute kidney injury and progression of diabetic kidney disease. Adv Chronic Kidney Dis. 2018;25:166–80.
138. Sabbisetti VS, Waikar SS, Antoine DJ, Smiles A, Wang C, Ravisankar A, et al. Blood kidney injury molecule-1 is a biomarker of acute and chronic kidney injury and predicts progression to ESRD in type I diabetes. J Am Soc Nephrol. 2014;25:2177–86.
139. Gilbert RE. Proximal tubulopathy: prime mover and key therapeutic target in diabetic kidney disease. Diabetes. 2017;66:791–800.
140. Ziyadeh FN, Snipes ER, Watanabe M, Alvarez RJ, Goldfarb S, Haverty TP. High glucose induces cell hypertrophy and stimulates collagen gene transcription in proximal tubule. Am J Physiol. 1990;259:F704–14.
141. Wilson PC, Wu H, Kirita Y, Uchimura K, Ledru N, Rennke HG, et al. The single-cell transcriptomic landscape of early human diabetic nephropathy. Proc Natl Acad Sci USA. 2019;116:19619–25.
142. Grgic I, Campanholle G, Bijol V, Wang C, Sabbisetti VS, Ichimura T, et al. Targeted proximal tubule injury triggers interstitial fibrosis and glomerulosclerosis. Kidney Int. 2012;82:172–83.
143. Hasegawa K, Wakino S, Simic P, Sakamaki Y, Minakuchi H, Fujimura K, et al. Renal tubular Sirt1 attenuates diabetic albuminuria by epigenetically suppressing Claudin-1 overexpression in podocytes. Nat Med. 2013;19:1496–504.
144. Alicic RZ, Johnson EJ, Tuttle KR. Inflammatory mechanisms as new biomarkers and therapeutic targets for diabetic kidney disease. Adv Chronic Kidney Dis. 2018;25:181–91.
145. Pichler R, Afkarian M, Dieter BP, Tuttle KR. Immunity and inflammation in diabetic kidney disease: translating mechanisms to biomarkers and treatment targets. Am J Physiol Renal Physiol. 2017;312:F716–31.
146. Nelson PJ, Rees AJ, Griffin MD, Hughes J, Kurts C, Duffield J. The renal mononuclear phagocytic system. J Am Soc Nephrol. 2012;23:194–203.

147. Nguyen D, Ping F, Mu W, Hill P, Atkins RC, Chadban SJ. Macrophage accumulation in human progressive diabetic nephropathy. Nephrology (Carlton). 2006;11:226–31.
148. Furuta T, Saito T, Ootaka T, Soma J, Obara K, Abe K, et al. The role of macrophages in diabetic glomerulosclerosis. Am J Kidney Dis. 1993;21:480–5.
149. Wintroub BU, Schechter NB, Lazarus GS, Kaempfer CE, Schwartz LB. Angiotensin I conversion by human and rat chymotryptic proteinases. J Invest Dermatol. 1984;83:336–9.
150. Reilly CF, Tewksbury DA, Schechter NM, Travis J. Rapid conversion of angiotensin I to angiotensin II by neutrophil and mast cell proteinases. J Biol Chem. 1982;257:8619–22.
151. Navarro-Gonzalez JF, Jarque A, Muros M, Mora C, Garcia J. Tumor necrosis factor-alpha as a therapeutic target for diabetic nephropathy. Cytokine Growth Factor Rev. 2009;20:165–73.
152. Awad AS, You H, Gao T, Cooper TK, Nedospasov SA, Vacher J, et al. Macrophage-derived tumor necrosis factor-alpha mediates diabetic renal injury. Kidney Int. 2015;88:722–33.
153. McCarthy ET, Sharma R, Sharma M, Li JZ, Ge XL, Dileepan KN, et al. TNF-alpha increases albumin permeability of isolated rat glomeruli through the generation of superoxide. J Am Soc Nephrol. 1998;9:433–8.
154. Gohda T, Niewczas MA, Ficociello LH, Walker WH, Skupien J, Rosetti F, et al. Circulating TNF receptors 1 and 2 predict stage 3 CKD in type 1 diabetes. J Am Soc Nephrol. 2012;23:516–24.
155. Brosius FC, Khoury CC, Buller CL, Chen S. Abnormalities in signaling pathways in diabetic nephropathy. Expert Rev Endocrinol Metab. 2010;5:51–64.
156. Lee EY, Chung CH, Khoury CC, Yeo TK, Pyagay PE, Wang A, et al. The monocyte chemoattractant protein-1/CCR2 loop, inducible by TGF-beta, increases podocyte motility and albumin permeability. Am J Physiol Renal Physiol. 2009;297:F85–94.
157. You H, Gao T, Raup-Konsavage WM, Cooper TK, Bronson SK, Reeves WB, et al. Podocyte-specific chemokine (C-C motif) receptor 2 overexpression mediates diabetic renal injury in mice. Kidney Int. 2017;91:671–82.
158. de Zeeuw D, Bekker P, Henkel E, Hasslacher C, Gouni-Berthold I, Mehling H, et al. The effect of CCR2 inhibitor CCX140-B on residual albuminuria in patients with type 2 diabetes and nephropathy: a randomised trial. Lancet Diabetes Endocrinol. 2015;3:687–96.
159. Tuttle KR, Brosius FC 3rd, Adler SG, Kretzler M, Mehta RL, Tumlin JA, et al. JAK1/JAK2 inhibition by baricitinib in diabetic kidney disease: results from a Phase 2 randomized controlled clinical trial. Nephrol Dial Transplant. 2018;33:1950–9.
160. Zeng C, Shi X, Zhang B, Liu H, Zhang L, Ding W, et al. The imbalance of Th17/Th1/Tregs in patients with type 2 diabetes: relationship with metabolic factors and complications. J Mol Med (Berl). 2012;90:175–86.

Diabetes and Sympathetic Nervous System

10

Gino Seravalle and Guido Grassi

10.1 Introduction

Epidemic is a word that is becoming more and more common for single pathophysiological conditions that ultimately underlie common mechanisms. In real life, pathophysiological conditions are associated thus favoring a recruiting of new mechanisms that lead to an increase in cardiovascular risk. Diabetes mellitus, as well as obesity, hypertension, renal diseases, and heart failure, is a pathophysiological condition that is developed through the activation of the sympathetic nervous system, one of the main culprits for their sustenance and progression. The last few decades have been devoted to the study of the pathophysiological mechanisms and possible remedies. This will be the argument of this chapter.

10.2 Epidemiology

Several evidences [1–4] and reports of the WHO [5] have clearly underlined the progressive increase in the prevalence of diabetes over recent decades. In the 1960s, it was estimated that 30 million people had diabetes [6], while in the new millennium, the WHO estimates that about 170 million people are affected by this pathophysiological condition [1]. Different is the estimation of the global prevalence of diabetes by the International Diabetes Federation rising from 151 million in 2000 to 382 million in 2013 [7, 8]. The numbers coming from the more recent 2019 IDF Diabetes Atlas (9th edition) are really impressive [9]: 1 in 11 adults (20–79 years old) have diabetes (463 million people), 1 in 2 adults with diabetes are undiagnosed

G. Seravalle (✉)
Cardiology Department, Istituto Auxologico Italiano, IRCCS S. Luca Hospital, Milan, Italy

G. Grassi
Clinica Medica, University Milano-Bicocca, Monza-Milano, Italy

A. E. Berbari, G. Mancia (eds.), *Blood Pressure Disorders in Diabetes Mellitus*, Updates in Hypertension and Cardiovascular Protection,
https://doi.org/10.1007/978-3-031-13009-0_10

(232 million people), 1 in 5 people with diabetes are above 65 years old (136 million people), 10% of global health expenditure is spent on diabetes (USD 760 billion), 1 in 6 live births (20 million) is affected by hyperglycemia in pregnancy and 84% of which have gestational diabetes, 3 in 4 (79%) people with diabetes live in low- and middle-income countries, over 1.1 million children and adolescents below 20 years old have type 1 diabetes, 1 in 13 adults (20–79 years old) have impaired glucose tolerance (374 million people), and 2 in 3 people with diabetes live in urban areas (310.3 million). All these evidences underline that this dramatic increase in diabetes is highlighting in all countries, in both urban and rural areas, and is associated with the progression of age. Of course the increase in diabetes is also observed very carefully by the economic study centers linked to the health departments of different nations due to the important increase in the health expenditure [3, 10, 11]. In 2040, it is estimated that 642 million (range 521–829 million) people aged 20–79 years will have diabetes with a total health expenditure amounting to 802 billion USD. It is also expected that the regions with the highest projected growth rates in the number of people with diabetes will be the areas of Africa, Southeast Asia, and Western Pacific due to the fact that a great number of subjects are actually undiagnosed.

10.3 Prediabetes and Diabetes

In many cases, the diagnosis of type 2 diabetes mellitus (T2DM) is preceded by a phase of "prediabetes" characterized by blood glucose levels above normal, but not so high as to lead to overt diabetes and high levels of circulating insulin (insulin resistance and hyperinsulinemia). Worldwide, many people have a so-called prediabetic condition without being aware of it.

There are several blood tests for prediabetes: (a) fasting blood sugar test, (b) oral glucose tolerance test, and (c) glycated hemoglobin (A1C) test.

For the fasting blood glucose test, a blood sample is taken after fasting for at least 8 hours or overnight. If the fasting blood glucose is normally higher than 110, but lower than 126 mg/dL (5.6–7.0 mmol/L), this is considered prediabetes or impaired fasting glucose. In this case, it is useful to carry out the oral glucose tolerance test which allows to ascertain the presence of reduced glucose tolerance (you will be intolerant to glucose with blood sugar levels after 2 h from the test up to 199 mg/dL) or diabetes (if values will be ≥200 mg/dL after 2 h of the glucose load test) (Fig. 10.1). It should be remembered that this load test should also be done periodically in subjects with other known risk factors for diabetes (e.g., over 50 years old, hypercholesterolemia, hypertriglyceridemia, visceral obesity, familial history).

The glycated hemoglobin (A1C) test shows the average blood sugar level for the past three months. The test measures the percentage of blood sugar attached to the oxygen-carrying protein in red blood cells called hemoglobin. The higher your blood sugar levels, the more hemoglobin you will have with sugar attached.

In general, an A1C level below 5.7% is considered normal, an A1C level between 5.7% and 6.4% is considered prediabetes, and an A1C level of 6.5% or higher on two separate tests indicates type 2 diabetes.

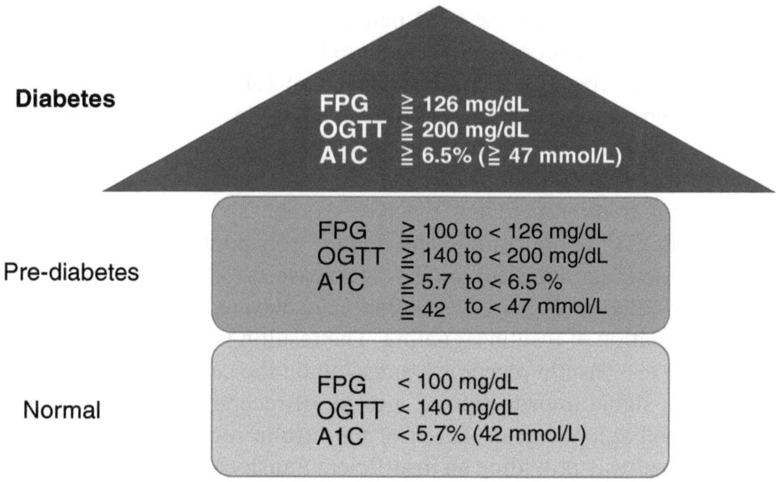

Fig. 10.1 Scheme of reference values of blood tests for the diagnosis of normalcy, prediabetes and diabetes

It has been widely demonstrated that if you start to control your hyperglycemia values from the prediabetes stage, you can delay or even prevent the onset of type 2 diabetes mellitus [12–16].

T2DM is the most common type of diabetes, accounting for around 90% of all diabetes cases. It is most commonly diagnosed in older adults, but is increasingly seen in children, adolescents, and younger adults due to rising levels of obesity, physical inactivity, and poor diet.

10.4 Pathophysiological Mechanisms

T2DM is a condition characterized by deficient insulin secretion by pancreatic islet β-cells, tissue insulin resistance (IR), and an inadequate compensatory insulin secretion response [17, 18]. IR contributes to increase glucose production in the liver and decrease glucose uptake in muscles, liver, and adipose tissue. Also in the early phase of the disease, β-cell dysfunction is usually more severe than IR. When both these conditions are present, hyperglycemia is amplified leading to the progression of T2DM [19, 20]. The dysfunction of β-cells in T2DM is due to a complex network of interactions between the environment and molecular pathways of cell biology [21]. An excess of food induces β-cell inflammation, inflammatory stress, stress in the endoplasmic reticulum (ER), metabolic/oxidative stress, and amyloid stress, with the potential loss of islet integrity [22]. An excess of free fatty acids (FFAs) and hyperglycemia lead to β-cell dysfunction by inducing ER stress through the activation of the apoptotic unfolded protein response (UPR) pathways [23]. This is evident in obesity and metabolic syndrome in which gluco- and lipotoxicity induce an oxidative stress and a β-cell damage [21]. Stress derived from high levels of saturated FFAs can activate the UPR pathway by several mechanisms including inhibition of the sarco-/endoplasmic reticulum Ca^{2+} ATPase (SERCA) responsible for the ER Ca^{2+} mobilization, activation of inositol 1,4,5-trisphospate (IP3) receptors, or direct impairment of ER homeostasis. High glucose levels may also favor proinsulin biosynthesis and islet amyloid polypeptides (IAAP) in β-cells, leading to the accumulation of misfolded insulin and IAAP and increasing the production of oxidative protein folding-mediated reactive oxygen species (ROS) [23]. These effects alter ER Ca^{2+} mobilization and induce proapoptotic signals, proinsulin mRNA degradation, and interleukin (IL)-1β release favoring local islet inflammation [21]. When cells are exposed to continuously elevated insulin levels, there is a partial downregulation of insulin signaling. The resulting "insulin resistance" is not primarily due to less insulin receptor expression on the cell surface but also due to impaired insulin signal transduction as a result of receptor dysfunction. Thus, we have a diminished autophosphorylation of the insulin receptor and impairment in the PI3K/AKT pathway providing an insufficient translocation of GLU4 for glucose uptake and deficient activation of eNOS [24, 25]. Insulin resistance can be seen as a protective mechanism for preventing excess activation of glucose transport from the blood despite chronically elevated insulin levels, to maintain glucose homeostasis and to mitigate oxidative stress [26, 27]. Other additional mechanisms linked to insulin toxicity are also activated (i.e., activation of mTORC1, MEK/ERK pathway), favoring cell proliferation, protein synthesis, and autophagy due to an impairment in oxygen radical defense [28–32] (Fig. 10.2).

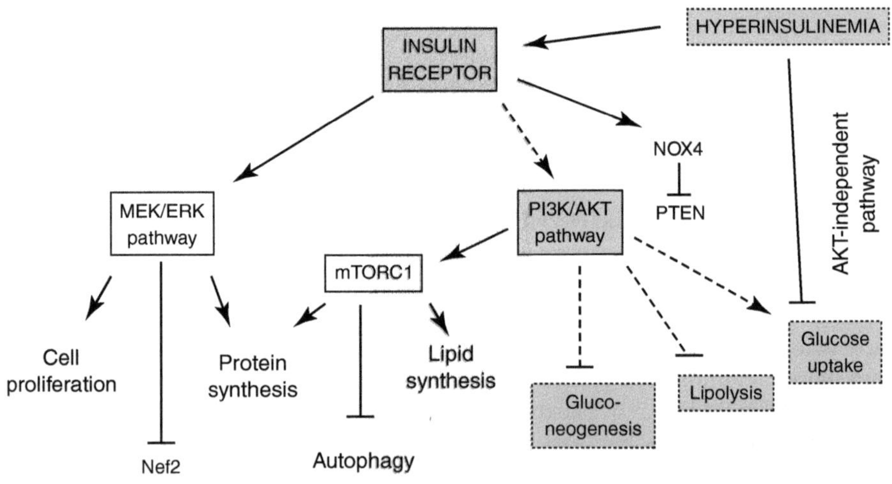

Fig. 10.2 During insulin resistance signaling through AKT kinases is partially impaired. Therefore, hyperinsulinemia, in the presence of insulin resistance, promotes anabolic cell activities via the MEK/ERK pathway and via TORC1. The net effect of these and other mechanisms is a mediation of cell constituent turnover and cell defense mechanisms to radical stress and a downregulation of glucose uptake

Several evidences have clearly shown that hypersecretion of insulin can precede and cause insulin resistance [33, 34] and that lowering insulin secretion in hyperinsulinemic individuals may be beneficial. This can be obtained through gastric surgery [35–38], loss of abdominal fat [39, 40], stimulating insulin clearance via exercise [41–43], or drug therapies [44–47].

10.5 Insulin Resistance and Sympathetic Nervous System

Dietary intake greatly influences plasma norepinephrine levels [48, 49]. An increase in plasma catecholamines and muscle sympathetic nerve traffic is also evident during euglycemic-hyperinsulinemic clamp-induced increases in plasma insulin levels [50–52]. A positive correlation was found between plasma insulin and muscle sympathetic nerve activity (MSNA) during OGTT [50]. This is true majorly in lean subjects, while a blunted MSNA response was observed in obese subjects [53, 54]. It has been reported [52] that increases in plasma insulin levels and MSNA are associated with vasodilation and increased muscle blood flow, thus promoting glucose uptake in the skeletal muscles. This action is impaired in obese subjects [55], justifying the reduced thermic effects of food in this population [56, 57]. From this hypothesis, several evidences in the next decades have shown that other mechanisms are involved in the relation between insulin, adrenergic tone, and pathophysiological conditions, contributing to increase the cardiovascular risk.

It has been shown that the blood pressure responses to hyperinsulinemia represent a complex interaction between the sympathetic nervous system, vessel characteristics, and biochemical mediators (for example, nitric oxide and leptin) [58–60]. It has been shown that insulin evokes both pressor (sympathoexcitatory) and depressor (vasodilation) actions; thus, a balance is maintained in healthy status. It may be that genetic factors, aging, structural vascular alterations, endothelial dysfunction, and concomitant pathophysiological conditions (increase in body weight, metabolic alterations, and preclinical alterations in blood pressure, renal function, and diabetes) would augment the pressor (sympathetic) action of insulin or attenuate the depressor (vasodilation) action, thus favoring the effects mediated by the hyperadrenergic tone [61–65]. Insulin resistance is usually associated with volume expansion, sodium retention, and enhanced adrenergic tone [58], thus justifying the role of the increase in blood pressure values. A relationship has been observed between insulin sensitivity and sympathetic activation mediated by factors like free fatty acids which cause insulin resistance [66] and increase sympathetic activity [67–69]. The idea that insulin resistance, hyperadrenergic tone, and the increase in blood pressure values are pathophysiologically linked may explain why these conditions coexist in the metabolic syndrome [70–74]. Several factors that are also involved are the activation of the renin-angiotensin system, the inflammatory status, and, more importantly, the impaired baroreflex sensitivity [36, 40, 70–76] (Fig. 10.3).

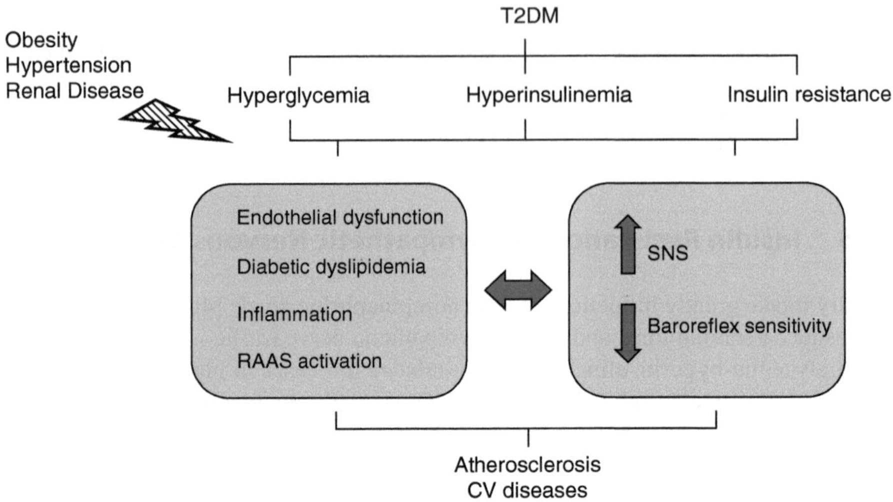

Fig. 10.3 Scheme of the pathophysiological mechanisms involved in the relationship between diabetes, insulin sensitivity, adrenergic tone, and cardiovascular risk

10.6 Adrenergic Tone and Diabetes

The first evidences of the influence of adrenergic tone in diabetes mellitus come from urinary or plasma norepinephrine levels or indirectly from the determination of heart rate variability [77–80]. Studies performed with new methodological approaches to investigate the adrenergic nervous system (i.e., microneurography, norepinephrine radiolabeled spillover) allowed to obtain information on the behavior of the regional sympathetic activity [81, 82]. It is important not to forget that some limitations could be present linked to the methodology itself and to the confounding effect of comorbidities associated with diabetes (obesity or hypertension). Prospective observational studies and meta-analysis have shown that prediabetes is associated with increased cardiovascular risk [83–85]. Only few studies addressed the issue whether an early increase in sympathetic drive may characterize the prediabetic state [65, 86]. Dell'Oro et al. [65] have clearly shown that prediabetes is characterized by a significant increase in muscle sympathetic nerve traffic, and this is associated by a significant impairment in the spontaneous baroreflex sensitivity. In this study the multivariate analysis showed that MSNA was directly and significantly related ($r = 0.41$, $P = 0.0374$) to the homeostatic model assessment (HOMA) index, an index of insulin resistance, and inversely and significantly related to baroreflex-MSNA sensitivity ($r = 0.84$, $P < 0.0001$). The important evidence of this study is that the relationship between HOMA-IR and MSNA is peculiar of prediabetic individuals. Thus, the major driver of the sympathetic overdrive characterizing the prediabetic state may depend on the hyperinsulinemia and the related insulin resistance state. This study has also an important clinical implication, that is, finding an early sympathetic activation in the early stages of the disease to implement interventions capable of reducing the sympathetic drive.

More recently, the same research group performed a systematic review and meta-analysis [87] on 11 microneurographic studies, with rigid selection criteria for inclusion and analysis, performed in about 300 diabetic patients. Results reveal that T1DM shows MSNA values superimposable to healthy individuals, T2DM was characterized by a significant increase in MSNA values. This sympathetic activation observed in T2DM does not show any relationship with anthropometric or metabolic variables with the exception of plasma insulin levels that are directly and significantly related to MSNA values. This confirms previous evidences that in diabetes adrenergic drive, plasma insulin and insulin resistance are closely related due to their reciprocal excitatory influence [58, 88, 89]. The effects of insulin are direct at the central level, while the sympathetic activity induces hyperinsulinemia and insulin resistance indirectly through its vasoconstrictive effects in the skeletal muscle areas and the impairment of the arterial baroreflex ability to restrain sympathetic drive [65, 90]. Factors other than insulin might contribute to the adrenergic activation in T2DM. The first factor is the renin-angiotensin system which stimulates the sympathetic nervous system through the direct action of angiotensin II at the central level [91], and the second factor is the increased level of leptin and ghrelin which have an excitatory effect on adrenergic drive [92, 93].

10.7 Drugs May Help to Reduce Adrenergic Tone?

The answer is positive. Sodium-glucose cotransporter type 2 inhibitors (SGLT2i) are new glucose-lowering agents that specifically target the kidney and promote glucosuria, independent of the action of insulin. This class of drugs is able to improve glucose control, without inducing hypoglycemia and with lower plasma insulin levels. It has been observed that they are able to promote weight reduction and to induce osmotic diuresis and natriuresis [94]. These actions therefore have favorable effects in hypertensive subjects [95, 96] but also in heart failure patients and in end-stage kidney disease [97–100]. Which are the mechanisms underlying these benefits? The renin-angiotensin system (RAS) plays a role in regulating BP and body fluids. This is usually activated in these pathophysiological conditions, and this is the case also for the sympathetic nervous system [63–65, 74, 91]. A cross-talk between the SNS and SGLT2 regulation at the level of the proximal tubules of the kidney has been also demonstrated [101]. Thus, treatment with SGLT2 results in sustained systolic and diastolic reduction through natriuresis and sympathoinhibition, without clinically relevant changes in heart rate [102, 103]. All these beneficial effects appear increased in heart failure patients that are characterized by an increased adrenergic tone and a marked impairment in baroreflex sensitivity, contributing to the reduction in hospitalization, favoring cardioprotection and reducing outcomes [104–107].

10.8 Conclusions

Hyperinsulinemia appears to be an important early factor capable of explaining the activation of the adrenergic tone in T2DM. Nonpharmacologic and pharmacologic approaches, in particular SGLT2 inhibitors, contribute, other than lowering hyperglycemia and plasma insulin levels, to a reduction in sympathetic nervous system and a better control of blood pressure and weight, a reduction in the risk of patients with advanced renal disease, and a reduction in hospitalization and outcome of heart failure patients.

References

1. Wild S, Roglic G, Green A, Sicree R, King H. Global prevalence of diabetes: estimates for the year 2000 and projections for 2030. Diabetes Care. 2004;27:1047–53.
2. Guariguata L, Whiting D, Weil C, Unwin N. The International Diabetes Federation diabetes atlas methodology for estimating global and national prevalence of diabetes in adults. Diabetes Res Clin Pract. 2011;94:322–32.
3. Da Rocha FJ, Ogurtsova K, Linnekamp U, Guariguata L, Seuring T, Zhang P, et al. IDF diabetes atlas estimates of 2014 global health expenditures on diabetes. Diabetes Res Clin Pract. 2016;117:48–54.
4. Ogurtsova K, da Rocha FJ, Huang Y, Linnekamp U, Guariguata L, Cho NH, et al. IDF diabetes atlas: global estimates for the prevalence of diabetes for 2015 and 2040. Diabetes Res Clin Prac. 2017;128:40–50.
5. World Health Organization. Global report on diabetes. Geneva, Switzerland; 2016.
6. Entmacher PS, Marks HH. Diabetes in 1964; a world survey. Diabetes. 1965;14:212–23.
7. International Diabetes Federation. IDF Diabetes Atlas. 1st ed. Brussels, Belgium: International Diabetes Federation; 2000.
8. International Diabetes Federation. IDF Diabetes Atlas. 6th ed. Brussels, Belgium: International Diabetes Federation; 2013.
9. International Diabetes Federation. IDF Diabetes Atlas. 9th ed. Brussels, Belgium: International Diabetes Federation; 2019.
10. Degli Esposti L, Saragoni S, Buda S, Sturani A, Degli EE. Glycemic control and diabetes-related health care costs in type 2 diabetes; retrospective analysis based on clinical and administrative databases. Clin Outcomes Res CEOR. 2013;5:193–201.
11. Diabetes UK. The cost of diabetes. London, United Kingdom: Diabetes UK; 2014.
12. Task Force on Diabetes and Cardiovascular Diseases of the European Society of Cardiology (ESC) and European Association for the Study on Diabetes (EASD). Guidelines on diabetes, pre-diabetes, and cardiovascular diseases: executive summary. Eur Heart J. 2007;28:88–136.
13. Skyler JS, Bergenstal R, Bonow RO, Buse J, Deedwania P, Gale EAM, et al. Intensive glycemic control and the prevention of cardiovascular events: implications of the ACCORD, ADVANCE, and VA diabetes trials: a position statement of the American Diabetes Association and a Scientific Statement of the American College of Cardiology Foundation and the American Heart Association. Circulation. 2009;119:351–7.
14. American Diabetes Association. Standards of medical care in diabetes--2011. Diabetes Care. 2011;34(Suppl 1):S11–61.
15. Williams B, Mancia G, Spiering W, Agabiti Rosei E, Azizi M, Burnier M, et al. 2018 ESC/ESH guidelines for the management of arterial hypertension. J Hypertens. 2018;36:1953–2041.
16. McCormack T, Boffa RJ, Jones NR, Carville S, McManus RJ. The 2018 ESC/ESH hypertension guidelines and the 2019 NICE hypertension guideline, how and why they differ. Eur Heart J. 2019;40:3456–8.

17. Chatterjee S, Khunti K, Davies MJ. Type 2 diabetes. Lancet. 2017;389:2239–51.
18. Roden M, Shulman GI. The integrative biology of type 2 diabetes. Nature. 2019;576:51–60.
19. Cerf ME. Beta cell dysfunction and insulin resistance. Front Endocrinol (Lausanne). 2013;4:37.
20. Zheng Y, Ley SH, Hu FB. Global etiology and epidemiology of type 2 diabetes mellitus and its complications. Nat Rev Endocrinol. 2018;14:88–98.
21. Halban PA, Polonsky KS, Bowden DW, Hawkins MA, Ling C, Mather KJ, et al. Beta cells failure in type 2 diabetes: postulated mechanisms and prospects for prevention and treatment. Diabetes Care. 2014;37:1751–8.
22. Christensen AA, Gannon M. The beta cell in type 2 diabetes. Curr Diabetes Rep. 2019;19:81.
23. Yamamoto WR, Bone RN, Sohn P, Syed F, Reissaus CA, Mosley AL, et al. Endoplasmatic reticulum stress alters ryanodine receptor function in the murine pancreatic beta cell. J Biol Chem. 2019;294:168–81.
24. Bertacca A, Ciccarone A, Cecchetti P, Vianello B, Laurenza I, Maffei M, et al. Continually high insulin levels impair Akt phosphorylation and glucose transport in human bioblasts. Metabolism. 2005;54:1687–93.
25. Catalano KJ, Maddux BA, Szary J, Youngren JF, Goldfine ID, Schaufele F. Insulin resistance induced by hyperinsulinemia coincides with a persistent alteration at the insulin receptor tyrosine kinase domain. PLoS One. 2014;9:e108693.
26. Hoehn KL, Salmon AB, Hohnen-Behrens C, Turner N, Hoy AJ, Maghzal GJ, et al. Insulin resistance is a cellular antioxidant defense mechanism. Proc Natl Acad Sci USA. 2009;106:17787–92.
27. Nolan CJ, Ruderman NB, Kahn SE, Pedersen O, Prentki M. Insulin resistance as a physiological defense against metabolic stress: implications for the management of subsets of type 2 diabetes. Diabetes. 2015;64:673–86.
28. Braccini L, Ciraolo L, Campa CC, Perino A, Dl L, Tibolla G, et al. PI3K-C2y is a Rab5 effector selectively controlling endosomal Akt2 activation downstream of insulin signalling. Nat Commun. 2015;6:7400.
29. Saxton RA, Sabatini DM. mTOR signaling in growth, metabolism, and disease. Cell. 2017;168:960–76.
30. Boden G, Cheung P, Kresge K, Homko C, Powers B, Ferrer L. Insulin resistance is associated with diminished endoplasmic reticulum stress responses in adipose tissue of healthy and diabetic subjects. Diabetes. 2014;63:2977–83.
31. Tan Y, Ichikawa T, Li J, Si Q, Yang H, Chen X, et al. Diabetic downregulation of Nrf2 activity via ERK contributes to oxidative stress-induced insulin resistance in cardiac cells in vitro and in vivo. Diabetes. 2011;60:625–33.
32. Bucris E, Beck A, Boura-Halfon S, Isaac R, Vinik Y, Rosenzweig T, et al. Prolonged insulin treatment sensitizes apoptosis pathways in pancreatic beta cells. J Endocrinol. 2016;230:291–307.
33. Corkey BE. Banting lecture 2011. Hyperinsulinemia: cause or consequence. Diabetes. 2012(61):4–13.
34. Czech MP. Insulin action and resistance in obesity and type 2 diabetes. Nat Med. 2017;23:804–14.
35. Reed MA, Pories WJ, Chapman W, Pender J, Bowden R, Bakarat H, et al. Roux-en-Y gastric bypass corrects hyperinsulinemia implications for the remission of type 2 diabetes. J Clin Endocrinol Metab. 2011;96:2525–31.
36. Seravalle G, Colombo M, Perego P, Giardini V, Volpe M, Dell'Oro R, et al. Long-term sympathoinhibitory effects of surgically induced weight loss in severe obese patients. Hypertension. 2014;64:431–7.
37. Purnell JQ, Johnson GS, Wahed AS, Dalla MC, Piccinini F, Cobelli C, et al. Prospective evaluation of insulin and incretin dynamics in obese adults with and without diabetes for 2 years after Roux-en-Y gastric bypass. Diabetologia. 2018;61:1142–54.
38. Thomas DD, Corkey BE, Istfan NW, Apovian CM. Hyperinsulinemia: an early indicator of metabolic dysfunction. J Endocr Soc. 2019;3:1727–47.

39. Aasen G, Fagertun H, Halse J. Effect of loss of regional fat assessed by DXA on insulin resistance and dyslipidemia in obese men. Scand J Clin Lab Invest. 2010;70:547–53.
40. Grassi G, Seravalle G, Colombo M, Bolla G, Cattaneo BM, Cavagnini F, et al. Body weight reduction, sympathetic nerve traffic, and arterial baroreflex in obese normotensive humans. Circulation. 1998;97:2037–42.
41. Perseghin G, Price TB, Petersen KF, Roden M, Cline GW, Gerow K, et al. Increased glucose transport-phosphorylation and muscle glycogen synthesis after exercise training in insulin-resistant subjects. N Engl J Med. 1996;335:1357–62.
42. Rabol R, Petersen KF, Dufour S, Flannery C, Shulman GI. Reversal of muscle insulin resistance with exercise reduces postprandial hepatic de novo lipogenesis in insulin resistant individuals. Proc Natl Acad Sci USA. 2011;108:13705–9.
43. Karauti MA, Freitas-Dias R, Ferreira SM, Vettorazzi JF, Nardelli TR, Araujo HN, et al. Acute exercise improves insulin clearance and increases the expression of insulin-degrading enzyme in the liver and skeletal muscle of Swiss mice. PLoS One. 2016;11:e0160239.
44. Greenwood RH, Mahler RF, Hales CN. Improvement in insulin secretion in diabetes after diazoxide. Lancet. 1976;1:444–7.
45. Alemzadeh R, Langley G, Upchurch L, Smith P, Slonim AE. Beneficial effect of diazoxide in obese hyperinsulinemic adults. J Clin Endocrinol Metab. 1998;83:1911–5.
46. American Diabetes Association. Pharmacologic approaches to glycemic treatment. Diabetes Care. 2017;40(Suppl 1):S64–74.
47. Bastin M, Andreelli F. Dual GIP-GLP1R agonists in the treatment of type 2 diabetes: a short review on emerging data and therapeutic potential. Diabetes Metab Syndr Obesity Targets Ther. 2019;12:1973–85.
48. O'Dea K, Esler M, Leonard P, Stockigt JR, Nestel P. Noradrenaline turnover during undereating and overeating in normal weight subjects. Metabolism. 1982;896-99
49. Welle S, Lilavivathana U, Campbell RG. Increased plasma norepinephrine concentrations and metabolic rates following glucose ingestion in man. Metabolism. 1980;29:806–9.
50. Berne C, Fagius J, Niklasson F. Sympathetic response to oral carbohydrate administration: evidence from microelectrode nerve recordings. J Clin Invest. 1989;84:1403–9.
51. Rowe JW, Young JB, Minaker KL, Stevens AL, Pallotta J, Landsberg L. Effect of insulin and glucose infusions on sympathetic nervous system activity in normal man. Diabetes. 1981;30:219–25.
52. Anderson EA, Hoffman RP, Balon TW, Sinkey CA, Mark AL. Hyperinsulinemia produces both sympathetic neural activation and vasodilation in normal humans. J Clin Invest. 1991;87:2246–52.
53. Bazelmans J, Nestel PJ, O'Dea K, Esler MD. Blunted norepinephrine responsiveness to changing energy states in obese subjects. Metabolism. 1985;34:154–60.
54. Astrup A, Andersen T, Christensen NJ, Bulow J, Madsen J, Breum L, et al. Impaired glucose-induced thermogenesis and arterial norepinephrine response persist after weight reduction in obese humans. J Clin Nutr. 1990;51:331–7.
55. Laakso M, Edelman SV, Brechtel G, Baron AD. Decreased effect of insulin to stimulate skeletal muscle blood flow in obese man: a novel mechanism for insulin resistance. J Clin Invest. 1991;87:2246–52.
56. Landsberg L. Diet, obesity and hypertension: an hypothesis involving insulin, the sympathetic nervous system, and adaptive thermogenesis. Q J Med. 1986;236:1081–90.
57. Ravussin E, Swinbum BA. Energy metabolism. In: Stunkard AJ, Wadden TA, editors. Obesity: theory and therapy. 2nd ed. Raven: New York; 1993. p. 97–123.
58. Landsberg L. Insulin-mediated sympathetic stimulation: role in the pathogenesis of obesity-related hypertension (or, how insulin affects blood pressure, and why). J Hypertens. 2001;19:523–8.
59. Sartori C, Scherrer U. Insulin, nitric oxide and the sympathetic nervous system: at the crossroads of metabolic and cardiovascular regulation. J Hypertens. 1999;17:1517–25.
60. Grassi G, Seravalle G, Dell'Oro R, Turri C, Pasqualinotto L, Colombo M, et al. Participation of the hypothalamus-hypophysis axis in the sympathetic activation of human obesity. Hypertension. 2001;38:1316–20.

61. Mark AL, Anderson EA. Genetic factors determine the blood pressure response to insulin resistance and hyperinsulinemia: a call to refocus the insulin hypothesis of hypertension. Proc Soc Exp Biol Med. 1995;208:330–6.
62. Hausberg M, Hoffman RP, Somers VK, Sinkey CA, Mark AL, Anderson EA. Contrasting autonomic and hemodynamic effects of insulin in healthy versus young subjects. Hypertension. 1997;29:700–5.
63. Seravalle G, Lonati L, Buzzi S, Cairo M, Quarti Trevano F, Dell'Oro R, et al. Sympathetic nerve traffic and baroreflex function in optimal, normal, and high-normal blood pressure states. J Hypertens. 2015;33:1411–7.
64. Grassi G, Quarti Trevano F, Seravalle G, Arenare F, Volpe M, Furiani S, et al. Early sympathetic activation in the initial stages of chronic renal failure. Hypertension. 2011;57:846–51.
65. Dell'Oro R, Quarti Trevano F, Gamba P, Ciuffarella C, Seravalle G, Mancia G, et al. Sympathetic and baroreflex abnormalities in the uncomplicated prediabetic state. J Hypertens. 2018;36:1195–200.
66. Boden G, Chen X, Ruiz J, White JV, Rossetti L. Mechanisms of fatty acid-induced inhibition of glucose uptake. J Clin Invest. 1994;93:2438–46.
67. Florian JP, Pawelczyk JA. Non-esterified fatty acids increase arterial pressure via central sympathetic activation in humans. Clin Sci. 2009;118:61–9.
68. Huggett RJ, Scott EM, Gilbey SG, Stoker JB, Mackintosh AF, Mary DASG. Impact of type 2 diabetes mellitus on sympathetic neural mechanisms in hypertension. Circulation. 2003;108:3097–101.
69. Curry TB, Hines CN, Barnes JN, Somaraju M, Basu R, Miles JM, et al. Relationship of muscle sympathetic nerve activity to insulin sensitivity. Clin Auton Res. 2014;24:77–85.
70. Grassi G, Biffi A, Seravalle G, Quarti Trevano F, Dell'oro R, Corrao G, et al. Sympathetic neural overdrive in the obese and overweight state: meta-analysis of published studies. Hypertension. 2019;74:349–58.
71. Lambert GW, Straznicky NE, Lambert EA, Dixon JB, Schlaich MP. Sympathetic nervous activation in obesity and metabolic syndrome – causes, consequences and therapeutic implications. Pharmacol Ther. 2010;126:159–72.
72. Grassi G, Dell'Oro R, Quarti Trevano F, Scopelliti F, Seravalle G, Paleari F, et al. Neuroadrenergic and reflex abnormalities in patients with metabolic syndrome. Diabetologia. 2005;48:1359–65.
73. Thorp AA, Schlaich MP. Relevance of sympathetic nervous system activation in obesity and metabolic syndrome. J Diabetes Res. 2015;2015:341583.
74. Esler M, Rumantir M, Wiesner G, Kaye D, Hastings J, Lambert G. Sympathetic nervous system and insulin resistance: from obesity to diabetes. Am J Hypertens. 2001;14:304S–9.
75. Sharma AM, Engeli S, Pischon T. New developments in mechanisms of obesity-induced hypertension. Curr Hypertens Rep. 2001;3:152–6.
76. Festa A, D'Agostino R Jr, Howard G, Mykkanen L, Tracy RP, Haffner SM. Chronic subclinical inflammation as part of the insulin resistance syndrome: the Insulin Resistance Atherosclerosis Study (IRAS). Circulation. 2000;102:42–7.
77. Christensen NJ. Catecholamines and diabetes mellitus. Diabetologia. 1979;16:211–24.
78. Frattola A, Parati A, Gamba P, Paleari F, Mauri G, Di Rienzo M, et al. Time and frequency domain estimates of spontaneous baroreflex sensitivity provide early detection of autonomic dysfunction in diabetes mellitus. Diabetologia. 1997;40:1470–5.
79. Sucharita S, Bantwal G, Idiculla J, Ayyar V, Vaz M. Autonomic nervous system function in type 2 diabetes using conventional clinical autonomic tests, heart rate and blood pressure variability measures. Indian J Endocrinol Metab. 2011;15:198–203.
80. Ziegler D, Strom A, Bonhof G, Puttgen S, Bodis M, Buckart V, et al. GDS Group. Differential associations of lower cardiac vagal tone with insulin resistance and insulin secretion in recently diagnosed type 1 and type 2 diabetes. Metabolism. 2018;79:1–9.
81. Malpas SC. Sympathetic nervous system overactivity and its role in the development of cardiovascular disease. Physiol Rev. 2010;90:513–57.

82. Miki K, Yoshomoto M. Sympathetic nerve activity during sleep, exercise, and mental stress. Auton Neurosci. 2013;174:15–20.
83. Yeboah J, Bertoni AG, Herrington DM, Post WS, Burke GL. Impaired fasting glucose and the risk of incident diabetes mellitus and cardiovascular events in an adult population: MESA (Multi-Ethnic Study of Atherosclerosis). J Am Coll Cardiol. 2011;58:140–6.
84. Anand SS, Dagenais GR, Mohan V, Diaz R, Probsfield J, Freeman R, et al. Glucose levels are associated with cardiovascular disease and death in an international cohort of normal glycaemic and dysglycaemic men and women: the EpiDREAM cohort study. Eur J Prev Cardiol. 2012;19:755–64.
85. Huang Y, Cai X, Mai W, Li M, Hu Y. Association between prediabetes and risk of cardiovascular disease and all-cause mortality: systematic review and meta-analysis. BMJ. 2016;355:i5953.
86. Straznicky NE, Grima AT, Sari CI, Eikelis N, Lambert EA, Nestel PJ, et al. Neuroadrenergic dysfunction along the diabetes continuum: a comparative study in obese metabolic syndrome subjects. Diabetes. 2012;61:2506–16.
87. Grassi G, Biffi A, Dell'Oro R, Quarti Trevano F, Seravalle G, Corrao G, et al. Sympathetic neural abnormalities in type 1 and type 2 diabetes: a systematic review and meta-analysis. J Hypertens. 2020;38:1436–42.
88. Jamerson KA, Julius S, Gudbrandsson T, Andersson O, Brand DO. Reflex sympathetic activation induces insulin resistance in the human forearm. Hypertension. 1993;21:618–23.
89. Scherrer U, Sartori C. Insulin is a vascular and sympathoexcitatory hormone: implications for blood pressure regulation, insulin sensitivity, and cardiovascular morbidity. Circulation. 1997;96:4104–13.
90. Wu JS, Lu FH, Yang YC, Chang SH, Huang YH, Jason Chen JJ, et al. Impaired baroreflex sensitivity in subjects with impaired glucose tolerance, but not isolated impaired fasting glucose. Acta Diabetol. 2014;51:535–41.
91. Zimmerman BG, Sybertz EJ, Wong PC. Interactions between sympathetic and renin-angiotensin system. J Hypertens. 1984;2:581–7.
92. Haynes WG, Sivitz WI, Morgan DA, Walsh SA, Mark AL. Sympathetic and cardiorenal action of leptin. Hypertension. 1997;30:619–23.
93. Lambert E, Lambert G, Ika-Sari C, Dawood T, Lee K, Chopra R, et al. Ghrelin modulates sympathetic nervous system and stress response in lean and overweight men. Hypertension. 2011;58:43–50.
94. Scheen AJ. Pharmacodynamics, efficacy and safety of sodium-glucose co-transporter type 2 (SGLT2) inhibitors for the treatment of type 2 diabetes mellitus. Drugs. 2015;75:33–59.
95. Mazidi M, Rezaie P, Gao HK, Kengne AP. Effect of sodium-glucose cotransport-2 inhibitors on blood pressure in people with type 2 diabetes mellitus: a systematic review and meta-analysis of 43 randomized control trials with 22528 patients. J Am Heart Assoc. 2017;6:e004007.
96. Baker WL, Buckley LF, Kelly MS, Bucheit JD, Pard ED, Brown R, et al. Effects of sodium-glucose cotransporter 2 inhibitors on 24-hour ambulatory blood pressure: a systematic review and meta-analysis. J Am Heart Assoc. 2017;6:e005686.
97. Sheen AJ, Delanaye P. Effects of reducing blood pressure on renal outcomes in patients with type 2 diabetes: focus on SGLT2 inhibitors and EMPA-REG OUTCOME. Diabetes Metab. 2017;43:99–109.
98. Neal B, Perkovic V, Mahaffey KW, de Zeeuw D, Fulcher G, Erondu N, et al. Canaglifozin and cardiovascular and renal events in type 2 diabetes. N Engl J Med. 2017;377:644–57.
99. Zelniker TA, Wiviott SD, Raz I, Im K, Goodrich EL, Bonaca MP, et al. SGLT2 inhibitors for primary and secondary prevention of cardiovascular and renal outcomes in type 2 diabetes: a systematic review and meta-analysis of cardiovascular outcome trials. Lancet. 2019;393:31–9.
100. Zannad F, Ferreira JP, Pocock SJ, Anker SD, Butler J, Filippatos G, et al. SGLT2 inhibitors in patients with heart failure with reduced ejection fraction: a meta-analysis of the EMPEROR-Reduced and DAPA-HF trials. Lancet. 2020;396:819–29.

101. Matthews VB, Elliot RH, Rudnicka C, Hricova J, Heart L, Schlaich MP. Role of the sympathetic nervous system in regulation of the sodium glucose cotransporter 2. J Hypertens. 2017;35:2059–68.
102. Briasoulis A, Al Dhaybi O, Bakris GL. SGLT2 inhibitors and mechanisms of hypertension. Curr Cardiol Rep. 2018;20:1.
103. Jordan J, Tank J, Heusser K, Heise T, Wanner C, Heer M, et al. The effect of empaglifozin on muscle sympathetic nerve activity in patients with type 2 diabetes mellitus. J Am Soc Hypertens. 2017;11:604–12.
104. Sano M. A new class of drugs for heart failure: SGLT2 inhibitors reduce sympathetic overactivity. J Cardiol. 2018;71:471–6.
105. Kiuchi S, Hisatake S, Kabuki T, Fujii T, Oka T, Dobashi S, et al. Long-term use of ipraglifozin improved cardiac sympathetic nerve activity in a patient with heart failure: a case report. Drug Discover Ther. 2018;12:51–4.
106. Verma S. Are the cardiorenal benefits of SGLT2 inhibitors due to inhibition of the sympathetic nervous system? JACC Basic Transl Sci. 2020;5:180–2.
107. Cowie MR, Fisher M. SGLT2 inhibitors: mechanisms of cardiovascular benefit beyond glycaemic control. Nature Rev Cardiol. 2020;17:2108–17.

Diabetes and Microcirculation

11

Damiano Rizzoni, Claudia Agabiti-Rosei,
Carolina De Ciuceis, and Enrico Agabiti Rosei

11.1 Introduction

Type 2 (T2DM) and type 1 diabetes mellitus (T1DM) are characterized by alterations of the microcirculation which are largely responsible for fatal and nonfatal cardiovascular and renal complications, affecting all vascular beds, particularly the renal and retinal, but also the coronary and cerebral districts, among others [1–3]. Dysfunction and damage of the microcirculation are hallmarks of the disease, and in fact the diagnosis of diabetes is defined by the level of hyperglycemia which causes microvascular complications [1–3]. Alterations of the microcirculation in diabetes involve all vessels with an internal diameter below about 350 micron and therefore include small resistance arteries, arterioles, capillaries, and postcapillary venules [1–5]. In this review we shall discuss (a) the mechanisms and characteristics of dysfunction and damage of microcirculation in diabetes, (b) the relation of microcirculation with organ damage and cardiovascular events, and (c) the effects of treatment.

11.2 Mechanisms of Microvascular Alterations in Diabetes

Diabetes is frequently associated to hypertension which is a very important hemodynamic and possibly neurohumoral cause of functional and structural alterations of microcirculation. However, several additional mechanisms may have a specific role in the development of microvascular dysfunction and damage in diabetes, including

The original version of the book has been revised. A correction to this book can be found at https://doi.org/10.1007/978-3-031-13009-0_30

D. Rizzoni · C. Agabiti-Rosei · C. De Ciuceis · E. Agabiti Rosei (✉)
Department of Clinical and Experimental Sciences, University of Brescia, Brescia, Italy
e-mail: enrico.agabitirosei@unibs.it

A. E. Berbari, G. Mancia (eds.), *Blood Pressure Disorders in Diabetes Mellitus*, Updates in Hypertension and Cardiovascular Protection,
https://doi.org/10.1007/978-3-031-13009-0_11

the following: (a) formation of reactive oxygen species (hydrogen peroxide, superoxide); (b) metabolic effects such as activation of polyol pathway, with consequent production of sorbitol and fructose which are unable to diffuse outside cells, thus inducing osmotic endothelial cell injury and protein kinase C activation; (c) glycosylation of proteins, including hemoglobin, with reduction of its affinity to oxygen and thus induction of micro-ischemia and endothelial damage; (d) glycosylation of collagen fibers with alterations of extracellular matrix, production of advanced glycosylation end products (AGE), involved in vascular damage (stimulation of cytokines, complement activation, upregulation of growth factor synthesis, induction of collagen cross-links), and depletion of basement membrane glycosaminoglycans; and (e) direct effect of growth factors, such as insulin or insulin-like growth factor-1 on vascular smooth muscle cells [1–5].

11.3 Endothelial Dysfunction

Endothelial cells are known to have important regulatory effects on the cardiovascular system through the release of vasodilator and vasoconstrictor factors. In addition, platelet aggregation as well as leukocyte extravasation through endothelium may be influenced by locally produced compounds. Therefore, endothelial dysfunction and damage may contribute to the inflammatory and thrombotic vascular lesions. An impairment of the endothelial function, as evaluated by the vasodilator response to acetylcholine, has been detected in human large and small arteries of patients with T1DM [6–10] as well as of those with T2DM [11–15]. We and others have previously demonstrated the presence of an impaired dilatation to acetylcholine and bradykinin in subcutaneous small resistance arteries of hypertensive and normotensive patients with T2DM [11, 12, 15].

In essential hypertensive patients, the relatively small vasodilator responses to acetylcholine and bradykinin infused into the brachial artery are not usually blocked by inhibitors of nitric oxide synthase (i.e., L-NMMA), while in normotensive subjects the inhibitory effect of L-NMMA is preserved. In subcutaneous small arteries of patients with essential hypertension, and also in those with T2DM, inhibitors of nitric oxide synthase are able to block about 50% of the vasodilator effect of acetylcholine or bradykinin, while the remaining vasodilatation is blocked by ouabain, thus suggesting that production of both nitric oxide and endothelium-derived hyperpolarizing factor may be involved. No effect has been observed when indomethacin was added to the organ bath; therefore, the production of cyclooxygenase-dependent substances seems to be of minor importance [11, 15].

It has been also proposed that insulin and insulin resistance may be involved in the genesis of endothelial and, in general, microvascular dysfunction in diabetes mellitus. Insulin is able to induce a vasodilating effect in the microcirculation (which is, at least in part, endothelium-dependent) in normal subjects [16, 17]. In addition, insulin may recruit skeletal muscle capillaries in vivo by a nitric oxide-dependent action, and this increased capillary recruitment may contribute to the subsequent glucose uptake [18]. However, part of these effects is lost in diabetes mellitus [16]. Hyperinsulinemia, as a result of insulin resistance, may have detrimental effects on microvascular function also in the prediabetic state [19]. On the other hand microvascular structural alterations may contribute to an impaired delivery of insulin to skeletal muscles. Endothelial dysfunction in microvasculature of T2DM may be related to increased permeability to large molecules, such as albumin [20]. Therefore, a complex interplay of structural and functional alterations of the microcirculation may, at least in part, explain the detrimental consequences of diabetes mellitus in terms of organ perfusion [21] and, ultimately, in terms of increased incidence of cardiovascular events.

11.4 Structural Alterations

11.4.1 Small Resistance Arteries

While there is a huge number of data about microangiopathy (capillary and arterioles), relatively few data about morphology of small resistance arteries (diameter ranging from 100 to 350 micron) in diabetes mellitus are presently available. In one study [6], no difference in subcutaneous small resistance arteries structure was observed between control subjects and patients with T1DM. On the contrary, it has been demonstrated that, in both hypertensive and normotensive patients with T2DM, marked alterations in small artery structure are present [11] and that these alterations are more pronounced in hypertensive patients with T2DM than in patients with essential hypertension or in normotensive diabetics (Fig. 11.1) [11]. In addition, in diabetic patients a clear increase in the media cross-sectional area of the vessels was observed, thus suggesting the presence of hypertrophic remodeling (vascular smooth muscle cell hypertrophy or hyperplasia) [11, 12] (Fig. 11.2). An increase of wall thickness and cross-sectional area has been also observed in retinal arterioles of hypertensive diabetic patients with a duration of diabetes longer than 6 months. This was not the case of patients with essential hypertension. A weak, but significant correlation between circulating levels of insulin and media-to-lumen ratio of subcutaneous small arteries was observed in diabetic patients, thus suggesting a possible role of insulin or insulin-like growth factor-1 in the genesis of hypertrophic remodeling in these patients [11]. However, an alternative explanation for the presence of hypertrophic remodeling in these vessels has been proposed [7]. In fact, a possible stimulus for hypertrophic remodeling could be the increased wall stress, as a consequence of the impaired myogenic response. Myogenic response is a pressure-induced vasoconstriction, which is the key component of blood flow autoregulation and stabilization of capillary pressure. The observation by Schofield et al. [12] of the lack of such a myogenic response in diabetic patients may therefore suggest a causal mechanism for the development of hypertrophic remodeling of small arteries. Diabetic patients with T2DM also show particularly evident alterations of the vascular extracellular matrix, as suggested by the observation of increased collagen to elastin ratio in their small arteries [11] (Fig. 11.1).

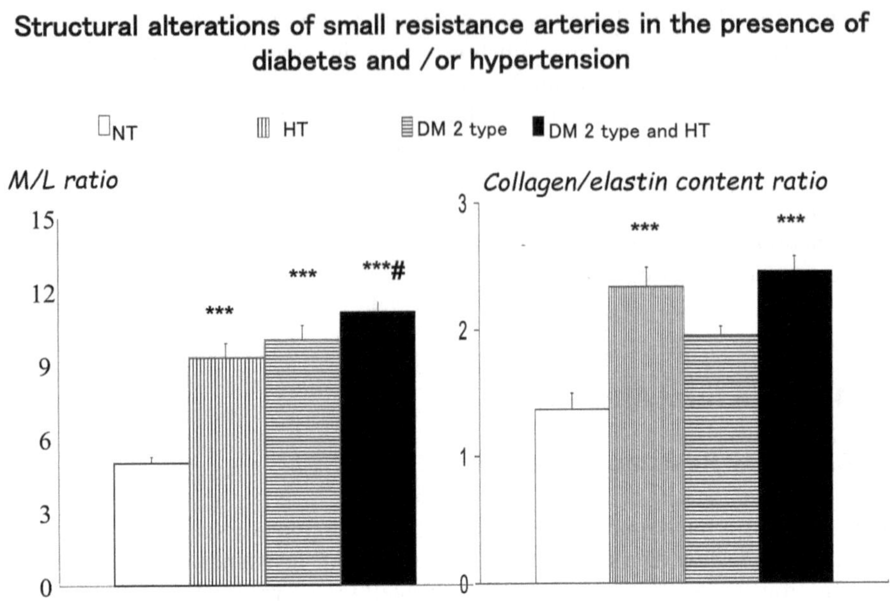

Fig. 11.1 Left: Media to lumen ratio in subcutaneous small resistance arteries from normotensive subjects (NT), essential hypertensive patients (HT), normotensive patients with non-insulin-dependent diabetes mellitus (NIDDM) (DM 2 type), and hypertensive patients with NIDDM (DM 2 type and HT). A clear increase may be observed in all the three pathologic groups, which is more evident in hypertensive patients with NIDDM. Right: collagen to elastin ratio (measured with electronic microscopy in the different groups. An increase was observed in essential hypertensive patients and in hypertensive patients with NIDDM. ***=$p < 0.001$ vs. normotensive subjects; #$p < 0.05$ vs essential hypertensive patients. Mean ± SEM (from reference 1, data from reference 11)

11.4.2 Capillaries

While small resistance arteries may undergo a remodeling process and fibrosis in pathological conditions, capillaries may undergo a functional or structural rarefaction. In fact, microvascular rarefaction can be due to a reduced number of perfused vessels (functional rarefaction) or to a reduced number of vessels in the tissue (structural rarefaction) [22]. Structural loss of vessels may follow progressive non-perfusion. In patients with hypertension and T2DM, rarefaction has been frequently reported in the myocardial and skeletal muscle microcirculatory bed [23].

On the contrary, in other vascular districts such as the retina, microvascular proliferation may be observed. In fact, diabetic retinopathy results either from capillary leakage or from new vessel formation (neovascularization, angiogenesis), caused by capillary closure and retinal ischemia. The capillaries leak lipid products and fluid in the area around the fovea and thicken the retina, which may lead to macular edema. Angiogenesis is the result of retinal ischemia, and retinal hemorrhages are the consequence of the fragility of neovessels. The hemorrhage can enter the

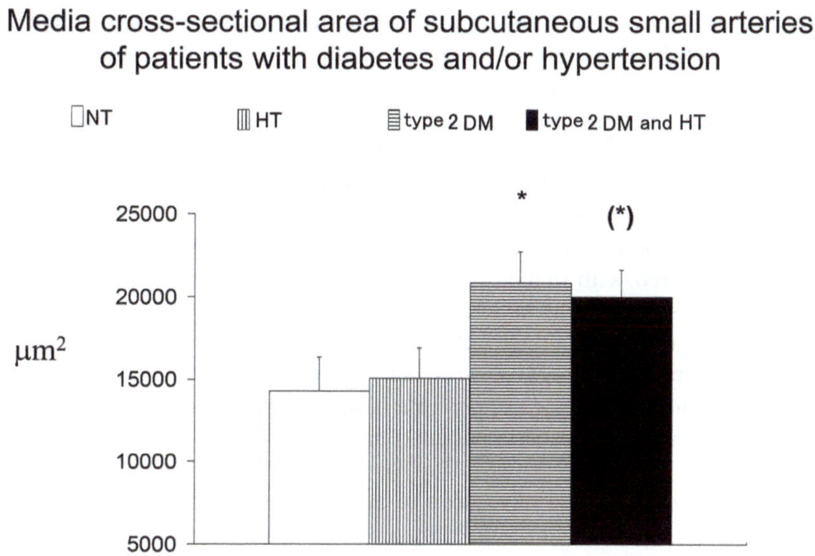

Fig. 11.2 Media cross-sectional area in subcutaneous small resistance arteries from normotensive subjects (NT), essential hypertensive patients (HT), normotensive patients with non-insulin-dependent diabetes mellitus (NIDDM) (DM 2 type), and hypertensive patients with NIDDM (DM 2 type and HT). An increase may be observed in the diabetic patients, which is more evident in normotensive patients with NIDDM. (*)$p = 0.06$, *$p < 0.05$ vs. normotensives. Mean ± SEM (from reference [1], data from reference [11])

vitreous and cause sudden loss of vision. Several mechanisms and metabolic abnormalities, acting alone or in concert with each other, may lead to capillary death, leakage, and occlusion and to the release of growth factors, finally resulting in new vessel formation and increase in vascular permeability. A relevant role is played by vascular endothelial growth factor (VEGF). Whereas VEGF is involved in vascular leakage and angiogenesis, growth hormones and the insulin-like growth factor-1 (IGF-1) may be also involved, as mediators, in angiogenesis. At present, inhibitors of these growth factors are under investigation in clinical trials in patients with diabetic retinopathy.

11.5 Vascular Structural Alterations, End-Organ Damage, and Cardiovascular Events

As previously mentioned, the extent of structural alterations in small resistance vessels is more pronounced in patients with both diabetes mellitus and hypertension, thus suggesting that clustering of risk factors may have synergistic deleterious effects on the vasculature [11, 12]. An important pathophysiological and clinical consequence of the presence of structural alterations in small resistance arteries and arterioles may be the impairment of vasodilator reserve [24]. In fact, remodeling of small resistance arteries is characterized by a narrowing of the lumen, which leads to an increase of flow resistance even at full dilatation, i.e., in the absence of vascular tone. A significant correlation between coronary flow reserve and subcutaneous small resistance artery remodeling has been observed in essential hypertensive patients, suggesting that structural alterations in small resistance arteries may be present at the same time in different vascular districts, including those of paramount clinical importance, such as the coronary circulation [25]. An impaired microvascular hyperemic response (which may reflect an altered flow reserve) has been observed in children with diabetes mellitus [26] as well as in adult patients with T2DM [27]. Thus, alterations in the microcirculation may play an important role in the development of organ damage not only in hypertension but also in diabetes mellitus. In fact, a relevant prognostic role of an increased media to lumen ratio of subcutaneous small resistance arteries in a high-risk population (including normotensive and hypertensive diabetic patients) has been previously demonstrated [28] (Fig. 11.3).

More recently, these data have been re-evaluated, taking into account also the characteristics of the vascular remodeling, i.e., eutrophic vs. hypertrophic remodeling. For the same values of internal diameter, those subjects who suffered cardiovascular events had a greater media cross-sectional area, in comparison with those without cardiovascular events [29]. Therefore, it seems that, for the same size of the vessels explored, a more consistent cell growth (hypertrophic remodeling, such as that observed in diabetic patients) means an even worse prognosis. It has been also

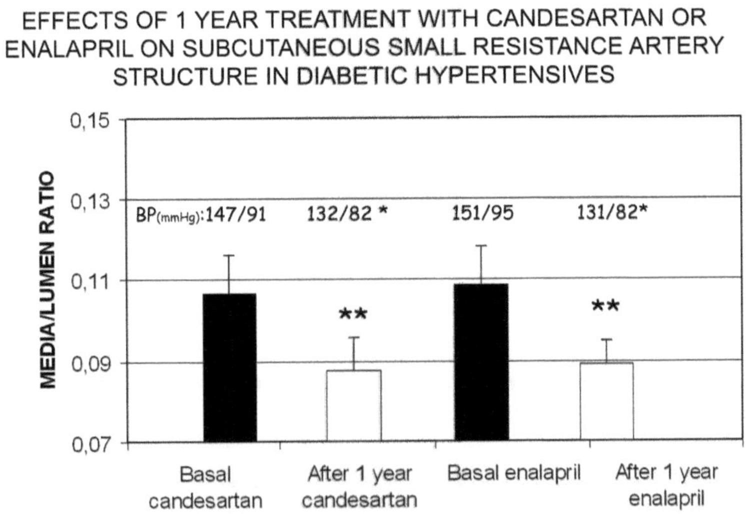

Fig. 11.3 Media to lumen ratio in subcutaneous small resistance arteries from hypertensive patients with non-insulin-dependent diabetes mellitus (NIDDM), before and after 1-year treatment with the ACE inhibitor enalapril or the angiotensin II receptor blocker candesartan. A significant and similar reduction was observed with both drugs. *BP* Blood pressure **=$p < 0.01$ vs. basal (from reference [1], data from [36])

suggested, as previously reported, that an impairment of myogenic response may have a relevant role in the development of hypertrophic remodeling in patients at high cardiovascular risk. In addition, an impaired myogenic response in small vessels may also induce an increase of high blood pressure flow to target organs and a downstream increase in capillary pressure, with consequent increased permeability and capillary leakage. Fluid extravasation may induce organ damage. Some data support the presence of an increased capillary pressure in patients with diabetes mellitus [30], especially if they have increased blood pressure values [31], although at present time there is no general agreement about this issue. The increase in capillary pressure seems to be related to the extent of clinical complications as well as to metabolic control [32]. Also vascular rarefaction may have important consequences in terms of tissue perfusion. In fact, it has been demonstrated that in patients with T2DM, the mechanisms through which insulin is able to increase total limb flow or achieve optimal microvascular perfusion are impaired [33].

11.6 Treatment

11.6.1 Effect of Antihypertensive Drugs

There is relatively few data about the effect of treatment on structural and functional alterations in the microcirculation of patients with diabetes mellitus. In the United Kingdom Prospective Diabetes Study (UKPDS), a large randomized controlled trial that included almost 5000 patients, it has been demonstrated that a tight hemodynamic and metabolic control is associated with a lower incidence of microvascular disease [33] and, in general, of clinical endpoints related to microvascular disease [34].

Even fewer data are presently available about the effects of antihypertensive dugs on small artery structure in hypertensive diabetic patients. Despite effective antihypertensive treatment, resistance arteries from hypertensive diabetic patients showed marked remodeling, greater than that of vessels from untreated, nondiabetic, hypertensive subjects, in agreement with the high cardiovascular risk of subjects suffering from both diabetes and hypertension [35]. Recently, a study has compared the effects of 1-year treatment with the ACE inhibitor (enalapril) or the angiotensin II receptor blocker (candesartan), on subcutaneous small artery structure in hypertensive patients with T2DM [36]. The two drugs were equally effective in reducing media-to-lumen ratio of small arteries (Fig. 11.4); however, candesartan was more effective than enalapril in normalizing vascular collagen content, probably through a more pronounced stimulation of the local production of metalloproteinase 9 (a collagen-degrading enzyme). At variance to what is observed in the majority of studies in normoglycemic hypertensive patients, media-to-lumen ratio of small arteries in treated diabetic patients did not reach the values observed in normotensive controls, therefore suggesting that a complete regression of vascular hypertrophic remodeling is probably more difficult to obtain [35]. Angiotensin II receptor blockers seem to be effective in diabetic hypertensive patients also when

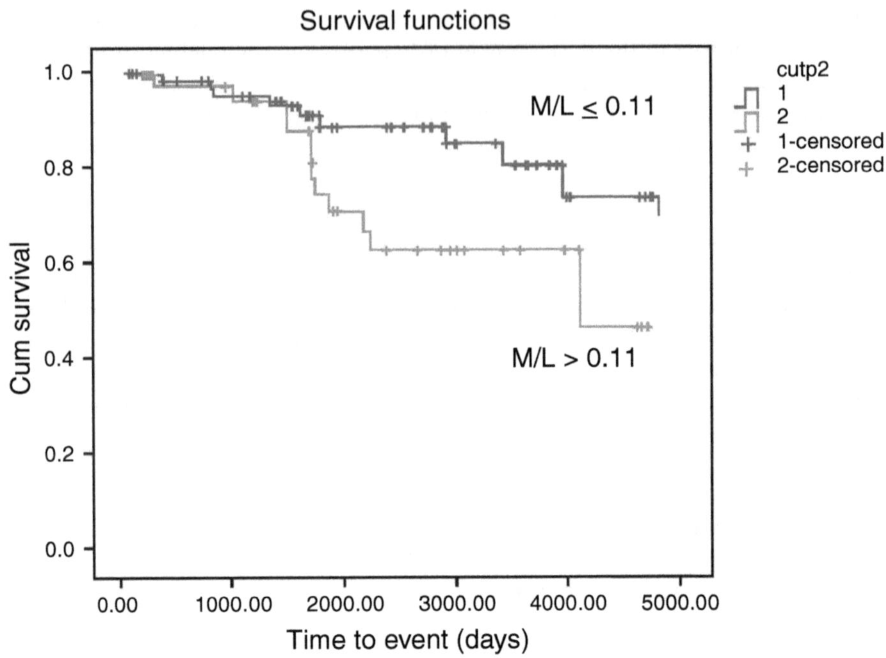

Fig. 11.4 Kaplan–Meier cum survival curves between normotensive and hypertensive diabetic patients with an M/L of subcutaneous small arteries below or above 0.11 (cutp2): log rank (Mantel–Cox test *P*¼0.034, Breslow–Wilcoxon test *P*¼0.057, Tarone–Ware test *P*¼0.041). Reanalysis of data, Cum, cumulative; M/L, media-to-lumen ratio (From Agabiti-Rosei E, Rizzoni D. Microvascular structure as a prognostically relevant endpoint. J Hypertens 2017; 35:914-921)

given on top of an ACE inhibitor treatment [37]. In addition, angiotensin II receptor blockers seem to be also particularly effective in terms of improvement of endothelial function in small resistance arteries [38]. Whether a regression of vascular structural or functional alterations in diabetic patients may be prognostically relevant, i.e., whether it is associated to a real protection from cardiovascular events, is not yet definitely established.

11.6.2 Effect of Antidiabetic Drugs

Experimental studies demonstrate early beneficial effects of DPP-4 inhibitors and GLP-1 agonists on diabetic microvascular complications; however clinical data are insufficient in this respect and need further studies for confirmation [39]. The SGLT-2 inhibitor dapagliflozin in a short-term study reduced retinal capillary flow and stabilized arteriolar structural remodeling [40]; however studies with other SGLT-2 inhibitors have given inconsistent results [39], and therefore additional studies are warranted to explore the effects of these drugs on the microcirculation.

11.7 Conclusions

Alterations in the microcirculation represent a common finding, and microangiopathy is one of the most important mechanisms involved in the development of organ damage as well as of clinical events in patients with diabetes mellitus. Both patients with essential hypertension and those with T2DM are characterized by alterations in the resistance vasculature, i.e., an increased media-to-lumen ratio, that in diabetics is the consequence of the the so-called hypertrophic remodeling. Structural alterations of small arteries are associated with an increased cardiovascular risk in hypertensive and diabetic patients, perhaps as a consequence of an impaired organ flow reserve in several vascular districts, including the coronary vascular bed. In fact, it has been observed that the presence of an increased wall to lumen ratio in the subcutaneous resistance arteries is associated with a worse prognosis in high-risk patients. Hypertrophic remodeling, such as that observed in diabetic patients, seems to be associated with an even worse prognosis. Data about the effect of therapy on microvascular structure in diabetic patients are scarce; however, renin–angiotensin system blockade seems to be effective in regressing, at least in part, the microvascular structure, although we do not know whether this improvement is associated with a better clinical prognosis.

References

1. Agabiti Rosei E, Rizzoni D. Small artery remodelling in diabetes. J Cell Mol Med. 2010;14:1030–6.
2. Rizzoni D, Agabiti-Rosei E. Small artery remodeling in hypertension and diabetes. Curr Hypertens Rep. 2006;8:90–5.
3. Rizzoni D, Agabiti-Rosei E. Small artery remodeling in diabetes mellitus. Nutr Metab Cardiovasc Dis. 2009;19:587–92.
4. De Ciuceis C. Microvascular alterations in diabetes: focus on small resistance arteries. In: Agabiti-Rosei E, Rizzoni D, Heagerty AM, editors. Microcirculation in cardiovascular disease. Springer Nature Switzerland AG; 2020. p. 149–64.
5. Agabiti-Rosei E, Rizzoni D. Hypertension and diabetes: how to predict end-organ damage from subcutaneous microcirculation morphofunctional studies? Microcirculation Cardiovasc Dis. 2009;23:15–23.
6. McNally PG, Watt PAC, Rimmer T, Burden AC, Hearnshaw JR, Thurston H. Impaired contraction and endothelium-dependent relaxation in isolated resistance vessels from patients with insulin-dependent diabetes mellitus. Clin Sci. 1994;87:31–6.
7. Johnstone MT, Creager SJ, Scales KM, Cusco JA, Lee BK, Creager MA. Impaired endothelium-dependent vasodilation in patients with insulin-dependent diabetes mellitus. Circulation. 1994;88:2510–6.
8. Clarkson P, Celermajer DS, Donald AE, Sampson M, Sorensen KE, Adams M, et al. Impaired vascular reactivity in insulin-dependent diabetes mellitus is related to disease duration and low density lipoprotein cholesterol levels. JACC. 1996;28:573–9.
9. Zenere BM, Arcaro G, Saggiani F, Rossi L, Muggeo M, Lechi A. Noninvasive detection of functional alterations of the arterial wall in IDDM patients with and without microalbuminuria. Diabetes Care. 1995;18:975–82.
10. Lambert J, Aarsen M, Donker AJ, Stehouwer CD. Endothelium-dependent and –independent vasodilation of large arteries in normoalbuminuric insulin-dependent diabetes mellitus. Arterioscler Thromb Vasc Biol. 1996;16:705–11.

11. Rizzoni D, Porteri E, Guelfi D, Muiesan ML, Valentini U, Cimino A, et al. Structural alterations in subcutaneous small arteries of normotensive and hypertensive patients with non-insulin-dependent diabetes mellitus. Circulation. 2001;103:1238–44.
12. Schofield I, Malik R, Izzard A, Austin C, Heagerty AM. Vascular structural and functional changes in type 2 diabetes mellitus. Evidence for the role of abnormal myogenic responsiveness and dyslipidemia. Circulation. 2002;106:3037–43.
13. Goodfellow J, Ramsey MW, Luddington LA, Jones CJ, Coates PA, Dunstan F, et al. Endothelium and inelastic arteries: an early marker of vascular dysfunction in non-insulin dependent diabetes. BMJ. 1996;312:744–5.
14. Parving HH, Nielsen FS, Bang LE, Smidt UM, Svedsen TL, Chen JW, et al. Macro-microangiopathy and endothelial dysfunction in NIDDM patients with and without diabetic nephropaty. Diabetologia. 1996;39:1590–7.
15. Rizzoni D, Porteri E, Guelfi D, Muiesan ML, Piccoli A, Valentini U, et al. Endothelial dysfunction in small resistance arteries of patients with non-insulin dependent diabetes mellitus. J Hypertens. 2001;19:913–9.
16. Rossi M, Cupisti A, Ricco R, Santoro G, Pentimone F, Carpi A. Skin vasoreactivity to insulin iontophoresis is reduced in elderly subjects and is absent in treated non-insulin-dependent diabetes patients. Biomed Pharmacother. 2004;58:560–5.
17. Clerk LH, Vincent MA, Lindner JR, Clark MG, Rattigan S, Barrett EJ. The vasodilatory actions of insulin on resistance and terminal arterioles and their impact on muscle glucose uptake. Diabetes Metab Res Rev. 2004;20:3–12.
18. Vincent MA, Clerk LH, Lindner JR, Klibanov AL, Clark MG, Rattigan S, et al. Microvascular recruitment is an early insulin effect that regulates skeletal muscle glucose uptake in vivo. Diabetes. 2004;53:1418–23.
19. Jaap AJ, Shore AC, Tooke JE. Relationship of insulin resistance to microvascular dysfunction in subjects with fasting hyperglycaemia. Diabetologia. 1997;40:238–43.
20. Scalia R, Gong Y, Berzins B. Hyperglycemia is a major determinant of albumin permeability in diabetic microcirculation: the role of mu-calpain. Diabetes. 2007;56:1842–9.
21. Scognamiglio R, Negut C, De Kreutzenberg SV, Tiengo A, Avogaro A. Postprandial myocardial perfusion in healthy subjects and in type 2 diabetic patients. Circulation. 2005;112:179–84.
22. Levy BI, Schiffrin EL, Mourad JJ, Agostini D, Vicaut E, Dafar ME, et al. Impaired tissue perfusion: a pathology common to hypertension, obesity and diabetes mellitus. Circulation. 2008;118:968–76.
23. Clark MG, Barrett EJ, Wallis MG, Vincent MA, Rattigan S. The microvasculature in insulin resistance and type 2 diabetes. Semin Vasc Med. 2002;2:21–31.
24. Folkow B. Physiological aspects of primary hypertension. Physiol Rev. 1982;62:347–504.
25. Rizzoni D, Palombo C, Porteri E, Muiesan ML, Kozàkovà M, La Canna G, et al. Relationships between coronary vasodilator capacity and small artery remodeling in hypertensive patients. J Hypertens. 2003;21:625–32.
26. Shore AC, Price KJ, Sandeman DD, Greeen EM, Tripp JH, Tooke JE. Impaired microvascular hyperaemic response in children with diabetes mellitus. Diabet Med. 1991;8:619–23.
27. Strain WD, Chaturvedi N, Nihoyannopoulos P, Bulpitt CJ, Rajkumar C, Shore AC. Differences in the association between type 2 diabetes and impaired microvascular function among Europeans and African Caribbeans. Diabetologia. 2005;48:2269–77.
28. Rizzoni D, Porteri E, Boari GEM, De Ciuceis C, Sleiman I, Muiesan ML, et al. Prognostic significance of small artery structure in hypertension. Circulation. 2003;108:2230–5.
29. Izzard AS, Rizzoni D, Agabiti-Rosei E, Heagerty AM. Small artery structure and hypertension: adaptive changes and target organ damage. J Hypertens. 2005;23:247–50.
30. Parving HH, Viberti GC, Keen H, Christensen JS, Lassen NA. Hemodynamic factors in the genesis of diabetic microangiopathy. Metabolism. 1883;32:943–9.
31. Fegan PG, Tooke JE, Gooding KM, Tullet JM, MacLeod KM, Shore AC. Capillary pressure in subjects with type 2 diabetes and hypertension and the effect of antihypertensive therapy. Hypertension. 2003;41:1111–7.

32. Sandeman DD, Shore AC, Tooke JE. Relation of skin capillary pressure in patients with insulin-dependent diabetes mellitus to complications and metabolic control. N Engl J Med. 1992;327:760–4.
33. Adler AI, Stratton IM, Neil HA, Yudkin JS, Matthews DR, Cull CA, et al. Association of systolic blood pressure with macrovascular and microvascular complications of type 2 diabetes (UKPDS 36): prospective observational study. BMJ. 2000;321:412–9.
34. UK Prospective Diabetes Study Group. Tight blood pressure control and risk of macrovascular and microvascular complications in type 2 diabetes: UKPDS 38. BMJ. 1998;317:703–13.
35. Endemann DH, Pu Q, De Ciuceis C, Savoia C, Virdis A, Neves MF, et al. Persistent remodeling of resistance arteries in type 2 diabetic patients on antihypertensive treatment. Hypertension. 2004;43:399–404.
36. Rizzoni D, Porteri E, De Ciuceis C, Sleiman I, Rodella L, Rezzani R, et al. Effect of treatment with candesartan or enalapril on subcutaneous small artery structure in hypertensive patients with non insulin-dependent diabetes mellitus. Hypertension. 2005;45:659–65.
37. Savoia C, Touyz RM, Endemann DH, Pu Q, Ko EA, De Ciuceis C, et al. Angiotensin receptor blocker added to previous antihypertensive agents on arteries of diabetic hypertensive patients. Hypertension. 2006;48:271–7.
38. Malik RA, Schofield IJ, Izzard A, Austin C, Bermann G, Heagerty AM. Effects of angiotensin type-1 receptor antagonism on small artery function in patients with type 2 diabetes mellitus. Hypertension. 2005;45:264–9.
39. Strain WD, Paldanius PM. Diabetes, cardiovascular disease and the microcirculation. Cardiovasc Diabetol. 2018;17:57.
40. Ott C, Jumar A, Striepe K, Friedrich S, Karg MV, Bramlage P, et al. A randomised study of the impact of the SGLT2 inhibitor dapagliflozin on microvascular and macrovascular circulation. Cardiovasc Diabetol. 2017;16:26.

Part V

Target Organ Damage in Hypertensive Diabetic Patient

Endothelial Dysfunction and Large Artery Stiffness

12

Rachel E. D. Climie

12.1 Introduction

Common to both diabetes and hypertension are abnormalities in blood vessel structure and function. While individuals with type 1 diabetes display abnormalities in vascular structure and function compared to their healthy counterparts [1], this chapter will predominantly focus on those with type 2 diabetes (T2D) due to the common coexistence (and bidirectional relationship) with hypertension.

Arterial ageing commences in early life and is a normal ageing phenomenon in most populations. However, pathological arterial ageing, as evident in conditions such as hypertension and T2D, results in accelerated vascular changes related to *atherosclerosis* in the arterial intima and *arteriosclerosis* in the arterial media. Exposure to adverse environmental and genetic factors as early as during childhood or even during foetal life promotes the development and accumulation of subclinical vascular changes that direct an individual towards a trajectory of early vascular ageing (EVA) [2]. Emerging evidence suggests that early life programming is also an important player in vascular remodelling mainly because the architecture of the vascular system is programmed in utero and elastin, the major structural component underlying arterial wall elasticity, is synthesised and deposited during this time. The EVA phenomenon is also evident among offspring with a positive family history of cardiovascular disease (CVD) or T2D [3, 4].

The ageing process affects the entire arterial wall and includes endothelial dysfunction, a decrease in nitric oxide (NO) production and local inflammation in the intima [5]; decreased levels of elastin and a relative increase in collagen content in the media [6]; and impairment of neuronal control, a loss of function of the vasa vasorum [7] and development of perivascular fat deposits that may increase local

R. E. D. Climie (✉)
Menzies Institute for Medical Research, University of Tasmania, Hobart, Australia
e-mail: Rachel.Climie@utas.edu.au

A. E. Berbari, G. Mancia (eds.), *Blood Pressure Disorders in Diabetes Mellitus*, Updates in Hypertension and Cardiovascular Protection,
https://doi.org/10.1007/978-3-031-13009-0_12

inflammation and adversely impact vasodilation in the adventitia [8]. This leads to structural changes in the arterial wall which manifest as an increase in intima-media thickness (IMT) [9–12], accompanied by lumen enlargement [10–12] and increased stiffness (*arteriosclerosis*) in the large, proximal elastic arteries [13]. The ageing process involves the entire vascular system including remodelling of the small arteries.

Alterations in vascular structure and function have been observed in patients with prediabetes or impaired fasting glucose as well as overt T2D, suggesting that the abnormalities in carbohydrate metabolism form a continuum that progressively worsens vascular health. An early feature of this adverse sequence of events that leads to atherosclerosis is believed to be endothelial dysfunction. Individuals with hypertension and T2D also display accelerated large artery stiffness compared to healthy individuals, of which endothelial dysfunction may be a key contributor [14].

In this chapter, literature on the association between T2D and hypertension with a particular focus on the changes that occur in relation to the endothelium and large arteries are summarised. The haemodynamic and biomechanical pathways involved in the bidirectional relationship between hypertension and T2D are discussed.

12.2 Endothelial Function and Large Artery Stiffness in Health and Disease

The vascular endothelial cells play an important role in maintaining vascular homeostasis. The endothelium provides a physical barrier between the vessel wall and lumen and actively secretes several mediators that regulate platelet aggregation, coagulation, fibrinolysis and vascular tone. The endothelial cells secrete mediators that cause vasoconstriction (endothelin-1 and thromboxane A2) or vasodilation (NO, prostacyclin and endothelium-derived hyperpolarising factor). NO plays a major role in endothelium-dependent relaxation in conduit arteries, while hyperpolarising factor predominates in the smaller, resistance vessels.

Endothelial dysfunction is characterised by a shift towards reduced vasodilation and a proinflammatory and prothrombotic state. Free radicals disrupt the balance of NO, damaging the endothelium leaving it permeable to toxins [15]. When NO action is impaired, endothelial signal is also impaired, leading to several systemic diseases. Endothelial dysfunction is associated with hypertension, coronary artery disease, heart failure, peripheral vascular disease, diabetes, kidney dysfunction as well as severe viral infections including the recent SARS-CoV-2 infection [16]. A number of factors can contribute to increased free radicals including obesity, hyperglycaemia, smoking, sleep deprivation and infection.

While the structural components within the arterial wall of large arteries (i.e. the aorta) such as elastin and collagen influence wall stiffness, arterial smooth muscle and locally derived, circulating factors also contribute to the regulation of large artery stiffness [17]. Vasoconstrictors (such as noradrenaline or angiotensin II) increase large artery stiffness, whereas vasodilators have an opposing effect [18]. In a healthy cardiovascular system, the compliant properties of the large arteries ensure that pulsations in pressure and flow generated by cyclic left ventricular contraction are dampened at the site of the ascending aorta into a continuous pressure (and flow) downstream at the site of arterioles. This allows for the delivery of a steady flow of blood during organ perfusion, and the microvasculature of target organs is protected from the damaging effects of pressure pulsatility [18]. The dampening of the pressure/flow wave is achieved via the windkessel effect whereby the aorta expands during systole and temporarily stores a portion of the stroke volume, which is then propelled into the systemic circulation during diastole via recoil of the elastic arterial wall. However, in response to ageing [19, 20], hypertension and other disease states such as diabetes mellitus [14, 21], arterial stiffening limits the buffering capacity of the elastic arteries. A reduction in NO availability may explain why patients with T2D demonstrate arterial stiffening before overt atherosclerosis is apparent.

The stiffness gradient between the proximal elastic arteries and distal muscular arteries leads to an impedance *mismatch*, generating backward pressure wave reflection (i.e. towards the heart) that reduces the forward transmission of pressure pulsatility to the small arteries of target organs. In the healthy vasculature, most of the backward wave travels at a low velocity and does not superimpose on the incident pressure wave and central blood pressure (BP) remains normal. However with increasing arterial stiffening and due to a lack of age-induced stiffening in the muscular arteries [22] , the stiffness gradient between the proximal and distal arteries is reduced, thus exposing the microvasculature to increased pulsatile stress [22, 23]. The backward travelling pulsatile energy travels at high velocity and superimposes on the incident pressure wave, increasing central systolic BP.

Arterial stiffening has a number of consequences for cardiovascular health. Firstly, the arterial pressure waveform is a composite of the forward and backward travelling pressure wave. In the case of stiff arteries, because the pressure wave propagation (i.e. pulse wave velocity, PWV) is high, the backward travelling wave arrives back at the central arteries sooner than if PWV was lower (i.e. in more compliant vessels) adding to the forward wave, augmenting pressure pulsatility and systolic BP. This results in isolated systolic hypertension at the central level and increased left ventricular afterload, ventricular remodelling, hypertrophy, dysfunction and failure [24, 25]. Secondly, arterial stiffening and the consequent loss of diastolic recoil and lower aortic diastolic BP reduce coronary perfusion pressure. Thirdly, the increased transmission of elevated pulsatile pressure/flow to the microvasculature of target organs may be particularly harmful to high flow/low resistance organs such as the brain and kidney, damaging capillary networks and resulting in target organ damage [26–32]. Indeed, arterial stiffness per se is a mechanism inducing cardiac, renal and brain microcirculatory damage, favouring CVD events [33]. Together, this may explain why the brain and kidney are more often affected by microvascular disease than are other organs in patients with both T2D and hypertension [34].

12.3 The Interplay Between Hypertension, Type 2 Diabetes, Endothelial Function and Large Artery Stiffness

Vascular abnormalities are common to both T2D and hypertension. A number of studies have shown that compared to their nondiabetic counterparts, patients with T2D display endothelial dysfunction [35–37] and accelerated arterial stiffness [38–41]. In patients with T2D, endothelial dysfunction is a consistent finding as hyperglycaemia and T2D lead to an impairment in NO production and bioavailability [42]. T2D exerts an additive deleterious effect on endothelial function, beyond other risk factors [43]. Individuals with both T2D and hypertension have elevated arterial stiffness compared to healthy controls or individuals with either T2D or hypertension alone [44]. In sub-Saharan populations, large artery abnormalities are significantly worse in those with coexistent T2D and hypertension but does not differ in those with either T2D or hypertension alone [45]. On the other hand, recent work has suggested that vascular changes may precede both T2D and hypertension [36, 46–54]. Thus, a bidirectional relationship between T2D and hypertension exists and is likely exacerbated by endothelial dysfunction and large artery stiffness [55] (Fig. 12.1). Importantly in people with T2D, large artery stiffness is independently related to CVD risk, mortality and all-cause mortality [56–58], and endothelial dysfunction is associated with adverse cardiovascular health and mortality [59–61].

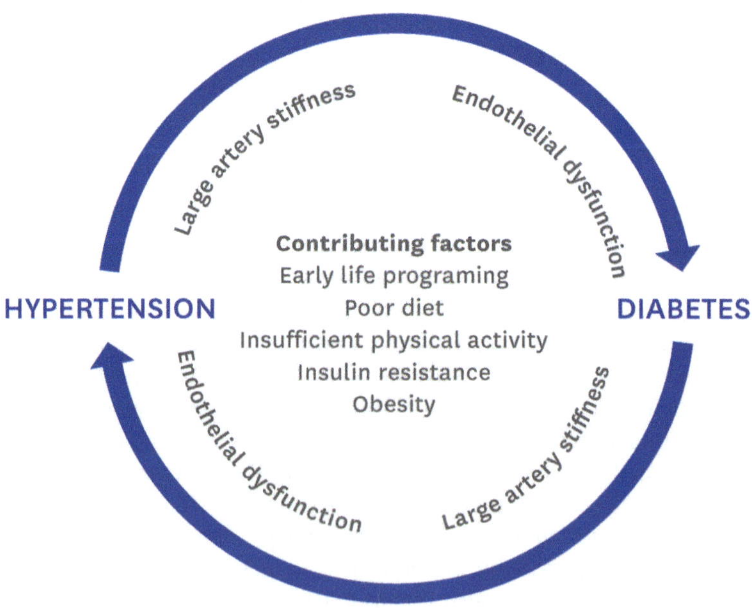

Fig. 12.1 The bidirectional relationship between diabetes and hypertension, perpetuated by endothelial dysfunction and large artery stiffness

12.3.1 Hypertension and Endothelial Dysfunction

Given that NO and endothelins are major regulators of vascular tone, they play a significant role in regulating BP. In hypertension, the balance between vasodilators and constrictors is disturbed, resulting in a predominance of vasoconstrictors such as endothelin-1. In patients with hypertension, impairment in vasodilation in the small resistance vessels in response to acetylcholine has been observed [62], and impaired flow-mediated dilation (FMD, a measure of endothelial function) distinguishes patients with hypertension at increased risk of fatal and non-fatal cardiovascular events [63]. Treatment with angiotensin-converting enzyme inhibitors, which act to increase NO bioavailability, improves endothelial function in patients with hypertension [64].

Whether endothelial dysfunction is a cause or a consequence of hypertension remains unclear [65]. Traditionally, it is believed that CVD risk factors including chronic inflammation, atherosclerosis, plaque instability and hypercoagulation preceded endothelial dysfunction. Normotensive offspring of parents with hypertension demonstrate impaired endothelial dysfunction [66], and the Cardiovascular Risk in Young Finns Study demonstrated that elevated BP in adolescence predicted future impaired endothelial function [67]. On the other hand, research in 952 postmenopausal women free from hypertension and risk factors showed that after 3.6 years of follow-up, there was a 5.77 increased risk of incident hypertension in those with the lowest flow-mediated dilation [68]. Interestingly, data from the Multi-Ethnic Study of Atherosclerosis cohort showed that FMD measured at baseline was not related to incident hypertension after 4.8 years of follow-up [69]. Furthermore, endothelial NO deficiency can occur via a number of non-hypertension-related insults that increase oxidative stress, such as hypercholesterolaemia. In the apolipoprotein E knockout mouse, where endothelial dysfunction results due to a hypercholesterolaemic diet, BP is not elevated.

12.3.2 Hypertension and Large Artery Stiffness

Hypertension is related to increased stiffness of the aorta for any given level of BP [70]. The enlargement of large proximal arteries is suggested to be a compensating mechanism, ensuring that a certain level of arterial compliance is maintained [18, 71, 72]. The effect of pulsatile mechanical load on arterial remodelling has been observed in large elastic arteries but not in more distal, muscular arteries (radial). The changes in the large arteries are generally due to the fracture of the load-bearing elastin fibres due to the fatiguing effect of both the steady and pulsatile tensile stress. Collagen replaces the loss of elastin, and advanced glycation end products (AGEs) formation is accelerated, promoting cross-linking of structural proteins [73]. Vascular smooth muscle cell (VSMC) growth and apoptosis may also be involved, as the cyclic, pulsatile strain on the vessels is also a determinant of gene expression and growth of VSMCs in vitro [74, 75]. The structural alterations associated with arterial stiffness may also impair the vasodilatory function and alter pulsatile haemodynamics, blood flow pattern and shear stress resulting in decreased NO bioavailability. Under conditions of increased oxidative stress, increased production of reactive oxygen species (ROS) leads to endothelial dysfunction and large elastic artery stiffening [76, 77]. Other molecular mechanisms associated with hypertension can also influence the stiffness of the arterial wall and are described in detail elsewhere [58]. Briefly, chronic activation of the renin-angiotensin system stimulates VSMC proliferation, low-grade inflammation, increased AGEs formation and collagen content which all promote arterial stiffening. Low-grade inflammation can lead to increased infiltration of VSMC, macrophages and mononuclear cells, media calcifications and cellular infiltration around the vasa vasorum which may result in ischaemia. Finally, sympathetic nervous system overdrive which occurs in individuals with hypertension [63] is an additional mechanism linking hypertension and increased large artery stiffness [64].

Although arterial stiffness has traditionally been viewed as a consequence of hypertension, the reverse may also be true, as recent studies have shown that arterial stiffness may contribute to the pathogenesis of hypertension [25, 46–49]. In mice who were fed a high-fat, high-sucrose diet and developed characteristics mirroring metabolic disease (insulin resistance, chronic inflammation and oxidative stress), aortic PWV increased within 2 months by 2.4-fold, while BP remained unchanged and only increased after 4–6 months [46]. In the Framingham offspring cohort, arterial stiffness (determined via carotid to femoral PWV) was associated with BP worsening and incident hypertension 4–10 years later [25]. Similarly, Zheng et al. [47] showed that after 27 months of follow-up, brachial to ankle PWV was associated with incident hypertension in Chinese adults, independent of traditional CVD risk factors. Furthermore, in young adults from the Young Finns Study, arterial stiffness (aortic arch to popliteal PWV) was independently associated with incident hypertension 4 years later [78].

12.3.3 Type 2 Diabetes and Endothelial Dysfunction

Hyperglycaemia, insulin resistance, dyslipidaemia, hyperuricaemia, increased dietary fructose and fat all predispose to endothelial dysfunction. People with T2D are particularly susceptible to the detrimental effects of endothelial dysfunction [36, 60]. T2D impairs the vasodilating properties of the endothelium via a number of mechanisms such as formation of AGEs and increased oxidative stress. Indeed, in patients with diabetes, exposure to acetylcholine causes vasoconstriction rather than vasodilation [79]. T2D may also amplify the detrimental effect of endothelial dysfunction on atherothrombosis via overproduction of ROS, inflammation, increased procoagulant activity and platelet aggregation [80]. Similar mechanisms have also been observed in those with impaired glucose metabolism or insulin resistance. Studies [60, 81] have shown that endothelial dysfunction is most strongly associated with incident CVD events in those with T2D compared to those without, suggesting the co-occurrence of T2D and endothelial dysfunction exacerbates CVD risk.

On the other hand, endothelial dysfunction exacerbates T2D by impairing the timely access of glucose and insulin in target tissues [54]. The Framingham Heart Study found that high levels of endothelial cell-derived Willebrand factor increased the risk of developing T2D, independently of other risk factors for T2D [81]. Similarly, in a large prospective study, higher levels of circulating E-selectin and intercellular adhesion molecule-1 (markers of endothelial dysfunction) were associated with increased risk of incident T2D after 5.9 years of follow-up [82]. Furthermore, hyperinsulinaemia and systemic insulin resistance stimulates the production of endothelin-1 (a vasoconstrictor) and, therefore, has been suggested to be a mechanism linking insulin resistance to the development of T2D. The combination of systematic insulin resistance and T2D accelerates endothelial cell dysfunction, thereby setting up a vicious, bidirectional cycle that promotes CVD.

12.3.4 Type 2 Diabetes and Large Artery Stiffness

While increased arterial stiffness is commonly observed in those with T2D, individuals with prediabetes also display arterial stiffening. A population-based cohort study (the Hoorn Study) in 747 individuals showed that prediabetes was associated with increased local femoral and brachial artery stiffness, but not carotid stiffness [83]. Others have also observed increased arterial stiffness in patients with prediabetes [41, 84] and accelerated progression of arterial stiffness over 4 years in non-diabetics but with elevated glycated haemoglobin or markers of insulin resistance [85]. The relationship between hyperglycaemia and arterial stiffening appears to be stronger in older, compared to younger adults [86]. Interestingly, endothelial dysfunction is related to aortic stiffness in those with hypertension and T2D, but not those without T2D, suggesting that diabetes-related metabolic alterations combined with hypertension may contribute to increased stiffness of large arteries via reduced endothelial function, independently of other confounders [43].

Recent work suggests there may be a bidirectional relationship between large artery stiffening and T2D, whereby arterial stiffening may contribute to the development of T2D. Indeed, Muhammad et al. [50] showed in 2450 individuals that after 4.5 years of follow-up, there was a stepwise increase in incidence of T2D across increasing tertiles of arterial stiffness independent of traditional risk factors. Another study recently showed that arterial stiffness measured via brachial-ankle PWV preceded increases in fasting blood glucose status [51]. Other haemodynamic markers related to large artery stiffness (pulse pressure, central systolic BP and augmentation index) have also been associated with increased risk of T2D [52, 53]. The relationship between arterial stiffness and incident diabetes may be explained via an increase in transmission of pressure and flow pulsatility to the microvasculature of the pancreas [6], which has a relatively high flow [79] and may be susceptible to the damaging effects of arterial stiffness. However, this is yet to be determined.

There are a number of mechanisms that may contribute to arterial changes in T2D which are discussed in detail elsewhere [14]. Briefly, hyperglycaemia contributes to blood vessel alterations early on in the progression of the disease [34], even prior to the diagnosis of T2D [87]. Hyperglycaemia modifies the structure of the vasa vasorum [88] and may stimulate VSMC proliferation, migration and altered reactivity. Hyperglycaemia also leads to various changes in the glycolytic pathway, the pentose phosphate pathway and tricarboxylic acid cycle, which all lead to the production of ROS and oxidative stress. Oxidative stress impairs endothelial NO synthase activation which reduces NO availability [89]. Chronic low-grade inflammation also leads to a reduction in the bioavailability and activation of NO [90] as well as releasing vasoconstrictor prostanoids, which can result in endothelial dysfunction and increased arterial stiffness [91]. AGEs encourage inflammation, inhibit NO release and further promote oxidative stress [92]. Furthermore, hyperinsulinaemia has direct deleterious effects on VSMCs and endothelial cells and may also induce vascular alterations by inducing sympathetic activation [93].

12.4 Summary and Conclusion

T2D is associated with an increased risk of CVD, which is exaggerated by the coexistence with hypertension. Many of the underlying molecular mechanisms that contribute to macrovascular and microvascular complications in patients with T2D such as oxidative stress, inflammation and fibrosis also cause vascular remodelling and dysfunction in hypertension. Endothelial dysfunction and large artery stiffening are key contributors to the bidirectional relationship between T2D and hypertension. While a genetic predisposition plays a critical role in the development of endothelial dysfunction and arterial stiffness, genetic markers do not seem to overlap between hypertension and T2D at least. Controlling hypertension in those with T2D and targeting strategies to promote vascular health may be especially important in reducing complications, CVD and premature death in patients with T2D.

References

1. Llauradó G, Ceperuelo-Mallafré V, Vilardell C, Simó R, Freixenet N, Vendrell J, et al. Arterial stiffness is increased in patients with type 1 diabetes without cardiovascular disease: a potential role of low-grade inflammation. Diabetes Care. 2012;35(5):1083–9.
2. Nilsson PM. Early vascular aging (EVA): consequences and prevention. Vasc Health Risk Manag. 2008;4(3):547–52.
3. Fatehali AA, Gottsäter M, Nilsson PM. Family history of cardiometabolic diseases and its association with arterial stiffness in the Malmö Diet Cancer cohort. J Hypertens. 2017;35(11):2262–7.
4. Uemura H, Katsuura-Kamano S, Yamaguchi M, Nakamoto M, Hiyoshi M, Arisawa K. Family history of stroke is potentially associated with arterial stiffness in the Japanese population. Arch Cardiovasc Dis. 2014;107(12):654–63.
5. Hansson GK, Robertson A-KL, Söderberg-Nauclér C. Inflammation and atherosclerosis. Annu Rev Pathol Mech Dis. 2006;1:297–329.
6. O'rourke MF, Hashimoto J. Mechanical factors in arterial aging: a clinical perspective. J Am Coll Cardiol. 2007;50(1):1–13.

7. Zeng Q, Dong S-Y, Wang M-L, Xiang H, Zhao X-L. Association of EZSCAN values with arterial stiffness in individuals without diabetes or cardiovascular disease. PLoS One. 2014;9(3):e90854.
8. Yudkin JS, Eringa E, Stehouwer CD. "Vasocrine" signalling from perivascular fat: a mechanism linking insulin resistance to vascular disease. Lancet. 2005;365(9473):1817–20.
9. Laurent S, Hayoz D, Trazzi S, Boutouyrie P, Waeber B, Omboni S, et al. Isobaric compliance of the radial artery is increased in patients with essential hypertension. J Hypertens. 1993;11(1):89–98.
10. Benetos A, Laurent S, Hoeks A, Boutouyrie P, Safar M. Arterial alterations with aging and high blood pressure. A noninvasive study of carotid and femoral arteries. Arterioscler Thromb. 1993;13(1):90–7.
11. Laurent S, Girerd X, Mourad J-J, Lacolley P, Beck L, Boutouyrie P, et al. Elastic modulus of the radial artery wall material is not increased in patients with essential hypertension. Arterioscler Thromb. 1994;14(7):1223–31.
12. Boutouyrie P, Bussy C, Lacolley P, Girerd X, Laloux B, Laurent S. Association between local pulse pressure, mean blood pressure, and large-artery remodeling. Circulation. 1999;100(13):1387–93.
13. Humphrey JD, Harrison DG, Figueroa CA, Lacolley P, Laurent S. Central artery stiffness in hypertension and aging: a problem with cause and consequence. Circ Res. 2016;118(3):379–81.
14. Stehouwer C, Henry R, Ferreira I. Arterial stiffness in diabetes and the metabolic syndrome: a pathway to cardiovascular disease. Diabetologia. 2008;51(4):527–39.
15. Rubanyi G, Vanhoutte P. Superoxide anions and hyperoxia inactivate endothelium-derived relaxing factor. Am J Physiol. 1986;250(5):H822–7.
16. Pons S, Fodil S, Azoulay E, Zafrani L. The vascular endothelium: the cornerstone of organ dysfunction in severe SARS-CoV-2 infection. Crit Care. 2020;24(1):1–8.
17. Kinlay S, Creager MA, Fukumoto M, Hikita H, Fang JC, Selwyn AP, et al. Endothelium-derived nitric oxide regulates arterial elasticity in human arteries in vivo. Hypertension. 2001;38(5):1049–53.
18. Nichols WW, O'Rourke MF. McDonald's blood flow in arteries: theoretical, experimental and clinical principles. London: Hodder Arnold Publishing; 2005.
19. McEniery CM, Yasmin HIR, Qasem A, Wilkinson IB, Cockcroft JR. Normal vascular aging: differential effects on wave reflection and aortic pulse wave velocity: the Anglo-Cardiff Collaborative Trial (ACCT). J Am Coll Cardiol. 2005;46(9):1753–60.
20. Vermeersch S. Reference values for arterial stiffness' collaboration. Determinants of pulse wave velocity in healthy people and in the presence of cardiovascular risk factors: Establishing normal and reference values. Eur Heart J. 2010;31(19):2338–50.
21. Franklin SS. Arterial stiffness and hypertension. Hypertension. 2005;45(3):349–51.
22. Laurent S, Boutouyrie P. The structural factor of hypertension: large and small artery alterations. Circ Res. 2015;116(6):1007–21.
23. Mitchell GF. Effects of central arterial aging on the structure and function of the peripheral vasculature: implications for end-organ damage. J Appl Physiol. 2008;105(5):1652–60.
24. Chirinos JA, Segers P. Noninvasive evaluation of left ventricular afterload: part 2: arterial pressure-flow and pressure-volume relations in humans. Hypertension. 2010;56(4):563–70.
25. Kaess BM, Rong J, Larson MG, Hamburg NM, Vita JA, Levy D, et al. Aortic stiffness, blood pressure progression, and incident hypertension. JAMA. 2012;308(9):875–81.
26. Leoncini G, Ratto E, Viazzi F, Vaccaro V, Parodi A, Falqui V, et al. Increased ambulatory arterial stiffness index is associated with target organ damage in primary hypertension. Hypertension. 2006;48(3):397–403.
27. Gómez-Marcos MÁ, Recio-Rodríguez JI, Patino-Alonso MC, Gómez-Sánchez L, Agudo-Conde C, Gómez-Sánchez M, et al. Ambulatory arterial stiffness indices and target organ damage in hypertension. BMC Cardiovasc Disord. 2012;12:1.
28. Katsi V, Vlachopoulos C, Souretis G, Baou K, Dagalaki I, Alexopoulos N, et al. Association between retinal microcirculation and aortic stiffness in hypertensive patients. Int J Cardiol. 2012;157(3):370–3.

29. Triantafyllidi H, Tzortzis S, Lekakis J, Ikonomidis I, Arvaniti C, Trivilou P, et al. Association of target organ damage with three arterial stiffness indexes according to blood pressure dipping status in untreated hypertensive patients. Am J Hypertens. 2010;23(12):1265–72.
30. Bruno RM, Cartoni G, Stea F, Armenia S, Bianchini E, Buralli S, et al. Carotid and aortic stiffness in essential hypertension and their relation with target organ damage: the CATOD study. J Hypertens. 2017;35(2):310–8.
31. Climie RE, Srikanth V, Keith LJ, Davies JE, Sharman JE. Exercise excess pressure and exercise-induced albuminuria in patients with type 2 diabetes mellitus. Am J Physiol Heart Circ Physiol. 2015;308(9):H1136–42.
32. Climie RE, Picone DS, Blackwood S, Keel SE, Qasem A, Rattigan S, et al. Pulsatile interaction between the macro-vasculature and micro-vasculature: proof-of-concept among patients with type 2 diabetes. Eur J Appl Physiol. 2018;118:2455–63.
33. Laurent S, Briet M, Boutouyrie P. Large and small artery cross-talk and recent morbidity-mortality trials in hypertension. Hypertension. 2009;54(2):388–92.
34. Zimmet P, Alberti K, Shaw J. Global and societal implications of the diabetes epidemic. Nature. 2001;414(6865):782–7.
35. Montero D, Walther G, Pérez-Martin A, Vicente-Salar N, Roche E, Vinet A. Vascular smooth muscle function in type 2 diabetes mellitus: a systematic review and meta-analysis. Diabetologia. 2013;56:2122–33.
36. Kim J-a, Montagnani M, Koh KK, Quon MJ. Reciprocal relationships between insulin resistance and endothelial dysfunction: molecular and pathophysiological mechanisms. Circulation. 2006;113(15):1888–904.
37. Xu J, Zou M-H. Molecular insights and therapeutic targets for diabetic endothelial dysfunction. Circulation. 2009;120(13):1266–86.
38. Woolam G, Schnur P, Vallbona C, Hoff H. The pulse wave velocity as an early indicator of atherosclerosis in diabetic subjects. Circulation. 1962;25(3):533–9.
39. Prenner SB, Chirinos JA. Arterial stiffness in diabetes mellitus. Atherosclerosis. 2015;238(2):370–9.
40. Chirinos JA, Segers P, Gillebert TC, De Buyzere ML, Khan ZA, Khawar U, et al. Central pulse pressure and its hemodynamic determinants in middle-aged adults with impaired fasting glucose and diabetes: the Asklepios study. Diabetes Care. 2013;36(8):2359–65.
41. Loehr LR, Meyer ML, Poon AK, Selvin E, Palta P, Tanaka H, et al. Prediabetes and diabetes are associated with arterial stiffness in older adults: the ARIC study. Am J Hypertens. 2016;29(9):1038–45.
42. Avogaro A, Albiero M, Menegazzo L, de Kreutzenberg S, Fadini GP. Endothelial dysfunction in diabetes: the role of reparatory mechanisms. Diabetes Care. 2011;34(Suppl 2):S285–90.
43. Bruno RM, Penno G, Daniele G, Pucci L, Lucchesi D, Stea F, et al. Type 2 diabetes mellitus worsens arterial stiffness in hypertensive patients through endothelial dysfunction. Diabetologia. 2012;55(6):1847–55.
44. Tedesco M, Natale F, Di Salvo G, Caputo S, Capasso M, Calabro R. Effects of coexisting hypertension and type II diabetes mellitus on arterial stiffness. J Hum Hypertens. 2004;18(7):469–73.
45. Yeboah K, Antwi DA, Gyan B, Govoni V, Mills CE, Cruickshank JK, et al. Arterial stiffness in hypertensive and type 2 diabetes patients in Ghana: comparison of the cardio-ankle vascular index and central aortic techniques. BMC Endocr Disord. 2016;16:53.
46. Weisbrod RM, Shiang T, Al Sayah L, Fry JL, Bajpai S, Reinhart-King CA, et al. Arterial stiffening precedes systolic hypertension in diet-induced obesity. Hypertension. 2013;62:1105–10.
47. Zheng X, Jin C, Liu Y, Zhang J, Zhu Y, Kan S, et al. Arterial stiffness as a predictor of clinical hypertension. J Clin Hypertens (Greenwich). 2015;17(8):582–91.
48. Takase H, Dohi Y, Toriyama T, Okado T, Tanaka S, Sonoda H, et al. Brachial-ankle pulse wave velocity predicts increase in blood pressure and onset of hypertension. Am J Hypertens. 2011;24(6):667–73.
49. Najjar SS, Scuteri A, Shetty V, Wright JG, Muller DC, Fleg JL, et al. Pulse wave velocity is an independent predictor of the longitudinal increase in systolic blood pressure and of incident hypertension in the Baltimore Longitudinal Study of Aging. J Am Coll Cardiol. 2008;51(14):1377–83.

50. Muhammad IF, Borné Y, Östling G, Kennbäck C, Gottsäter M, Persson M, et al. Arterial stiffness and incidence of diabetes: a population-based cohort study. Diabetes Care. 2017;40(12):1739–45.
51. Zheng M, Zhang X, Chen S, Song Y, Zhao Q, Gao X, et al. Arterial stiffness preceding diabetes: a longitudinal study. Circ Res. 2020;127(12):1491–8.
52. Yasuno S, Ueshima K, Oba K, Fujimoto A, Hirata M, Ogihara T, et al. Is pulse pressure a predictor of new-onset diabetes in high-risk hypertensive patients?: A subanalysis of the Candesartan Antihypertensive Survival Evaluation in Japan (CASE-J) trial. Diabetes Care. 2010;33(5):1122–7.
53. Chen J-Y, Chou C-H, Lee YL, Tsai W-C, Lin C-C, Huang Y-Y, et al. Association of central aortic pressures indexes with development of diabetes mellitus in essential hypertension. Am J Hypertens. 2010;23(10):1069–73.
54. Muris DM, Houben AJ, Schram MT, Stehouwer CD. Microvascular dysfunction is associated with a higher incidence of type 2 diabetes mellitus: a systematic review and meta-analysis. Arterioscler Thromb Vasc Biol. 2012;32(12):3082–94.
55. Climie RE, van Sloten TT, Bruno R-M, Taddei S, Empana J-P, Stehouwer CD, et al. Macrovasculature and microvasculature at the crossroads between type 2 diabetes mellitus and hypertension. Hypertension. 2019;73(6):1138–49.
56. Mansour AS, Yannoutsos A, Majahalme N, Agnoletti D, Safar ME, Ouerdane S, et al. Aortic stiffness and cardiovascular risk in type 2 diabetes. J Hypertens. 2013;31(8):1584–92.
57. Shoji T, Emoto M, Shinohara K, Kakiya R, Tsujimoto Y, Kishimoto H, et al. Diabetes mellitus, aortic stiffness, and cardiovascular mortality in end-stage renal disease. J Am Soc Nephrol. 2001;12(10):2117–24.
58. Cruickshank K, Riste L, Anderson SG, Wright JS, Dunn G, Gosling RG. Aortic pulse-wave velocity and its relationship to mortality in diabetes and glucose intolerance: an integrated index of vascular function? Circulation. 2002;106(16):2085–90.
59. van Sloten TT, Henry RM, Dekker JM, Nijpels G, Unger T, Schram MT, et al. Endothelial dysfunction plays a key role in increasing cardiovascular risk in type 2 diabetes: the Hoorn study. Hypertension. 2014;64(6):1299–305.
60. de Jager J, Dekker JM, Kooy A, Kostense PJ, Nijpels G, Heine RJ, et al. Endothelial dysfunction and low-grade inflammation explain much of the excess cardiovascular mortality in individuals with type 2 diabetes: the Hoorn Study. Arterioscler Thromb Vasc Biol. 2006;26(5):1086–93.
61. Quyyumi AA. Prognostic value of endothelial function. Am J Cardiol. 2003;91(12):19–24.
62. Deng L-Y, Jin-Sheng L, Schiffrin EL. Endothelium-dependent relaxation of small arteries from essential hypertensive patients: mechanisms and comparison with normotensive subjects and with responses of vessels from spontaneously hypertensive rats. Clin Sci (Lond). 1995;88(6):611–22.
63. Muiesan ML, Salvetti M, Paini A, Monteduro C, Galbassini G, Poisa P, et al. Prognostic role of flow-mediated dilatation of the brachial artery in hypertensive patients. J Hypertens. 2008;26(8):1612–8.
64. Aznaouridis K, Stamatelopoulos K, Karatzis E, Protogerou A, Papamichael C, Lekakis J. Acute effects of renin-angiotensin system blockade on arterial function in hypertensive patients. J Hum Hypertens. 2007;21(8):654–63.
65. Quyyumi AA, Patel RS. Endothelial dysfunction and hypertension: cause or effect? Hypertension. 2010;55:1092–4.
66. Gkaliagkousi E, Douma S, Zamboulis C, Ferro A. Nitric oxide dysfunction in vascular endothelium and platelets: role in essential hypertension. J Hypertens. 2009;27(12):2310–20.
67. Juonala M, Viikari JS, Rönnemaa T, Helenius H, Taittonen L, Raitakari OT. Elevated blood pressure in adolescent boys predicts endothelial dysfunction: the cardiovascular risk in young Finns study. Hypertension. 2006;48(3):424–30.
68. Rossi R, Chiurlia E, Nuzzo A, Cioni E, Origliani G, Modena MG. Flow-mediated vasodilation and the risk of developing hypertension in healthy postmenopausal women. J Am Coll Cardiol. 2004;44(8):1636–40.

69. Shimbo D, Muntner P, Mann D, Viera AJ, Homma S, Polak JF, et al. Endothelial dysfunction and the risk of hypertension: the multi-ethnic study of atherosclerosis. Hypertension. 2010;55(5):1210–6.
70. Mattace-Raso FUS, Hofman A, Verwoert GC, Wittemana JCM, Wilkinson I, Cockcroft J, et al. Reference Values for Arterial Stiffness' Collaboration. Determinants of pulse wave velocity in healthy people and in the presence of cardiovascular risk factors:'establishing normal and reference values'. Eur Heart J. 2010;31(19):2338–50.
71. Guala A, Camporeale C, Ridolfi L. Compensatory effect between aortic stiffening and remodelling during ageing. PLoS One. 2015;10(10):e0139211.
72. Guala A, Rodriguez-Palomares J, Dux-Santoy L, Teixido-Tura G, Maldonado G, Galian L, et al. Influence of aortic dilation on the regional aortic stiffness of bicuspid aortic valve assessed by 4-dimensional flow cardiac magnetic resonance: comparison with Marfan syndrome and degenerative aortic aneurysm. JACC Cardiovasc Imaging. 2019;12(6):1020–9.
73. Semba RD, Nicklett EJ, Ferrucci L. Does accumulation of advanced glycation end products contribute to the aging phenotype? J Gerontol A Biol Sci Med Sci. 2010;65(9):963–75.
74. Leung D, Glagov S, Mathews MB. Cyclic stretching stimulates synthesis of matrix components by arterial smooth muscle cells in vitro. Science. 1976;191(4226):475–7.
75. Lehoux S, Tedgui A. Cellular mechanics and gene expression in blood vessels. J Biomech. 2003;36(5):631–43.
76. Ungvari Z, Tarantini S, Donato AJ, Galvan V, Csiszar A. Mechanisms of vascular aging. Circ Res. 2018;123(7):849–67.
77. Donato AJ, Eskurza I, Silver AE, Levy AS, Pierce GL, Gates PE, et al. Direct evidence of endothelial oxidative stress with aging in humans: relation to impaired endothelium-dependent dilation and upregulation of nuclear factor-kappaB. Circ Res. 2007;100(11):1659–66.
78. Koivistoinen T, Lyytikäinen L-P, Aatola H, Luukkaala T, Juonala M, Viikari J, et al. Pulse wave velocity predicts the progression of blood pressure and development of hypertension in young adults novelty and significance. Hypertension. 2018;71(3):451–6.
79. Nitenberg A, Valensi P, Sachs R, Dali M, Aptecar E, Attali JR. Impairment of coronary vascular reserve and ACh-induced coronary vasodilation in diabetic patients with angiographically normal coronary arteries and normal left ventricular systolic function. Diabetes. 1993;42(7):1017–25.
80. Luscher TF, Creager MA, Beckman JA, Cosentino F. Diabetes and vascular disease: pathophysiology, clinical consequences, and medical therapy: Part II. Circulation. 2003;108(13):1655–61.
81. Frankel DS, Meigs JB, Massaro JM, Wilson PW, O'Donnell CJ, D'Agostino RB, et al. Von Willebrand factor, type 2 diabetes mellitus, and risk of cardiovascular disease: the framingham offspring study. Circulation. 2008;118(24):2533–9.
82. Song Y, Manson JE, Tinker L, Rifai N, Cook NR, Hu FB, et al. Circulating levels of endothelial adhesion molecules and risk of diabetes in an ethnically diverse cohort of women. Diabetes. 2007;56(7):1898–904.
83. Henry RM, Kostense PJ, Spijkerman AM, Dekker JM, Nijpels G, Heine RJ, et al. Arterial stiffness increases with deteriorating glucose tolerance status: the Hoorn Study. Circulation. 2003;107(16):2089–95.
84. Li C-H, Wu J-S, Yang Y-C, Shih C-C, Lu F-H, Chang C-J. Increased arterial stiffness in subjects with impaired glucose tolerance and newly diagnosed diabetes but not isolated impaired fasting glucose. J Clin Endocrinol Metab. 2012;97(4):E658–62.
85. McEniery CM, Wilkinson IB, Johansen NB, Witte DR, Singh-Manoux A, Kivimaki M, et al. Nondiabetic glucometabolic status and progression of aortic stiffness: the Whitehall II Study. Diabetes Care. 2017;40(4):599–606.
86. Taimour S, Gottsäter A, Jujic A, Nilsson PM. Hyperglycemia and arterial stiffness across two generations. J Hypertens. 2021;39(3):471–5.
87. Rahman S, Rahman T, Ismail AAS, Rashid ARA. Diabetes-associated macrovasculopathy: pathophysiology and pathogenesis. Diabetes Obes Metab. 2007;9(6):767–80.
88. Veerman K, Venegas-Pino D, Shi Y, Khan M, Gerstein H, Werstuck G. Hyperglycaemia is associated with impaired vasa vasorum neovascularization and accelerated atherosclerosis in apolipoprotein-E deficient mice. Atherosclerosis. 2013;227(2):250–8.

89. Gage MC, Yuldasheva NY, Viswambharan H, Sukumar P, Cubbon RM, Galloway S, et al. Endothelium-specific insulin resistance leads to accelerated atherosclerosis in areas with disturbed flow patterns: a role for reactive oxygen species. Atherosclerosis. 2013;230(1):131–9.
90. Clapp BR, Hingorani AD, Kharbanda RK, Mohamed-Ali V, Stephens JW, Vallance P, et al. Inflammation-induced endothelial dysfunction involves reduced nitric oxide bioavailability and increased oxidant stress. Cardiovasc Res. 2004;64(1):172–8.
91. Vlachopoulos C, Dima I, Aznaouridis K, Vasiliadou C, Ioakeimidis N, Aggeli C, et al. Acute systemic inflammation increases arterial stiffness and decreases wave reflections in healthy individuals. Circulation. 2005;112(14):2193–200.
92. Stirban A, Gawlowski T, Roden M. Vascular effects of advanced glycation endproducts: clinical effects and molecular mechanisms. Mol Metab. 2014;3(2):94–108.
93. Masuo K, Rakugi H, Ogihara T, Esler MD, Lambert GW. Cardiovascular and renal complications of type 2 diabetes in obesity: role of sympathetic nerve activity and insulin resistance. Curr Diabetes Rev. 2010;6(2):58–67.

The Heart in Diabetic Hypertensive Patients

13

Amera Halabi and Thomas H. Marwick

Abbreviations

ACEi	Angiotensin-converting enzyme inhibitor
AMPK	Adenosine monophosphate-activated protein kinase
ARB	Angiotensin-II receptor blocker
BP	Blood pressure
CAD	Coronary artery disease
CAN	Cardiac autonomic neuropathy
CVD	Cardiovascular disease
DD	Diastolic dysfunction
ECM	Extracellular matrix
eNOS	Endothelial nitric oxide synthetase
EF	Ejection fraction
GLP-1 RA	Glucagon like protein-1 receptor agonist
GLS	Global longitudinal strain
HbA1c	Haemoglobin A1c

A. Halabi
Baker Heart and Diabetes Institute, Melbourne, VIC, Australia

School of Public Health and Preventive Medicine, Monash University, Melbourne, VIC, Australia

T. H. Marwick (✉)
Baker Heart and Diabetes Institute, Melbourne, VIC, Australia

School of Public Health and Preventive Medicine, Monash University, Melbourne, VIC, Australia

Menzies Institute for Medical Research, Imaging Research, Hobart, Tasmania, Australia
e-mail: tom.marwick@bakeridi.edu.au

A. E. Berbari, G. Mancia (eds.), *Blood Pressure Disorders in Diabetes Mellitus*, Updates in Hypertension and Cardiovascular Protection,
https://doi.org/10.1007/978-3-031-13009-0_13

HF	Heart failure
HFpEF	Heart failure with preserved ejection fraction
HFrEF	Heart failure with reduced ejection fraction
IGFR-1	Insulin-like growth factor receptor I
IR	Insulin receptor
LA	Left atrium
LV	Left ventricle
LVH	Left ventricular hypertrophy
RAAS	Renin-angiotensin-aldosterone system
SGLT2	Sodium glucose cotransporter-2
STE	Speckle tracking imaging
T2DM	Type 2 diabetes mellitus

13.1 Introduction

Heart disease remains the most frequent complication of long-standing hypertension and diabetes [1]. When the two conditions co-exist, coupled with other cardiovascular risk factors such as older age and dyslipidaemia, the development of heart disease accelerates.

Cardiac complications primarily manifest in two ways: as coronary artery disease (CAD) or as heart failure, with hallmarks of myocardial fibrosis and hypertrophy [1]. Typically, both cardiac complications present in the later stages of the disease, with consequent morbidity and mortality. However, in recent times, with sensitive tools and wider availability of cardiac diagnostic testing, a paradigm shift has ensued towards early detection and management.

13.2 Epidemiology

Cardiovascular disease (CVD) is a common complication of long-term type 2 diabetes mellitus (T2DM), even in the absence of hypertension. In a systematic review of over 4 million patients with established T2DM, prevalence rates of CVD in males and females were reported at 32% [2]. Although the prevalence of CAD (21%) exceeds that of HF (15%) [2], the latter is likely to be underestimated – as indeed it is an underestimated CV outcome in clinical trials of diabetes.

In hypertension, CVD risk is associated with increasing blood pressure (BP). In younger individuals, it was shown that grade 2 hypertension had a significantly higher risk of CAD (HR 2.27 [95% CI 1.86–2.78]) and all-cause mortality (HR 2.01 [95% CI 1.38–2.93]) than normal BP [3]. Similarly, the risk of developing HF increases in a direct relationship with rising BP [4].

In patients with both hypertension and T2DM, there is a significantly higher incidence of CV complications, such as stroke and acute myocardial infarction (AMI) than patients with hypertension but no T2DM (stroke RR 6.1 [95% CI 1.3–27.7], $p = 0.007$; AMI RR 12.2 [95% CI 1.6–95], $p = 0.002$) [5]. Furthermore,

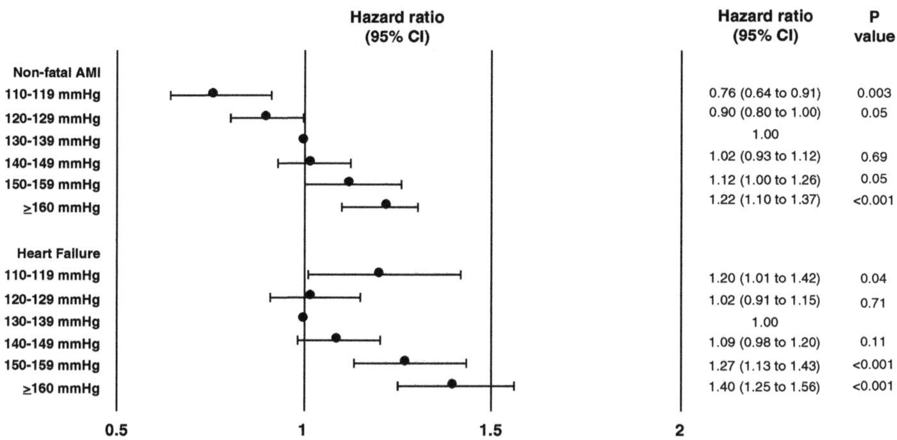

Fig. 13.1 Hazard ratio of non-fatal acute myocardial infarction (AMI) and heart failure across different levels of systolic blood pressure in T2DM individuals. Adapted from Adamsson Eryd, S. et al. (2016). BMJ; 354:i4070 [6]

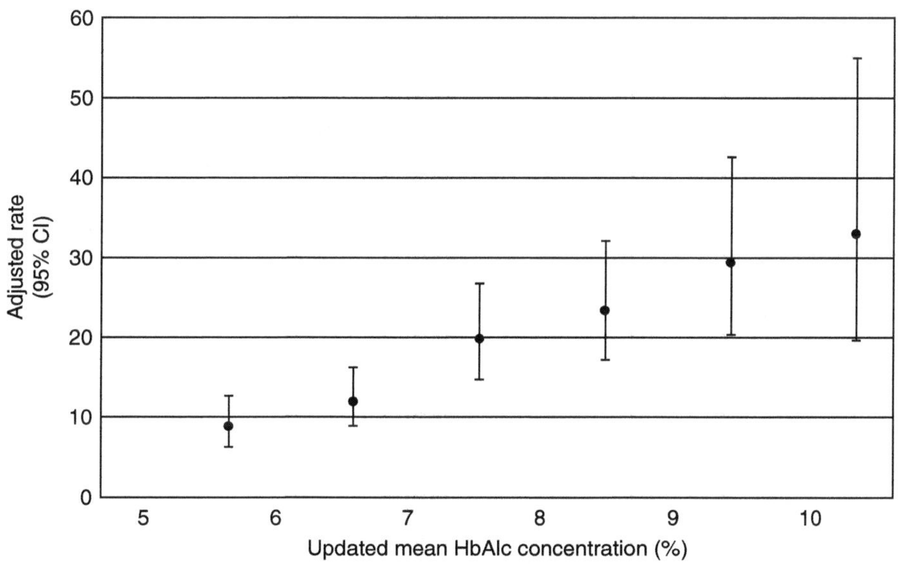

Fig. 13.2 Adjusted rates and corresponding 95% confidence intervals for the endpoint of diabetes-related death at corresponding haemoglobin A1c (HbA1c) concentration. Adapted from Stratton, IM. et al. (2002). BMJ; 321(7258): 405–412 [8]

in a Swedish analysis of 187,106 individuals with T2DM, the incidence of AMI and HF was higher in individuals with systolic BP ≥160 mmHg (Fig. 13.1) [6]. Likewise diabetes-related deaths were 1.82 times more frequent in hypertensive compared to non-hypertensive individuals [7], and for every 1% decrease in haemoglobin A1c (HbA1c), diabetes-related deaths decrease by 21% (Fig. 13.2) [8].

13.3 Mechanisms of Myocardial Dysfunction in Type 2 Diabetes Mellitus and Hypertension

13.3.1 Type 2 Diabetes Mellitus

Type 2 diabetes mellitus is hallmarked by the development of insulin resistance, systemic inflammation and autonomic dysfunction ultimately leading to micro- and macrovascular end-organ damage (Fig. 13.3) [9].

Chronic low-grade inflammation is a key feature of T2DM [9]. Adipose tissue acts as a major source of inflammation, which fits with the prominence of central obesity in T2DM and its role as a CVD risk factor. Systemic inflammation is driven by macrophages that reside within adipose tissue, releasing inflammatory factors such as tumour necrosis factor (TNF) and other cytokines [9]. These macrophages are upregulated with increasing body weight [9]. Furthermore, hyperinsulinaemia and insulin resistance amplify inflammation by causing changes in energy utilisation and metabolism within adipocytes inducing the release of adipokines and free fatty acids [10]. The end result is a systemic inflammatory state that further propagates insulin resistance within localised adipocyte tissue and other organs, such as the heart [10].

Cardiac autonomic neuropathy (CAN) is another complication of the diabetic state that likely contributes to CVD. CAN is often misconstrued as a late complication of DM, and its pathophysiology is poorly understood but is thought to result from the accumulation of glycated end products of protein, nucleic acids and lipids that cross-link with corresponding receptors [11]. This changes the intricate

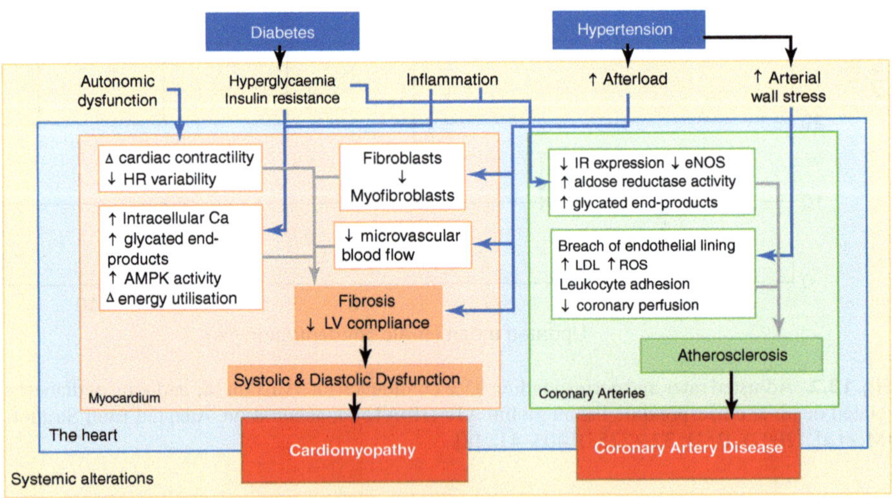

Fig. 13.3 Pathophysiological mechanisms in type 2 diabetes mellitus and hypertension that contribute to cardiomyopathy and coronary artery disease *AMPK* Adenosine monophosphate-activated protein kinase, *eNOS* Endothelial nitric oxide synthetase, *HR* Heart rate, *IR* Insulin receptor, *LDL* Low-density lipoprotein, *LV* Left ventricle, *ROS* Reactive oxygen species

extracellular matrix (ECM) leading to the neuropathy. Alterations in autonomic function create an imbalance in sympathetic and parasympathetic tone within the myocardium [11]. Over time, sympathetic tone is augmented primarily due to parasympathetic denervation leading to loss of heart rate variability, alterations in cardiac contractility and vascular function [11].

13.3.2 Hypertension

Long-term hypertension is a major cause of CVD morbidity and mortality and is primarily manifested in the heart as left ventricular hypertrophy (LVH) and diastolic dysfunction (DD) [12]. In older patients arterial stiffness, α-adrenoreceptor activity and release of endothelial agents, such as angiotensin and endothelin, cause an increase in systemic vascular resistance and vascular tone [12]. This promotes the accumulation of cytosolic calcium within vascular smooth muscle cells causing vasoconstriction. Furthermore, due to aortic stiffening, pulse pressure within the LV shifts from early diastole to late systole resulting in decreased coronary perfusion [13]. These processes combined increase the afterload on the LV and result in LVH and DD.

13.4 Coronary Artery Disease in Hypertensive Diabetic Patients

T2DM and hypertension are well-known drivers of atherosclerosis. Prevalence estimates of hypertension amongst T2DM patients are significantly higher than the general population (55% vs. 2–4%, respectively) [14]. Coupled with 'silent ischaemia' due to autonomic neuropathy, undetected events translate into elevated rates of mortality. Thus, understanding the pathogenesis of this higher CAD risk and providing earlier diagnosis are important.

13.4.1 Pathophysiology

Several key factors in T2DM promote the development of atherosclerosis. Insulin resistance, hyperglycaemia and inflammation alter metabolic pathways and energy handling increasing the atherogenic potential of coronary vasculature [15]. In the normal state, insulin receptor (IR) activation leads to the recruitment of phosphoinositide 3 (PI3)-kinase resulting in upregulation of 2-phophoinositide-dependent protein kinase 1 (PDK1). The end result is glycogen synthesis and protein translation [15]. In T2DM, the presence of insulin resistance and hyperinsulinaemia causes endothelial cells, vascular smooth muscle cells and macrophages to downregulate the IR and its downstream signalling pathway [15].

Atherogenesis is promoted by several changes. Within endothelial cells, insulin resistance causes reduced levels of endothelial nitric oxide synthetase (eNOS) causing vasoconstriction and adhesion of leucocytes [16]. Systemic and localised inflammation increases macrophage activity and atherosclerosis. Furthermore, increased flux of glucose through the aldose reductase/polyol pathway leads to accumulation of sorbitol and by-products that are pro-atherogenic [17]. Finally, increased glycation and formation of glycated end products alter cellular and extracellular molecular function causing atherosclerosis [18].

In hypertension, atherosclerosis is promoted by increased pulse pressure of the LV resulting in reduced coronary perfusion [13]. Hypertension also induces and suppresses vasomotor activity of the arterial tree. This direct mechanical shear stress on the arterial wall can breach the endothelial lining promoting the accumulation of low-density lipoproteins (LDL), oxidation by reactive oxygen species (ROS), leucocyte adhesion and the development of an atherosclerotic plaque [1]. Another key player is the renin-angiotensin-aldosterone system (RAAS) which through increased angiotensin-II activity causes vasoconstriction. RAAS is also pro-inflammatory by upregulating cytokines, chemokines and growth factors promoting recruitment of macrophages and other leucocytes into the plaque [19].

13.4.2 Clinical Features

The most typical manifestation of CAD is angina that limits exertion. Unfortunately, atypical anginal variants, sex differences and 'silent' myocardial ischaemia make the diagnosis challenging [20]. In a large prospective study, shoulder and arm pain occurred nearly twice as frequently in women than in men and shortness of breath was predictive of non-ACS in men [21].

13.4.3 Imaging Findings

Non-invasive testing should precede invasive testing in the assessment of suspected coronary disease, unless symptoms and clinical signs carry a high pre-test probability warranting invasive coronary angiography as the first test.

Non-invasive coronary imaging incorporates several validated modalities in the assessment of CAD (Table 13.1). Technetium-99m single-photon emission computed tomography (SPECT) is a commonly used modality to assess myocardial perfusion defects. Ischaemic defects have lesser degrees of hyperaemia (induced by exercise or pharmacologic stimuli such as adenosine) than normal segments. 'Fixed defects' (reduced regional perfusion at rest and stress) reflect infarcted myocardium (Fig. 13.4) [20]. Both exercise and adenosine SPECT carry a high sensitivity and specificity in the assessment of CAD [22], but it needs to be kept in mind that LVH and CAD influence coronary flow reserve, and as both DM and hypertension are drivers of LVH, this may be an important confounder.

Stress echocardiography is a widespread and readily available modality to assess CAD. Stress is induced via exercise or administration of dobutamine. Wall-motion abnormalities are evaluated in a 16- or 17-segment model, with induced or worsened abnormalities reflecting CAD [23]. Diagnostic accuracy is improved with the administration of contrast (Fig. 13.5).

Table 13.1 Predictive value of imaging modalities in the detection of coronary artery disease

Modality	Sensitivity (%)	Specificity (%)	Reference
SPECT			
– Exercise	87	73	[22]
– Adenosine	90	85	
Stress echocardiography			
– Exercise	85	77	[29, 30]
– Dobutamine	80	86	
Stress perfusion MRI	90	81	[31]
64-slice CTCA	88	90	[27]

CTCA Computed tomography coronary angiography, *MRI* Magnetic resonance imaging, *SPECT* Single-positron emission computed tomography

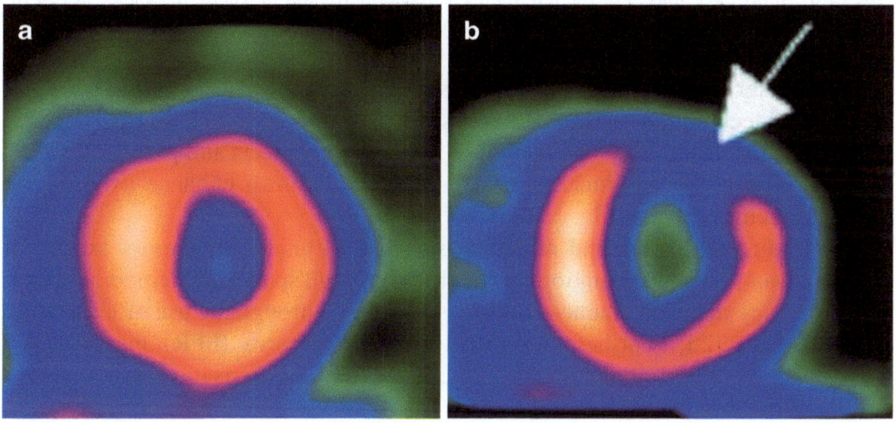

Fig. 13.4 Short-axis image of the left ventricle during SPECT imaging at rest (**a**) and after stress (**b**). A reversible perfusion defect is observed in the anterolateral wall (white arrow) indicative of coronary ischaemia. Reproduced from Ghersin et al. (2006). Circulation; 114:e237–239 [32]

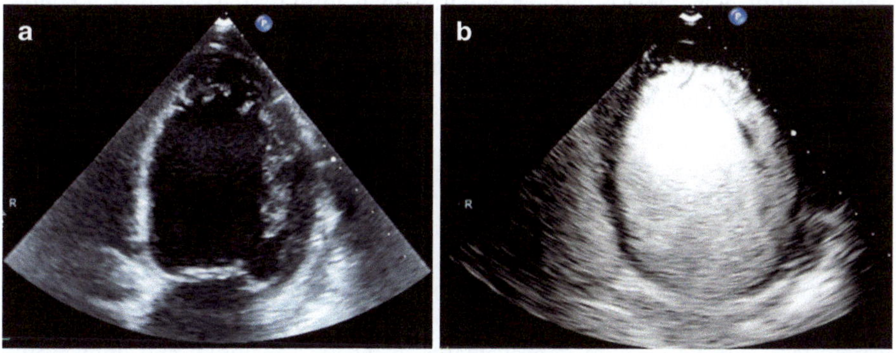

Fig. 13.5 Apical four-chamber view of the heart, illustrating trabeculations and poor endocardial definition of the left ventricle (**a**) which improves with administration of contrast agent (**b**)

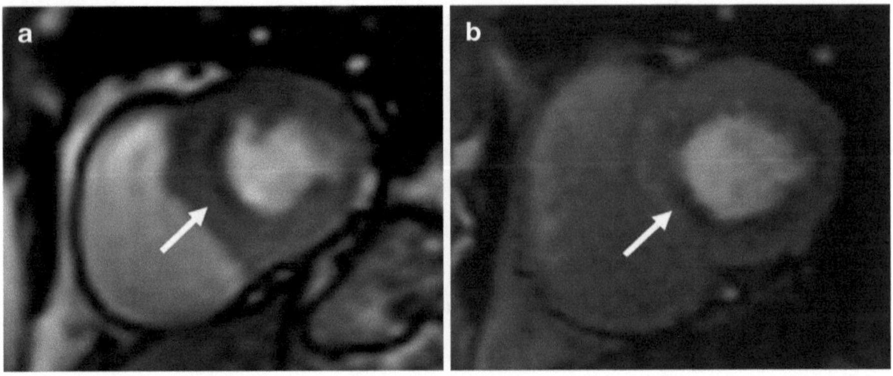

Fig. 13.6 Short-axis images of the left ventricle during perfusion magnetic resonance at rest (**a**) and during stress (**b**) with a fixed anterior/septum wall defect seen (white arrows)

Myocardial perfusion by magnetic resonance imaging (MRI) is another commonly used technique. Pharmacological stress is most commonly administered by adenosine [24]. Both visual estimation of wall motion defects and perfusion abnormalities assessed by administration of gadolinium contrast enhance its ability to detect ischaemic defects (Fig. 13.6).

The traditional anatomical reference standard technique in the assessment of CAD is invasive coronary angiography, which has high spatial and temporal resolution. Accuracy in lesion characterisation is improved through the use of intravascular ultrasound [25]. Furthermore, fractional flow reserve (FFR) measures the trans-stenotic gradient at maximal hyperaemia with revascularisation recommended at FFR <0.8 [26].

Computed tomography coronary angiography (CTCA) has emerged as a reliable and safe imaging modality [27]. Coronary arteries are evaluated by the use of peripherally injected contrast and are reconstructed by multi-slice imaging of the LV. With increasing spatial resolution, CTCA has a high detection rate of atherosclerotic lesions (Table 13.1) [27]. However, high heart rate and ectopy can affect image quality. Nonetheless, this test is extremely helpful for the detection of nonobstructive plaque, the recognition of which may lead to better control of risk factors, especially LDL cholesterol, with favourable impacts on outcomes [28]. Coronary flow reserve calculations are also possible with CT (Fig. 13.7).

13.4.4 Treatment

13.4.4.1 Lifestyle Modifications

Weight loss and dietary modifications are important in preventing and managing CAD in T2DM and hypertension. Obesity is a major driving factor of CVD, with weight loss correlating with improvements in insulin sensitivity and lipid profile [33]. In obese patients, metabolic surgery was associated with a 39% reduction in

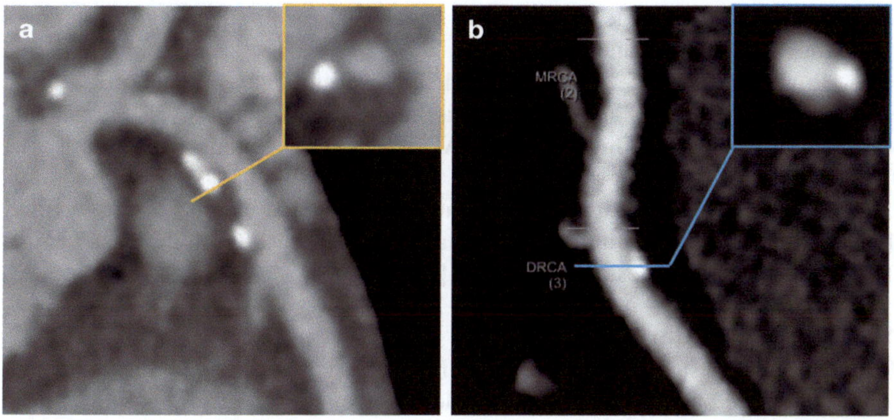

Fig. 13.7 CT coronary angiogram showing mixed (**a**) and calcified (**b**) atherosclerotic plaques

the primary endpoint of all-cause mortality, MI, stroke, HF, nephropathy and atrial fibrillation compared to nonsurgical patients (HR 0.61 [95% CI 0.55–0.69], $p < 0.001$) [34]. Low salt, reduced fat, low carbohydrate and limiting red meat intake are the key messages in dietary modifications [33]. Physical activity, recommended as 30 minutes of moderate intensity exercise at least five times a week, has been shown to reduce both HbA1c and waist circumference [33]. Finally, smoking cessation is paramount in reducing CVD risk.

13.4.4.2 Primary Prevention

Screening for atherosclerotic CAD is not recommended in asymptomatic T2DM. In the DIAD study, diabetic patients without prior CVD were randomised to screening with myocardial perfusion imaging or no screening [35]. There was no significant reduction in the primary outcome of cardiac death of non-fatal MI between the two groups (HR 0.88 [95% CI 0.44–1.88], $p = 0.73$).

The American Diabetes Association (ADA) recommends a fasting lipid profile upon diagnosis of T2DM [33]. Moderate-dose statin therapy is recommended in those with elevated cholesterol, aged 40–75 years. A weaker recommendation of high-dose statin is suggested for those with multiple CVD risk factors.

Low-dose aspirin therapy in T2DM patients with high CVD risk is also recommended [33]. The ASCEND trial randomised T2DM patients without prior CVD to aspirin 100mg daily or placebo [36]. Aspirin reduced the primary endpoint of vascular death, MI and stroke/transient ischaemic attack (TIA) by 12% ($p = 0.01$). However, there was no difference in non-fatal MI between the two groups (RR 0.98 [95% CI 0.80–1.19]), and there was higher rate major bleeding in the aspirin group (RR 1.29 [95% CI 1.09–1.52], $p = 0.003$).

A BP target of <140/90 mmHg is recommended in patients with T2DM [33]. However, those at high CVD risk are suggested to have tighter control at <130/80 mmHg. First-line agents recommended are angiotensin-converting enzyme inhibitors (ACEi) or angiotensin-II receptor blocker (ARB), particularly in those with proteinuria. These agents reduce BP but also have anti-atherosclerotic properties through an anti-oxidant effect [37].

A HbA1c target of 6.5% is recommended; however a relaxed target of 7.5–8.0% is advised for the elderly and those with a limited life expectancy [38]. In patients without established or a high risk of CAD, the ADA recommends metformin as first-line therapy of hyperglycaemia [39]. Metformin is the most widely used anti-diabetic drug, is relatively inexpensive and has few side effects. In the UKPDS 10-year follow-up, metformin was associated with reduced CVD death and MI in T2DM patients without established CVD [40].

13.4.4.3 Secondary Prevention

In patients with established CAD, high-intensity statin therapy is recommended with emphasis on lowering LDL cholesterol by ≥50% from baseline [41]. Antiplatelet therapy is also recommended. Guideline recommendations for target BP in established CAD stand at <130/80 mmHg; however recent evidence suggests that intensive BP control might not be safe in T2DM and treatment targets need to be individualised [42].

Upfront combination antidiabetic therapy is recommended in T2DM patients deemed at high CVD risk or have established atherosclerotic CVD. Metformin in combination with either a glucagon-like protein-1 receptor agonist (GLP-1 RA) or sodium glucose co-transporter-2 (SGLT-2) inhibitor is suggested in this patient group [39].

GLP-1 is a component of the incretin hormonal system [43]. It enhances the release of insulin from the pancreas, delays gastric emptying and has beneficial effects on BP. The GLP-1 RA has shown to not only improve HbA1c levels but also has beneficial effects on weight and BP control. A meta-analysis showed that GLP-1 RA reduced the outcomes of fatal or non-fatal myocardial infarction by 9% (HR 0.91 [95% CI 0.84–1.00], $p = 0.043$) [44].

The SGLT2 inhibitors promote glucose excretion via the kidneys, by inhibiting its reuptake at the proximal convoluted tubules [45]. The SGLT2 inhibitors have beneficial effects on glycaemic control and weight. Furthermore, empagliflozin reduced both systolic and diastolic BP by 2.46 mmHg and 1.46 mmHg, respectively [46]. A meta-analysis of three major CV outcome trials of SGLT2 inhibitors showed a 14% reduction in the composite endpoint of MI, stroke and cardiovascular death (HR 0.86 [95% CI 0.90–0.93]) [45].

13.4.4.4 Invasive Management

There is a large evidence base comparing coronary artery bypass grafting (CABG) and percutaneous coronary intervention (PCI) in T2DM patients. In those with stable CAD, CABG compared to PCI is associated with lower rates of MI and repeat revascularisation months post-procedure [47]. Furthermore, in the FREEDOM follow-on study with a median follow-up of 7.5 years, the PCI drug-eluting stent group had a higher rate of all-cause mortality compared to the CABG group (HR 1.36 [95% CI 1.07–1.74], $p = 0.01$) [48].

In the setting of ST-segment elevation MI (STEMI), guidelines clearly recommend primary PCI as the revascularisation strategy of choice in all patients [47]. However, in patients with non-STEMI, controversy exists in which treatment is optimal in T2DM patients with multi-vessel disease (MVD). Current evidence suggests that CABG is superior to PCI in reducing long-term major adverse cardiac outcomes and all-cause mortality [49].

13.5 Cardiomyopathy in Hypertensive Diabetic Patients

Heart failure is a well-documented complication of T2DM and hypertension. When the latter conditions occur simultaneously, the resultant cardiomyopathy often occurs earlier and is a severe phenotype [1]. With hypertension, both systolic and diastolic BP are associated with an increased risk of HF. In fact, there is a linear relationship between systolic BP and risk of HF in the elderly [4]. In T2DM, HF is the most common CV complication and occurs four times more frequently than in the general population [50]. Furthermore, sex differences were observed in the Framingham study, with the risk of HF in T2DM increasing by more than twofold in men and fivefold in women [51].

13.5.1 Pathophysiology

Diabetic cardiomyopathy refers to the development of HF in the absence of ischaemic CAD [50]. The systemic effects of T2DM influence metabolic pathways within the myocardium and extracellular matrix (ECM) resulting in the cardiomyopathy.

Myocardial stiffening in T2DM is caused by increased intracellular calcium [52]. This results from decreased activity of the calcium pump on the sarcoplasmic reticulum due to reductions in glucose uptake, glucose transporter type-4 (GLUT-4) expression on the plasma membrane and eNOS activity in the endothelium [52]. Cardiomyocyte hypertrophy due to activation of the insulin-like growth factor-1 receptor is caused by hyperinsulinaemia [52]. Furthermore, intracellular and extracellular fibrosis as a result collagen and fibrin deposition are classic pathological findings [53]. Fibrosis in T2DM is driven by activation of the RAAS and sympathetic nervous systems, increase in advanced glycated end products, hyperinsulinaemia and altered degradation of the ECM [53].

Adenosine monophosphate-activated protein kinase (AMPK) is a ubiquitously expressed enzyme that acts as a master energy sensor [54]. In energy-depleted states, it is activated by AMP. In T2DM, in the presence of hyperglycaemia, lipid and amino acid accumulation, insulin resistance and inflammation, AMPK is inhibited resulting in reduced glucose utilisation within cardiomyocytes and a switch to free fatty acids as the primary energy source. This causes impaired oxidative phosphorylation and an increase in the production of ROS by the mitochondria [54].

In the cardiomyopathy associated with hypertensive diabetic subjects, the major pathological findings are myocardial fibrosis and hypertrophy. Fibrosis develops in response to the constant stress imposed on the myocardium by persistent hypertension [55]. It is initiated by the activation and transformation of cardiac fibroblasts to myofibroblasts increasing the deposition of proteins, fibrin and collagen and disrupting ECM turnover. Furthermore, hypertension also enhances inflammation further promoting ECM fibrosis [55].

LV remodelling is another key finding of hypertensive heart disease. Increased LV wall stress causes elevated cavity pressure and radius resulting in increased myocardial oxygen demand and impaired myocardial shortening; subsequently a compensatory hypertrophy develops. The increase in myocardial workload causes increased myocardial blood flow; however maximum flow is reduced [56]. This reduction in hyperaemic response is driven by external compression by fibrosis and coronary microvascular dysfunction. Impairment in coronary blood flow ultimately results in microvascular ischaemia further propagating cardiac fibrosis and dysfunction [56].

13.5.2 Clinical Features

The American College of Cardiology and American Heart Association define HF as a disease that progresses depending on clinical signs and evidence of structural heart disease (Table 13.2) [57]. Although it is a continuum, the number of people within each stage decreases as the severity increases. In fact, the prevalence of stage B HF is four times that of stage C and D [58]. Thus, risk factor management is key in preventing disease progression.

HF can present with a vast array of clinical signs and symptoms. Its diagnosis can be challenging particularly given that patients can present with non-specific symptoms [59]. Shortness of breath is the most sensitive symptom of HF; however, orthopnoea is more specific (Table 13.3). Physical examination findings can range from tachycardia to fluid overload, evidenced as elevated jugular venous pressure or crepitations on respiratory examination [59].

Table 13.2 The American College of Cardiology/American Heart Association stages of heart failure definitions. Adapted from Yancy et al. (2013). JACC; 62(16): e147–239 [57]

Stage	Definition
A	CVD risk factors for the development of HF No symptoms or clinical signs of HF No evidence of structural heart disease
B	Presence of structural heart disease (e.g. LV systolic impairment, diastolic dysfunction) No symptoms or clinical signs of HF
C	Present or prior symptoms or signs of HF Evidence of structural heart disease
D	End-stage HF with refractory symptoms and signs despite maximal tolerate medical therapy Require specialised treatment

Table 13.3 Sensitivity and specificity of clinical signs and symptoms of HF. Reproduced from Watson et al. (2000). BMJ;320:236–239 [59]

Clinical feature	Sensitivity (%)	Specificity (%)
History		
Shortness of breath	66	52
Orthopnoea	21	81
PND	33	76
Oedema	23	80
Examination		
Tachycardia	7	99
Crepitations	13	91
Oedema	10	93
S3 heart sound	31	95
Elevated JVP	10	97

JVP Jugular venous pressure, *PND* Paroxysmal nocturnal dyspnoea

13.5.3 Imaging Findings

Echocardiography is the gold-standard imaging modality in diagnosing HF. The primary goal is to assess LV function, which is dependent on both contractility of the myocardium and loading conditions which can be altered in T2DM, but particularly in hypertension.

Clinically, stage B HF is hallmarked by subclinical LV dysfunction in the absence of HF symptoms. In hypertensive diabetic cardiomyopathy, changes in geometry and diastolic function are early manifestations of LV dysfunction. LVH can be identified on two-dimensional echocardiography and it is usually concentric [1]. It is indexed to body surface area (BSA); however BSA can underestimate LVH in obese patients [60]. Thus, other methods used for indexation are height$^{1.7}$ or height$^{2.7}$ [60]. Three-dimensional (3D) echocardiography has optimised the assessment of LV volume and mass.

A structural sign of diastolic dysfunction (DD) is left atrial (LA) enlargement measured as volume indexed to BSA [60]. Diastolic function is also evaluated with Doppler imaging which assesses movement based on frequency shifts in the ultrasound signal; therefore, it can study blood flow through structures of the heart. Transmitral Doppler flow is seen as an E- and A-wave, representing early passive and active LV filling by atrial contraction, respectively (Fig. 13.8). Early features of impaired relaxation are a reduced E-wave and elevated A-wave [60]. Tissue Doppler imaging (TDI) is a technique that quantifies velocity of blood through myocardial tissue and effectively measures motion through the cardiac cycle. Two key measurements of velocity at the mitral valve annulus are e' (early diastolic) and a' (atrial contraction) (Fig. 13.9) [61]. The E/e' ratio is derived and is a measure of LV filling pressure. Elevated LV filling pressure is suggested when E/e' is greater than 14 [61].

Pulmonary vein (PV) flow is another modality used in the assessment of diastolic function [60]. Normal PV flow has two positive deflections, the S- and D-components representing atrial relaxation and flow into the LA during LV

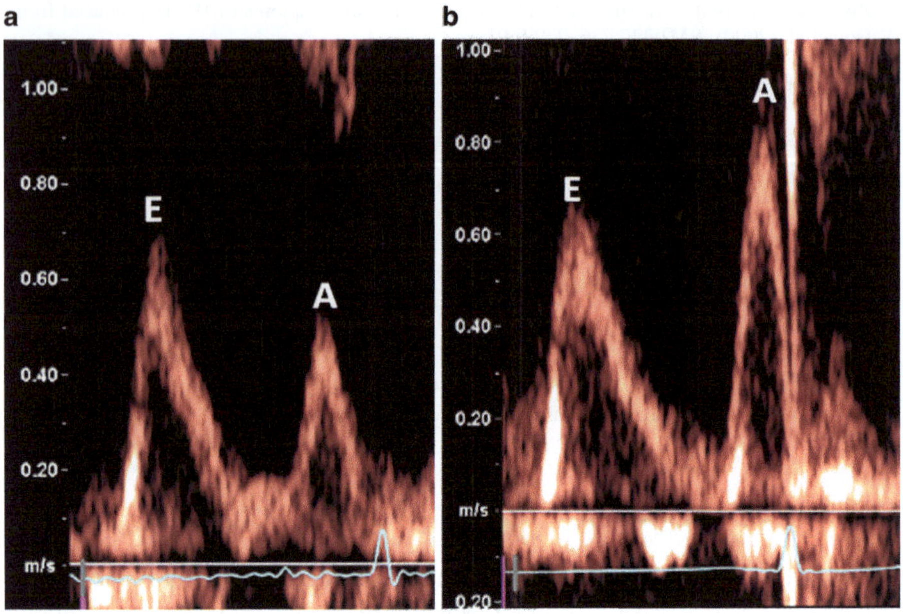

Fig. 13.8 Transmitral flow with normal (**a**) and impaired relaxation (**b**)

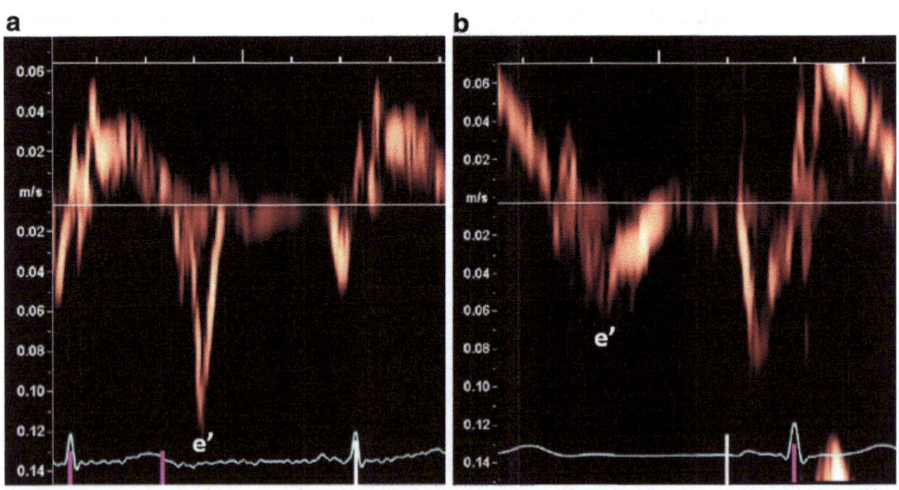

Fig. 13.9 Tissue Doppler imaging at the medial mitral valve annulus lateral showing normal velocity (**a**) and reduced velocity (**b**) through the cardiac cycle

diastole, respectively (Fig. 13.10). A negative deflection (A reversal) represents blood flow into the PV during atrial contraction. With rising LA pressure, the amplitude of the S-component is reduced and the D-component and duration of A are both increased [60].

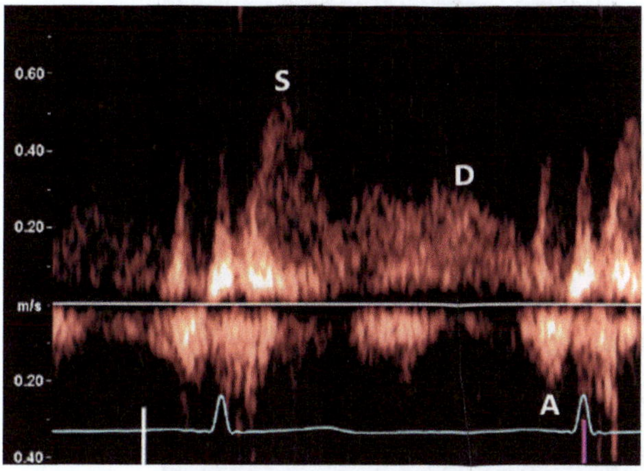

Fig. 13.10 Pulmonary vein flow hallmarked by the S-component (atrial relaxation), D-component (flow into the left atrium) and A (reversal of flow into the pulmonary vein due to atrial contraction)

LV systolic function can be measured in multiple ways. Ejection fraction (EF) is the most commonly used approach; however it lacks reproducibility, is insensitive to minor changes in LV function and has geometric assumptions [62]. Its measurement can be improved with 3D echocardiography, but its limitations are not completely resolved. Speckle tracking echocardiography (STE) assesses myocardial deformation and LV strain. It is a dimensionless index that measures change in length between two points; thus, a negative number is derived due to myocardial shortening during systole (Fig. 13.11). Global longitudinal strain (GLS) is a reproducible, sensitive and reliable measure of LV function. Compared to EF, GLS can detect early impairment of systolic function particularly in stage B HF [62].

The two primary manifestations of overt HF are defined by EF: either reduced (HFrEF) or preserved (HFpEF) [63]. HFpEF is defined as a normal EF coupled with diastolic impairment. However, implying normal systolic function can be misleading as GLS can be reduced despite a diagnosis of HFpEF [61].

Cardiac MRI is another imaging modality that can be used in the diagnosis of hypertensive diabetic cardiomyopathy [61]. It has greater temporal and spatial resolution than echocardiography. Therefore, it is more accurate in the measurement of chamber size, LV mass, volume and ejection fraction. Tissue characterisation can be assessed with the use of T1- and T2-weighted imaging [61]. Administration of gadolinium contrast can be used to evaluate myocardial scarring patterns to differentiate the cause of the cardiomyopathy. Furthermore, adenosine stress perfusion cardiac MRI is useful in the assessment of microvascular disease in diabetic cardiomyopathy. Coronary flow reserve is reduced in this cohort and is related to increased major adverse cardiovascular outcomes [64].

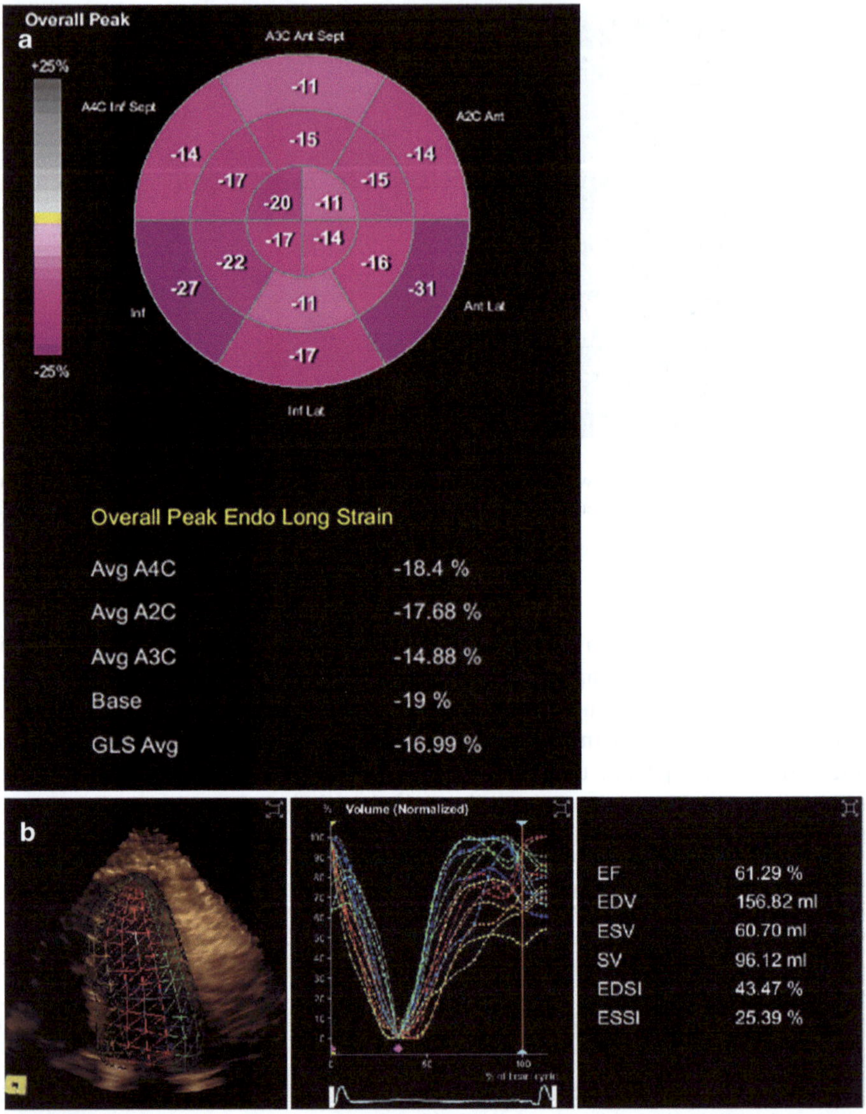

Fig. 13.11 Reduced global longitudinal strain (**a**) despite normal left ventricular ejection fraction (EF) (**b**) in an asymptomatic patient with type 2 diabetes mellitus and hypertension

13.5.4 Treatment

Many of the pillars of lifestyle and risk factor management discussed above hold true for the management of a hypertensive diabetic cardiomyopathy [1]. However, particular importance is directed towards a low-sodium diet and weight loss in this group of patients.

13.5.4.1 Blood Pressure Management

Control of BP is important in managing LVH. Studies have shown that adequately controlled BP with the use of an ACEi/ARB or diuretic therapy can cause LV mass regression [65]. Furthermore, in the TOMHS study BP reduction with combination antihypertensive therapy coupled with weight loss showed LV mass regression at 4 years [66].

13.5.4.2 Diabetes Management

In observational studies metformin has shown mortality benefits in diabetic HF patients and particularly in the HFpEF group [67]. In a study on progression of echocardiographic parameters over time, metformin had no effect on GLS, but deterioration in E/e' and e' was avoided in the metformin group [68].

The SGLT2 inhibitors have shown benefit in HF in several randomised controlled trials. In a meta-analysis of the three seminal SGLT2 inhibitor CV outcome trials, in patients with atherosclerotic CVD, hospitalisation for HF and CV death was reduced by 24% (HR 0.76 [95% CI 0.69–0.84]) [45]. Furthermore, in the DAPA-HF trial, in patients with symptomatic HF with an LVEF <40%, dapagliflozin 10mg daily was shown to reduce the primary endpoint of hospitalisation from HF and CV death by 26% (HR 0.74 [95% CI 0.65–0.85], $p < 0.001$) [69].

The use of GLP-1 RA in HF has been studied in three small randomised controlled trials, all with patients with reduced ejection fraction. Results were neutral on HF outcomes [70]. However, these studies did show that GLP-1 RA is safe to use in HF patients. There is no study to date on the effects of GLP-1 RA in HFpEF.

13.5.4.3 Heart Failure Management

Management of stage B HF centralises around risk factor management; however, ACEi/ARB is recommended in those with reduced EF [57]. In established HFrEF, medications with a class I-A recommendation should be initiated to reduce morbidity and mortality outcomes [63]. These are added sequentially and up-titrated to the maximal tolerated doses. Traditionally these include ACEi/ARB, cardio-selective beta blocker and aldosterone receptor agonists. Newer therapies such as sinoatrial node modulators (ivabradine) and angiotensin receptor-neprilysin inhibitors (ARNI) are also suggested but carry a recommendation level of IIa-B and I-B, respectively [63]. In HFpEF treatment options are limited; however symptom control with diuretic therapy and management of risk factors is advised [57].

13.6 Conclusions

Hypertension and T2DM are strong risk factors for heart disease. This is driven by several deranged mechanical, inflammatory and metabolic processes that alter the normal functioning of the myocardium and coronary arteries. When hypertension and T2DM co-exist, the development of heart disease is accelerated and more severe. Therefore, emphasis on early diagnosis and risk factor management is important in preventing the development of cardiac complications.

References

1. Grossman E, Messerli FH. Hypertension and diabetes. Adv Cardiol. 2008;45:82–106.
2. Einarson TR, Acs A, Ludwig C, Panton UH. Prevalence of cardiovascular disease in type 2 diabetes: a systematic literature review of scientific evidence from across the world in 2007-2017. Cardiovasc Diabetol. 2018;17(1):83.
3. Luo D, Cheng Y, Zhang H, Ba M, Chen P, Li H, et al. Association between high blood pressure and long term cardiovascular events in young adults: systematic review and meta-analysis. BMJ. 2020;370:m3222.
4. Butler J, Kalogeropoulos AP, Georgiopoulou VV, Bibbins-Domingo K, Najjar SS, Sutton-Tyrrell KC, et al. Systolic blood pressure and incident heart failure in the elderly. The Cardiovascular Health Study and the Health, Ageing and Body Composition Study. Heart. 2011;97(16):1304–11.
5. Sousa AC, Jardim TV, Costa TO, Magalhães FG, Montelo MPM, Souza WKB, et al. Hypertensive diabetic patients: incidence of cardiovascular and renal outcomes in a historical cohort over 11 years. Diabetol Metab Syndr. 2017;9:98.
6. Eryd SA, Gudbjörnsdottir S, Manhem K, Rosengren A, Svensson A, Miftaraj M, et al. Blood pressure and complications in individuals with type 2 diabetes and no previous cardiovascular disease: national population based cohort study. BMJ. 2016;354:i4070.
7. Hypertension in Diabetes Study (HDS): II. Increased risk of cardiovascular complications in hypertensive type 2 diabetic patients. J Hypertens. 1993;11(3):319–25.
8. Stratton IM, Adler AI, Neil HA, Matthews DR, Manley SE, Cull CA, et al. Association of glycaemia with macrovascular and microvascular complications of type 2 diabetes (UKPDS 35): prospective observational study. BMJ. 2000;321(7258):405–12.
9. Donath MY, Shoelson SE. Type 2 diabetes as an inflammatory disease. Nat Rev Immunol. 2011;11(2):98–107.
10. de Luca C, Olefsky JM. Stressed out about obesity and insulin resistance. Nat Med. 2006;12(1):41–2; discussion 42.
11. Vinik AI, Erbas T, Casellini CM. Diabetic cardiac autonomic neuropathy, inflammation and cardiovascular disease. J Diabetes Investig. 2013;4(1):4–18.
12. Oparil S, Acelajado MC, Bakris GL, Berlowitz DR, Cífková R, Dominiczak AF, et al. Hypertension. Nat Rev Dis Primers. 2018;4:18,014.
13. Franklin SS, Khan SA, Wong ND, Larson MG, Levy D. Is pulse pressure useful in predicting risk for coronary heart Disease? The Framingham heart study. Circulation. 1999;100(4):354–60.
14. Sowers JR, Epstein M, Frohlich ED. Diabetes, hypertension, and cardiovascular disease: an update. Hypertension. 2001;37(4):1053–9.
15. Boucher J, Kleinridders A, Kahn CR. Insulin receptor signaling in normal and insulin-resistant states. Cold Spring Harb Perspect Biol. 2014;6(1):a009191.
16. Yu Q, Gao F, Ma XL. Insulin says NO to cardiovascular disease. Cardiovasc Res. 2011;89(3):516–24.
17. Tang WH, Martin KA, Hwa J. Aldose reductase, oxidative stress, and diabetic mellitus. Front Pharmacol. 2012;3:87.
18. Bornfeldt KE, Tabas I. Insulin resistance, hyperglycemia, and atherosclerosis. Cell Metab. 2011;14(5):575–85.
19. Endtmann C, Ebrahimian T, Czech T, Arfa O, Laufs U, Fritz M, et al. Angiotensin II impairs endothelial progenitor cell number and function in vitro and in vivo: implications for vascular regeneration. Hypertension. 2011;58(3):394–403.
20. DeVon HA, Mirzaei S, Zegre-Hemsey J. Typical and atypical symptoms of acute coronary syndrome: time to retire the terms? J Am Heart Assoc. 2020;9(7):e015539.
21. Devon HA, Rosenfeld A, Steffen AD, Daya M. Sensitivity, specificity, and sex differences in symptoms reported on the 13-item acute coronary syndrome checklist. J Am Heart Assoc. 2014;3(2):e000586.

22. Underwood SR, Anagnostopoulos C, Cerqueira M, Ell PJ, Flint EJ, Harbinson M, et al. Myocardial perfusion scintigraphy: the evidence. Eur J Nucl Med Mol Imaging. 2004;31(2):261–91.
23. Marwick TH. Stress echocardiography. Heart. 2003;89(1):113–8.
24. Jerosch-Herold M, Seethamraju RT, Swingen CM, Wilke NM, Stillman AE. Analysis of myocardial perfusion MRI. J Magn Reson Imaging. 2004;19(6):758–70.
25. Nissen S. Coronary angiography and intravascular ultrasound. Am J Cardiol. 2001;87(4A):15A–20A.
26. Balanescu S. Fractional flow reserve assessment of coronary artery stenosis. Eur Cardiol. 2016;11(2):77–82.
27. Meijboom WB, Meijs MFL, Schuijf JD, Cramer MJ, Mollet NR, van Mieghem CAG, et al. Diagnostic accuracy of 64-slice computed tomography coronary angiography: a prospective, multicenter, multivendor study. J Am Coll Cardiol. 2008;52(25):2135–44.
28. Newby DE, Adamson PD, Berry C, Boon NA, Dweck MR, Flather M, et al. SCOT-HEART Investigators. Coronary CT angiography and 5-year risk of myocardial infarction. N Engl J Med. 2018;379(10):924–33.
29. Fleischmann KE, Hunink MGM, Kuntz KM, Douglas PS. Exercise echocardiography or exercise SPECT imaging? A meta-analysis of diagnostic test performance. JAMA. 1998;280(10):913–20.
30. Senior R, Monaghan M, Becher H, Mayet J, Nihoyannopoulos P, British Society of Echocardiography. Stress echocardiography for the diagnosis and risk stratification of patients with suspected or known coronary artery disease: a critical appraisal. Supported by the British Society of Echocardiography. Heart. 2005;91(4):427–36.
31. Hamon M, Fau G, Née G, Ehtisham J, Morello R, Hamon M. Meta-analysis of the diagnostic performance of stress perfusion cardiovascular magnetic resonance for detection of coronary artery disease. J Cardiovasc Magn Reson. 2010;12:29.
32. Ghersin E, Keidar Z, Rispler S, Litmanovich D, Bar-Shalom R, Roguin A, et al. Images in cardiovascular medicine. Hybrid cardiac single photon emission computed tomography/computed tomography imaging with myocardial perfusion single photon emission computed tomography and multidetector computed tomography coronary angiography for the assessment of unstable angina pectoris after coronary artery bypass grafting. Circulation. 2006;114(6):e237–9.
33. American Diabetes Association. 10. Cardiovascular disease and risk management: standards of medical care in diabetes-2020. Diabetes Care. 2020;43(Suppl 1):S111–34.
34. Aminian A, Zajichek A, Arterburn DE, Wolski KE, Brethauer SA, Schauer PR, et al. Association of metabolic surgery with major adverse cardiovascular outcomes in patients with type 2 diabetes and obesity. JAMA. 2019;322(13):1271–82.
35. Young LH, Wackers FJT, Chyun DA, Davey JA, Barrett EJ, Raymond Tailleferet R, et al. Cardiac outcomes after screening for asymptomatic coronary artery disease in patients with type 2 diabetes: the DIAD study: a randomized controlled trial. JAMA. 2009;301(15):1547–55.
36. ASCEND Study Collaborative Group, Louise Bowman L, Mafham M, Wallendszus K, Stevens W, Buck G, Barton J, et al. Effects of aspirin for primary prevention in persons with diabetes mellitus. N Engl J Med. 2018;379(16):1529–39.
37. Hurtubise J, McLellan K, Durr K, Onasanya O, Nwabuko D, Ndisang JF. The different facets of dyslipidemia and hypertension in atherosclerosis. Curr Atheroscler Rep. 2016;18(12):82.
38. American Diabetes Association. 9. Cardiovascular disease and risk management: standards of medical care in diabetes-2018. Diabetes Care. 2018;41(Suppl 1):S86–104.
39. American Diabetes Association. 9. Pharmacologic approaches to glycemic treatment: standards of medical care in diabetes-2020. Diabetes Care. 2020;43(Suppl 1):S98–110.
40. Holman RR, Paul SK, Bethel MA, Matthews DR, Neil HAW. 10-year follow-up of intensive glucose control in type 2 diabetes. N Engl J Med. 2008;359(15):1577–89.
41. Grundy SM, Stone NJ, Bailey AL, Craig Beam C, Birtcher KK, Blumenthal RS, et al. 2018 AHA/ACC/AACVPR/AAPA/ABC/ACPM/ADA/AGS/APhA/ASPC/NLA/PCNA Guideline on the Management of Blood Cholesterol: A Report of the American College of Cardiology/

American Heart Association Task Force on Clinical Practice Guidelines. J Am Coll Cardiol. 2019;73(24):e285–350.
42. Deedwania P. The ongoing saga of optimal blood pressure level in patients with diabetes mellitus and coronary artery disease. J Am Heart Assoc. 2018;7(20):e010752.
43. Del Olmo-Garcia MI, J.F. Merino-Torres JF. GLP-1 receptor agonists and cardiovascular disease in patients with type 2 diabetes. J Diabetes Res. 2018;2018:4020492.
44. Kristensen SL, Rørth R, Jhund PS, Docherty KF, Sattar N, Preiss D, et al. Cardiovascular, mortality, and kidney outcomes with GLP-1 receptor agonists in patients with type 2 diabetes: a systematic review and meta-analysis of cardiovascular outcome trials. Lancet Diabetes Endocrinol. 2019;7(10):776–85.
45. Zelniker TA, Wiviott SD, Raz I, Im K, Goodrich EL, Bonaca MP, et al. SGLT2 inhibitors for primary and secondary prevention of cardiovascular and renal outcomes in type 2 diabetes: a systematic review and meta-analysis of cardiovascular outcome trials. Lancet. 2019;393(10166):31–9.
46. Tentolouris A, Vlachakis P, Tzeravini E, Eleftheriadou I, Tentolouris N. SGLT2 inhibitors: a review of their antidiabetic and cardioprotective effects. Int J Environ Res Public Health. 2019;16(16):2965–90.
47. Godoy LC, Rao V, Farkouh ME. Coronary revascularization of patients with diabetes mellitus in the setting of acute coronary syndromes. Circulation. 2019;140(15):1233–5.
48. Farkouh ME, Domanski M, Dangas GD, Godoy LC, Mack MJ, Siami FS, et al. Long-term survival following multivessel revascularization in patients with diabetes: the FREEDOM follow-on study. J Am Coll Cardiol. 2019;73(6):629–38.
49. Ramanathan K, Abel JG, Park JE, Fung A, Mathew V, Taylor CM, et al. Surgical versus percutaneous coronary revascularization in patients with diabetes and acute coronary syndromes. J Am Coll Cardiol. 2017;70(24):2995–3006.
50. Rosano GM, Vitale C, Seferovic P. Heart failure in patients with diabetes mellitus. Card Fail Rev. 2017;3(1):52–5.
51. Kannel WB, Hjortland M, Castelli WP. Role of diabetes in congestive heart failure: the Framingham study. Am J Cardiol. 1974;34(1):29–34.
52. Jia G, DeMarco VG, Sowers JR. Insulin resistance and hyperinsulinaemia in diabetic cardiomyopathy. Nat Rev Endocrinol. 2016;12(3):144–53.
53. Jia G, Hill MA, Sowers JR. Diabetic cardiomyopathy: an update of mechanisms contributing to this clinical entity. Circ Res. 2018;122(4):624–38.
54. Haye A, Ansari MA, Rahman SO, Shamsi Y, Ahmed D, Sharma M. Role of AMP-activated protein kinase on cardio-metabolic abnormalities in the development of diabetic cardiomyopathy: a molecular landscape. Eur J Pharmacol. 2020;888:173376.
55. Nwabuo CC, Vasan RS. Pathophysiology of hypertensive heart disease: beyond left ventricular hypertrophy. Curr Hypertens Rep. 2020;22(2):11.
56. Camici PG, Olivotto I, Rimoldi OE. The coronary circulation and blood flow in left ventricular hypertrophy. J Mol Cell Cardiol. 2012;52(4):857–64.
57. Yancy CW, Jessup M, Bozkurt B, Butler J, Casey DE Jr, Drazner MH, et al. 2013 ACCF/AHA guideline for the management of heart failure: a report of the American College of Cardiology Foundation/American Heart Association Task Force on Practice Guidelines. J Am Coll Cardiol. 2013;62(16):e147–239.
58. Frigerio M, Oliva F, Turazza FM, Bonow RO. Prevention and management of chronic heart failure in management of asymptomatic patients. Am J Cardiol. 2003;91(9A):4F–9F.
59. Watson RD, Gibbs CR, Lip GY. ABC of heart failure. Clinical features and complications. BMJ. 2000;320(7229):236–9.
60. Wang Y, Marwick TH. Update on echocardiographic assessment in diabetes mellitus. Curr Cardiol Rep. 2016;18(9):85.
61. Lorenzo-Almoros A, Tuñón J, Orejas M, Cortés M, Egido J, Lorenzo Ó. Diagnostic approaches for diabetic cardiomyopathy. Cardiovasc Diabetol. 2017;16(1):28.

62. Potter E, Marwick TH. Assessment of left ventricular function by echocardiography: the case for routinely adding global longitudinal strain to ejection fraction. JACC Cardiovasc Imaging. 2018;11(2 Pt 1):260–74.
63. Yancy CW, Jessup M, Bozkurt B, Butler J, Casey DE Jr, Colvin MM, et al. 2017 ACC/AHA/HFSA focused update of the 2013 ACCF/AHA guideline for the management of heart failure: a report of the American College of Cardiology/American Heart Association Task Force on Clinical Practice Guidelines and the Heart Failure Society of America. J Am Coll Cardiol. 2017;70(6):776–803.
64. Kato S, Fukui K, Kodama S, Azuma M, Iwasawa T, Kimura K, et al. Incremental prognostic value of coronary flow reserve determined by phase-contrast cine cardiovascular magnetic resonance of the coronary sinus in patients with diabetes mellitus. J Cardiovasc Magn Reson. 2020;22(1):73.
65. Diamond JA, Phillips RA. Hypertensive heart disease. Hypertens Res. 2005;28(3):191–202.
66. Neaton JD, Grimm RH Jr, Prineas RJ, Stamler J, Grandits GA, Elmer PJ, et al. Treatment of Mild Hypertension Study. Final results. Treatment of Mild Hypertension Study Research Group. JAMA. 1993;270(6):713–24.
67. Halabi A, Sen J, Huynh Q, Marwick TH. Metformin treatment in heart failure with preserved ejection fraction: a systematic review and meta-regression analysis. Cardiovasc Diabetol. 2020;19(1):124–34.
68. Halabi A, Yang H, Wright L, Potter E, Huynh Q, Negishi K, et al. Evolution of myocardial dysfunction in asymptomatic patients at risk of heart failure. JACC Cardiovasc Imaging. 2021;14(2):350–61.
69. McMurray JJV, Docherty KF, Jhund PS. Dapagliflozin in patients with heart failure and reduced ejection fraction. Reply. N Engl J Med. 2020;382(10):973.
70. Khan MS, Fonarow GC, McGuire DK, Hernandez AF, Vaduganathan M, Rosenstock J, et al. Glucagon-like peptide 1 receptor agonists and heart failure: the need for further evidence generation and practice guidelines optimization. Circulation. 2020;142(12):1205–18.

14 Cerebrovascular Structural Alterations/Dysautonomic Disorders in Diabetes Mellitus

Damiano Rizzoni and Paolo Desenzani

14.1 Introduction

Diabetes mellitus has long been known to be able to determinate consequences on the structure and function of the brain. Since the early twentieth century, it has been observed that diabetic patients frequently complained of poor memory and attention [1]. In 1922, Miles and Root [2] showed that people with diabetes performed poorly on cognitive tasks, namely, those involving memory and attention. The term "diabetic encephalopathy" was proposed in the 1950s to describe central nervous system-related complications of diabetes [3]. Other terms like "functional cerebral impairment" and "central neuropathy" have also been proposed to describe diabetes-related cognitive impairment, and the term "diabetes-associated cognitive decline" was proposed to describe diabetes-related mild to moderate reductions in cognitive functions [4].

Since the prevalence of diabetes mellitus is growing rapidly throughout the world, diabetes-related cognitive dysfunction could have challenging future public health implications [5]. In this chapter we will cover available data concerning how diabetes affects the central nervous system, in particular brain function and structure. In addition, we will also address pathophysiologic characteristics of diabetic autonomic disorders.

D. Rizzoni (✉)
Division of Medicine, Spedali Civili di Brescia, Montichiari, Brescia, Italy

Clinica Medica, Department of Clinical and Experimental Sciences, University of Brescia, Brescia, Italy
e-mail: damiano.rizzoni@unibs.it

P. Desenzani
Division of Medicine, Spedali Civili di Brescia, Montichiari, Brescia, Italy

A. E. Berbari, G. Mancia (eds.), *Blood Pressure Disorders in Diabetes Mellitus*, Updates in Hypertension and Cardiovascular Protection,
https://doi.org/10.1007/978-3-031-13009-0_14

14.2 Cerebrovascular Structural Alterations

14.2.1 Atherosclerosis and Stroke

Atherosclerotic disease often involves the intracranial and extracranial arteries [6]. Age, hypertension, and diabetes mellitus are independent risk factors for intracranial as well as extracranial atherosclerosis [6], which can result in thromboembolism with or without hypoperfusion leading to transient or permanent cerebral ischemic events [7], thus possibly having functional consequences, including cognitive decline, vascular dementia, and even depression [6, 8].

Diabetes is also a well-established independent risk factor for stroke. In the INTERSTROKE study, a 22-nation case-control study, the presence of diabetes increased the risk of stroke by 36% [9]. In the Framingham Study, diabetic males who were in their fifth and sixth decades of life had a fourfold increase in the incidence of stroke, while females in the sixth decade had a fourfold increase and in the seventh decade a threefold increase [9]. In a large biracial population from the Cincinnati/Northern Kentucky area of the Unites States, there was a five- to 14-fold increased risk of stroke in diabetic subjects who were between the ages of 20 and 65 years [9]. A prospective Japanese study showed that for both male and female diabetic subjects, there was two- to fourfold higher rate of all types of ischemic stroke without an association with intraparenchymal or subarachnoid hemorrhage [9]. In type 1 diabetes mellitus (T1DM), the increase in the incidence of stroke is even greater than in the type 2 diabetes mellitus (T2DM). In the prospective Nurses' Study, those with T2DM had a 2.3-fold increase in the incidence of stroke, whereas those with T1DM had a 6.3-fold increase when compared with nondiabetic individuals [9]. Unlike T2DM, T1DM was associated with a 3.8-fold increased risk of hemorrhagic stroke. The major source of extracranial embolism causing an ischemic stroke in the diabetic patient is the extracranial portion of the internal carotid artery. Furthermore, diffuse atherosclerotic disease (multiple atherosclerotic lesions in the coronary, carotid, and iliofemoral arteries) is more prevalent in those subjects with T2DM who have a stroke, especially when atherosclerosis is accompanied by hypertension [9].

14.2.2 Imaging Studies on Diabetes and Brain Structure

Type 1 diabetes Structural magnetic resonance imaging (MRI) techniques are commonly used to examine the possible consequences of diabetes on the brain structure, in particular on total and regional brain volumes [5]. Structural MRI studies have shown lower gray and white volumes in subject with T1DM compared to nondiabetic controls [5]. Diffusion tensor imaging (DTI) can identify white matter microstructural deficits by measuring the directionally restrained diffusion of water (anisotropy) within fiber tracts [5]. When fiber bundles are damaged, a reduction in fractional anisotropy (due to the loss of restriction of water movement) is to be expected. Kodl et al. [10] reported white matter microstructural deficits in the posterior corona radiata and the optic radiation in a DTI study in subjects who had diabetes for at least 15 years [9]; these changes correlated with lower performance in cognitive tests, probably as a consequence of an impairment of white matter function [5].

In vivo brain magnetic resonance spectroscopy may be used to noninvasively quantify concentration of various metabolites, and lower N-acetylaspartate (probably a marker of neuronal dysfunction) and glutamate concentration in gray matter-rich occipital lobe of patients with T1DM was observed [11].

Type 2 diabetes People with T2DM have also been shown to have brain atrophy [12] including lower total and regional white and gray matter volumes, as compared to nondiabetic controls [5]. Moran et al. [13] showed that subjects with T2DM had lower total gray, white, and hippocampal volumes; in the medial temporal, anterior cingulate, and medial frontal lobes, a loss of gray matter was clearly observed, while white matter loss was found mainly in the frontal and temporal regions [5, 13]. In this study it was also observed that brain volume loss was associated with poor performance in cognitive testing [13]. Other studies have suggested that atrophy may be particularly pronounced in the hippocampal region [14]. In people with long-standing, less strictly controlled type 2 diabetes, white matter hyperintensity volumes were associated with decreased processing speed [15]. This suggests that cerebral small vessel disease may be a mechanism underlying cognitive dysfunction in these individuals [15].

In a systematic review of DTI studies, the presence of brain microstructural abnormalities in T2DM was confirmed [16]. Twenty-nine studies have demonstrated widespread brain microstructural impairment and topological network disorganization in patients with T2DM; microstructural abnormalities were correlated with pathological derangements in the endocrine profile as well as deficits in cognitive performance in the domains of memory, information-processing speed, executive function, and attention [16]. Therefore, microvascular alterations and dysfunction may play a major role in the development of brain damage in diabetes mellitus and cardiometabolic disease [17, 18]. Also in T2DM altered brain metabolites were detected, to be possibly regarded as noninvasive biomarkers for diabetes-induced brain metabolic changes during progression of the disease [19].

14.3 Cognitive Function

14.3.1 Type 1 Diabetes

A meta-analysis by Brands et al. [20] examined the nature and extent of cognitive impairment in T1DM. Thirty-three studies were included; participants were mostly less than 50 years of age. Compared to nondiabetic controls, patients with T1DM had mild to moderate declines in multiple domains, including intelligence, speed of information processing, psychomotor efficiency, attention, cognitive flexibility, and visual perception [5, 20]. This lower cognitive performance appeared to be associated with the presence of microvascular complications but not with the occurrence of severe hypoglycemic episodes or with poor metabolic control [5, 20]. Also the pediatric setting was explored in this regard; in fact, Gaudieri et al. [21] preformed a meta-analysis including data from 19 studies in children with T1DM. A decrement in a broad range of domains was found; however the magnitude of decrement was greater in children with an early diagnosis of diabetes (less than 7 years of age) [5, 21]. Therefore, early age of onset may be an important variable of cognitive dysfunction in children with T1DM [5]. In the Diabetes Control and Complications Trial (DCCT) and its follow-up Epidemiology of Diabetes Interventions and Complications (EDIC) study, it was demonstrated that T1DM patients with worse metabolic control (glycated hemoglobin values >8.8%) showed moderate declines in motor speed and psychomotor efficiency, but this was not the case for those with better control (glycated hemoglobin <7.4%) [22]. Frequency of severe hypoglycemia was not associated with decline in any cognitive domain in this population [5]. Similar results were seen in the Stockholm Diabetes Intervention Study (SDIS), where at 10-year follow-up cognitive function was similar in both treatment groups and was not related to the number of severe hypoglycemic episodes [23].

In summary, T1DM seems to be associated with mild to modest decrements in cognitive function. Domains of psychomotor speed, mental flexibility, attention, and general intelligence are most commonly affected [5].

14.3.2 Type 2 Diabetes

Longitudinal and cross-sectional studies have consistently demonstrated an association between T2DM and mild to moderate cognitive dysfunction, but less is known about the strength of association between T2DM and dementia [5].

Dementia due to both Alzheimer's disease and vascular disease has also been linked to T2DM in longitudinal studies. In the ARIC (Atherosclerosis Risk in Communities) study cohort, Rawkings and colleagues [24] observed that diabetes in midlife was associated with a 19% greater cognitive decline over 20 years. Cognitive decline was noted primarily in the domains of processing speed and executive function and was associated with duration of diabetes [5, 24]. In the Rotterdam Study, a prospective population-based cohort study of more than 6000 elderly subjects, T2DM almost doubled the risk of dementia [25].

Investigators have also performed systematic reviews and meta-analyses to address in more details the problem of the possible association between T2DM and dementia. Biessels et al. [1] reported that risk of dementia was increased by 50–100% in people with T2DM relative to people without diabetes. Processing speed, attention, memory, and cognitive flexibility were the most commonly effected domains in subjects with T2DM [26]. Palta et al. [27] in a meta-analyses of data from 24 studies found small to moderate reductions in the domains of motor function executive function, processing speed verbal memory, and visual memory in people with T2DM.

T2DM or insulin resistance frequently co-occurs with bipolar disorders and is associated with negative psychiatric clinical outcomes and compromised brain health [8, 28].

There are several pathophysiological mechanisms through which diabetes could influence the onset and progress of the various pathologies associated with dementia. Some of these are common to Alzheimer's and vascular dementia, as well as the aging process. In some people with diabetes, vascular damage may be predominant leading to the development of a form of dementia that can be clinically classified as "pure vascular dementia"; in other patients, on the other hand, the mechanisms associated with the formation of beta amyloid plaques predominate, which will lead to the development of a clinical picture that can be classified as "pure Alzheimer's". The majority of patients, on the other hand, present an intermediate clinical picture between these two forms of dementia that can be classified as "mixed."

In synthesis, both T1DM and T2DM have been associated with reduced performance on multiple domains of cognitive function and with evidence of abnormal structure and function of the brain [5, 29]. There are significant differences in the underlying pathophysiology of cognitive impairment between T1DM and T2DM. T1DM is usually diagnosed at an early age and may have effects on brain development [30]. Chronic hyperglycemia and microvascular complications [17, 18] are important risk factors common to both T1DM and T2DM. T2DM is usually diagnosed at an older age and is commonly associated with obesity, insulin resistance, hypertension, and dyslipidemia, all of which can have negative impact on the brain [18].

The pathophysiology underlying the cognitive decline and brain structural changes in subjects with diabetes is poorly understood [5]. Poor glycemic control, microvascular disease [31, 32], oxidative stress, genetic predisposition, insulin resistance, and amyloid disposition have been proposed as possible contributors [5, 33]. Also blood-brain barrier injuries [34, 35] and changes in brain metabolism [36] have been advocated as contributors to the development of brain functional and structural damage and cognitive alterations. Another pathogenetic factor that could be involved in determining the presence of cognitive deficits in diabetes mellitus is the hyperglycemia-related production of advanced glycosylation terminal products, which may induce vascular and endothelial damage, inflammatory reactions, and deposition of amyloid. The detrimental effects of cerebral microvascular dysfunction in this regard are described in Fig. 14.1 [8].

Cognitive damage may also result from recurrent strokes or transient ischemic attacks that are, as previously mentioned, more frequent and with worse outcomes in the diabetic population [37]. Large longitudinal studies, especially in older people with diabetes, are however needed to better understand the impact, progression, and risk factors that drive the development of diabetes-related cognitive dysfunctions [5].

14.3.3 Depression

Observational studies strongly suggest that depression is more prevalent among adults with diabetes than among the general population. Patients with both T1DM and T2DM have a risk of developing a depressive disorder that is more than twice

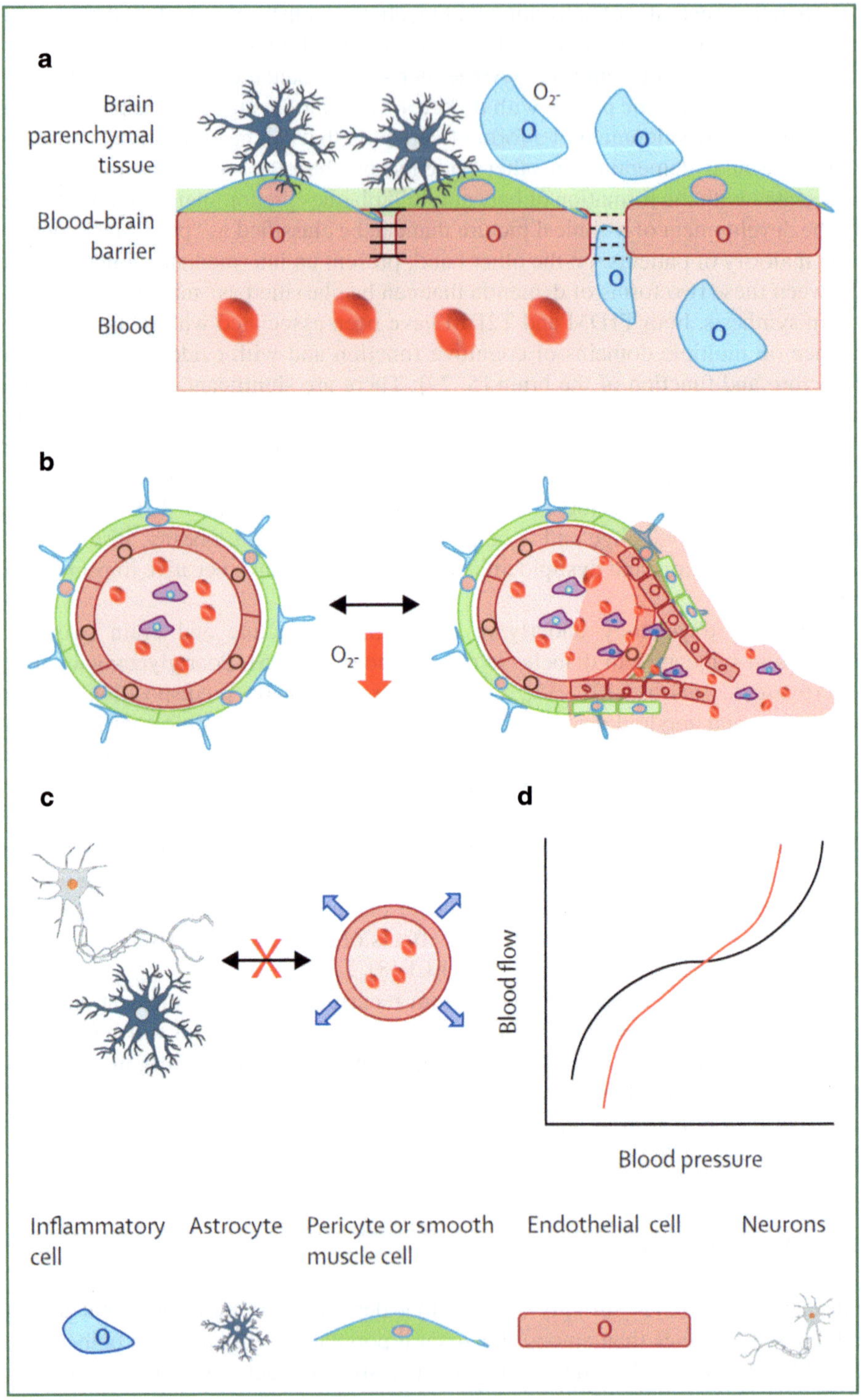
a
Brain parenchymal tissue
Blood–brain barrier
Blood
O_2^-
b
O_2^-
c
d
Blood flow
Blood pressure
Inflammatory cell
Astrocyte
Pericyte or smooth muscle cell
Endothelial cell
Neurons

Fig. 14.1 Detrimental effects of cerebral microvascular dysfunction. (**a**) Type 2 diabetes-related microvascular dysfunction is related to increased oxidative stress, inflammatory and immune responses, and increased blood-brain barrier permeability, resulting in leakage of proteins and other plasma constituents into the perivascular space. (**b**) Microvascular dysfunction might lead to perfusion defects, hypoxia, and increased angiogenesis. Angiogenesis is associated with formation of capillaries that are leaky and poorly perfused and have reduced pericyte support. (**c**) Microvascular dysfunction might contribute to impaired neurovascular coupling, leading to compromised neuronal function. Neurovascular coupling is the mechanism that links transient local neural activity to the subsequent increase in blood flow. (**d**) Microvascular dysfunction might impair cerebral autoregulation, leading to greater vulnerability of brain tissue to the harmful effects of blood pressure changes. With impaired autoregulation, the normal autoregulation curve that shows the relation between cerebral blood flow and mean blood pressure (black curve) might become more linear and steeper, with perfusion becoming pressure dependent (red curve). From Ref. [8]

that that of the healthy control population [38]. About 20–30% of diabetic patients experience depression; individuals withT2DMs have a doubled risk for depression, and individuals with depression have a one to five times increased risk of presenting a T2DM [38]. The reasons for these high prevalence rates of depression in diabetic patients are not yet fully understood. The two dominant hypotheses are the following: depression may result from biochemical changes directly due to the illness or its treatment, or it may be explained by psychosocial demands or psychological factors related to the illness or its treatment [38]. This may contribute to explain the higher recurrence and longer duration of major depressive disorders and related symptoms. The link between diabetes and depression might also include shared risk factors (obesity, physical inactivity, or psychosocial stress related to any chronic disorder) and shared underlying mechanisms (inflammation, alterations in hypothalamic-pituitary-adrenal axis, vascular damage) [38]. The vascular depression hypothesis proposes that vascular damage in frontal and subcortical brain regions, which are involved in mood regulation, might lead to depression at least in some individuals [38]. Major depressive disorders in diabetic individuals represent, therefore, a multifaceted phenomenon, resulting from interactions between various biologic and psychosocial factors [38].

14.4 Dysautonomic Disorders

14.4.1 Definition

Diabetes mellitus represents the main cause of neuropathy [39, 40]. Being one of the major diabetic complications [41], it plays a relevant role in morbidity and mortality in diabetic patients. Diabetic neuropathy may be defined as "the presence of symptoms and/or signs of peripheral nerve dysfunction in people with diabetes after the exclusion of other causes" [42]. Sensory, motor, or autonomic nerves can be involved, even at the same time [40]. Generalized symmetric polyneuropathies and focal/multifocal neuropathies may be present [40, 43]; diabetic autonomic neuropathy (DAN) belongs to the first group. DAN was wrongly considered for a long time as a rare condition, while it should be regarded as a serious and often underestimated complication of diabetes, potentially affecting any part of the autonomic nervous system [40], and possibly leading to a significant increase in morbidity and mortality [40].

Early stages of DAN may be even asymptomatic, especially in young T1DM patients, and may represent, therefore, a diagnostic and therapeutic challenge. Subclinical DAN can occur within a year of diagnosis in T2DM and within 2 years in T1DM, while clinical symptoms may appear even after years [40].

14.4.2 Cardiovascular Autonomic Neuropathy

Cardiovascular autonomic neuropathy (the impairment of autonomic control of the cardiovascular system) [43] is the most common manifestation of DAN and may be associated with severe and even life-threatening complications (arrhythmias, silent myocardial ischemia, and sudden death) [40].

Cardiovascular autonomic neuropathy may be detected in the first years after diabetes onset mainly by means of cardiovascular reflex tests [44] supported recently by newer procedures [40].

Clinical indicators of cardiovascular autonomic neuropathy are reduced heart rate variability during deep breath, a prolongation of QT interval, temporally followed by resting tachycardia, an impaired exercise tolerance, and a decreased baroreflex sensitivity with consequent abnormal blood pressure regulation and orthostatic hypotension [40, 45].

Cardiovascular autonomic neuropathy prevalence tends progressively to increase; however, diabetes duration is not a good predictor of its severity [46]. Initially, there is a relative increase of the sympathetic tone, since diabetic neuropathy firstly impairs longest fibers as those of the parasympathetic system (e.g., vagal fibers) [40]; the following stage is represented by sympathetic denervation [45].

14.4.3 Other Clinical Manifestations of DAN

DAN may affect the central control of breathing and the sympathetic bronchial innervation. Peripheral and central chemosensitivity to hypoxia may be altered, as well as the bronchomotor tone in the lung [40]. Sleep apnea syndrome is highly prevalent in diabetic patient [47], with consequent decrease in quality of life and to an increased risk of sudden death [48].

Also the enteric nervous system may be affected, with loss in inhibitory and increase in excitatory enteric neurons, and, therefore, gastrointestinal symptoms may appear, such as gastroparesis, esophageal dysmotility, constipation, diarrhea, fecal incontinence, or gallbladder atony [40, 49]. Gastroparesis correlates weakly with upper gastrointestinal autonomic symptoms (nausea, vomiting, early satiety, postprandial fullness, bloating, and abdominal pain) which are common in T1DM and T2DM patients [40]. However, alterations in gastric motility may have an impact in acute glycemic control by delaying glucose absorption [50].

Sacral parasympathetic fibers may be damaged even in early stages of diabetes; thus genitourinary dysfunction may occur (impaired bladder sensation with increase in urine retention to dysuria, nicturia, incomplete bladder emptying, and urgency up to overflow incontinence due to the progressive involvement of motor sympathetic and somatic nerves) [40, 43]. Bladder dysfunction may predispose to recurrent urinary tract infections. Also the sexual sphere may be affected: diabetic autonomic neuropathy together with other concomitant conditions including vascular alterations, connective tissue damage, and psychological, endocrine, nutritional, and pharmacological factors may cause erectile dysfunction, retrograde ejaculation, and decreased sexual desire in female, dyspareunia, or inadequate lubrication [40].

DAN may have consequence on the eye: sympathetic predominance in pupil control decreases its diameter at rest [51]. A preserved pupil miotic reaction to accommodation convergence without the miotic reaction to light is named "Argyll Robertson pupil," which is a clinical sign shared with neurosyphilis (40). Sudomotor function may be also affected: sweat gland denervation may result in skin dryness, which is a risk factor for the development of foot ulcerations [40, 52].

The prevalence of DAN is highly dependent on the criteria used to define autonomic dysfunction (type of tests performed, application of age-related normative values, presence or absence of clinical signs and symptoms, different patient cohorts studied) [40]. A meta-analysis of adult patients including 15 studies from 1966 to 2001 reported prevalence rates of cardiovascular autonomic neuropathy ranging from 1 to 90% [40, 53]. Similarly, Dimitropoulos reported prevalences between 1 and 90% in patients with T1DM and 20–70% in patients with T2DM [54]. In a community-based population study, the prevalence of autonomic neuropathy, as defined by the presence of one or more abnormal heart rate variability test, was around 17% [40, 55].

Using other definitions, Ziegler et al. reported prevalences of cardiovascular autonomic neuropathy in T1DM and T2DM patients of 25.3 and 34.3%, respectively [40, 56]. Finally, using more conservative criteria (alterations of at least three of six autonomic function tests), the prevalence of cardiovascular autonomic neuropathy was 16.8% in T1DM and 22.1% in T2DM [40, 53].

Dealing with the time of onset of DAN, it should be remarked that cardiovascular autonomic neuropathy may be detected in about 7% of both T1DM and T2DM at the time of diagnosis [40], and the yearly increase in its prevalence has been reported to be around 6% in T2DM and 2% in T1DM [40]. The incidence of the single symptoms related to DAN is highly variable, and indicative values are the following: delayed esophageal transit, 50%; gastroparesis, 40%; disordered small and large intestinal motility with diarrhea, 20% or constipation, 25% [40, 53]; erectile dysfunction, 35–90%; and retrograde ejaculation, 32% [40, 53]; bladder dysfunction may be present in 43–85% of patients with T1DM and in 25% of T2DM [40, 53].

Glycemic control and longer diabetes duration may be among the predictors of autonomic test abnormalities in young people [51]; however, only few studies have addressed the possible associations between DAN and other microvascular complications, although some association with retinopathy and nephropathy seems to be present [51].

14.4.4 Pathogenesis

The genesis of DAN is probably multifactorial (Fig. 14.2). A key role is played by hyperglycemia, oxidative stress, and insulin resistance [40, 57]. In addition, the role of inflammation in the pathogenesis of DAN has increasingly been highlighted (Fig. 14.2) [40]. With reference to T1DM, the possible role of autoimmunity has also been postulated. Autoantibodies against sympathetic ganglia vagus nerve and adrenal medulla were found in T1DM patients [58]. Also nerve growth factors may be involved in the pathogenesis of DAN: insulin-like growth factor-1 and neurotrophin-3 have been demonstrated, in an animal model, to be able to reverse diabetic neuropathy [59]. The role of hyperglycemia in the pathogenesis of diabetic autonomic neuropathy as the cause of inflammation and oxidative stress is described in Fig. 14.2 [40].

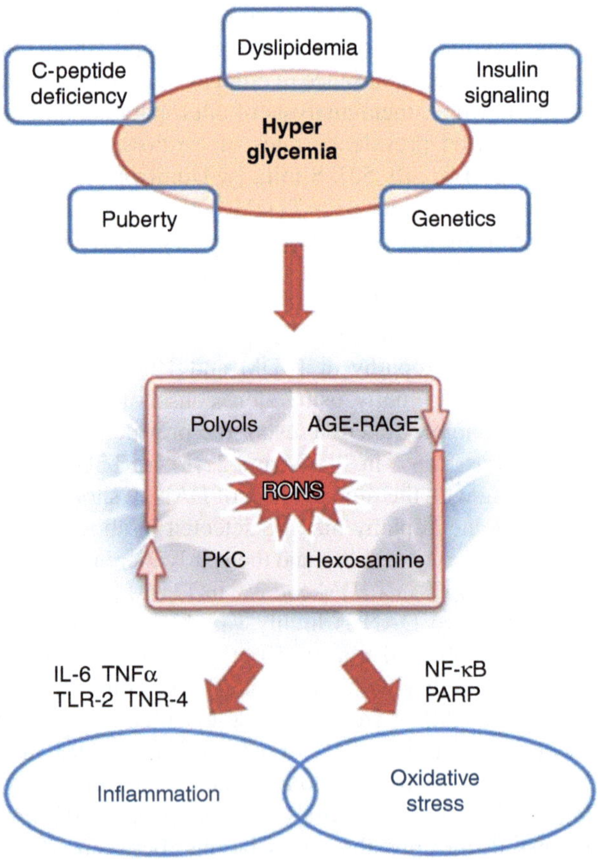

Fig. 14.2 Pathogenesis of diabetic autonomic neuropathy: the role of hyperglycemia as the cause of inflammation and oxidative stress. *RONS* Reactive oxygen and nitrogen species (mitochondrial overproduction), *AGE* Advanced glycation end products, *RAGE* AGE receptors, *IL* Interleukin, *TNF* Tumor necrosis factor, *NF* Nuclear factor, *PKC* Protein kinase C, *TLR* Toll-like receptors, *PARP* Poly-ADP ribose polymerase. From Ref. [40]

14.4.5 Prevention and Treatment

Intensive glycemic control seems to be the most effective way to prevent or delay the onset and slow the progression of autonomic dysfunction in patients with T1DM [40, 53, 54]. Once DAN becomes clinically evident, there is no specific treatment which was proved to be able to stop or reverse it. The most recent studies confirmed the efficacy of intensive insulin therapy in slowing the progression of both diabetic peripheral neuropathy [60] and DAN [61].

14.5 Conclusions

According to existing scientific evidence, both T1DM and T2DM are associated with mild to modest decrements in cognitive function [5]. Domains of psychomotor speed, mental flexibility, attention, and general intelligence are those most frequently affected [5]. Hypoglycemia is not usually risk factor for cognitive decline; however, this may not be true for children with young age at onset of diabetes [5]. Relevant risk factors for the development of cognitive decline are an early age of onset and the presence of microvascular complications. Since age and duration of diabetes are important contributors to the changes in cognitive function, we need longitudinal studies looking at cognitive function, especially in elderly subject with T1DM. In addition, more information is needed in order to better understand the clinical implications of these mild-moderate decrements in cognitive function, also in terms of impact on daily lives and habits. In addition, the underlying mechanism and the risk factors that may lead to the development of more severe cognitive dysfunction like dementia in some, but not all diabetic patients are not clear [5].

DAN represents a particular aspect of diabetic neuropathy, which may lead impairment of several organs, including the heart, both in T1DM and in T2DM patients. The pathogenesis of DAN is not entirely clear, but metabolic, genetic, and hormonal factors may be involved; however, the final pathway probably involves oxidative stress and inflammation caused by hyperglycemia [40]. Since no therapy was demonstrated to effectively reverse DAN, prevention with close glycemic control, multifactorial intervention, and lifestyle modification remain crucial [40].

References

1. Biessels GJ. Risk of dementia in diabetes mellitus: a systematic review. Lancet Neurol. 2006;5:64–74.
2. Miles WR, Root HF. Psychologic tests applied to diabetic patients. Arch Intern Med. 1922;30:767.
3. Dejong R. The nervous system complications of diabetes mellitus, with special reference to cerebrovascular changes. J Nerv Ment Dis. 1950;111:181–206.
4. Mijnhout GS, Scheltens P, Diamant M, Biessels GJ, Wessels AM, Simsek S, et al. Diabetic encephalopathy: a concept in need of a definition. Diabetologia. 2006;49:1447–8.

5. Moheet A, Mangia S, Seaquist ER. Impact of diabetes on cognitive function and brain structure. Ann N Y Acad Sci. 2015;1353:60–71.
6. Qureshi AI, Caplan LR. Intracranial atherosclerosis. Lancet. 2014;383(9921):984–98.
7. Ergul A, Kelly-Cobbs A, Abdalla M, Fagan SC. Cerebrovascular complications of diabetes: focus on stroke. Endocr Metab Immune Disord Drug Targets. 2012;12:148–58.
8. van Sloten TT, Sedaghat S, Carnethon MR, Launer LJ, Stehouwer CDA. Cerebral microvascular complications of type 2 diabetes: stroke, cognitive dysfunction, and depression. Lancet Diabetes Endocrinol. 2020;8:325–36.
9. Bell DSH, Goncalves E. Stroke in the patient with diabetes (Part 1)—epidemiology, etiology, therapy and prognosis. Diabetes Res Clin Pract. 2020;164:108193.
10. Kodl C, Franc D, Rao J, et al. Diffusion tensor imaging identifies deficits in white matter microstructure in subjects with type 1 diabetes that correlate with reduced neurocognitive function. Diabetes. 2008;57:3083–9.
11. Mangia S, Kumar AF, Moheet AA, Roberts RJ, Eberly LE, Seaquist ER, et al. Neurochemical profile of patients with type 1 diabetes measured by H-1-MRS at 4 T. J Cereb Blood Flow Metab. 2013;33:754–9.
12. Fang F, Zhan YF, Zhuo YY, Yin DZ, Li KA, Wang YF. Brain atrophy in middle-aged subjects with type 2 diabetes mellitus, with and without microvascular complications. J Diabetes. 2018;10:625–32.
13. Moran C, Phan TG, Chen J, Blizzard L, Beare R, Venn A, et al. Brain atrophy in type 2 diabetes regional distribution and influence on cognition. Diabetes Care. 2013;36:4036–42.
14. den Heijer T, Vermeer SE, van Dijk EJ, Prins ND, Koudstaal PJ, Hofman A, et al. Type 2 diabetes and atrophy of medial temporal lobe structures on brain MRI. Diabetologia. 2003;46:1604–10.
15. Mankovsky B, Zherdova N, van den Berg E, Biessels GJ, de Bresser J. Cognitive functioning and structural brain abnormalities in people with Type 2 diabetes mellitus. Diabet Med. 2018;35:1663–70.
16. Sanjari Moghaddam H, Ghazi Sherbaf F, Aarabi MH. Brain microstructural abnormalities in type 2 diabetes mellitus: A systematic review of diffusion tensor imaging studies. Front Neuroendocrinol. 2019;55:100782.
17. Horton WB, Barrett EJ. Microvascular dysfunction in diabetes mellitus and cardiometabolic disease. Endocr Rev. 2021;42:29–55.
18. Manolis AJ, Kallistratos MS, Vlahakos DS, Mitrakou A, Poulimenos LE. Comorbidities often associated with brain damage in hypertension: diabetes, coronary artery disease, chronic kidney disease and obstructive sleep apnea. In: Coca A, editor. Hypertension and brain damage. Springer Switzerland; 2016. p. 35–46.
19. Zhao X, Han Q, Gang X, Wang G. Altered brain metabolites in patients with diabetes mellitus and related complications—evidence from ^{1}H MRS study. Biosci Rep. 2018;38(5):BSR20180660.
20. Brands AM, Biessels GJ, de Haan EH, Kappelle LJ, Kessels RPC. The effects of type 1 diabetes on cognitive performance: a meta-analysis. Diabetes Care. 2005;28:726–35.
21. Gaudieri PA. Cognitive function in children with type 1 diabetes: a meta-analysis. Diabetes Care. 2008;31:1892–7.
22. Jacobson A, Musen G, Ryan C, Silvers N, Cleary P, Waberski B, et al. Long-term effect of diabetes and its treatment on cognitive function. N Engl J Med. 2007;356:1842–52.
23. Reichard P, Pihl M, Rosenqvist U, Sule J. Complications in IDDM are caused by elevated blood glucose level: the Stockholm Diabetes Intervention Study (SDIS) at 10-year follow up. Diabetologia. 1996;39:1483–8.
24. Rawlings AM, Sharrett AR, Schneider ALC, Coresh J, Albert M, Couper D, et al. Diabetes in midlife and cognitive change over 20 years: a cohort study. Ann Intern Med. 2014;161:785–93.
25. Ott A, Stolk RP, van Harskamp F, Pols HA, Hofman A, Breteler MM. Diabetes mellitus and the risk of dementia—the Rotterdam study. Neurology. 1999;53:1937–42.
26. van den Berg E, Kloppenborg RP, Kessels RPC, Kappelle LJ, Biessels GJ. Type 2 diabetes mellitus, hypertension, dyslipidemia and obesity: a systematic comparison of their impact on cognition. Biochim Biophys Acta. 2009;1792:470–81.

27. Palta P, Schneider ALC, Biessels GJ, Touradji P, Hill-Briggs F. Magnitude of cognitive dysfunction in adults with type 2 diabetes: a meta-analysis of six cognitive domains and the most frequently reported neuropsychological tests within domains. J Int Neuropsychol Soc. 2014;20:278–91.
28. Hajek T, McIntyre R, Alda M. Bipolar disorders, type 2 diabetes mellitus, and the brain. Curr Opin Psychiatry. 2016;29:1–6.
29. Zilliox LA, Chadrasekaran K, Kwan JY, Russell JW. Diabetes and cognitive impairment. Curr Diab Rep. 2016;16:87.
30. Cameron FJ, Northam EA, Ryan CM. The effect of type 1 diabetes on the developing brain. Lancet Child Adolesc Health. 2019;3:427–36.
31. Agabiti-Rosei E, Rizzoni D, Cunha P. Pathophysiology of brain damage in hypertension. In: Coca A, editor. Hypertension and brain damage. Springer Switzerland; 2016. p. 47–60.
32. De Ciuceis C. Microvascular alterations in diabetes: focus on small resistance arteries. In: Agabiti-Rosei E, Heagerty AM, Rizzoni D, editors. Microcirculation in cardiovascular diseases. Springer Switzerland; 2020. p. 149–64.
33. Muriach M, Flores-Bellver M, Romero FJ, Barcia JM. Diabetes and the brain: oxidative stress, inflammation, and autophagy. Oxid Med Cell Longev. 2014;2014:102158.
34. Bogush M, Heldt NA, Persidsky. Blood brain barrier injury in diabetes: unrecognized effects on brain and cognition. J Neuroimmune Pharmacol. 2017;12:593–601.
35. Goldwaser EL, Acharya NK, Sarkar A, Godsey G, Nagele RG. Breakdown of the cerebrovasculature and blood-brain barrier: a mechanistic link between diabetes mellitus and Alzheimer's disease. J Alzheimers Dis. 2016;54:445–56.
36. Li W, Risacher SL, Huang E, Saykin AJ, Alzheimer's Disease Neuroimaging Initiative. Type 2 diabetes mellitus is associated with brain atrophy and hypometabolism in the ADNI cohort. Neurology. 2016;87:595–600.
37. Biessels GJ. Cerebral complications of diabetes: clinical findings and pathogenetic mechanism. Neth J Med. 1999;54:35–45.
38. Talbot F, Nouwen A. A review of the relationship between depression and diabetes in adults. Diabetes Care. 2000;23:1556–62.
39. Said G. Diabetic neuropathy. Handb Clin Neurol. 2013;115:579–89.
40. Verrotti A, Prezioso G, Scattoni R, Chiarelli F. Autonomic neuropathy in diabetes mellitus. Front Endocrinol (Lausanne). 2014;5:205.
41. Pasnoor M, Dimachkie MM, Kluding P, Barohn RJ. Diabetic neuropathy part1:overview and symmetric phenotypes. Neurol Clin. 2013;31:425–45.
42. Boulton AJ, Gries FA, Jervell JA. Guidelines for diagnosis and outpatient management of diabetic peripheral neuropathy. Diabetes Metab. 1998;15:508–14.
43. Tesfaye S, Boulton AJ, Dyck PJ, Freeman R, Horowitz M, Kempler P, et al. Diabetic neuropathies: update on definitions, diagnostic criteria, estimation of severity, and treatments. Diabetes Care. 2010;33:2285–93.
44. Ewing DJ, Martyn CN, Young RJ, Clarke BF. The value of cardiovascular autonomic function tests: 10 years' experience in diabetes. Diabetes Care. 1985;8:491–8.
45. Pop-Busui R. Cardiac autonomic neuropathy in diabetes: a clinical perspective. Diabetes Care. 2010;33:434–41.
46. Pavy-LeTraon A, Fontaine S, Tap G, Guidolin B, Senard JM, Hanaire H. Cardiovascular autonomic neuropathy and other complications in type 1 diabetes. Clin Auton Res. 2010;20:153–60.
47. Tantucci C, Scionti L, Bottini P, Dottorini ML, Puxeddu E, Casucci G, et al. Influence of autonomic neuropathy of different severities on the hypercapnic drive to breathing in diabetic patients. Chest. 1997;112:145–53.
48. Fujihara K, Kodama S, Horikawa C, Yoshizawa S, Sugawara A, Hirasawa R, et al. The relationship between diabetic neuropathy and sleep apnea syndrome: a meta-analysis. Sleep Disord. 2013;2013:150371.
49. Chandrasekharan B, Srinivasan S. Diabetes and the enteric nervous system. Neurogastroenterol Motil. 2007;19:951–60.

50. Chang J, Rayner CK, Jones KL, Horowitz M. Diabetic gastroparesis—backwards and forwards. J Gastroenterol Hepatol. 2011;26(Suppl 1):46–57.
51. Tang M, Donaghue KC, Cho YH, Craig ME. Autonomic neuropathy in young people with type 1 diabetes: a systematic review. Pediatr Diabetes. 2013;14:239–48.
52. Tentolouris N, Marinou K, Kokotis P, Karanti A, Diakoumopoulou E, Katsilambros N. Sudomotor dysfunction is associated with foot ulceration in diabetes. Diabet Med. 2009;26:302–5.
53. Vinik AI, Erbas T. Diabetic autonomic neuropathy. Handb Clin Neurol. 2013;117:279–94.
54. Dimitropoulos G, Tahrani AA, Stevens MJ. Cardiac autonomic neuropathy in patients with diabetes mellitus. World J Diabetes. 2014;5:17–39.
55. Maser RE, Mitchell BD, Vinik AI, Freeman R. The association between cardiovascular autonomic neuropathy and mortality in individuals with diabetes: a meta-analysis. Diabetes Care. 2003;26:1895–901.
56. Ziegler D, Gries FA, Spüler M, Lessmann F. The epidemiology of diabetic neuropathy. J Diabetes Complications. 1992;6:49–57.
57. Frontoni S, Bracaglia D, Gigli F. Relationship between autonomic dysfunction, insulin resistance and hypertension, in diabetes. Nutr Metab Cardiovasc Dis. 2005;15:441–9.
58. Ejskjaer N, Arif S, Dodds W, Zanone MM, Vergani D, Watkins PJ, et al. Prevalence of autoantibodies to autonomic nervous tissue structures in type 1diabetes mellitus. Diabet Med. 1999;16:544–9.
59. Schmidt RE, Dorsey DA, Beaudet LN, Plurad SB, Parvin CA, Ohara S. Effect of IGF-I and neurotrophin-3 on gracile neuroaxonal dystrophy in diabetic and aging rats. Brain Res. 2000;876:88–94.
60. Callaghan BC, Little AA, Feldman EL, Hughes RA. Enhanced glucose control for preventing and treating diabetic neuropathy. Cochrane Database Syst Rev. 2012;6:CD007543.
61. Lee SS, Han HS, Kim H. A 5-yr follow-up nerve conduction study for the detection of subclinical diabetic neuropathy in children with newly diagnosed insulin-dependent diabetes mellitus. Pediatr Diabetes. 2010;11:521–8.

Diabetic Nephropathy in Type 1 Diabetes Mellitus

15

Peter Rossing

15.1 Epidemiology

The overall prevalence of microalbuminuria and macroalbuminuria is around 30–35%. The cumulative incidence of persistent proteinuria in patients whose type 1 diabetes was diagnosed before 1942 was about 40–50% after diabetes of 25 to 30 years' duration, but it declined to 15–30% in patients receiving a diagnosis of type 1 diabetes after 1953 [1]. The reason for the declining cumulative incidence of proteinuria in type 1 diabetic patients is unknown, but improved diabetes care and control, in addition to a decline in the prevalence of smoking and a general decline in nondiabetic glomerulopathies, have been suggested as factors.

Diabetic nephropathy rarely develops in patients with type 1 diabetes before 10 years after diagnosis, whereas approximately 3% of patients with newly diagnosed type 2 diabetes already have overt nephropathy. The incidence peak (3% per year) is usually found in those who have had diabetes for 10–20 years, thereafter a progressive decline in incidence takes place. Thus, the risk of developing diabetic nephropathy is reduced for a normoalbuminuric patient who has had diabetes for longer than 30 years is reduced [2].

Studies have demonstrated impaired renal function (CKD stage 3: estimated GFR <60 mL/min/1.73 m^2) in many patients with normoalbuminuria [3, 4]. It is being discussed if this is due to aging, rather than kidney disease, or if it is due to treatment-induced remission of albuminuria in patients with diabetic nephropathy, or even a non-albuminuric phenotype of diabetic nephropathy. In a 19-year follow-up of the Diabetes Control and Complications Study in type 1 diabetic patients, 24% of patients developing eGFR below 60 mL/min/1.73 m^2 had

P. Rossing (✉)
Steno Diabetes Center Copenhagen (SDCC), Herlev, Denmark

Institute of Clinical Medicine, University of Copenhagen, Copenhagen, Denmark
e-mail: Peter.Rossing@RegionH.dk

A. E. Berbari, G. Mancia (eds.), *Blood Pressure Disorders in Diabetes Mellitus*, Updates in Hypertension and Cardiovascular Protection,
https://doi.org/10.1007/978-3-031-13009-0_15

normoalbuminuria on all prior measurements [5]. In a Finnish study of type 1 diabetes, non-albuminuric chronic kidney disease did not increase the risk of albuminuria (hazard ratio [HR] 2.0 [95% CI 0.9–4.4]) or end-stage renal disease (HR 6.4 [0.8–53.0]) but did increase the risk of cardiovascular events (HR 2.0 [1.4–3.5]) and all-cause mortality (HR 2.4 [1.4–3.9]) [6].

The subpopulation of patients with type 1 diabetes who are at risk for nephropathy may be identified fairly accurately by the detection of microalbuminuria [3]. Several longitudinal studies have shown that microalbuminuria strongly predicts the development of diabetic nephropathy in type 1 diabetic patients with a predictive power of 80%. It has been suggested that 58% of microalbuminuric patients revert to normoalbuminuria, but in contrast to treatment-induced regression, long-lasting spontaneous normalization is seen in 16% of microalbuminuric patients with type 1 diabetes [4].

15.1.1 Prognosis of Microalbuminuria

Microalbuminuria is a strong predictor of total and cardiovascular mortality and cardiovascular morbidity in diabetic patients. In the guideline from the Kidney Disease: Improving Global Outcomes for chronic kidney disease, elevated albuminuria was included as a marker of ESKD and death [7]. The Chronic Kidney Disease Epidemiology consortium also demonstrated that increase in albuminuria compared to normal albuminuria, conferred a similar increase in relative risk for death and ESKD in patients with and without diabetes. In people with diabetesic the risk is however at a higher level [8]. The mechanisms linking microalbuminuria to death from cardiovascular disease are poorly understood. Microalbuminuria has been proposed to be a marker of widespread endothelial dysfunction which might predispose to enhanced penetrations of atherogenic lipoprotein particles [9], into the arterial wall, as well as a marker of established cardiovascular disease. In addition, the cardio renal link is evident both for risk markers and for therapeutic targets [10]. Raised blood pressure, dyslipoproteinemia, increased platelet aggregability, endothelial dysfunction, insulin resistance, and hyperinsulinemia have all been demonstrated in microalbuminuric diabetic patients. Autonomic neuropathy, which is also associated with microalbuminuria, predicts death (often sudden) from cardiovascular disease in diabetic patients [10]. Echocardiographic studies have revealed impaired diastolic function and cardiac hypertrophy in microalbuminuric patients with type 1 diabetes [11].

15.1.2 Prognosis of Diabetic Nephropathy

In three early studies that described the natural course of diabetic nephropathy patients with type 1 diabetes, the cumulative death rate 10 years after onset of nephropathy ranged from 50% to 77%. Studies have demonstrated how excess mortality in type 1 diabetes compared to the background population is almost entirely seen in patients with elevated albumin excretion [12–14].

The overall decrease in relative mortality in diabetes from 1933 to 1972 was 40% and is partly explained by the decrease in the cumulative incidence of proteinuria. ESKD was a major cause of mortality, accounting for 59–66% of all deaths, in type 1 diabetic patients with nephropathy. The cumulative incidence of ESKD 10 years after onset of persistent proteinuria in type 1 diabetic patients was 50% but has been suggested to level off. In addition, the survival of diabetic patients with ESKD has been improved [15]. In addition to mortality related to ESKD, cardiovascular disease is a major cause of death (15–25%) in type 1 diabetic patients with nephropathy.

15.2 Clinical Course and Pathophysiology

15.2.1 Normoalbuminuria

Approximately one third of type 1 diabetic patients will have a GFR above the upper normal range for age-matched healthy nondiabetic subjects. The GFR elevation is particularly pronounced in patients with newly diagnosed diabetes and during other intervals with poor metabolic control. Intensified insulin treatment and control to near-normal blood glucose levels reduces GFR toward normal levels after a period of days to weeks [16].

Longitudinal studies suggest that hyperfiltration is a risk factor for subsequent development of diabetic nephropathy in type 1 diabetic patients, but conflicting results have also been reported. A meta-analysis based on ten cohort studies following 780 patients found a hazard ratio of 2.71 (95% confidence interval [CI] = 1.20–6.11) for progression to microalbuminuria in patients with hyperfiltration. These authors also found evidence of heterogeneity [17].

15.2.2 Microalbuminuria

The day-to-day variation in urinary albumin excretion is high, 30–50%. Persistent microalbuminuria is not detected in children with type 1 diabetes younger than 12 years of age and, in general, is exceptional in the first 5 years of diabetes. Changes in tubular function take place early in diabetes and are related to the degree of glycemic control. The proximal tubular reabsorption of fluid, sodium, and glucose is enhanced [18]. This process could diminish distal sodium delivery and thereby modify tubuloglomerular feedback signals, which would result in enhancement of GFR. A direct effect of insulin in increasing distal sodium reabsorption has also been demonstrated. The consequences of these alterations in tubular transport for overall kidney function are unknown but has been suggested to be important for the renal effect of SGLT2 inhibitors [19]. Markers of acute tubular damage have also been investigated in relation to prediction and progression of diabetic nephropathy [20].

Several studies have demonstrated blood pressure elevation in children and adults with type 1 diabetes and microalbuminuria [21]. The prevalence of arterial hypertension in adults with type 1 diabetes increases with urine albumin level, and prevalence rates are 42%, 52%, and 79% in individuals with normo-, micro-, and macroalbuminuria, respectively.

15.2.3 Diabetic Nephropathy

A close correlation between blood pressure and the rate of decline in GFR has been documented. This suggests that systemic blood pressure accelerates the progression of diabetic nephropathy. Previously, the adverse impact of systemic hypertension on renal function and structure was thought to be mediated through vasoconstriction and arteriolar nephrosclerosis. However, evidence from rat models shows that systemic hypertension is transmitted to the single glomerulus, which results in increases in glomerular hydrostatic pressure in such a way as to lead to hyperperfusion and increased capillary pressure. Intraglomerular hypertension has also been documented directly in rats with streptozotocin-induced diabetes and has been estimated to prevail in human diabetic patients particularly those whose diabetes is complicated by kidney disease. Impaired or abolished renal autoregulation of GFR and renal plasma flow as demonstrated in type 1 and type 2 diabetic patients with nephropathy increases vulnerability to hypertension or ischemic injury of glomerular capillaries [16].

Nocturnal blood pressure elevation ("nondipping") occurs more frequently in patients with nephropathy [21]. Exaggerated blood pressure response to exercise has also been reported in patients with long-standing type 1 diabetes who have microangiopathy.

Several components of the RAAS are elevated and considered to contribute to the progression of diabetic nephropathy. Accordingly blocking the RAAS has been demonstrated to be reno-protective. Initially focus was on the damaging effect of angiotensin II. Aldosterone represents another component of the RAAS that should be considered important in the pathophysiology of diabetic nephropathy. Aldosterone is regulating electrolyte and fluid homeostasis and has widespread actions through genomic and nongenomic effects both in the kidney and in tissues not originally considered target tissue for aldosterone, such as the vasculature, central nervous system, and heart.

It has been suggested that uric acid level is related to hypertension, metabolic syndrome, and renal disease. Recently elevated serum uric acid was found to be a predictor of the development of diabetic nephropathy in type 1 diabetic patients [22, 23], and a multicenter study was initiated to study if lowering uric acid with allopurinol compared to placebo in 530 type 1 diabetes patients with early diabetic nephropathy would preserve renal function, but after 3 years there was no difference in decline in GFR(24).

Several gene variants have been investigated as candidate genes for risk factors for diabetic nephropathy. One of the initially studied is the insertion/deletion (I/D) polymorphism of the ACE gene (*ACE*/ID), which is strongly associated with the level of circulating ACE and increased risk of coronary heart disease in nondiabetic and diabetic patients. Recently genome-wide association studies have been performed in the search for genes linked to diabetic nephropathy, and although several areas of the genome have attracted attention, no major susceptibility genes have been identified [25, 26].

Urinary proteomic profiles characteristic for diabetic nephropathy have been identified [27]. These changes reflect extracellular matrix components and are partly normalized during renoprotective intervention. In plasma a profile related to inflammation has been identified [28]. Furthermore the urinary proteomic-retinopathy was observed dubased profile was also able to identify normoalbuminuric patients with elevated risk for later development of diabetic nephropathy, independent of other risk factors [29].

15.3 Treatment

15.3.1 Glycemic Control

A meta-analysis documented a beneficial effect on the progression from normoalbuminuria to microalbuminuria in type 1 diabetes [30]. The odds ratio for progressing from normoalbuminuria to microalbuminuria ranged from 0.22 to 0.40 in the intensified treatment groups. A worsening of diabetic retinopathy was observed during the initial months of intensive therapy, but in the longer term the rate of deterioration was slower than it was in the type 1 diabetic patients receiving conventional treatment. Side effects are a major concern with intensive therapy, and the frequency of severe hypoglycemia and diabetic ketoacidosis was greater in several studies. In the Diabetes Control and Complications Trial (DCCT) [31], intensive therapy reduced the occurrence of microalbuminuria by 39% (95% CI = 21–52%) and that of albuminuria by 54% (95% CI = 19–74%). With further follow up of the patients from DCCT, it was demonstrated that the reduction in development of microalbuminuria and albuminuria translated into a 50% (95% confidence interval, 18–69; $P = 0.006$) reduced risk of development of impaired renal function (eGFR <60) [32]. Despite this, 16% in the primary prevention cohort and 26% in the secondary prevention cohort developed microalbuminuria during the 9 years of intensive treatment.

15.3.1.1 Nephropathy

The impact of improved metabolic control on progression of kidney function in type 1 diabetic patients with nephropathy has been disappointing. Studies have not found the rate of decline in GFR, and the rise in proteinuria and systemic blood pressure to be affected by improved glycemic control. However, it should be stressed that none of the trials was randomized and the number of patients included was small. It was demonstrated that insulin pump therapy compared to multiple insulin injections in an open randomized trial reduced progression of albuminuria over 12 months [33] in line with observational data [34] which were not explained by improvement in mean glycemic levels, but perhaps less glycemic variability, as increased time in optimal glucose range was associated with the improved albuminuria [35].

15.3.2 Blood Pressure Control

15.3.2.1 Primary Prevention

Originally, Zatz et al. [36] showed that prevention of glomerular capillary hypertension in normotensive insulin-treated rats with streptozotocin-induced diabetes effectively protects against proteinuria and focal and segmental glomerular structural lesions. A randomized placebo-controlled trial in normotensive type 1 diabetes with normal AER has suggested a beneficial effect of ACE inhibitors on the development of microalbuminuria [37].

The Renin Angiotensin System Study (RASS) compared, the effect of ACE inhibition, angiotensin II receptor blockade, and placebo on the primary renal structural endpoint of mesangial volume fraction, in type 1 diabetic patients who were normotensive (blood pressure of <135/85 mmHg) and normoalbuminuric. This 5-year randomized controlled trial did not find any benefit of RAS blockade on the progression of nephropathy as measured in terms of the primary endpoint and other secondary renal structural parameters [38]. In contrast, the odds for progression of retinopathy were significantly reduced by 65–70% with the RAS blocking agents compared with placebo. The DIRECT study evaluated the effect of angiotensin II receptor blockade with candesartan versus placebo on the development or progression of retinopathy in a randomized controlled trial lasting 5 years involving 3326 patients with type 1 diabetes and 1905 patients type 2 diabetes. Most patients were normotensive, and all had normoalbuminuria. In type 1 diabetic patients, the incidence of new retinopathy in patients without retinopathy was reduced by candesartan treatment, but progression of established retinopathy was not affected. The study did not show any significant effect on the incidence of microalbuminuria [39].

In conclusion, RAS blockade has been effective in reducing the frequency of development of microalbuminuria in hypertensive normoalbuminuric patients, whereas the effect has not been significant in normotensive patients. The use of ACE inhibitors or other antihypertensive agents for primary prevention of nephropathy in normotensive normoalbuminuric patients is not recommended in guidelines [40].

15.3.2.2 Secondary Prevention

A meta-analysis of 12 trials encompassing 698 type 1 diabetic patients with microalbuminuria who were followed for at least 1 year revealed that treatment with ACE inhibitors reduced the risk of progression to macroalbuminuria compared with placebo (odds ratio = 0.38; 95% CI = 0.25–0.57) [41]. At 2 years, the urinary AER was 50% lower in patients taking ACE inhibitors than in those receiving placebo. Furthermore, the beneficial effect of ACE inhibitors in preventing progression from microalbuminuria to overt nephropathy is long-lasting (8 years), and, more importantly, it is associated with preservation of normal GFR [42].

Current guidelines recommend "Either ACE inhibitors or ARBs (but not both in combination) are recommended for the treatment of the nonpregnant patient with modestly elevated (30–299 mg/24 h) or higher levels (>300 mg/24 h) of urinary albumin excretion" [40].

15.3.2.3 Nephropathy

In 1982, Mogensen described a beneficial effect of long-term antihypertensive treatment in five hypertensive men with type 1 diabetes and nephropathy. A prospective study of nine patients initiated in 1976 demonstrated that early and aggressive antihypertensive treatment reduces albuminuria and the rate of decline in GFR in young men and women with type 1 diabetes and nephropathy.

In 1992, Björck and colleagues suggested that the use of ACE inhibitors in patients with diabetic nephropathy confers renoprotection; that is, it has a beneficial effect on renal function and structure above and beyond that expected from the blood-pressure-lowering effect alone [43].

The first information regarding the effect of antihypertensive treatment on progression of nephropathy to come from a randomized, double-blind, placebo-controlled trial was presented by the Collaborative Study Group of Angiotensin-Converting Enzyme Inhibition, which examined the use of captopril in type 1 diabetic patients with diabetic nephropathy [44]. In this study which lasted on average 2.7 years, the risk of death or progression to dialysis or transplantation was reduced by 61% (95% CI = 26–80%, $P = 0.002$) in the subgroup of 102 captopril-treated patients with a baseline serum creatinine concentration of more than 133 μmol/L and 46% (95% CI = 22–76%; $P = 0.14$) in the 307 patients with a baseline serum creatinine concentration below 133 μmol/L, compared with placebo-treated patients.

Short-term studies indicated that the combination of ACE inhibition and angiotensin II receptor blockade may offer additional renal and cardiovascular protection in diabetic patients with elevated AER. In a meta-analysis it was concluded that the combination reduced albuminuria approximately 25% more than monotherapy [45]. Subsequent studies have not been able to document long-term benefits and this is not recommended [40].

From a clinical point of view the ability to predict the long-term effect on kidney function of a recently initiated treatment modality (e.g., antihypertensive therapy) would be of great value because this could allow for early identification of patients in need of an intensified or alternative therapeutic regimen. Two prospective studies found that the initial reduction in albuminuria (surrogate endpoint) predicted a beneficial long-term treatment effect on rate of decline in GFR (principal endpoint) in diabetic nephropathy [1]. These findings have been confirmed and extended in recent analyses of both observational and interventional studies [46, 47].

In recent years it has become clear that aldosterone should be considered a hormone with widespread unfavorable effects on the vasculature, the heart, and the kidneys. It has been demonstrated that elevated plasma aldosterone level during long-term treatment with losartan is associated with an enhanced decline in GFR in type 1 diabetic patients with diabetic nephropathy [48]. Consequently, aldosterone blockade could be considered in patients with suboptimal renoprotection during conventional RAS blockade. Short-term studies in type 1 and type 2 proteinuric diabetic patients have demonstrated that spironolactone adds to the renal and cardiovascular protective benefits of treatment with maximally recommended dosages of ACE inhibitors or ARBs by reducing albuminuria and blood pressure [49]. As hyperkalemia has been a concern, this has not been tested in long-term studies, but with the recent development of selective non-steroidal mineralocorticoid receptor antagonists like finerenone, demonstrating long-term benefit on renal and cardiac outcome in type 2 diabetic CKD with manageable hyperkalemia, this will hopefully also be tested in type 1 diabetes [50].

Early studies describing the prognosis for overt diabetic nephropathy observed a median patient survival time of 5–7 years after the onset of persistent proteinuria. Fortunately, survival improved with implementation of antihypertensive therapy, a median survival time of 21 years after the onset of diabetic nephropathy was demonstrated [51], and further with control of multiple risk factors a further 50% reduction in age-adjusted mortality was seen [15].

15.3.3 Lipid-Lowering Therapy

In albuminuric patients with diabetes, the risk of cardiovascular disease is enhanced. Consequently these patients should be treated with statins according to current guidelines for patients at high risk targeting all risk factors for progression of cardiovascular disease [52]. The renoprotective effect of 3-hydroxy-3-methylglutaryl-coenzyme A reductase inhibitors in patients with type 1 or type 2 diabetes who have microalbuminuria or macroalbuminuria appears to be highly variable [16].

15.3.4 Dietary Protein Restriction

Short-term studies in type 1 diabetic patients with normoalbuminuria, microalbuminuria, or macroalbuminuria have shown that low-protein diet (0.6–0.8 g/kg/day) reduces urinary albumin excretion and hyperfiltration, independently of changes in glucose control and blood pressure. A 4-year prospective randomized controlled trial with concealed randomization compared the effects of a low-protein diet with a usual-protein diet in 82 type 1 diabetic patients with progressive diabetic nephropathy. The endpoint of ESKD or death occurred in 27% of patients consuming a usual-protein diet compared with 10% consuming a low-protein diet (log-rank test, $P = 0.04$) [53]. The relative risk of ESKD or death was 0.23 (95% CI = 0.07–0.72) for patients assigned to a low-protein diet, after an adjustment for the presence of cardiovascular disease at baseline. Currently a dietary protein intake of 0.8 g/kg body weight per day is recommended in guidelines for diabetes with CKD [52].

15.3.5 New Treatment Options

New options are needed to treat diabetic nephropathy despite the success of antihypertensive therapies. There have been no successful studies with hard endpoints in diabetic kidney disease since the studies with ARBs in 2001 until recently, where several studies have found positive effects in type 2 diabetes with CKD. Only few studies have been conducted in type 1 diabetes, and a rare example was the uric acid-lowering trial mentioned above [24]. It will briefly be discussed if these options could be relevant for diabetic nephropathy in type 1 diabetes.

Most positive data are in relation to the sodium glucose cotransporter 2 inhibitors (SGLT2i) initially launched to treat type 2 diabetes by inducing glucosuria. This mechanism has also been tested in type 1 diabetes, and although the effect on hba1c is modest, there is benefit on glucose variability with a small but significant risk for ketoacidosis with normal glucose levels. In Europe this have led to approval of some SGLT2is for treatment of obese type 1 diabetes. The kidney benefit seems independent of the glucose effect, as it is seen even in low eGFR subjects with no benefit on glucose and also in nondiabetic CKD [54]. Although important pathophysiological studies of SGLT2is suggesting a benefit via reduction of intraglomerular pressure were done in type 1 diabetes [19], we are lacking renal outcome studies in type 1. Post hoc analyses suggest that maybe there could be a benefit [55].

Atrasentan is a selective endothelin receptor A antagonist with antiproteinuric effects. This was tested in the SONAR study in type 2 diabetes, and was stopped early because of low event rates, but turned out to have significant benefit on the primary renal outcome of progression of CKD or ESKD [56]. Whether this has a future in type 1 or 2 CKD is currently not known.

Fibrosis and inflammation is important for progression of nephropathy, and as mentioned aldosterone-mediated mineralocorticoid receptor (MR) overactivation is damaging. Blockade of MR overactivation with new agents like the non-steroidal mineralocorticoid receptor antagonist finerenone reduced progression of CKD in type 2 diabetes with significant reduction in the primary renal and secondary cardiovascular endpoints in FIDELIO DKD [50] and FIGARO-DKD [57].

Finally correction of the hyperglycemia with closed-loop insulin-glucose sensor systems, or insulin producing new beta cells with islet cells, stem cells, or whole pancreas transplantations, may become important.

After the seminal double transplantation by Lillehei [58] in Minneapolis, the results of simultaneous pancreas and kidney transplantation (SPK) remained disappointing for a long time. The breakthrough came with the introduction of calcineurin inhibitors and low-steroid protocols. The current regimens usually include initial induction therapy (anti-thymocyte globulin, alemtuzumab, or interleukin2 receptor antagonists) and mycophenolate mofetil, tacrolimus, and steroids. This regimen reduced acute rejections after combined kidney-pancreas transplantation from 30% to 18%. The graft survival has improved considerably and the 5-year survival was in 2010 about 70% [16]. There are no controlled randomized studies, but some evaluations suggest a benefit on diabetic complications after transplantation, but also risks [59].

Conflicts of Interest PR: Steno Diabetes Center Copenhagen has received fee for consultancy and/or speaking from AstraZeneca, Bayer, Boehringer Ingelheim, Gilead, Eli Lilly, Mundi, Novo Nordisk, Vifor, MSD MERCK, and Sanofi Aventis.

References

1. Rossing P. Prediction, progression and prevention of diabetic nephropathy. The Minkowski Lecture 2005. Diabetologia. 2006;49(1):11–9.
2. Rossing P, Hougaard P, Parving HH. Progression of microalbuminuria in type 1 diabetes: ten-year prospective observational study. Kidney Int. 2005;68(4):1446–50.
3. Vistisen D, Andersen GS, Hulman A, Persson F, Rossing P, Jorgensen ME. Progressive decline in estimated glomerular filtration rate in patients with diabetes after moderate loss in kidney function-even without albuminuria. Diabetes Care. 2019;42:1886–94.
4. MacIsaac RJ, Jerums G. Diabetic kidney disease with and without albuminuria. Curr Opin Nephrol Hypertens. 2011;20(3):246–57.
5. Molitch ME, Steffes M, Sun W, Rutledge B, Cleary P, de Boer IH, et al. Development and progression of renal insufficiency with and without albuminuria in adults with type 1 diabetes in the diabetes control and complications trial and the epidemiology of diabetes interventions and complications study. Diabetes Care. 2010;33(7):1536–43.
6. Thorn LM, Gordin D, Harjutsalo V, Hägg S, Masar R, Saraheimo M, et al. The presence and consequence of nonalbuminuric chronic kidney disease in patients with type 1 diabetes. Diabetes Care. 2015;38(11):2128–33.
7. Kidney Disease: Improving Global Outcomes (KDIGO) CKD Work Group. KDIGO. Clinical practice guideline for the evaluation and management of chronic kidney disease. Kidney Int Suppl. 2012;2013(3):1–150.
8. Fox CS, Matsushita K, Woodward M, Bilo HJ, Chalmers J, Heerspink HJ, et al. Associations of kidney disease measures with mortality and end-stage renal disease in individuals with and without diabetes: a meta-analysis. Lancet. 2012;380:1662–73.
9. Deckert T, Feldt-Rasmussen B, Borch-Johnsen K, Jensen T, Kofoed-Enevoldsen A. Albuminuria reflects widespread vascular damage. The Steno hypothesis. Diabetologia. 1989;32:219–26.
10. Rossing P, Persson F, Frimodt-Moller M, Hansen TW. Linking kidney and cardiovascular complications in diabetes-impact on prognostication and treatment: the 2019 Edwin Bierman Award Lecture. Diabetes. 2021;70(1):39–50.
11. Jensen MT, Sogaard P, Andersen HU, Bech J, Hansen TF, Galatius S, et al. Prevalence of systolic and diastolic dysfunction in patients with type 1 diabetes without known heart disease: the Thousand & 1 Study. Diabetologia. 2014;57:672–80.
12. Groop PH, Thomas MC, Moran JL, Waden J, Thorn LM, Makinen VP, et al. The presence and severity of chronic kidney disease predicts all-cause mortality in type 1 diabetes. Diabetes. 2009;58(7):1651–8.
13. Orchard TJ, Secrest AM, Miller RG, Costacou T. In the absence of renal disease, 20 year mortality risk in type 1 diabetes is comparable to that of the general population: a report from the Pittsburgh Epidemiology of Diabetes Complications Study. Diabetologia. 2010;53(11):2312–9.
14. Jorgensen ME, Almdal TP, Carstensen B. Time trends in mortality rates in type 1 diabetes from 2002 to 2011. Diabetologia. 2013;56(11):2401–4.
15. Andresdottir G, Jensen ML, Carstensen B, Parving HH, Hovind P, Hansen TW, et al. Improved prognosis of diabetic nephropathy in type 1 diabetes. Kidney Int. 2015;87(2):417–26.
16. Rossing PF, Feldt-Rasmussen B, Parving HH. Diabetic nephropathy. Brenner and Rector's The Kidney. 2. 10th ed: Elsevier; 2016. pp. 1283–321.
17. Magee GM, Bilous RW, Cardwell CR, Hunter SJ, Kee F, Fogarty DG. Is hyperfiltration associated with the future risk of developing diabetic nephropathy? A meta-analysis. Diabetologia. 2009;52(4):691–7.
18. Skøtt P. Lithium clearance in the evaluation of segmental renal tubular reabsorption of sodium and water in diabetes mellitus. Dan Med Bull. 1993;41:23–37.
19. Cherney DZ, Perkins BA, Soleymanlou N, Maione M, Lai V, Lee A, et al. Renal hemodynamic effect of sodium-glucose cotransporter 2 inhibition in patients with type 1 diabetes mellitus. Circulation. 2014;129(5):587–97.
20. Nielsen SE, Sugaya T, Hovind P, Baba T, Parving HH, Rossing P. Urinary liver-type fatty acid-binding protein predicts progression to nephropathy in type 1 diabetic patients. Diabetes Care. 2010;33(6):1320–4.

21. Theilade S, Lajer M, Hansen TW, Joergensen C, Persson F, Andresdottir G, et al. 24-hour central aortic systolic pressure and 24-hour central pulse pressure are related to diabetic complications in type 1 diabetes - a cross-sectional study. Cardiovasc Diabetol. 2013;12:122.
22. Pilemann-Lyberg S, Hansen TW, Tofte N, Winther SA, Theilade S, Ahluwalia TS, et al. Uric acid is an independent risk factor for decline in kidney function, cardiovascular events, and mortality in patients with type 1 diabetes. Diabetes Care. 2019;42(6):1088–94.
23. Hovind P, Rossing P, Tarnow L, Johnson RJ, Parving H-H. Serum uric acid as a predictor for development of diabetic nephropathy in type 1 diabetes: an inception cohort study. Diabetes. 2009;58(7):1668–71.
24. Doria A, Galecki AT, Spino C, Pop-Busui R, Cherney DZ, Lingvay I, et al. Serum urate lowering with allopurinol and kidney function in type 1 diabetes. N Engl J Med. 2020;382(26):2493–503.
25. Sandholm N, Van Zuydam N, Ahlqvist E, Juliusdottir T, Deshmukh HA, Rayner NW, et al. The genetic landscape of renal complications in type 1 diabetes. J Am Soc Nephrol. 2017;28(2):557–74.
26. Salem RM, Todd JN, Sandholm N, Cole JB, Chen WM, Andrews D, et al. Genome-wide association study of diabetic kidney disease highlights biology involved in glomerular basement membrane collagen. J Am Soc Nephrol. 2019;30(10):2000–16.
27. Rossing K, Mischak H, Dakna M, Zurbig P, Novak J, Julian BA, et al. Urinary proteomics in diabetes and CKD. J Am Soc Nephrol. 2008;19(7):1283–90.
28. Niewczas MA, Pavkov ME, Skupien J, Smiles A, Md Dom ZI, Wilson JM, et al. A signature of circulating inflammatory proteins and development of end-stage renal disease in diabetes. Nat Med. 2019;25(5):805–13.
29. Zurbig P, Jerums G, Hovind P, MacIsaac RJ, Mischak H, Nielsen SE, et al. Urinary proteomics for early diagnosis in diabetic nephropathy. Diabetes. 2012;61(12):3304–13.
30. Wang PH, Lau J, Chalmers TC. Meta-analysis of effects of intensive blood-glucose control on late complications of type I diabetes. Lancet. 1993;341:1306–9.
31. The Diabetes Control and Complications Trial Research Group. Effect of intensive therapy on the development and progression of diabetic nephropathy in the diabetes control and complications trial. Kidney Int. 1995;47:1703–20.
32. de Boer IH, Sun W, Cleary PA, Lachin JM, Molitch ME, Steffes MW, et al. Intensive diabetes therapy and glomerular filtration rate in type 1 diabetes. N Engl J Med. 2011;365(25):2366–76.
33. Rosenlund S, Hansen TW, Rossing P, Andersen S. Effect of sensor-augmented pump treatment versus multiple daily injections on albuminuria: a 1-year randomized study. J Clin Endocrinol Metab. 2015;100(11):4181–8.
34. Rosenlund S, Hansen TW, Andersen S, Rossing P. Effect of 4 years subcutaneous insulin infusion treatment on albuminuria, kidney function and HbA1c compared with multiple daily injections: a longitudinal follow-up study. Diabet Med. 2015;32(11):1445–52.
35. Ranjan AG, Rosenlund SV, Hansen TW, Rossing P, Andersen S, Norgaard K. Improved time in range over 1 year is associated with reduced albuminuria in individuals with sensor-augmented insulin pump-treated type 1 diabetes. Diabetes Care. 2020;43:2882–5.
36. Zatz R, Dunn BR, Meyer TW, Anderson S, Rennke HG, Brenner BM. Prevention of diabetic glomerulopathy by pharmacological amelioration of glomerular capillary hypertension. J Clin Invest. 1986;77:1925–30.
37. The Euclid Study Group. Randomised placebo-controlled trial of lisinopril in normotensive patients with insulin-dependent diabetes and normoalbuminuria or microalbuminuria. Lancet. 1997;349:1787–92.
38. Mauer M, Zinman B, Gardiner R, Suissa S, Sinaiko A, Strand T, et al. Renal and retinal effects of enalapril and losartan in type 1 diabetes. N Engl J Med. 2009;361(1):40–51.
39. Bilous R, Chaturvedi N, Sjolie AK, Fuller J, Klein R, Orchard T, et al. Effect of candesartan on microalbuminuria and albumin excretion rate in diabetes: three randomized trials. Ann Intern Med. 2009;151(1):11–4.

40. de Boer IH, Bangalore S, Benetos A, Davis AM, Michos ED, Muntner P, et al. Diabetes and hypertension: a position statement by the American Diabetes Association. Diabetes Care. 2017;40(9):1273–84.
41. The ACE Inhibitors in Diabetic Nephropathy Trialist Group. Should all type 1 diabetic microalbuminuric patients receive ACE inhibitors? A meta-regression analysis. Ann Intern Med. 2001;134:370–9.
42. Mathiesen ER, Hommel E, Hansen HP, Smidt UM, Parving HH. Randomised controlled trial of long term efficacy of captopril on preservation of kidney function in normotensive patients with insulin dependent diabetes and microalbuminuria. BMJ. 1999;319(7201):24–5.
43. Björck S, Mulec H, Johnsen SA, Nordén G, Aurell M. Renal protective effect of enalapril in diabetic nephropathy. BMJ. 1992;304:339–43.
44. Lewis EJ, Hunsicker LG, Bain RP, Rohde RD. The effect of angiotensin-converting-enzyme inhibition on diabetic nephropathy. The Collaborative Study Group. N Engl J Med. 1993;329:1456–62.
45. Kunz R, Friedrich C, Wolbers M, Mann JF. Meta-analysis: effect of monotherapy and combination therapy with inhibitors of the renin angiotensin system on proteinuria in renal disease. Ann Intern Med. 2008;148(1):30–48.
46. Coresh J, Heerspink HJL, Sang Y, Matsushita K, Arnlov J, Astor BC, et al. Change in albuminuria and subsequent risk of end-stage kidney disease: an individual participant-level consortium meta-analysis of observational studies. Lancet Diabetes Endocrinol. 2019;7(2):115–27.
47. Heerspink HJL, Greene T, Tighiouart H, Gansevoort RT, Coresh J, Simon AL, et al. Change in albuminuria as a surrogate endpoint for progression of kidney disease: a meta-analysis of treatment effects in randomised clinical trials. Lancet Diabetes Endocrinol. 2019;7(2):128–39.
48. Schjoedt KJ, Andersen S, Rossing P, Tarnow L, Parving HH. Aldosterone escape during blockade of the renin-angiotensin-aldosterone system in diabetic nephropathy is associated with enhanced decline in glomerular filtration rate. Diabetologia. 2004;47(11):1936–9.
49. Currie G, Taylor AH, Fujita T, Ohtsu H, Lindhardt M, Rossing P, et al. Effect of mineralocorticoid receptor antagonists on proteinuria and progression of chronic kidney disease: a systematic review and meta-analysis. BMC Nephrol. 2016;17(1):127.
50. Bakris GL, Agarwal R, Anker SD, Pitt B, Ruilope LM, Rossing P, et al. Effect of finerenone on chronic kidney disease outcomes in type 2 diabetes. N Engl J Med. 2020;383(23):2219–29.
51. Astrup AS, Tarnow L, Rossing P, Pietraszek L, Riis Hansen P, Parving HH. Improved prognosis in type 1 diabetic patients with nephropathy: a prospective follow-up study. Kidney Int. 2005;68(3):1250–7.
52. de Boer IH, Caramori ML, Chan JCN, Heerspink HJL, Hurst C, Khunti K, et al. Executive summary of the 2020 KDIGO Diabetes Management in CKD Guideline: evidence-based advances in monitoring and treatment. Kidney Int. 2020;98(4):839–48.
53. Hansen HP, Tauber-Lassen E, Jensen BR, Parving HH. Effect of dietary protein restriction on prognosis in patients with diabetic nephropathy. Kidney Int. 2002;62(1):220–8.
54. Heerspink HJL, Stefansson BV, Correa-Rotter R, Chertow GM, Greene T, Hou FF, et al. Dapagliflozin in patients with chronic kidney disease. N Engl J Med. 2020;383:1436–46.
55. van Raalte DH, Bjornstad P, Persson F, Powell DR, de Cassia CR, Wang PS, et al. The impact of sotagliflozin on renal function, albuminuria, blood pressure, and hematocrit in adults with type 1 diabetes. Diabetes Care. 2019;42(10):1921–9.
56. Heerspink HJL, Parving HH, Andress DL, Bakris G, Correa-Rotter R, Hou FF, et al. Atrasentan and renal events in patients with type 2 diabetes and chronic kidney disease (SONAR): a double-blind, randomised, placebo-controlled trial. Lancet. 2019;393(10184):1937–47.
57. Pitt B, Filippatos G, Agarwal R, Anker SD, Bakris GL, Rossing P, et al. Cardiovascular events with finerenone in kidney disease and type 2 diabetes. N Engl J Med. 2021;385:2252–63.
58. Kelly WD, Lillehei RC, Merkel FK, Idezuki Y, Goetz FC. Allotransplantation of the pancreas and duodenum along with the kidney in diabetic nephropathy. Surgery. 1967;61(6):827–37.
59. Aref A, Zayan T, Pararajasingam R, Sharma A, Halawa A. Pancreatic transplantation: brief review of the current evidence. World J Transplant. 2019;9(4):81–93.

Diabetic Chronic Kidney Disease in Type 2 Diabetes Mellitus (Albuminuric/Non-albuminuric)

16

Stefanos Roumeliotis, Francesca Mallamaci, and Carmine Zoccali

16.1 Overview of Clinical Epidemiology

The global diabetes prevalence has reached epidemic proportions and is projected to rise from 9.3% (463 million people) in 2019 to 10.9% (700 million people) by the year 2045 [1]. Approximately 40% of people with diabetes will eventually develop chronic kidney disease (CKD) over lifetime. Type 2 diabetes mellitus (T2DM) is the leading cause of end-stage kidney disease (ESKD) in the USA [2] and worldwide [1]. Since 33% of ESKD patients in the USA have received no prior nephrology care [3], and because renal biopsies in diabetics with ESKD are infrequently performed, causation for T2DM is difficult to assess which makes difficult the true prevalence and incidence of ESKD by T2DM. Diabetic kidney disease (DKD) is associated with increased risks for all-cause and cardiovascular (CV) mortality, and it is well known that most DKD patients die before development of ESKD requiring dialysis. The annual incidence rates of ESKD attributed to DKD are gradually increasing worldwide and vary from 10 to 67 per million patients [2].

DKD is a heterogenous disease. The Developing Education on Microalbuminuria for Awareness of reNal and cardiovascular risk in Diabetes (DEMAND) study assessed the prevalence of DKD in 32,308 T2DM patients from 33 countries without known kidney disease and found that the prevalence of albuminuria was 39% and that of reduced glomerular filtration rate (GFR) 22% [4]. This study reported a wide variation of albuminuria prevalence across different ethnic groups, with

S. Roumeliotis
Division of Nephrology and Hypertension, 1st Department of Internal Medicine, School of Medicine, AHEPA Hospital, Aristotle University of Thessaloniki, Thessaloniki, Greece

F. Mallamaci · C. Zoccali (✉)
CNR-IFC (National Research Council of Italy), Clinical Epidemiology of Renal Diseases and Hypertension Unit, Centre of Clinical Physiology, Reggio Calabria, Italy

A. E. Berbari, G. Mancia (eds.), *Blood Pressure Disorders in Diabetes Mellitus*, Updates in Hypertension and Cardiovascular Protection,
https://doi.org/10.1007/978-3-031-13009-0_16

Hispanic and Asian patients presenting a higher prevalence than Caucasians. A cross-sectional study of a representative sample of Chinese adults found a 5.5-fold higher prevalence of albuminuria (9.4%) than of impaired kidney function (1.7%) [5]. Over the past two decades the proportion of people with T2DM has increased by 4% in the USA, while the prevalence of DKD has reached a plateau of approximately 26–29% [6]. During this period the proportion of patients with albuminuria declined by 5%, whereas the prevalence of patients with decreased eGFR increased by 5% [6]. However, testing for albuminuria in high-risk populations remains low; in 2017, only 43% of patients with T2DM and hypertension in the USA were tested for albuminuria [2] (Box 16.1). The National Kidney Foundation's Kidney Early Evaluation Program (KEEP) study enrolled patients with preserved GFR with and without albuminuria that were followed for a median of 4.8 years, with outcome the development of ESKD requiring dialysis. During the follow-up period, the crude incidence for developing kidney failure among T2DM patients was 11.5 times higher in those with albuminuria, compared to those without albuminuria at baseline. Moreover, among non-albuminuric participants, compared to nondiabetics, T2DM patients exhibited eight times higher risk for developing ESKD [7]. These findings changed the perspective that diabetic nephropathy is a process where albuminuria is an obligatory step preceding the eGFR decline. Microalbuminuria—urinary albumin to creatinine ratio (ACR) of 30–300 mg/g KDIGO stage A2—was long regarded to reflect an initial and potentially reversible stage of DKD. However, and it is now clear that the decline in eGFR might occur independently of albuminuria, and non-albuminuric nephropathy is considered as the main clinical phenotype underlying the global ESKD burden by DKD [8]. The Chronic Renal Insufficiency Cohort (CRIC) study showed that 28% of diabetic patients with CKD patients do not present albuminuria. Compared to albuminuric diabetics, these patients have a significant reduced risk for CKD progression and ESKD [9]. Similarly in the United Kingdom Prospective Diabetes Study (UKPDS), 28% developed eGFR decline, 38% albuminuria, and 14% both conditions over a 15-year follow-up [10]. Sixty-four percent of the diabetic patients who displayed albuminuria did not develop renal impairment, and 51% of patients that developed renal impairment over time remained normoalbuminuric. A high prevalence of non-albuminuric DKD was also observed in the Action in Diabetes and Vascular disease: preterAx and diamicroN-MR Controlled Evaluation (ADVANCE) study [11] and in the Renal Insufficiency And Cardiovascular Events (RIACE) Italian Multicenter Study [12] as well as in the National Evaluation of the Frequency of Renal Impairment cO-existing with Noninsulin-dependent diabetes mellitus (NEFRON) study [13].

In type 1 diabetes (T1DM), the absence of albuminuria is more common than in T2DM (about 50%) and carries a lower risk for CKD progression, but still 10% of non-albuminuric diabetics might present a more than 30% loss of eGFR after 4 years of follow-up [14]. In disagreement with these findings, a cohort study in 600 T2DM patients with hypertension and albuminuria below 200 μg/min reported similar trends of eGFR decline among albuminuric and non-albuminuric patients, over a median follow-up period of 4 years [15]. A longitudinal cohort study in 1984 T2DM patients showed that non-albuminuric T2DM patients might also manifest pathological eGFR loss and even progression to ESKD. In this study the authors reported that the presence and degree of albuminuria affects the eGFR loss rate, with macroalbuminuric patients displaying the steepest eGFR decline, during the follow-up. However, the normoalbuminuric group still experienced rates of renal function loss above the anticipated age-related eGFR decline, and about 20% of the patients who developed ESKD did not manifest transition to macroalbuminuria [16]. Data from the large Joslin Kidney studies also suggest that a 20% of T2DM normoalbuminuric patients might manifest an early, progressive loss of renal function [17]. Therefore, it is important to screen for both albuminuria and eGFR trajectories in T2DM patients.

It was hypothesized that the high prevalence of non-albuminuric DKD might reflect the changes in therapeutic agents and treatment and the use of angiotensin-converting enzyme inhibitors (ACEi) or angiotensin receptor blockers. However, data from the CRIC study and two small studies in T2DM patients [18, 19] suggest that the shift of the DKD clinical course to non-albuminuric pattern cannot be attributed to treatment with these agents. In the study by Vistisen et al., it was shown that in T2DM patients developing CKD3 stage, the annual loss rate of eGFR across categories of albuminuria (normo-, micro-, and macroalbuminuria) was 1.9, 2.1, and 3.0 ml/min, even after adjustment for treatment with renin-angiotensin system (RAS) inhibitors [16]. In this cohort of normoalbuminuric T2DM patients, the vast majority (90%) manifested the classical initial increase in renal function, followed by a progressive linear decrease in eGFR, whereas the rest (10%) presented an accelerated eGFR decline, followed by a small increase. This progression pattern was associated with significant less treatment with RAS inhibitors and other antihypertensive agents.

Box 16.1

- T2DM is the leading cause of ESKD worldwide.
- The annual incidence rates of ESKD attributed to DKD are gradually increasing worldwide and vary from 10 to 67 per million patients.
- Among T2DM patients, the prevalence of albuminuria is higher than the prevalence of reduced eGFR.
- In the USA, during the past 20 years, the prevalence of DKD has reached a plateau of approximately 26–29%.
- During this period the proportion of patients with albuminuria declined by 5%, whereas the prevalence of patients with decreased eGFR increased by 5%.
- Non-albuminuric nephropathy is considered as the main clinical phenotype underlying the global ESKD burden by DKD.

16.2 Pathophysiology, Risk Factors, and Novel Biomarkers

Risk factors for DKD and DKD progression do not coincide in albuminuric and non-albuminuric patients. First and foremost, albuminuria per se induces kidney damage [20], and this phenomenon in large part accounts for the much slower progression toward kidney failure in non-albuminuric patients as compared to albuminuric ones. In albuminuric T2DM patients, the prevalence of diabetic retinopathy increases progressively across CKD stages, while in non-albuminuric patients, the prevalence of low ankle-brachial index (an indicator of macrovascular disease) goes along with the eGFR decline [21]. These observations suggest that the main mechanism that drives progression in non-albuminuric DKD individuals might be macroangiopathy, as opposed to microangiopathy in albuminuric individuals. Repeated episodes of acute kidney injury of various severities have also been suspected as responsible for the evolution of non-albuminuric DKD toward renal failure [22]. In line with this hypothesis, a nonlinear eGFR decline pattern is more frequent among DKD patients than in nondiabetic CKD patients [23]. Urinary concentration tumor necrosis factor alpha (TNF-a), an inflammatory mediator implicated in the progression of DKD, was strictly associated with the ACR in the whole population of patients with DKD and was much lower among non-albuminuric T2DM patients [24] than among albuminuric diabetics pointing to different degrees of inflammation among the two clinical phenotypes of DKD.

Non-albuminuric DKD is more prevalent in T2DM women than in men, probably due to the action of estrogens [10, 12, 25]. Even at late CKD stages (stage 4), despite the low eGFR, female gender has been independently associated with preservation of normoalbuminuria [26]. Data from the Swedish National Diabetes Register [25] showed that advanced age, increased systolic blood pressure (BP), low body mass index (BMI), poor glycemic control, and high triglycerides are independently associated with both decline of renal function and development of albuminuria, whereas female gender was an independent predictor of the eGFR decline only. In the Atherosclerosis Risk in Communities (ARIC) Study, high glycated hemoglobin (HbA1c) predicted incident CKD (defined as a eGFR < 60 ml/min/1.73 m^2) and this relationship was independent of albuminuria [27]. In a diverse high-risk population of T2DM patients with preserved renal function, higher systolic BP and black race were risk factors for developing treated ESKD, irrespective of the degree of albuminuria [7]. In the UK Prospective Diabetes Study, development of incident CKD or albuminuria was independently associated with Indian-Asian race and high systolic BP, whereas female sex, smoking, and decreased waist circumference predicted renal dysfunction independently of albuminuria. Therefore, these risk factors for CKD apply to both, albuminuric and non-albuminuric DKD patients [10]. Overall, high HbA1c and high systolic BP appear to be coherent risk factors for non-albuminuric DKD.

Box 16.2

- The main mechanism that drives progression of non-albuminuric DKD is macroangiopathy, as opposed to microangiopathy in albuminuric DKD.
- High HbA1c and high systolic BP appear to be coherent risk factors for non-albuminuric DKD.
- The biological pathways that promote progression of DKD include the following:
  - Production of advanced glycation end products (AGEs).
  - Reactive oxygen species (ROS).
  - Activation of protein kinase C (PKC).
  - Stimulation of the hexosamine and polyol pathway.
  - Systemic hypertension and alterations in renal hemodynamics.
  - Autophagy.
  - SGLT and cell hypoxia.
  - Urinary microRNAs and the mitochondria.

Several biological pathways may induce and promote the progression of DKD. Hyperglycemia is central to renal damage both in albuminuric and non-albuminuric DKD, and this applies to both, type 1 and 2 diabetes. The hyperglycemia-derived glycolysis triggers several metabolic pathways in DKD, including production of advanced glycation end products (AGEs), reactive oxygen species (ROS), activation of protein kinase C (PKC), and stimulation of the hexosamine and polyol pathway (Box 16.2).

16.2.1 Hyperglycemia, AGEs, Asymmetric Dimethyl Arginine, and the PKC Pathway

Glucose causes slow, non-enzymatic glycation of protein and the products are compounds characterized by an imine (C=N) bond (Schiff bases). Further molecular arrangements of these bases generate reversible production of Amadori compounds that can undergo oxidation, dehydration, cyclization, and condensation reactions that produce protein-bound compounds, the AGEs. This process is slow at normal glucose levels, but it is much accelerated in hyperglycemia, like in diabetes. AGEs typically alter the structure and function of cytosolic molecules and intracellular proteins and upregulate several signaling genes and proinflammatory and profibrotic pathways. High levels of AGEs induce dose-dependent increases of fibronectin, collagen, vascular endothelial growth factor (VEGF), and the inflammatory mediators, transforming growth factor beta 1 (TGF-β1) and TNF-a. VEGF associates with alterations in the capillary permeability and intrarenal blood flow and contributes to the development of albuminuria [28, 29].

In the early stages of experimental diabetic nephropathy, hyperglycemia upregulates the activity of nitric oxide (NO) synthase, and the resulting increase in NO bioavailability at kidney level dilatates the afferent arteriole and magnifies angiotensin II effects on the efferent arteriole [30]. On the other hand, the diabetic milieu in the kidney decreases the activity of dimethylarginine dimethylaminohydrolase (DDAH), an enzyme which metabolizes asymmetric dimethylarginine (ADMA), thereby increasing the levels ADMA at kidney level. This effect contributes to inflammation, oxidative stress (OS), and albuminuria and can be reversed by intrarenal injection of DDAH-1 [31]. At more advanced stages of nephropathy, accumulation of the endogenous inhibitor of NO, ADMA, reduces NO bioavailability triggering eGFR decline, severe albuminuria, and hypertension [32].

Hyperglycemia also upregulates the PKC pathway and by this pathway stimulates the expression of VEGF, fibronectin, collagen, and TGF-β, all effects leading to accumulation of extracellular matrix (ECM) and thickening of the basal membrane.

16.2.2 Phosphofructokinase and the Hexosamine Pathway

Glucose is fundamental for the production of energy in the cell. This normally occurs by phosphorylation of this molecule by the enzyme hexokinase. However, in the presence of sustained hyperglycemia, hexokinase is overwhelmed and excess glucose is diverted to the polyol pathway where it is converted to sorbitol by aldose reductase and then to fructose by sorbitol dehydrogenase. Fructose is then metabolized by fructokinase, a reaction triggering ATP depletion, proinflammatory cytokine expression, and OS. Wild-type mice with streptozotocin-induced diabetes exhibit high renal expression of aldose reductase; high levels of sorbitol, fructose, and uric acid; and low levels of ATP, all changes pointing to activation of the fructokinase pathway. Experimental data in mice indicate that enhanced fructokinase activity is toxic to the proximal tubule, triggering kidney injury and proteinuria and kidney dysfunction which are in large part prevented in fructokinase-deficient mice [33].

The hexosamine pathway is activated by the third step of glycolysis (phosphorylation of fructose-6-phosphate, catalyzed by the enzyme phosphofructokinase, see above) and produces sugar molecules in which a hydroxyl group is replaced by an amine group (amino sugars), and the most abundant of these sugars is *N*-acetyl-D-glucosamine. In this pathway, fructose-6-phosphate is converted to glucosamine-6-phosphate (GlucNAc-6-P) by the rate-limiting enzyme glutamine: fructose-6-phosphate aminotransferase (GFAT), which uses glutamine as an amino donor. GlucNAc-6-P is further converted in a rapid manner to uridine-5-diphosphate-*N*-acetylglucosamine (UDP-GlucNAc), the precursor for all other amino sugars that are necessary for the biosynthesis of glycoproteins, glycolipids, proteoglycans, and glycosaminoglycans. Because glucosamine levels of extracellular fluids are below the limit of detection (i.e., <0.02 mmol/L), cellular uptake of glucosamine is negligible under physiologic conditions. However, in the presence of excess glucosamine, this compound is avidly taken up by the glucose transporter and phosphorylated by hexokinase yielding GlucNAc-6-P, thereby bypassing the rate-limiting enzyme GFAT. The activation of the hexosamine pathway upregulates the transcription and expression of TGF-β1 and TNF-a associated with endothelial apoptosis, thickening of the basement membrane, and kidney injury [34, 35]. The causal role of TGF-β1 in diabetic nephropathy in experimental models is supported by the observation that the administration of a neutralizing anti-TGF-β prevents renal damage in the same models [36].

16.2.3 Systemic Hypertension and Alterations in Renal Hemodynamics

Systemic hypertension is a risk factor of primary importance for the risk of CKD in the diabetic population. In newly diagnosed T2DM patients, every 10 mm Hg increase in systolic BP portends a 15% risk excess for the incidence DKD and albuminuria [10].

The hyperglycemic environment activates the RAS and several other metabolic and hormonal mediators, resulting in kidney hypertrophy and glomerular hyperfiltration both at single nephron and whole kidney level. Vasodilators, such as nitric oxide, cyclooxygenase-2 (COX-2) prostanoids, and atrial natriuretic peptide, reduce vascular renal resistances and dilate the afferent arteriole [37]. On the other hand, the role of angiotensin II, an efferent arteriole vasoconstrictor, in renal hemodynamics is of paramount importance [38]. Other glomerular vasoconstrictors with a prevailing action on the efferent side of the microcirculation of the kidney such as thromboxane A2 and endothelin-1 (ET-1) contribute to increase the GFR in experimental models and in human disease [37]. In type 1 normoalbuminuric and normotensive diabetic adolescents, the renal hemodynamic response to hyperglycemia is gender dependent [39]. Indeed, in a Canadian study testing the effect of hyperglycemia on renal hemodynamics, during clamped euglycemia, effective renal plasma flow (ERPF) and renal blood flow (RBF) were higher and renal vascular resistance (RVR) lower in males than in females. During clamped hyperglycemia, females presented increases in RVR and the filtration fraction (FF) and reductions in RBF and ERPF, whereas no significant renal hemodynamic changes occurred in males. Furthermore, in the face of similar changes in blood pressure after ACE inhibition, this intervention reduced the eGFR and the filtration fraction only in females [39]. Thus, females exhibit an unfavorable renal response to hyperglycemia but a protective renal hemodynamic response to ACE inhibition.

Like angiotensin II, also ET-1 promotes efferent arteriolar vasoconstriction as well as inflammation, fibrosis, endothelial dysfunction, and hypertension in kidney diseases. Moreover, this autacoid triggers mesangial hypertrophy and ECM accumulation and increases glomerular permeability, thus resulting in increased albuminuria and deterioration of kidney function [40].

The prevalence of glomerular hyperfiltration is largely dependent on the duration of hyperglycemia. Probably due to advanced age, hypertension-induced glomerulosclerosis, and age-dependent kidney senescence, the prevalence of hyperfiltration among T2DM patients is lower than that in T1DM (6–23% and 34–67%, respectively) [37]. Glomerular hyperfiltration has been repeatedly associated with subsequent eGFR reduction and albuminuria worsening. Among T2DM patients with hyperfiltration at baseline, those who maintained hyperfiltration after treatment with ACE inhibitors presented a higher risk for developing albuminuria and an accelerated eGFR loss (5.2 ml/min and 2.4 respectively) as compared to those in whom hyperfiltration was corrected by ACE inhibition [15]. Thus, early correction of whole kidney hyperfiltration mitigates the progression of DKD.

16.2.4 Autophagy

Autophagy is a regulated biological process in which a special type of newly formed vesicles, the autophagosomes, phagocytize and degrade cytoplasmic content. This phenomenon is important for cell biology because it serves to eliminate aging cells and long-lived proteins and damaged organelles. The optimal level of cell autophagy depends on tissues, age, and contingent physiology needs. To maintain their homeostasis, podocytes have an increased basal autophagy level. Exposure of podocytes to hyperglycemia leads to decreased autophagy and induces severe podocyte injury, and studies in obese T2DM patients documented defective autophagy in proximal tubular cells in these patients. This alteration has long been implicated in podocyte injury and death and in the progression of DKD [41, 42]. Impaired tubular autophagy in patients with DKD triggers tubular hypertrophy, inflammation, and fibrosis, through the pathway of p53/microRNA-214 [43].The causal role of disturbed autophagy is supported by the observation in experimental models with T2DM that dietary restriction exerts anti-inflammatory effects and restores both autophagy and kidney injury [44]. However, a recent biopsy study in T1DM, 10 years after pancreas transplantation and restoration of euglycemia, showed a significant reversal of DKD (assessed by reduction in basal membrane width and ECM accumulation) despite the fact that the injury of podocytes remained unchanged or even deteriorated [45].

16.2.5 Sodium Glucose Cotransporter (SGLT) and Cell Hypoxia

Due to enhanced proximal sodium reabsorption mainly mediated by the SGLT2, sodium delivery to the macula densa is reduced in diabetic patients. This causes a reflex reduction of afferent arteriole resistance and glomerular hyperfiltration. SGLT2 inhibition reduces proximal glucose reabsorption and glomerular hyperfiltration and mitigates OS and fibrosis in the kidney [46]. Along with the hypothesis that the macula densa is key to the hemodynamic alterations induced by hyperglycemia, randomized controlled trials testing the effect of SGLT2 on renal function coherently detected a small, initial eGFR decrease followed by a substantial attenuation of DKD progression in the long term [47, 48]. In this regard, it should be noted that among T2DM patients with eGFR below 45 ml/min, the long-term renoprotective effects of SGLT2 inhibitors occur without causing the early short-term eGFR decline, thus suggesting that the mechanisms affected by SGLT2 inhibition might be other than hyperfiltration [49].

Chronic cell hypoxia has been suggested to be a primary driver of DKD. T2DM causes oxygen imbalance by compromising oxygen delivery (due to diabetes-induced microvascular injury) in the face of a high oxygen demand by enhanced kidney sodium reabsorption coupled with glucose reabsorption, a process mainly mediated by SGLT2. The hyperglycemia-associated hypoxic damage mediates capillary injury, inflammation, fibrosis, and nephron loss in diabetes [50], and the renoprotective effect of SGLT2 inhibitors might be at least partially attributed to improvement of kidney hypoxic status allowed by these drugs.

16.2.6 Urinary microRNAs and the Mitochondria

In recent years, urinary microRNAs (miRNAs) have been associated with clinical and histopathologic parameters in DKD and are now implicated in the progression of this disease. In both non-albuminuric and albuminuric T2DM patients, urinary miRNA-192 is strongly associated with the expression of TGF-β, and the degree of albuminuria [51] and urinary exosomal miRNA-29 is a marker of kidney fibrosis [52]. Moreover, in diabetic animals, the increase of miRNA-451-5p levels in urine exosomes precedes albuminuria and kidney fibrosis and is a potential biomarker of early DKD [53]. miRNA dysregulation in diabetes is extensive, and two recent meta-analyses reported that seven miRNAs (miR-21-5p, miR-29a-3p, miR-126-3p, miR-192-5p, miR-214-3p, miR-342-3p, and the hsa-miR-770 family) are substantially dysregulated in blood or urine from DKD patients compared to controls [54, 55].

The mitochondria are considered the powerhouse of the cell because these cell organelles generate most of the cell's supply of ATP which is used as a source of chemical energy. Interestingly, increased mitochondrial oxidation might be both the cause and the effect of hyperglycemia, and, once established, such an alteration activates proinflammatory, profibrotic, and apoptotic mediators. Mitochondrial DNA changes have been detected in blood, urine, and other tissues of DKD patients. Monitoring the molecular alterations in mitochondrial DNA might predict incident DKD and might also serve as a potential therapeutic target [56], an issue intensively investigated in experimental studies. Figure 16.1 summarizes the main and novel pathophysiologic mechanisms underlying development of DKD.

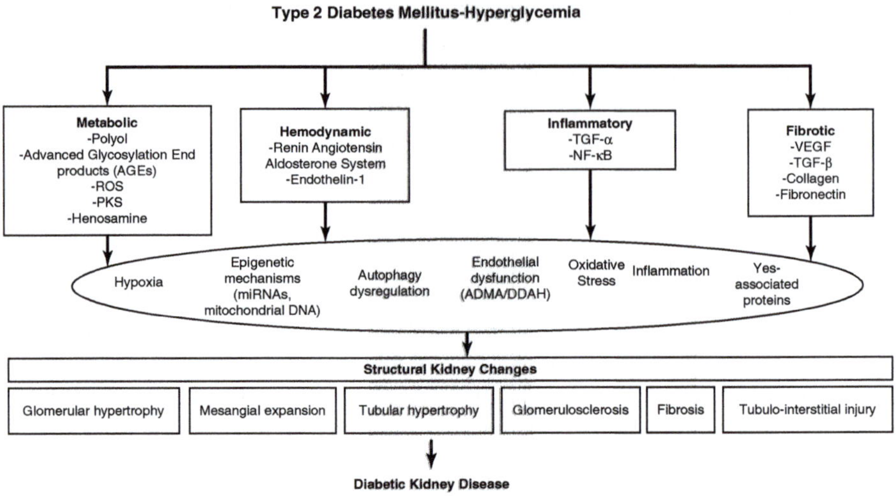

Fig. 16.1 Main and novel pathophysiologic mechanisms underlying development of DKD

16.3 Novel Biomarkers of DKD

Both albuminuria (which is believed to be the first sign of DKD) and eGFR are characterized by significant variability and lack of accuracy in the detection and prediction of DKD progression. This is attributed to the fact that these two biomarkers are not linked to the molecular alterations responsible for DKD but are the actual result of kidney injury. Developing novel biomarkers that reflect pathophysiologic alterations at a preclinical stage is now perceived as an unmet clinical need. To improve the prediction of DKD, "omics" studies identified novel proteins and metabolites that may predict the course of this disease. Among those, the CKD273 urinary proteome-based classifier that consists of collagen fragments and proteins involved in inflammation and fibrosis is now considered the most accurate predictor of DKD progression in longitudinal and cross-sectional studies [57]. In a longitudinal study of T2DM patients, the CKD273 classifier was a stronger and more accurate predictor of macroalbuminuria (AUC, area under the curve, = 0.93) as compared to microalbuminuria (AUC = 0.67). Moreover, this classifier predicted the occurrence of macroalbuminuria 4.9 years before the actual occurrence of this alteration, compared with only 3.4 years for microalbuminuria [58]. The Proteomic prediction and Renin angiotensin aldosterone system Inhibition prevention Of early diabetic nephRopathy In TYpe 2 diabetic patients with normoalbuminuria (PRIORITY) study showed that various clinical risk factors for DKD were associated with the CKD273 score, including old age, male gender, longer duration of T2DM, lower eGFR, and higher albuminuria [59]. A post hoc analysis of the Diabetic Retinopathy Candesartan Trials (DIRECT-Protect 2 study) in T2DM patients showed that this classifier predicts the development of microalbuminuria independently of age, gender, albuminuria, eGFR, and HBA1c, with hazard ratio of 2.5 and AUC of 0.79 [60].

Both in type 1 and 2 diabetes, the CKD273 identifies patients who experience a decline of eGFR to below 60 mL/min, even in the absence of albuminuria [61]. Since the CKD273 classifier is thought to predict the response of mineralo-receptor blockade in T2DM, the ongoing PRIORITY trial [62] will use this score to stratify treatment response (spironolactone-derived prevention of albuminuria). Thus, the potential of urinary "omics" markers like the CKD273 classifier in DKD extends from the early detection of DKD to progression, prognosis, and prediction of response to treatment (Box 16.3).

Box 16.3
- CKD273 classifier is a novel biomarker of DKD.
- It includes several collagen fragments and proteins involved in inflammation and fibrosis.
- It predicts macroalbuminuria more accurately, as compared to microalbuminuria.
- CKD273 score correlates with old age, male gender, long duration of T2DM, low eGFR, and high albuminuria.

16.4 Therapeutic Advancements

Diabetic subjects without renal dysfunction and without albuminuria do not exhibit any excess risk for renal function loss over time as compared to individuals in the general population matched for age and gender. The question whether the lack of albuminuria may afford the same protection in diabetic individuals with established renal dysfunction (CKD stage 3) was examined by Vistisen in 935 persons with T1DM and 1984 with T2DM during up to 16 years of follow-up at the Steno Diabetes Center in Copenhagen [16]. In this study, the yearly eGFR loss over the following 10 years was dose-dependently associated with the presence and the magnitude of albuminuria both in T1DM (normoalbuminuria 1.9 ml/min/1.73 m^2, microalbuminuria 2.3 ml/min/1.73m^2, and 3.3 mL/min/1.73 m^2 for macroalbuminuria) and T2DM (1.9 ml/min/1.73m^2, 2.1 ml/min/1.73m^2, and 3.0 ml/min/1.73m^2). The 14% of T1DM and the 10% of T2DM individuals with CKD and normoalbuminuria developed an early decline in the eGFR. These subgroups were characterized by a lower use of lipid-lowering drugs, RAS blockers, and other antihypertensive treatment suggesting that these interventions may slow CKD progression in non-albuminuric DKD. Remarkably, in this contemporary cohort the rate of eGFR loss in micro- and macroalbuminuric T1DM and T2DM patients (between 2.1 and 3.3 mL/min/1.73 m^2 per year) was substantially less than in historical cohorts in Denmark [63, 64] and in England [65] which was in the 10–20 mL/min/1.73 m^2 per year range. This spectacular improvement in kidney outcomes underlines the achievements of primary and secondary prevention of DKD of the last three decades.

As to **primary prevention of DKD**, a trial of caloric restriction in non-albuminuric obese individuals with T2DM and high or normal eGFR showed that this intervention reduced the high eGFR in hyperfiltering patients, improved insulin sensitivity, and reduced albuminuria even though this parameter was already within the normal range at baseline [66]. However, glomerular hyperfiltration per se, i.e., unassociated with albuminuria, is a surrogate of uncertain clinical relevance. Therefore, the renal effect of calorie restriction and other non-pharmacologic or pharmacologic interventions in these patients should be assessed in trials based on classical clinical endpoints like eGFR loss >50%, dialysis and transplantation, or by detailed studies of the rate of eGFR loss over time [67]. Given the very low rate of eGFR fall registered in normoalbuminuric individuals with diabetes without renal dysfunction, these trials should be done in normoalbuminuric patients with established DKD, particularly in the subset of patients (about 10%, see above) manifesting an early decline in eGFR.

Four drug trials, the BErgamo NEphrologic DIabetes Complications Trial (BENEDICT) [68], the Action in Diabetes and Vascular disease: preterAx and diamicroN-MR Controlled Evaluation (ADVANCE) [69], the Randomized Olmesartan And Diabetes MicroAlbuminuria Prevention (ROADMAP) [70], and the DIabetic REtinopathy Candesartan Trial and the progression of retinopathy in type 2 diabetes-Prevent 2 (DIRECT Protect-2) [71], reported that ACEi like perindopril in BENEDICT and angiotensin II receptor blockers (ARBs) like olmesartan and candesartan in the other two trials prevent the onset of albuminuria in hypertensive, normoalbuminuric patients with T2DM. However, none of these trials were based on established clinical renal endpoints and/or the rate of the eGFR decline. Furthermore, olmesartan in ROADMAP was associated with increased mortality risk, despite albuminuria reduction. Overall, for the lack of studies based on clinical endpoints, ACEis and ARBs are not recommended for primary prevention of DKD in T2DM in the clinical practice guidelines by the American Diabetes Association current (11. Microvascular Complications and Foot Care: Standards of Medical Care in Diabetes 2019) which is in line with the recent recommendation by KDIGO (Kidney Disease: Improving Global Outcomes Diabetes Work Group, 2020).

As to **secondary prevention of DKD**, RAS inhibitors are established agents for the treatment of albuminuric DKD in T2DM. This is because of landmark trials published in 2001, the Irbesartan Diabetic Nephropathy Trial (IDNT) [72] and the Reduction of End Points in Non-Insulin-Dependent Diabetes with the Angiotensin II Antagonist Losartan (RENAAL) [73] in DKD patients with ACR over 300 mg/g. In both trials RAS blockade was associated with a reduction in the risk for the classical combined renal endpoint (serum creatinine doubling or progression to ESKD). However, the residual risk in these studies was still substantial, ranging from 6 to 8/100 patient-years for individual outcomes and 11/100 patient-years for the composite outcome. Given the global burden of diabetes in the world population, the search for novel therapies to prevent DKD progression is a public health priority. Over the last decade new antidiabetic agents (SGLT2 inhibitors, GLP-1RA, and DDP-4 inhibitors) and new antihypertensive agents with unique nephroprotective properties have enlarged the armamentarium applied to treat DKD. Furthermore, new K-binders allow a better control of hyperkalemia, a relevant side effect of RAS blockers and aldosterone antagonists.

16.4.1 SGLT2 Inhibitors

SGLT2 inhibitors are glucose-lowering agents endowed with relevant protective effects for the kidney and the CV system. The Empagliflozin Cardiovascular Outcome Event Trial in Type 2 Diabetes Mellitus Patients (EMPA-REG OUTCOME) was the first of a series of randomized controlled trials showing that treatment with a SGLT2 inhibitor, empaglifozin, improves CV outcomes and reduces DKD progression both in non-albuminuric and albuminuric patients [47, 74, 75]. In this trial, empagliflozin substantially reduced the eGFR decline across all albuminuria strata. In the same vein, the Canagliflozin and Renal Events in Diabetes with Established Nephropathy Clinical Evaluation (CREDENCE) trial showed that canagliflozin decreases the risks for doubling of serum creatinine, progression to ESKD, death from kidney causes, or CV disease in patients with DKD [76]. Importantly, these agents reduced proteinuria, and canagliflozin slowed DKD progression also in patients with severe DKD (eGFR < 30 ml/min) [77]. In both, EMPA-REG and CREDENCE, initiation of treatment with these drugs was followed by an acute drop in eGFR in more than 50% of patients. However, the long-term clinical benefit of treatment was independent of this initial renal-hemodynamic effect [74, 78]. Besides nephroprotection, empaglifozin [79] and canagliflozin [80] stimulate erythropoiesis via increased erythropoietin levels. A third SGLT2 inhibitor, dapaglifozin (DAPA), exhibits the same cardioprotective and nephroprotective effects of empaglifozin and canagliflozin also in nondiabetic CKD patients. The Dapagliflozin and Prevention of Adverse Outcomes in Chronic Kidney Disease (DAPA-CKD) trial randomized 4304 patients with eGFR between 25 and 75 ml/min and ACR ranging from 200 to 5000 mg/g to either 10 mg per day of dapagliflozin or placebo. About 1/3 of participants had nondiabetic CKD. After a median follow-up of 2.4 years, dapagliflozin significantly decreased total mortality, progression to ESKD, and the risk for a ≥ 50% reduction in baseline eGFR, in both DKD and nondiabetic CKD patients [81]. In patients with DKD stage 3b-4, dapagliflozin caused clinically significant reductions in BP, albuminuria, and body weight, but failed to decrease HbA1c [49]. Therefore, the beneficial effects of this drug are independent of glycemic control. Even though affording the same beneficial effects for renal and CV prevention of the previously discussed SGLT2 inhibitors, another drug of this class, sotagliflozin, increased the risk of volume depletion, diarrhea, and diabetic ketoacidosis [82]. This trial, the Sotagliflozin in Patients with Diabetes and Chronic Kidney Disease (SCORED), was interrupted for the lack of funding after 14 months. Longer trials with sotagliflozin are still needed to evaluate the safety of this compound in patients with DKD.

The previously discussed large CV and renal outcome trials in patients with T2DM have shown that SGLT2 inhibitors improve CV and renal outcomes, and, in particular, they are quite effective for reducing the risk of hospitalization for heart failure [83–85]. Other trials with the same agents focusing on diabetic and nondiabetic patients with heart failure have now shown that they are unquestionably beneficial in this population. Indeed, a meta-analysis [86] of two large trials in nondiabetic and diabetic patients with heart failure, the Dapagliflozin and Prevention of Adverse Outcomes in Heart Failure (DAPA-HF) [87] and the Empagliflozin Outcome Trial in Patients with Chronic Heart Failure and a Reduced Ejection Fraction (EMPEROR-Reduced) [88] showed that these drugs reduce the risk of CV death or hospitalization for heart failure (composite outcome). However, neither trial had sufficient power to assess the effects on all-cause or CV death or adverse renal events (secondary outcomes). Overall, based on the very positive effects of SGLT2 inhibitors for CV and renal protection, the new KDIGO guideline for the treatment of T2DM with DKD recommends SGLT2 inhibitors as first-line therapy [89] in patients with eGFR above 30 ml/min. Even though the previously mentioned post hoc analysis of the CREDENCE study by Bakris [77] demonstrated that canagliflozin may prevent CKD progression in patients with eGFR < 30 ml/min/1.73m^2, this analysis was based on 170 patients only. Ongoing studies, namely, the Effects of Dapagliflozin in Nondiabetic Patients with Proteinuria (DIAMOND) trial that recruited participants with eGFR down to 25 ml/min per 1.73 m^2 [90] and the Study of Heart and Kidney Protection with Empagliflozin (EMPA-Kidney) trial [91] that includes patients with an eGFR down to 20 ml/min per 1.73 m^2, will clarify whether the benefit of SGLT2 inhibition apply also to patients with eGFR < 30 ml/min/1.73m^2.

A recent observational study based on electronic healthcare databases from seven Canadian provinces and the UK reported that, compared to dipeptidyl peptidase 4 (DPP-4) inhibitors, SGLT2 inhibitors are associated with a 2.7-fold increased risk for incident diabetic ketoacidosis events [92]. Therefore, the use of SGLT2 needs caution in patients with risk factors for diabetic ketoacidosis, such as alcoholism, drug abuse, and pancreatic insufficiency. Other risks of SGLT2 inhibitors include volume depletion and genital mycotic infections.

16.4.2 GLP-1RA and DDP-4 Inhibitors

Glucagon-like peptide-1 receptor agonists (GLP-1 RA) or incretin mimetics are of proven value for the management of T2DM, because they can reduce body weight, appetite, and HbA1c while having a decreased risk of hypoglycemia. In patients with T2DM who were at high CV risk, the rate of CV death, nonfatal myocardial infarction, or nonfatal stroke was significantly lower among patients receiving semaglutide than among those receiving placebo in the Semaglutide and Cardiovascular Outcomes in Patients with Type 2 Diabetes (SUSTAIN) trial [93]. As for SGLT2 inhibitors, the benefit of this drug went beyond CV outcomes. The Liraglutide Effect and Action in Diabetes: Evaluation of Cardiovascular Outcome Results (LEADER) trial was indeed the first of a series of GLP-1 analogues showing that liraglutide reduces (−22% in this trial) the risk of new-onset persistent macroalbuminuria, serum creatinine doubling, progression to ESKD, or death [94]. Interestingly, the renoprotective effect of liraglutide was driven almost completely by a decrease in new-onset macroalbuminuria and not by effects on ESKD or doubling serum creatinine. A recent meta-analysis of seven trials including 56,000 T2DM patients [95] confirmed that diverse GLP-1RA (a class effect) causes a 17%

decrease in the same composite renal outcome, which was largely driven by a significant decrease in macroalbuminuria (HR, 0.76, 95% CI 0.68–0.86, $p = 0.003$). However, GLP-1 RA failed to show any beneficial effect on microalbuminuria, eGFR decline, and progression of DKD toward kidney failure. On the other hand, post hoc analyses of the SUSTAIN-6 and the Peptide Innovation for Early Diabetes Treatment-6 (PIONEER-6), two large trials in T2DM patients at high CV risk, showed that semaglutide mitigated the reduction of the eGFR over time [96]. Of note, this renoprotective effect was documented in all patients and across different eGFR strata, and patients with baseline eGFR ranging from 30 to 60 ml/min were those who mostly benefited from the treatment. Based on these data, the recent KDIGO guidelines recommend use of GLP-1 RA in T2DM patients with DKD unable to achieve optimal glycemic control despite treatment with metformin or SGLT2 inhibitors or when these drugs are contraindicated [89].

DPP-4 inhibitors are hypoglycemic agents that stimulate the endogenous production of GLP-1. Data from four randomized controlled trials—the Saxagliptin Assessment of Vascular Outcomes Recorded in Patients with Diabetes Mellitus (SAVOR)-Thrombolysis in Myocardial Infarction (TIMI) 53 (SAVOR-TIMI 53) [97], the Examination of Cardiovascular Outcomes with Alogliptin versus Standard of Care (EXAMINE) [98], the Trial Evaluating Cardiovascular Outcomes with Sitagliptin (TECOS) [99], and the Cardiovascular and Renal Microvascular Outcome Study With Linagliptin (CARMELINA) [100]—pointed that among T2DM patients with CV disease, DDP-4 inhibitors have just a minor effect in albuminuria reduction, but no effect on renal endpoints and eGFR decline. Compared to canagliflozin, semaglutide induces a more pronounced weight loss (−1.1 kg) and a greater decrease in HbA1c (−0.5% at 1 year) [101]. However, a recent network meta-analysis of trials comparing new antidiabetic agents showed that SGLT2 inhibitors exhibit a much stronger renoprotective effect than GLP-1RA. Indeed, in this analysis dapagliflozin caused a 47% risk reduction of a composite kidney outcome (kidney death and clinical end-stage kidney disease, represented by progression to kidney transplantation, initiation of maintenance dialysis, or an eGFR < 15 mL/min/1.73 m^2 sustained for at least 30 days, and a third variable to represent marked worsening in kidney function, by any one or combination of new-onset macroalbuminuria, a pre-specified percent reduction in eGFR, and doubling of serum creatinine), followed by empagliflozin, canagliflozin, and then semaglutide and liraglutide, whereas linagliptin failed to show a significant beneficial effect [102].

16.4.3 Endothelin-1 Antagonists

Evidence that antagonism of endothelin-1 has beneficial effects in experimental models of kidney diseases is well established [103]. The Avosentan on Time to Doubling of Serum Creatinine, End Stage Renal Disease or Death (ASCEND) trial demonstrated that this drug causes a dose-dependent reduction in albuminuria in patients with DKD [104]. However the trial was prematurely stopped due to an excessive incidence of congestive heart failure in the treatment group, caused by fluid retention [105]. The Reducing Residual Albuminuria in T2DM patients Treated With the Maximum Tolerated Labeled Dose of a Renin Angiotensin System Inhibitor (RADAR) showed that addition of atrasentan to treatment with RAS inhibitors dose-dependently reduced residual albuminuria [106]. Although body weight, a surrogate marker of fluid retention, was significantly increased in the treatment group, there was no difference in the incidence of CV events among groups in this trial. Making treasure of the risk of heart failure triggered by fluid retention in ASCEND and RADAR, the atrasentan and renal events in patients with type 2 diabetes and chronic kidney disease (SONAR) adopted a special design and enrolled only patients exhibiting early reduction in albuminuria and no substantial fluid overload. This individualized approach excluded approximately 50% of the patients that were initially screened. In the patients that were finally included in the study, the addition of atrasentan to pre-existing treatment with a RAS inhibitor resulted in a 35% reduction of a composite renal outcome of serum creatinine doubling or progression to ESKD [107] and reduced albuminuria status, independently of eGFR and hemoglobin levels [108]. Notwithstanding the strict preselection, edema and anemia, well-known side effects of ET-1, were more frequent in the treatment group but no excess risk for CV outcomes and hospitalizations due to heart failure.

16.4.4 Patiromer

International guidelines recommend the use of spironolactone as a fourth-line, add-on therapy in patients with uncontrolled resistant hypertension. Although the prevalence of resistant hypertension is much higher in advanced CKD (stages 3b-4) compared to the general hypertensive population, the use of spironolactone in CKD is limited by the risk of hyperkalemia. Potassium binding agents represent an interesting means for mitigating hyperkalemia by aldosterone antagonists. In this regard, the Patiromer (a K-binder) versus placebo to enable spironolactone use in patients with resistant hypertension and chronic kidney disease (AMBER) trial [109] showed that among patients with uncontrolled resistant hypertension and advanced CKD (eGFR of 25–45 ml/min), the drug meaningfully reduced the risk of hyperkalemia and increased the proportion of patients who continued treatment with spironolactone during a 12-week follow-up, an effect that was independent of diabetes status [110].

16.4.5 Finerenone

Finerenone, a nonsteroidal, selective, oral mineralocorticoid receptor antagonist (MRA), has a better safety profile for the risk of hyperkalemia as compared to spironolactone. Furthermore, this drug maintains the beneficial properties of MRAs including suppression of fibrosis and inflammation. The minerAlocorticoid Receptor antagonist Tolerability Study (ARTS) trial in DKD patients showed that the addition of finerenone to standard treatment with a RAS inhibitor results in a significant, dose-dependent improvement in albuminuria [111]. However, in this study, there was no effect of finerenone in the secondary renal outcome (≥30% reduction on eGFR), which might have been due to the small power of this study for this outcome. This issue was more recently addressed in the Finerenone in Reducing Kidney Failure and Disease Progression in Diabetic Kidney Disease (FIDELIO-DKD) trial. In this trial 5734 T2DM patients with DKD and moderately increased albuminuria (30–300 mg/g ACR) and diabetic retinopathy or severely increased albuminuria (300–5000 mg/g ACR), that were being treated with ACEi or ARBS, were randomized to either finerenone or placebo. Remarkably, patients in the finerenone group presented a slower decline of eGFR rate, a lower rate of CV mortality and morbidity, and a nonsignificant reduction in mortality and progression to ESKD [112]. Until now no study focused on the possible additive beneficial effect of finerenone in DKD patients already treated with ACEi and SGLT2 inhibitors, which is a question of obvious importance for exploiting in full the new drugs which entered into the therapeutic scenario of DKD in the recent years (Table 16.1).

Table 16.1 Summary of randomized controlled trials investigating the effects of novel therapeutic agents for management of DKD

Drug	Trial	Study population	Outcome	Result
SGLT2				
Empagliflozin	EMPA-REG OUTCOME [75, 83]	4124 T2DM patients with eGFR ≥ 30 ml/min	Progression to macroalbuminuria, doubling of the serum creatinine level, ESKD, or death from renal causes	6.1% reduction
			Incident albuminuria	No difference among groups
		7020 T2DM with high CV risk	Death from CV event, nonfatal stroke, or nonfatal myocardial infarction	14% reduction
			Hospitalization for unstable angina	35% reduction
	EMPEROR-REDUCED [88]	3730 patients with heart failure and EF ≤ 40%	CV death or hospitalization for heart failure	25% reduction

(continued)

Table 16.1 (continued)

Drug	Trial	Study population	Outcome	Result
Canagliflozin	CREDENCE [76, 77, 80]	4401 T2DM patients with 30 < eGFR < 90 ml/min and UACR of >300–5000 mg/g treated with RASi	Major CV events, CV death	20% reduction
			ESKD, doubling of serum creatinine, or death from renal or CV causes	Reduction
			Anemia events or initiation of treatment for anemia	35% reduction
		170 T2DM patients with eGFR < 30 ml/min and UACR of >300–5000 mg/g treated with RASi	Rate of eGFR decline	66% reduction
			AKI and kidney-related adverse events	No difference among groups
Dapagliflozin	DAPA-CKD [49, 81]	4304 T2DM patients with 25 < eGFR < 75 ml/min and UACR of >200–5000 mg/g	ESKD, ≥50% eGFR reduction, or death from renal or CV causes	39% reduction
			CV death or hospitalization for heart failure	29% reduction
	DECLARE-TIMI 58 [47]	17,160 T2DM patients with atherosclerotic CV disease OR Multiple risk factors and eGFR > 60 mL/min	ESKD, ≥40% eGFR reduction to less than 60 ml/min, kidney transplantation, or death from renal or CV causes	24% reduction, including 46% reduction in ≥40% eGFR decline
	DAPA-HF [87]	4744 patients with heart failure and EF ≤ 40%	CV death, hospitalizations/urgent visits for heart failure resulting in intravenous therapy for heart failure	26% reduction
Sotagliflozin	SCORED [82]	10,584 T2DM patients with 25 < eGFR < 60 ml/min	CV death, hospitalizations/urgent visits for heart failure	26% reduction
			Diarrhea, genital mycotic infections, volume depletion, and diabetic ketoacidosis	Increase

Table 16.1 (continued)

Drug	Trial	Study population	Outcome	Result
GLP-1RA				
Semaglutide	SUSTAIN [93]	3297 T2DM patients, with 83% having pre-existing CV disease or CKD or both	Death from CV event, nonfatal stroke, or nonfatal myocardial infarction	Reduction
			New onset of CKD or worsening pre-existing CKD	Reduction
Liraglutide	LEADER [94]	9340 T2DM patients with Age > 50 years and CV disease or CKD OR Age > 60 years and other specified risk factors of CV disease	New-onset persistent macroalbuminuria, doubling of the serum creatinine level, ESKD, or death from renal causes	22% reduction (26% reduction in albuminuria, similar rates in doubling of the serum creatinine level, ESKD, or death from renal causes)
			AKI	No difference among groups
Semaglutide	SUSTAIN-6 PIONEER-6 [96]	6480 T2DM	Annual eGFR decline	Reduction by 0.60 ml/min
DDP-4 inhibitors				
Saxagliptin	SAVOR-TIMI 53 [97]	16,492 T2DM patients (58.8% with normoalbuminuria, 26.8% with microalbuminuria, 9.9% with macroalbuminuria)	Doubling of serum creatinine, ESKD, renal transplantation, or serum creatinine >6.0 mg/dL	No difference among groups
			eGFR	No difference among groups
			UACR	Minor reduction in all categories of albuminuria
Alogliptin	EXAMINE [98]	5380 T2DM patients with a recent acute coronary syndrome	Death from CV event, nonfatal stroke, or nonfatal myocardial infarction	No difference among groups
			HbA1c	Reduction
			ESKD	No difference among groups
Sitagliptin	TECOS [99]	14,671 T2DM patients with pre-existing CV disease	CV events	No difference among groups
			eGFR decline	No difference among groups

(continued)

Table 16.1 (continued)

Drug	Trial	Study population	Outcome	Result
Linagliptin	CARMELINA [100]	6991 T2DM patients type 2 diabetes, with a history of vascular disease and UACR > 30 mg/g OR 45 < eGFR < 75 ml/min and UACR > 200 mg/g OR 15 < eGFR < 45 ml/min	CV death, nonfatal myocardial infarction, or nonfatal stroke	No difference among groups
			ESKD, ≥40% eGFR reduction or death from renal causes	No difference among groups
Endothelin-1 antagonists				
Avosentan	ASCEND [104, 105]	1392 DKD patients treated with RASi	UACR	Dose-dependent reduction
			CV events	Increase (reason for premature termination of the study)
			ESKD, doubling of serum creatinine, or death	No difference among groups
Atrasentan	RADAR [106]	211 T2DM patients, with UACR of 300–3500 mg/g, and 30 < eGFR < 75 ml/min treated with RASi	UACR	Dose-dependent reduction
			eGFR, office BP measurements, heart failure, peripheral edema, CV events	No difference among groups
			24-h systolic and diastolic BP, LDL cholesterol, triglycerides	Reduction
			Body weight	Increase
Atrasentan	SONAR [107, 108]	2648 T2DM patients, with UACr of 300–5000 mg/g, and 25 < eGFR < 75 ml/min treated with RASi	ESKD or doubling of serum creatinine or death from renal causes	35% reduction
			UACR	Reduction, independently of eGFR and Hb
			Hospitalizations for heart failure	No difference among groups
Potassium binding agents				

Table 16.1 (continued)

Drug	Trial	Study population	Outcome	Result
Patiromer	AMBER [109]	295 CKD with uncontrolled resistant hypertension and 25 < eGFR < 45 ml/min	Difference in the proportion of patients on spironolactone	Increase in treatment group (16% increase in patients with HF, 22.4% increase in patients without HF), independently of diabetes
			Change in systolic AOBP	No difference among groups
			Risk of hyperkalemia	Reduction
Mineralocorticoid receptor antagonist				
Finerenone	ARTS [111]	821 T2DM treated with RASi	UACR change	Dose-dependent reduction
			≥30% eGFR reduction	No difference among groups
Finerenone	FIDELIO-DKD [112]	5734 T2DM with DKD treated with RASi and 30–300 mg/g UACR, 25 < eGFR < 60 ml/min and diabetic retinopathy OR 300–5000 mg/g UACR, 25 < eGFR < 75 ml/min	ESKD, ≥40% eGFR reduction, or death from renal causes	18% reduction
			CV death, CV events, hospitalization for heart failure	14% reduction

T2DM type 2 diabetes mellitus, *CV* cardiovascular, *ESKD* end-stage kidney disease, *EF* ejection fracture, *eGFR* estimated glomerular filtration rate, *UACR* urinary albumin to creatinine ratio, *RASi* renin-angiotensin system inhibitors, *AKI* acute kidney injury, *CKD* chronic kidney disease, *HBA1c* glycated hemoglobin, *BP* blood pressure, *LDL* low-density lipoprotein, *AOBP* automated office blood pressure, *DKD* diabetic kidney disease

References

1. Saeedi P, Petersohn I, Salpea P, Malanda B, Karuranga S, Unwin N, et al. Global and regional diabetes prevalence estimates for 2019 and projections for 2030 and 2045: results from the international diabetes federation diabetes atlas, 9th edition. Diabetes Res Clin Pract. 2019;157:107843.
2. Saran R, Robinson B, Abbott KC, Bragg-Gresham J, Chen X, Gipson D, et al. US renal data system 2019 annual data report: epidemiology of kidney disease in the United States. Am J Kidney Dis. 2020;75:A6–7.
3. Gillespie BW, Morgenstern H, Hedgeman E, Tilea A, Scholz N, Shearon T, et al. Nephrology care prior to end-stage renal disease and outcomes among new ESRD patients in the USA. Clin Kidney J. 2015;8(6):772.

4. Parving HH, Lewis JB, Ravid M, Remuzzi G, Hunsicker LG. Prevalence and risk factors for microalbuminuria in a referred cohort of type II diabetic patients: a global perspective. Kidney Int. 2006;69(11):2057–63.
5. Zhang L, Wang F, Wang L, Wang W, Liu B, Liu J, et al. Prevalence of chronic kidney disease in China: a cross-sectional survey. Lancet. 2012;379(9818):815–22.
6. Afkarian M, Zelnick LR, Hall YN, Heagerty PJ, Tuttle K, Weiss NS, et al. Clinical manifestations of kidney disease among US adults with diabetes, 1988–2014. JAMA. 2016;316(6):602–10.
7. Chang TI, Li S, Chen SC, Peralta CA, Shlipak MG, Fried LF, et al. Risk factors for ESRD in individuals with preserved estimated GFR with and without albuminuria: results from the kidney early evaluation program (KEEP). Am J Kidney Dis. 2013;61(4 Suppl 2):S4–11.
8. Bolignano D, Zoccali C. Non-proteinuric rather than proteinuric renal diseases are the leading cause of end-stage kidney disease. Nephrol Dial Transplant. 2017;32(Suppl 2):ii194–9.
9. Koye DN, Magliano DJ, Reid CM, Jepson C, Feldman HI, Herman WH, et al. Risk of progression of nonalbuminuric CKD to end-stage kidney disease in people with diabetes: the CRIC (chronic renal insufficiency cohort) study. Am J Kidney Dis. 2018;72(5):653–61.
10. Retnakaran R, Cull CA, Thorne KI, Adler AI, Holman RR. Risk factors for renal dysfunction in type 2 diabetes: U.K. prospective diabetes study 74. Diabetes. 2006;55(6):1832–9.
11. Ninomiya T, Perkovic V, De Galan BE, Zoungas S, Pillai A, Jardine M, et al. Albuminuria and kidney function independently predict cardiovascular and renal outcomes in diabetes. J Am Soc Nephrol. 2009;20(8):1813–21.
12. Penno G, Solini A, Bonora E, Fondelli C, Orsi E, Zerbini G, et al. Clinical significance of nonalbuminuric renal impairment in type 2 diabetes. J Hypertens. 2011;29(9):1802–9.
13. Thomas MC, MacIsaac RJ, Jerums G, Weekes A, Moran J, Shaw JE, et al. Nonalbuminuric renal impairment in type 2 diabetic patients and in the general population (national evaluation of the frequency of renal impairment cO-existing with NIDDM [NEFRON] 11). Diabetes Care. 2009;32(8):1497–502.
14. Lamacchia O, Viazzi F, Fioretto P, Mirijello A, Giorda C, Ceriello A, et al. Normoalbuminuric kidney impairment in patients with T1DM: insights from annals initiative. Diabetol Metab Syndr. 2018;10:60.
15. Ruggenenti P, Porrini EL, Gaspari F, Motterlini N, Cannata A, Carrara F, et al. Glomerular hyperfiltration and renal disease progression in type 2 diabetes. Diabetes Care. 2012;35(10):2061–8.
16. Vistisen D, Andersen GS, Hulman A, Persson F, Rossing P, Jørgensen ME. Progressive decline in estimated glomerular filtration rate in patients with diabetes after moderate loss in kidney function-even without albuminuria. Diabetes Care. 2019;42(10):1886–94.
17. Krolewski AS, Skupien J, Rossing P, Warram JH. Fast renal decline to end-stage renal disease: an unrecognized feature of nephropathy in diabetes. Kidney Int. 2017;91:1300–11.
18. Ekinci EI, Jerums G, Skene A, Crammer P, Power D, Cheong KY, et al. Renal structure in normoalbuminuric and albuminuric patients with type 2 diabetes and impaired renal function. Diabetes Care. 2013;36(11):3620–6.
19. An JH, Cho YM, Yu HG, Jang HC, Park KS, Kim SY, et al. The clinical characteristics of normoalbuminuric renal insufficiency in Korean type 2 diabetic patients: a possible early stage renal complication. J Korean Med Sci. 2009;24(Suppl):1:S75–81.
20. Abbate M, Zoja C, Remuzzi G. How does proteinuria cause progressive renal damage? J Am Soc Nephrol. 2006;17:2974–84.
21. Wu D, Xuan Y, Ruan Y, Feng X, Zhu Y, Jia C, et al. Prevalence of macro- and microvascular complications in patients with type 2 diabetes and kidney disease with or without albuminuria in a single Chinese diabetes centre. Diabetes Vasc Dis Res. 2016;13(1):21–30.
22. Johnson RJ, Rodriguez-Iturbe B. Rethinking progression of CKD as a process of punctuated equilibrium. Nat Rev Nephrol. 2018;14:411–2.
23. Weldegiorgis M, de Zeeuw D, Li L, Parving HH, Hou FF, Remuzzi G, et al. Longitudinal estimated GFR trajectories in patients with and without type 2 diabetes and nephropathy. Am J Kidney Dis. 2018;71(1):91–101.

24. Lampropoulou IT, Stangou M, Papagianni A, Didangelos T, Iliadis F, Efstratiadis G. TNF- α and microalbuminuria in patients with type 2 diabetes mellitus. J Diabetes Res. 2014;2014:394206.
25. Afghahi H, Cederholm J, Eliasson B, Zethelius B, Gudbjrnsdottir S, Hadimeri H, et al. Risk factors for the development of albuminuria and renal impairment in type 2 diabetes-the Swedish National Diabetes Register (NDR). Nephrol Dial Transplant. 2011;26(4):1236–43.
26. Boronat M, García-Cantón C, Quevedo V, Lorenzo DL, López-Ríos L, Batista F, et al. Non-albuminuric renal disease among subjects with advanced stages of chronic kidney failure related to type 2 diabetes mellitus. Ren Fail. 2014;36(2):166–70.
27. Bash LD, Selvin E, Steffes M, Coresh J, Astor BC. Poor glycemic control in diabetes and the risk of incident chronic kidney disease even in the absence of albuminuria and retinopathy: atherosclerosis risk in communities (ARIC) study. Arch Intern Med. 2008;168(22):2440–7.
28. Menne J, Park JK, Boehne M, Elger M, Lindschau C, Kirsch T, et al. Diminished loss of proteoglycans and lack of albuminuria in protein kinase C-α-deficient diabetic mice. Diabetes. 2004;53(8):2101–9.
29. Noh H, King GL. The role of protein kinase C activation in diabetic nephropathy. Kidney Int Suppl. 2007;106:S49–53.
30. Nagahama T, Hayashi K, Ozawa Y, Takenaka T, Saruta T. Role of protein kinase C in angiotensin II-induced constriction of renal microvessels. Kidney Int. 2000;57(1):215–23.
31. Wetzel MD, Gao T, Stanley K, Cooper TK, Morris SM, Awad AS. Enhancing kidney DDAH-1 expression by adenovirus delivery reduces ADMA and ameliorates diabetic nephropathy. Am J Physiol Renal Physiol. 2020;312(2):F509–17.
32. Tessari P. Nitric oxide in the normal kidney and in patients with diabetic nephropathy. J Nephrol. 2015;28:257–68.
33. Lanaspa MA, Ishimoto T, Cicerchi C, Tamura Y, Roncal-Jimenez CA, Chen W, et al. Endogenous fructose production and fructokinase activation mediate renal injury in diabetic nephropathy. J Am Soc Nephrol. 2014;25(11):2526–38.
34. Navarro JF, Mora C, Muros M, García J. Urinary tumour necrosis factor-α excretion independently correlates with clinical markers of glomerular and tubulointerstitial injury in type 2 diabetic patients. Nephrol Dial Transplant. 2006;21(12):3428–34.
35. Navarro-González JF, Mora-Fernández C. The role of inflammatory cytokines in diabetic nephropathy. J Am Soc Nephrol. 2008;19(3):433–42.
36. Chen S, Jim B, Ziyadeh FN. Diabetic nephropathy and transforming growth factor-β: transforming our view of glomerulosclerosis and fibrosis build-up. Semin Nephrol. 2003;23(6):532–43.
37. Tonneijck L, Muskiet MHA, Smits MM, Van Bommel EJ, Heerspink HJL, Van Raalte DH, et al. Glomerular hyperfiltration in diabetes: mechanisms, clinical significance, and treatment. J Am Soc Nephrol. 2017;28:1023–39.
38. Steinhausen M, Kucherer H, Parekh N, Weis S, Wiegman DL, Wilhelm KR. Angiotensin II control of the renal microcirculation: effect of blockade by saralasin. Kidney Int. 1986;30(1):56–61.
39. Cherney DZI, Sochett EB, Miller JA. Gender differences in renal responses to hyperglycemia and angiotensin-converting enzyme inhibition in diabetes. Kidney Int. 2005;68(4):1722–8.
40. Benz K, Amann K. Endothelin in diabetic renal disease. Contrib Nephrol. 2011;172:139–48.
41. Yamahara K, Kume S, Koya D, Tanaka Y, Morita Y, Chin-Kanasaki M, et al. Obesity-mediated autophagy insufficiency exacerbates proteinuria-induced tubulointerstitial lesions. J Am Soc Nephrol. 2013;24(11):1769–81.
42. Fang L, Zhou Y, Cao H, Wen P, Jiang L, He W, et al. Autophagy attenuates diabetic glomerular damage through protection of hyperglycemia-induced podocyte injury. PLoS One. 2013;8(4):e60546.
43. Ma Z, Li L, Livingston MJ, Zhang D, Mi Q, Zhang M, et al. P53/microRNA-214/ULK1 axis impairs renal tubular autophagy in diabetic kidney disease. J Clin Invest. 2020;130(9):5011–26.
44. Kitada M, Takeda A, Nagai T, Ito H, Kanasaki K, Koya D. Dietary restriction ameliorates diabetic nephropathy through anti-inflammatory effects and regulation of the autophagy

via restoration of sirt1 in diabetic wistar fatty (fa/fa) rats: a model of type 2 diabetes. Exp Diabetes Res. 2011;2011:908185.
45. Najafian B, Mauer M, Fioretto P. From mechanisms to treatment reversal of diabetic nephropathy after 10 years of pancreas transplantation occurs despite parallel podocyte loss. J Am Soc Nephrol. 2020;31
46. Kawanami D, Matoba K, Takeda Y, Nagai Y, Akamine T, Yokota T, et al. SGLT2 inhibitors as a therapeutic option for diabetic nephropathy. Int J Mol Sci. 2017;18:1083.
47. Neal B, Perkovic V, Mahaffey KW, de Zeeuw D, Fulcher G, Erondu N, et al. Canagliflozin and cardiovascular and renal events in type 2 diabetes. N Engl J Med. 2017;377(7):644–57.
48. Perkovic V, Jardine MJ, Neal B, Bompoint S, Heerspink HJL, Charytan DM, et al. Canagliflozin and renal outcomes in type 2 diabetes and nephropathy. N Engl J Med. 2019;380(24):2295–306.
49. Dekkers CCJ, Wheeler DC, Sjöström CD, Stefansson BV, Cain V, Heerspink HJL. Effects of the sodium-glucose co-transporter 2 inhibitor dapagliflozin in patients with type 2 diabetes and stages 3b-4 chronic kidney disease. Nephrol Dial Transplant. 2018;33(11):2005–11.
50. Hesp AC, Schaub JA, Prasad PV, Vallon V, Laverman GD, Bjornstad P, et al. The role of renal hypoxia in the pathogenesis of diabetic kidney disease: a promising target for newer renoprotective agents including SGLT2 inhibitors? Kidney Int. 2020;98:579–89.
51. Jia Y, Guan M, Zheng Z, Zhang Q, Tang C, Xu W, et al. MiRNAs in urine extracellular vesicles as predictors of early-stage diabetic nephropathy. J Diabetes Res. 2016;2016:7932765.
52. Lv LL, Cao YH, Ni HF, Xu M, Liu D, Liu H, et al. MicroRNA-29c in urinary exosome/microvesicle as a biomarker of renal fibrosis. Am J Physiol Ren Physiol. 2013;305(8):F1220–7.
53. Mohan A, Singh RS, Kumari M, Garg D, Upadhyay A, Ecelbarger CM, et al. Urinary exosomal microRNA-451-5p is a potential early biomarker of diabetic nephropathy in rats. PLoS One. 2016;11(4):e0154055.
54. Park S, Moon S, Lee K, Park IB, Lee DH, Nam S. Urinary and blood MicroRNA-126 and -770 are potential noninvasive biomarker candidates for diabetic nephropathy: a meta-analysis. Cell Physiol Biochem. 2018;46(4):1331–40.
55. Assmann TS, Recamonde-Mendoza M, de Souza BM, Bauer AC, Crispim D. MicroRNAs and diabetic kidney disease: systematic review and bioinformatic analysis. Mol Cell Endocrinol. 2018;477:90–102.
56. Huang Y, Chi J, Wei F, Zhou Y, Cao Y, Wang Y. Mitochondrial DNA: a new predictor of diabetic kidney disease. Int J Endocrinol. 2020;2020:3650937.
57. Pontillo C, Mischak H. Urinary peptide-based classifier CKD273: towards clinical application in chronic kidney disease. Clin Kidney J. 2017;10:192–201.
58. Zürbig P, Jerums G, Hovind P, MacIsaac RJ, Mischak H, Nielsen SE, et al. Urinary proteomics for early diagnosis in diabetic nephropathy. Diabetes. 2012;61(12):3304–13.
59. Tofte N, Lindhardt M, Adamova K, Beige J, Beulens JWJ, Birkenfeld AL, et al. Characteristics of high- and low-risk individuals in the PRIORITY study: urinary proteomics and mineralocorticoid receptor antagonism for prevention of diabetic nephropathy in type 2 diabetes. Diabet Med. 2018;35(10):1375–82.
60. Lindhardt M, Persson F, Zürbig P, Stalmach A, Mischak H, De Zeeuw D, et al. Urinary proteomics predict onset of microalbuminuria in normoalbuminuric type 2 diabetic patients, a sub-study of the DIRECT-protect 2 study. Nephrol Dial Transplant. 2017;32(11):1866–73.
61. Zürbig P, Mischak H, Menne J, Haller H. CKD273 enables efficient prediction of diabetic nephropathy in nonalbuminuric patients. Diabetes Care. 2019;42:e4–5.
62. Lindhardt M, Persson F, Currie G, Pontillo C, Beige J, Delles C, et al. Proteomic prediction and renin angiotensin aldosterone system inhibition prevention of early diabetic nephRopathy in TYpe 2 diabetic patients with normoalbuminuria (PRIORITY): essential study design and rationale of a randomised clinical multicentre trial. BMJ Open. 2016;6(3):e010310.
63. Mogensen CE. Progression of nephropathy in long-term diabetics with proteinuria and effect of initial anti-hypertensive treatment. Scand J Clin Lab Invest. 1976;36(4):383–8.
64. Parving HH, Smidt UM, Friisberg B, Bonnevie-Nielsen V, Andersen AR. A prospective study of glomerular filtration rate and arterial blood pressure in insulin-dependent diabetics with diabetic nephropathy. Diabetologia. 1981;20(4):457–61.

65. Viberti GC, Bilous RW, Mackintosh D, Keen H. Monitoring glomerular function in diabetic nephropathy. Am J Med. 1983;74(2):256–64.
66. Ruggenenti P, Abbate M, Ruggiero B, Rota S, Trillini M, Aparicio C, et al. Renal and systemic effects of calorie restriction in patients with type 2 diabetes with abdominal obesity: a randomized controlled trial. Diabetes. 2017;66(1):75–86.
67. Greene T, Ying J, Vonesh EF, Tighiouart H, Levey AS, Coresh J, et al. Performance of GFR slope as a surrogate end point for kidney disease progression in clinical trials: a statistical simulation. J Am Soc Nephrol. 2019;30(9):1756–69.
68. Ruggenenti P, Fassi A, Ilieva AP, Bruno S, Iliev IP, Brusegan V, et al. Preventing microalbuminuria in type 2 diabetes. N Engl J Med. 2004;351(19):1941–51.
69. Patel A. Effects of a fixed combination of perindopril and indapamide on macrovascular and microvascular outcomes in patients with type 2 diabetes mellitus (the ADVANCE trial): a randomised controlled trial. Lancet. 2007;370(9590):829–40.
70. Haller H, Ito S, Izzo JL, Januszewicz A, Katayama S, Menne J, et al. Olmesartan for the delay or prevention of microalbuminuria in type 2 diabetes. N Engl J Med. 2011;364(10):907–17.
71. Bilous R, Chaturvedi N, Sjølie AK, Fuller J, Klein R, Orchard T, et al. Effect of candesartan on microalbuminuria and albumin excretion rate in diabetes: three randomized trials. Ann Intern Med. 2009;151(1):11–20.
72. Lewis EJ, Hunsicker LG, Clarke WR, Berl T, Pohl MA, Lewis JB, et al. Renoprotective effect of the angiotensin-receptor antagonist irbesartan in patients with nephropathy due to type 2 diabetes. N Engl J Med. 2001;345(12):851–60.
73. Brenner BM, Cooper ME, de Zeeuw D, Keane WF, Mitch WE, Parving HH, et al. Effects of losartan on renal and cardiovascular outcomes in patients with type 2 diabetes and nephropathy. N Engl J Med. 2001;345(12):861–9.
74. Wanner C, Inzucchi SE, Lachin JM, Fitchett D, von Eynatten M, Mattheus M, et al. Empagliflozin and progression of kidney disease in type 2 diabetes. N Engl J Med. 2016;375(4):323–34.
75. Mosenzon O, Wiviott SD, Cahn A, Rozenberg A, Yanuv I, Goodrich EL, et al. Effects of dapagliflozin on development and progression of kidney disease in patients with type 2 diabetes: an analysis from the DECLARE–TIMI 58 randomised trial. Lancet Diabetes Endocrinol. 2019;7(8):606–17.
76. Mahaffey KW, Jardine MJ, Bompoint S, Cannon CP, Neal B, Heerspink HJL, et al. Canagliflozin and cardiovascular and renal outcomes in type 2 diabetes mellitus and chronic kidney disease in primary and secondary cardiovascular prevention groups: results from the randomized CREDENCE trial. Circulation. 2019;140(9):739–50.
77. Bakris G, Oshima M, Mahaffey KW, Agarwal R, Cannon CP, Capuano G, et al. Effects of canagliflozin in patients with baseline eGFR <30 ml/min per 1.73 m^2. Clin J Am Soc Nephrol. 2020;15(12):1705–14.
78. Oshima M, Jardine MJ, Agarwal R, Bakris G, Cannon CP, Charytan DM, et al. Insights from CREDENCE trial indicate an acute drop in estimated glomerular filtration rate during treatment with canagliflozin with implications for clinical practice. Kidney Int. 2020;99:999–1009.
79. Ferrannini E, Baldi S, Frascerra S, Astiarraga B, Barsotti E, Clerico A, et al. Renal handling of ketones in response to sodium-glucose cotransporter 2 inhibition in patients with type 2 diabetes. Diabetes Care. 2017;40(6):771–6.
80. Oshima M, Neuen BL, Jardine MJ, Bakris G, Edwards R, Levin A, et al. Effects of canagliflozin on anaemia in patients with type 2 diabetes and chronic kidney disease: a post-hoc analysis from the CREDENCE trial. Lancet Diabetes Endocrinol. 2020;8(11):903–14.
81. Heerspink HJL, Stefánsson BV, Correa-Rotter R, Chertow GM, Greene T, Hou F-F, et al. Dapagliflozin in patients with chronic kidney disease. N Engl J Med. 2020;383(15):1436–46.
82. Bhatt DL, Szarek M, Pitt B, Cannon CP, Leiter LA, McGuire DK, et al. Sotagliflozin in patients with diabetes and chronic kidney disease. N Engl J Med. 2021;384(2):129–39.
83. Zinman B, Wanner C, Lachin JM, Fitchett D, Bluhmki E, Hantel S, et al. Empagliflozin, cardiovascular outcomes, and mortality in type 2 diabetes. N Engl J Med. 2015;373(22):2117–28.

84. Thomson SC, Rieg T, Miracle C, Mansoury H, Whaley J, Vallon V, et al. Acute and chronic effects of SGLT2 blockade on glomerular and tubular function in the early diabetic rat. Am J Physiol Regul Integr Comp Physiol. 2012;302(1):R75–83.
85. Heerspink HJL, Perkins BA, Fitchett DH, Husain M, Cherney DZI. Sodium glucose cotransporter 2 inhibitors in the treatment of diabetes mellitus: cardiovascular and kidney effects, potential mechanisms, and clinical applications. Circulation. 2016;134(10):752–72.
86. Zannad F, Ferreira JP, Pocock SJ, Anker SD, Butler J, Filippatos G, et al. SGLT2 inhibitors in patients with heart failure with reduced ejection fraction: a meta-analysis of the EMPEROR-reduced and DAPA-HF trials. Lancet. 2020;396(10254):819–29.
87. McMurray JJV, Solomon SD, Inzucchi SE, Køber L, Kosiborod MN, Martinez FA, et al. Dapagliflozin in patients with heart failure and reduced ejection fraction. N Engl J Med. 2019;381(21):1995–2008.
88. Packer M, Anker SD, Butler J, Filippatos G, Pocock SJ, Carson P, et al. Emperor-reduced Trial Investigators. Cardiovascular and renal outcomes with empagliflozin in heart failure. N Engl J Med. 2020;383:1413–24.
89. KDIGO. 2020 clinical practice guideline for diabetes management in chronic kidney disease. Kidney Int. 2020;98(4):S1–115.
90. Cherney DZI, Dekkers CCJ, Barbour SJ, Cattran D, Abdul Gafor AH, Greasley PJ, et al. Effects of the SGLT2 inhibitor dapagliflozin on proteinuria in non-diabetic patients with chronic kidney disease (DIAMOND): a randomised, double-blind, crossover trial. Lancet Diabetes Endocrinol. 2020;8(7):582–93.
91. Herrington WG, Preiss D, Haynes R, Von Eynatten M, Staplin N, Hauske SJ, et al. The potential for improving cardio-renal outcomes by sodium-glucose co-transporter-2 inhibition in people with chronic kidney disease: a rationale for the EMPA-KIDNEY study. Clin Kidney J. 2018;11:749–61.
92. Douros A, Lix LM, Fralick M, Dell'Aniello S, Shah BR, Ronksley PE, et al. Sodium-glucose Cotransporter-2 inhibitors and the risk for diabetic ketoacidosis: a multicenter cohort study. Ann Intern Med. 2020;173(6):417–25.
93. Marso SP, Bain SC, Consoli A, Eliaschewitz FG, Jódar E, Leiter LA, et al. Semaglutide and cardiovascular outcomes in patients with type 2 diabetes. N Engl J Med. 2016;375(19):1834–44.
94. Mann JFE, Ørsted DD, Brown-Frandsen K, Marso SP, Poulter NR, Rasmussen S, et al. Liraglutide and renal outcomes in type 2 diabetes. N Engl J Med. 2017;377(9):839–48.
95. Giugliano D, Maiorino MI, Bellastella G, Longo M, Chiodini P, Esposito K. GLP-1 receptor agonists for prevention of cardiorenal outcomes in type 2 diabetes: an updated meta-analysis including the REWIND and PIONEER 6 trials. Diabetes Obes Metab. 2019;21(11):2576–80.
96. Tuttle KR, Cherney DZ, Hadjadj S, Idorn T, Mosenzon O, Perkovic V, et al. Reduction in the rate of eGFR decline with Semaglutide vs. placebo: a post hoc pooled analysis of SUSTAIN 6 and PIONEER 6. Nephrol Dial Transplant. 2020;35(Suppl 3):gfaa141.TO002. https://doi.org/10.1093/ndt/gfaa141.TO002.
97. Mosenzon O, Leibowitz G, Bhatt DL, Cahn A, Hirshberg B, Wei C, et al. Effect of saxagliptin on renal outcomes in the SAVOR-TIMI 53 trial. Diabetes Care. 2017;40(1):69–76.
98. White WB, Cannon CP, Heller SR, Nissen SE, Bergenstal RM, Bakris GL, et al. Alogliptin after acute coronary syndrome in patients with type 2 diabetes. N Engl J Med. 2013;369(14):1327–35.
99. Cornel JH, Bakris GL, Stevens SR, Alvarsson M, Bax WA, Chuang LM, et al. Effect of sitagliptin on kidney function and respective cardiovascular outcomes in type 2 diabetes: outcomes from TECOS. Diabetes Care. 2016;39(12):2304–10.
100. Rosenstock J, Perkovic V, Johansen OE, Cooper ME, Kahn SE, Marx N, et al. Effect of linagliptin vs placebo on major cardiovascular events in adults with type 2 diabetes and high cardiovascular and renal risk: the CARMELINA randomized clinical trial. JAMA. 2019;321(1):69–79.
101. Lingvay I, Catarig AM, Frias JP, Kumar H, Lausvig NL, le Roux CW, et al. Efficacy and safety of once-weekly semaglutide versus daily canagliflozin as add-on to metformin in

patients with type 2 diabetes (SUSTAIN 8): a double-blind, phase 3b, randomised controlled trial. Lancet Diabetes Endocrinol. 2019;7(11):834–44.

102. Cha AS, Chen Y, Fazioli K, Rivara MB, Devine EB. Microvascular benefits of new antidiabetic agents: a systematic review and network meta-analysis of kidney outcomes. J Clin Endocrinol Metab. 2021;106(4):1225–34.
103. Dhaun N, Webb DJ, Kluth DC. Endothelin-1 and the kidney - beyond BP. Br J Pharmacol. 2012;167(4):720–31.
104. Mann JFE, Green D, Jamerson K, Ruilope LM, Kuranoff SJ, Littke T, et al. Avosentan for overt diabetic nephropathy. J Am Soc Nephrol. 2010;21(3):527–35.
105. Hoekman J, Lambers Heerspink HJ, Viberti G, Green D, Mann JFE, De Zeeuw D. Predictors of congestive heart failure after treatment with an endothelin receptor antagonist. Clin J Am Soc Nephrol. 2014;9(3):490–8.
106. De Zeeuw D, Coll B, Andress D, Brennan JJ, Tang H, Houser M, et al. The endothelin antagonist atrasentan lowers residual albuminuria in patients with type 2 diabetic nephropathy. J Am Soc Nephrol. 2014;25(5):1083–93.
107. Heerspink HJL, Parving HH, Andress DL, Bakris G, Correa-Rotter R, Hou FF, et al. Atrasentan and renal events in patients with type 2 diabetes and chronic kidney disease (SONAR): a double-blind, randomised, placebo-controlled trial. Lancet. 2019;393(10184):1937–47.
108. Koomen JV, Stevens J, Bakris G, Correa-Rotter R, Hou FF, Kitzman DW, et al. Inter-individual variability in atrasentan exposure partly explains variability in kidney protection and fluid retention responses: a post hoc analysis of the SONAR trial. Diabetes Obes Metab. 2021;23(2):561–8.
109. Rossignol P, Williams B, Mayo MR, Warren S, Arthur S, Ackourey G, et al. Patiromer versus placebo to enable spironolactone use in patients with resistant hypertension and chronic kidney disease (AMBER): results in the pre-specified subgroup with heart failure. Eur J Heart Fail. 2020;22(8):1462–71.
110. Agarwal R, Rossignol P, Arthur S, Conrad A, White WB, Williams B. Patiromer to enable spironolactone in patients with resistant hypertension and chronic kidney disease (AMBER): results in the prespecified subgroup with diabetes. Diabetes. 2020;69(Suppl 1):1054–P.
111. Bakris GL, Agarwal R, Chan JC, Cooper ME, Gansevoort RT, Haller H, et al. Effect of finerenone on albuminuria in patients with diabetic nephropathy. JAMA. 2015;314(9):884–94.
112. Bakris GL, Agarwal R, Anker SD, Pitt B, Ruilope LM, Rossing P, et al. Effect of finerenone on chronic kidney disease outcomes in type 2 diabetes. N Engl J Med. 2020;383(23):2219–29.

Diabetic Retinopathy

17

Andrea Grosso

17.1 Epidemiology

Diabetes mellitus (DM) is a global epidemic [1], and diabetic retinopathy (DR) is one of the major causes of visual impairment in working middle-aged adults [2–5]. As outlined by Prof. Tien Yin Wong during the Euretina Lecture "Improving awareness and knowledge about the natural history of diabetes and the risk of complications, including diabetic retinopathy, is recognized as an important public health strategy. However, awareness of DR in diabetes patients continues to be suboptimal [3].

Early detection of retinopathy in individuals with diabetes is critical for preventing visual loss. Nonproliferative diabetic retinopathy (NPDR) is an early stage of DR. Moreover, NPDR can be classified into mild, moderate, and severe based on extension and severity of retinal lesions and vascular abnormalities [6, 7]. Vision loss from DR can be prevented [8–10] with broad-level public health strategies, DR screening programs, and using cost-effective treatments for vision-threatening levels of DR based on resource settings. The therapeutical armamentarium for ocular treatment was largely implemented in the last 10 years (laser, anti-VEGF, novel agents), and the ophthalmologists, particulary in high-income countries, have focused their efforts on tertiary prevention and have effective measures to treat the DR. However, the "weak rings" in the global strategy for tackling the epidemic of diabetic retinopathy are the primary and secondary prevention. In order to effectively tackle DR at a global level, we agree that a major paradigm shift is necessary

A. Grosso (✉)
Santo Spirito Hospital and ASL AL, Casale Monferrato, Italy

Centre for Macular Research, San Mauro Torinese, Italy

Former Fellow Centre for Eye Research Australia, Royal Victorian Eye and Ear Hospital, Melbourne, Australia

A. E. Berbari, G. Mancia (eds.), *Blood Pressure Disorders in Diabetes Mellitus*, Updates in Hypertension and Cardiovascular Protection,
https://doi.org/10.1007/978-3-031-13009-0_17

from tertiary towards secondary and primary prevention measures, particularly in low- and middle-income countries [3, 4]. A strict collaboration between diabetologists, family physicians, and ophthalmologists is essential: for example, national diabetic registries may enhance this collaboration and the implementation of guidelines to improve the quality of diabetes care.

Noteworthy there is a particular population of patients with type 1 diabetes who are completely spared from diabetic retinal complications [11, 12].

17.2 Hypertension: The Risk Factor for Retinopathy in Diabetics

The achievement of near-good glycemia is the main goal of diabetes patients to prevent the onset of diabetic retinopathy; nevertheless multiple studies since the 1980s have shown the crucial role of high blood pressure as a risk factor for retinopathy in diabetics.

West et al. [13] did not find any correlations between blood pressure levels and incidence of diabetic retinopathy in type 2 diabetes when blood pressure levels were below 170 mmHg, but when this cutoff was overwhelmed the incidence of retinopathy increased.

In Pima Indians Knowler et al. [14] demonstrated a clear association between blood pressure levels higher than 145 mmHg and the incidence of retinopathy.

In a population-based study in patients with type 1 diabetes, a bad control in blood pressure played a role in the severity of retinopathy [15].

Interestingly Rand et al. [16] demonstrated that diseases characterized by a low retinal flow, such as glaucoma, myopia, and chorioretinal scars, may delay the features of retinopathy. All these conditions share as a common pathological mechanism—a reduction in the perfusion as in the argon laser treatment.

High blood pressure is detrimental to each aspect of diabetic retinopathy, from microaneurysms to visual loss: the UKPDS 38 showed that a tight control of blood pressure in type 2 diabetics leads to a significant reduction in the diabetes-related mortality risk and a reduction in the progression of diabetic retinopathy. The good blood pressure control must be continued to maintain the benefits in terms of protection in the onset and progression of microvascular and macrovascular complications [17–20].

In 1998, the Euclid [21] study was the first to demonstrate a clear beneficial effect of lisinopril in the prevention of nephropathy and diabetic retinopathy: since the last 20 years we have known the pleiotropic effects of antihypertensive drug classes beyond their blood pressure-lowering effect.

Findings from the DIRECT [22] study showed that diabetic retinopathy regresses with control of hypertensive retinopathy, glucose, and lipids. Particularly renin-angiotensin blockade with candesartan may reduce diabetic retinopathy by 35% in type 2 diabetes mellitus with mild to moderate nonproliferative diabetic retinopathy.

17.3 Similarities and Differences in Early Retinal Phenotypes in Diabetes and Hypertension

17.3.1 The Morphological Correlations

Ophthalmologists need to work in close collaboration with diabetologists and specialists in internal medicine because an early and sustained improvement in blood pressure levels may protect diabetic patients from diabetic retinopathy onset and progression [3, 4, 23].

Retinopathy, particularly at its early stage, shares a number of similar morphological features representing small vessel damage by hypertensive or diabetic processes [23–28].

Further population-based studies have shown that approximately 5–10% of nondiabetic persons may have retinopathy signs similar to diabetic persons with mild retinopathy [29–32].

Therefore, understanding the clinical meaning of the retinal vascular microvascular abnormalities may provide insights into the microvasculature involved in systemic vascular disease [27, 33].

What is still under investigation is the separate contribution of hypertension and diabetes in the pathophysiology of retinopathy [6, 28].

An acute raise in systemic blood pressure may induce retinal vascular changes that are very similar to the retinal vascular changes seen in moderate nonproliferative diabetic retinopathy [6, 28, 34–40] (Figs.17.1 and 17.2).

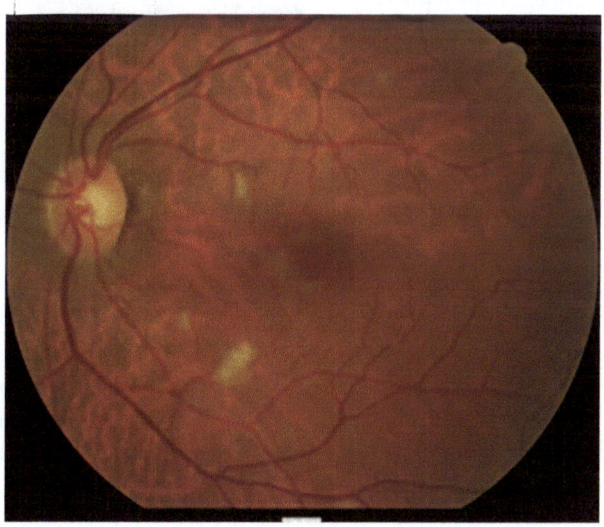

Fig. 17.1 The fundus retinal photograph shows retinal vascular abnormalities in a patient with acute rise in blood pressure (acute hypertensive retinopathy). (Courtesy of Centre for Eye Research Australia, Department of Retinal Imaging)

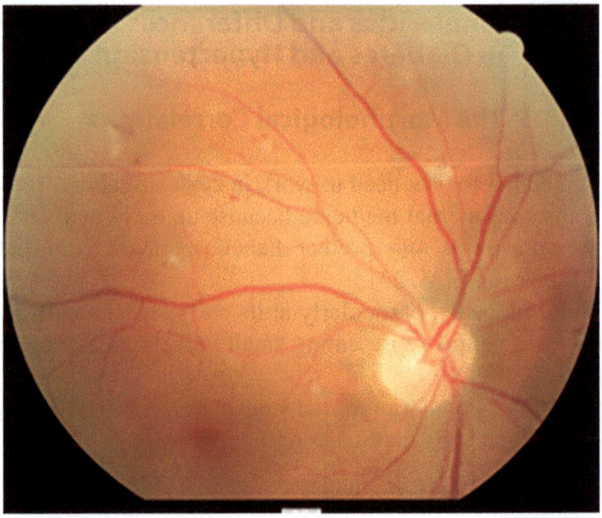

Fig. 17.2 The fundus retinal photograph shows moderate hypertensive retinopathy. (Courtesy of Centre for Eye Research Australia, Department of Retinal Imaging)

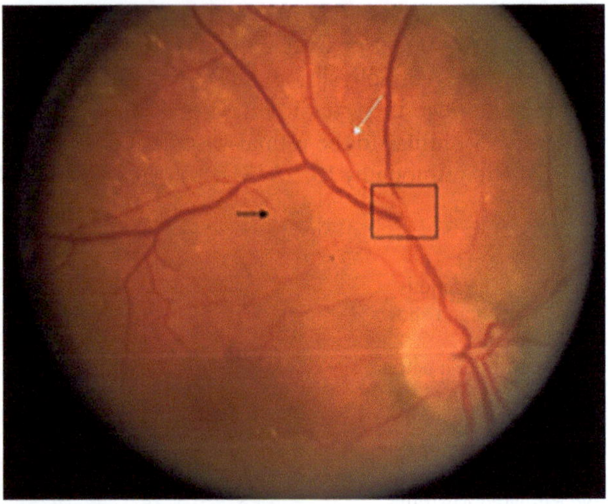

Fig. 17.3 The fundus retinal photograph shows isolated retinal microaneurysm in association with focal vascular signs in a patient with systemic blood pressure. (Courtesy of Centre for Eye Research Australia, Department of Retinal Imaging)

The cotton-wool spots may be detected in people with diabetes or hypertension with no specific differences in number, size, or location and are more common when both conditions are associated [28].

However there are some retinal vascular changes with distinct morphological differences. For example, retinal arteriolar abnormalities, such as generalized or focal arteriolar narrowing and arteriovenous nicking, are preferentially seen in people with hypertension, whereas these arteriolar changes are less commonly present in diabetic individuals without hypertension [28, 41–45].

Clustering of microaneurysms [46–48] may be a feature pointing more towards diabetes and has been shown to predict diabetic retinopathy progression (Fig. 17.2).

Isolated retinal microaneurysms may indicate hypertensive retinopathy [28] (Fig. 17.3) in association with focal arteriolar signs [49].

Hemorrhagic signs may also demonstrate subtle morphological differences in hypertensive and diabetic retinopathy as retinal hemorrhages in diabetes are normally intra-retinal hemorrhages (Fig. 17.4), whereas retinal hemorrhages induced by hypertension are superficial or nerve fiber layer hemorrhages (Fig. 17.5) [28].

As retinopathy progresses, additional idiosyncratic signs may develop. Retinal swelling has been shown in both diabetic and hypertensive retinopathies, but macular edema is a hallmark of blood-retinal barrier impairment in diabetes. On the contrary, in hypertensive retinopathy optic disk swelling is a specific sign [28].

Driven by hypoperfusion the new vessel formation is a specific sign associated with chronic not well-compensated diabetes and is not seen in long-standing hypertensive retinopathy [4, 5].

Fig. 17.4 The fundus retinal photograph shows intraretinal hemorrhages in a patient with moderate NPDR. (Courtesy of Centre for Eye Research Australia, Department of Retinal Imaging)

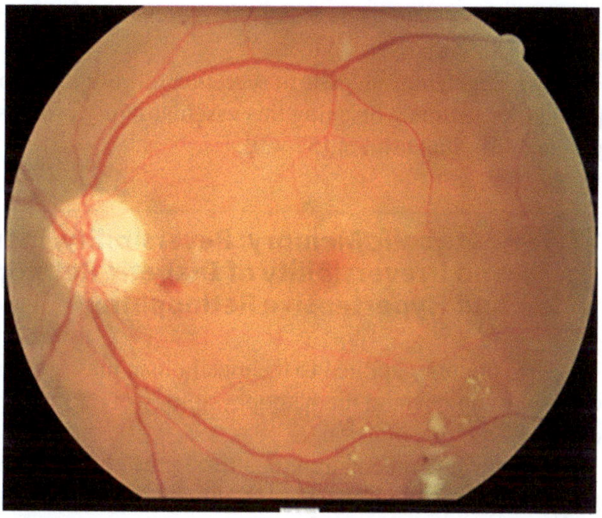

Fig. 17.5 The fundus retinal photograph shows retinal hemorrhages in a patient with systemic hypertension. (Courtesy of Centre for Eye Research Australia, Department of Retinal Imaging)

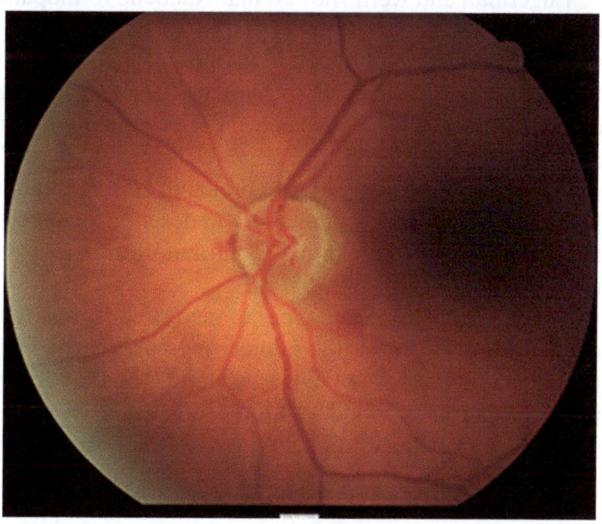

17.3.2 The Pathophysiology

The internal blood-retinal barrier is impaired in both diabetes and hypertension; however the mechanistic stress signaling pathways are different [28, 50].

Retinal blood flow is steadily maintained by autoregulation. Incremental changes in blood pressure usually have little effects on retinal flow until mean arterial blood pressure is raised by 40%, when the retinal vascular autoregulation system is impaired. As a consequence, uncontrolled increase in retinal blood flow occurs and damages the endothelial cells through increased shear stress [51].

On the opposite side, diabetes exerts its deleterious effects by increasing the expression of permeabilizing molecules [4, 52–54].

Circulating macrophages, antibodies, inflammatory cytokines, and excitotoxic amino acids or fatty acids may enter into the retina and promote damage to the neural cells [55, 56].

Neurodegeneration leads to secretion of growth factors (e.g., VEGF) and loss of pro-barrier factors worsening this vascular injury process by capillary occlusion and permeability impairment [57–60].

17.4 Metabolic Memory: Reversibility, Inertia, and Irreversibility of Diabetic Retinopathy and Hypertensive Retinopathy

The term memory applied to the metabolism may appear misleading, but it is a core concept to understand the pathophysiology of early retinal changes in patients with diabetes and hypertension.

It is known that acute retinopathy signs induced by arterial hypertension may be generally reversible [28, 51, 61, 62], whereas retinal changes correlated to diabetes are generally progressive with time despite tight metabolic control [4, 5, 28, 63, 64].

Engerman and Kern showed that "diabetic retinopathy tends to resist arrest even in its incipient stages" in an animal model in 1987 [64]. Other experimental data in support of the concept of a sort of "memory" come from the research group headed by Renu Kowluru: "although hyperglycemia is the main initiator, progression of diabetic retinopathy continues even after re-institution of normal glycemic control in diabetic patients" [65].

The group headed by Mara Lorenzi in Harvard published in 1990 the first paper [66] to introduce the term memory to describe an abnormal gene expression among the mechanisms that might contribute to the poor reversibility of diabetic retinopathy.

We can distinguish two types of memory in the tissues that are targets of complications [28, 67]. One is the salutary memory of good glycemic control; the other is the damaging memory of hyperglycemia. The Edic Study [67, 68] showed that early implementation of good glycemic control may produce long-lasting protective effects on diabetic retinopathy, by slowing the rate of progression of vascular changes.

The Diabetes Control and Complications Trial (DCCT) results and the UK Prospective Diabetes Study (UKPDS) and their follow-up studies [69–72] have documented that the duration of diabetes is a key factor in preventing retinopathy: when the glycemic control is started early in the course of diabetes, it is possible to obtain greater protection from retinopathy. These data support the concept that the progression of diabetic retinopathy incorporates memory of the years of hyperlgycemia that preceded interventional near-normoglycemia [28].

The years of poor control in glycemia may have determined marks in multiple ways [73–75]. The effects of hyperglycemia induce changes in gene expression and cellular functions, and some of the changes persist when high glucose is removed, even in cells that have gone through rounds of replication [67, 73, 74].

Histone modifications may be one of the mechanisms for persistence of altered cellular phenotypes since they can be inherited during cell division [73, 74]. The investigation of molecular features and mechanisms that may account for apparently irreversible marks left on tissues by hyperglycemia has been to date in short-term models. These models have documented that there is inertia in returning to the original state when hyperglycemia is corrected, but have not investigated inertia versus irreversibility [28]. Failure to reverse retinal inflammatory mediators shown in the animal models by the group of Renu Kowluru emphasizes their important role in the resistance of retinopathy to arrest despite restitution of near-normoglycemia [76].

One point that needs to be addressed is the question of reversibility of retinal microvascular abnormalities: with the advent of new imaging technologies and computer-assisted fundus image analysis [77–79], the clinical interest is focused on the early subclinical vascular signs. In hypertensive retinopathy the hemodynamic changes are reversible at the early stages before developing the vascular remodeling. The damage to the vascular cells, the apoptosis, and the deposition of extracellular matrix lead to vascular remodeling and progress even when hypertension is improved with therapy [28, 80].

There is some indication that the type of antihypertensive medication has a role in the improvement of hypertensive retinopathy with clinical case series showing regression of some acute retinopathy signs (hemorrhages, cotton-wool spots, retinal edema) but not chronic (generalized arteriolar narrowing, arteriovenous nicking, increased wall-to-lumen ratio) with control of blood pressure [28, 61, 62, 80, 81].

Ongoing studies about bariatric surgery [82–87] and the analysis of the vascular effects after pancreas islet cell transplantation [88, 89] may better clarify the concept of reversibility of diabetic retinopathy. Young age, male gender, high preoperative HbA1c, and presence of preoperative retinopathy were the significant predictors of worsening postoperatively in patients who underwent bariatric surgery [83]. A meta-analysis of only controlled studies showed that bariatric surgery can prevent appearance of retinopathy, but is unable to prevent deterioration of pre-existing retinopathy [90].

Another clinical scenario where it is possible to demonstrate the effects of the improvement of metabolic control to near-normoglycemia is represented by the clinical follow-up in patients who underwent islet transplantation. Islet transplantation has been reported to restore normoglycemia and the overall metabolic control in type 1 diabetes mellitus (DM) [88, 89, 91]. Clinical studies and laboratory investigations showed improvement or stabilization of the diabetic retinopathy following islet transplantation. Further, the progression of diabetic retinopathy was more likely to occur during medical therapy than after islet cell transplantation [89, 91–93].

In conclusion the cumulative glycemic exposure plays a critical role in the development of micro- and macrovascular complications in diabetic patients. It is of fundamental importance to remind ophthalmologists that a prompt diagnosis and a prompt therapeutical management may save the sight in diabetic patients.

17.5 Diabetic Choroidopathy

The choroid plays a pivotal role in the retinal function by supplying continuous perfusion into the outer retina, crucial for the thermoregulation and the secretion of growth factors [94, 95].

The advent of indocyanine green (ICG) dye fluorescence in our clinical activity has demonstrated the early involvement of the choriocapillaris in diabetics patients with and without diabetic retinopathy [96].

The retinal imaging by ICG dye fluorescence was shown to allow a more precise quantification of the extension of abnormalities in the permeability of the capillary bed compared to traditional fluorescein angiography essential for tailored laser treatments [97–99].

The advancements in fundus imaging by structural optical coherence tomography (OCT) and recently by Angio OCT (OCT-A) allowed a standardized classification of early abnormalities of the choriocapillaris in diabetics without diabetic retinopathy [100–103].

We know the characteristics of the choroidal vasculopathy from previous histological studies, and they include basement membrane thickening, vascular luminal narrowing, periodic acid-Schiff-positive homogeneous acellular nodules similar to nodules described in Kimmelstiel-Wilson glomerulosclerosis, capillary dropout, aneurysmal changes, choroidal neovascularization with subretinal fibrovascular membranes, and leakage of proteinaceous fluid into the choroidal stroma [104–106].

In the recent literature the term "diabetic choroidopathy" was used to describe both the vascular and tissue abnormalities in the choroid in diabetic patients [107–111].

In patients with Stargardt disease and concomitant diabetic retinopathy, the early abnormalities in the choriocapillaris in patients with diabetes are clearly showed in the posterior pole (Figs. 17.6 and 17.7).

It is also known that hypertensive patients have abnormalities in choroidal flow: choroidal flow impairment was documented by luminal narrowing of the capillaries, capillary dropout, and focal scarring [112–114].

Although the early histopathological abnormalities in the choriocapillaris in diabetes and hypertension share many similarities, the choroidal changes secondary to

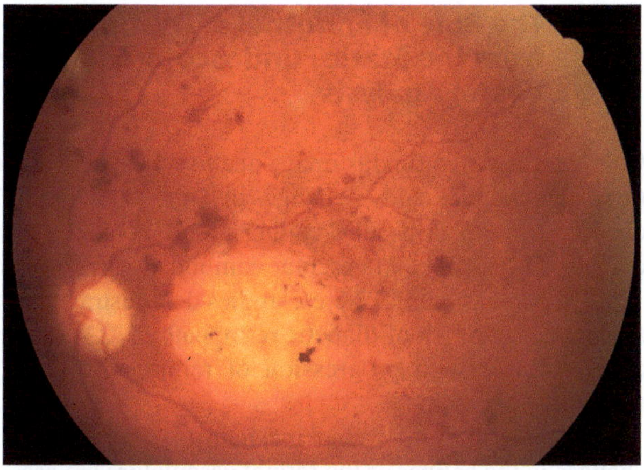

Fig. 17.6 The fundus retinal photograph documents the abnormalities in the choriocapillaris in the macular area: the macular atrophy creates a unique window beyond the retina layers in a patient with Stargardt disease. (Courtesy of Dr Eric Sigler, New York)

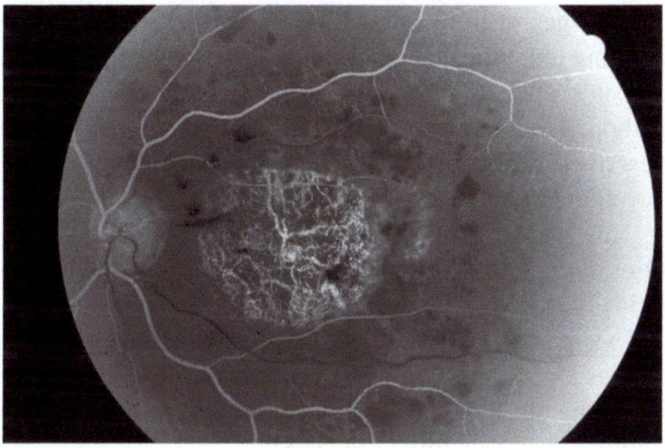

Fig. 17.7 The FFA shows choroidal abnormalities at the posterior pole in a patient with Stargardt disease and diabetic retinopathy: the window defects in the macular area clearly demonstrate the microvascular changes in the choriocapillaris. (Courtesy of Dr Eric Sigler, New York)

diabetes may be not reversible as we have discussed in the section focused to the concept of metabolic memory [28].

Studies from Prof. Gerard A. Lutty, at the Wilmer Ophthalmological Institute, Johns Hopkins Hospital, Baltimore show that diabetic choroidopathy is an inflammatory disease because there are many indicators of an inflammatory process: among them the leukocyte adhesion molecules are elevated in the choroidal vasculature and polymorphonuclear neutrophils are often isolated in the nonperfusion areas [115, 116].

The analysis of the choroidal thickness in diabetic eyes without diabetic retinopathy is not conclusive.

A recent meta-analysis [117] focused on this subject showed that diabetic eyes without diabetic retinopathy had significantly thinner choroidal thickness compared to control eyes. In addition, a sub-analysis of axial length, HbA1c, and duration of diabetes revealed that these were factors affecting choroid thickness.

In conclusion the diabetic choroidopathy (DC) should be considered in future clinical trials of drugs targeting DR because vascular changes similar to those in diabetic retinopathy are occurring in diabetic choroidopathy.

17.6 The Role of Endothelial Dysfunction: A Journey from the Static Fundoscopy to the Dynamic Vessel Analysis

Computer-assisted fundus image analysis has allowed precise measurement of subtle retinal vascular caliber changes in large populations [118]. It has been shown that changes in retinal vascular caliber are associated with the development of type 2 diabetes [119–121] and vascular complications of both type 1 and 2 diabetes [122–129]. In persons with diabetes, studies demonstrated that wider retinal arterioles are associated with risk of diabetic retinopathy [123–125], while wider retinal venules are associated with progression of retinopathy [128] and diabetic nephropathy [126, 127].

However, the underlying mechanisms for these relationships and why subtle changes in the caliber of the retinal vasculature are associated with both macro- and microvascular complications in diabetes remain unclear [42, 118].

Changes in retinal vascular caliber, as measured from fundus photographs and imaging techniques, may reflect underlying endothelial dysfunction in persons with diabetes [27, 28, 42]. Endothelial dysfunction has been suggested as a possible pathophysiogical mechanism in the pathogenesis of retinopathy beyond the well-described effects of hyperglycemia and other stress signaling pathways and the development of subsequent microvascular complications [130–133].

However clinical and epidemiological data have not found consistent associations of diabetic retinopathy with indirect serum markers of endothelial dysfunction [134–142].

In support of endothelial dysfunction in diabetic retinopathy [132, 143], there are studies showing relationships of diabetic retinopathy with cardiovascular diseases, including stroke, coronary heart disease, obesity, and heart failure, independent of traditional risk factors [144–148].

A major obstacle to clinical research of endothelial dysfunction is the difficulty in assessing its function level in vivo. Most measurements of endothelial function are time-consuming and require highly specialized personnel and equipment. In contrast, it is possible to analyze the behavior of retinal arterioles and venules non-invasively through retinal imaging techniques [28, 77]. Blood flow in the retina is in large part regulated by the diameter of retinal vessels. These vessels are not supplied with autonomic innervation and their vascular tone is mostly regulated by endocrine and paracrine factors [132]. Retinal neuronal stimulation by flicker light results in retinal vessel dilation (neurovascular coupling) and may reflect endothelial function of the retinal circulation [149–151]. The evidence that the retinal circulatory response to diffuse flicker light is related to endothelial function [152] is based on the documented role of NO in flickering light-induced vasodilation [151–154]. In fact it has been showed that nitric oxide is released in the retinal vasculature when it is stimulated by flicker light [153]. In a study by Dorner et al. [153], N^{G}-monomethyl-L-arginine (LNMMA), an inhibitor of NO synthase, blunted this flicker-induced vasodilation in healthy individuals. Furthermore, impaired response to flicker-light stimulation in persons with hypertension could be restored by angiotensin II subtype 1 receptor blockade [51], similar to a study which found improvement in the retinal arteriolar architecture with successful treatment of hypertension [155]. For example, it has been demonstrated previously that systemic administration of valsartan (angiotensin II type 1 receptor blockers) has little effect on the retinal blood flow in healthy humans [156], whereas treatment with either an angiotensin-converting enzyme inhibitor or an angiotensin II type 1 receptor blocker normalized retinal blood flow in diabetic rats [157].

It was showed that individuals with diabetes and diabetic retinopathy have reduced flicker-induced retinal vasodilation [158].

The research team headed by Prof. Tien Wong in Melbourne investigated among the firsts whether flicker light-induced vasodilation was impaired in patients with diabetes without diabetic retinopathy independent of major risk factors since 2006. The hypothesis was that a reduced vasodilation response (vasodilation reserve) in the retinal capillary bed in diabetic subjects was an *early (trailing) indicator* of subclinical retinal pathology and it was predictive *(biomarker)* of subsequent development of retinopathy and other microvascular complications.

The assessment of flicker-induced vasodilation was made possible by a specific retinal imaging technology, the Dynamic Vessel Analyzer^{R} (DVA, IMEDOS, Jena, Germany): the DVA does not require much training, and the measurement can be performed noninvasively in less than 15 min. Thanh Nguyen and associates at the Melbourne University demonstrated that among patients with diabetes, those with reduced flicker induced-dilation were more likely to have diabetic retinopathy (ORs 2.2 and 2.5, respectively, for arteriolar and venular dilation) [78, 159]. Similar results were found in other studies [160, 161]. However, the use of flickering light may be biased by a defective function of photorecpetors [132].

A different way to analyze the endothelial function is the drug delivery to the skin by iontophoresis accompanied by laser Doppler technology [162]. Responses of the skin microcirculation to sodium nitroprusside (SNP) and acetylcholine (ACh) are measures of endothelium-independent and endothelium-dependent responses, respectively: it is known that ACh stimulates nitric oxide (NO) production in endothelial cells (endothelium-dependent vasodilation), and SNP is a NO donor to vascular smooth muscle cells (endothelium-independent vasodilation). A reduction in vascular response in ACh with no concurrent reduction in SNP response would be indicative of endothelial dysfunction. The observation of reduction in responses to endothelial-dependent vasodilatation may therefore reflect endothelial dysfunction [163, 164].

Tien Wong, Thanh Nguyen, and associates at Melbourne University in collaboration with the International Diabetes Institute examined the relationship of diabetic retinopathy (DR) with skin microvascular dysfunction as measured by iontophoresis and laser Doppler flowmetry in a clinical sample of patients with diabetes. The purpose of their analysis was to establish whether diabetic retinopathy was associated with systemic microvascular dysfunction evidenced in the skin and whether this was primarily driven by endothelial dysfunction. This clinical study demonstrated that among patients with diabetes, those with DR had a reduction in the skin microvascular responses to iontophoresis of both SNP (endothelium-independent response) andACh (endothelium-dependent response). Patients with a reduction in responses to SNP or ACh were two times more likely to have diabetic retinopathy, whereas those with a reduction in responses to both SNP and ACh were four times more likely to have diabetic retinopathy. These associations were independent of major risk factors for diabetes and cardiovascular diseases, including duration of diabetes, glycemia, and blood pressure. The findings of this study suggested that diabetic retinopathy is closely linked with systemic vascular disease processes, as evidenced in the skin, that reflect a combination of endothelium-dependent dysfunction and endothelium-independent mechanisms. The paper by Thanh Nguyen and colleagues was the first published paper that examined DR and changes in skin microcirculation, as measured by laser Doppler flowmetry in response to iontophoresis of SNP and Ach [164].

At the time time of that research, another consecutive interesting issue was to establish whether an impaired retinal vasodilation response in diabetic patients without retinopathy was associated with systemic microvascular dysfunction evidenced in the skin. In an unpublished study by Prof. Wong Tien and Dr. Thanh Nguyen at Melbourne University, the relationships of skin microvascular dysfunction, as measured by laser Doppler flowmetry in response to iontophoresis of SNP and ACh, to static retinal vessel diameter and dynamic flicker light-induced retinal vasodilation were measured in a sample of patients with diabetes. The hypothesis was that reduced skin microvascular responses to iontophoresis of both SNP and ACh were related to wider retinal venular diameter and a reduced dynamic vasodilatory response to flicker light. In their study, it was shown that diabetic patients with reduced responses to iontophoresis of both SNP and ACh have wider static retinal venules. These associations were independent of the major risk factors including duration of diabetes, glycemia, and blood pressure level. The strongest associations were seen with response to ACh, which suggest that wider static retinal venular diameter may be considered a measure of endothelial dysfunction. Flicker light-induced retinal vessel dilation was also reduced in those with reduced responses to SNP or ACh, although this was not significant. The association of wider retinal venules with a reduction to ACh responses provides an explanation for previously observed associations of wider venules with other systemic diabetic complications and cardiovascular disease [165, 166]. Nguyen and colleagues were unable to demonstrate strong evidence of impaired responses to iontophoresis of SNP or ACh in those with reduced flicker-induced retinal vasodilation. Although it was previously demonstrated a correlation between the dynamic response of retinal circulation to flicker light and retinal vessel diameter in persons with diabetes [167], it was unclear then whether these associations were due to endothelial dysfunction or could also simply reflect a reduced "vasodilatory reservoir" or the inability of vessels to further dilate in already dilated retinal arterioles and venules in people with diabetes and diabetic retinopathy. In light of the lack of the association between flicker-induced vasodilation and responses to SNP and ACh, it was hypothesized that the previously observed correlation between dynamic and static vessel diameters [159, 164, 167] may reflect a reduced "vasodilatory reservoir" in persons with diabetes (Courtesy of Dr. Thanh T. Nguyen MBBS PhD, *Melbourne University*).

17.7 Diabetic Retinopathy Seeing Beyond Glucose-Induced Microvascular Disease, New Imaging Technologies, and Digital Models of Care

All cell types in the retina are affected in diabetic retinopathy as shown by several experimental and clinical studies [168–176].

The clinical goal is to identify patients with diabetes mellitus before they develop diabetic retinopathy (DR). In the past 10 years computer-assisted fundus image analysis has allowed reliable measurements of subtle retinal vascular caliber changes in large populations and correlations with systemic micro- and macrovascular complications [3, 27, 28, 77].

Recently, new imaging technologies have enabled early identification of retinal structural and functional changes, such as thinning of the inner retinal layers, even before DR is clinically evident [169]. Optical coherence tomography angiography (OCT-A), a noninvasive dye-free imaging modality, provides a highly detailed view of the retinal and choroidal vasculature. The multimodal imaging allows the physician to combine different techniques to increase the sensitivity in the detection of early retinal pathology (Fig. 17.8 and Table 17.1).

Optimized OCT-A algorithms may be used to detect early retinal and choriocapillaris (CC) microvascular flow alterations, which may be seen even before the DR presentation and may potentially result in irreversible retinal damage. The group of De Carlo et al. [184] showed OCT-A ability to detect foveal avascular zone (FAZ)

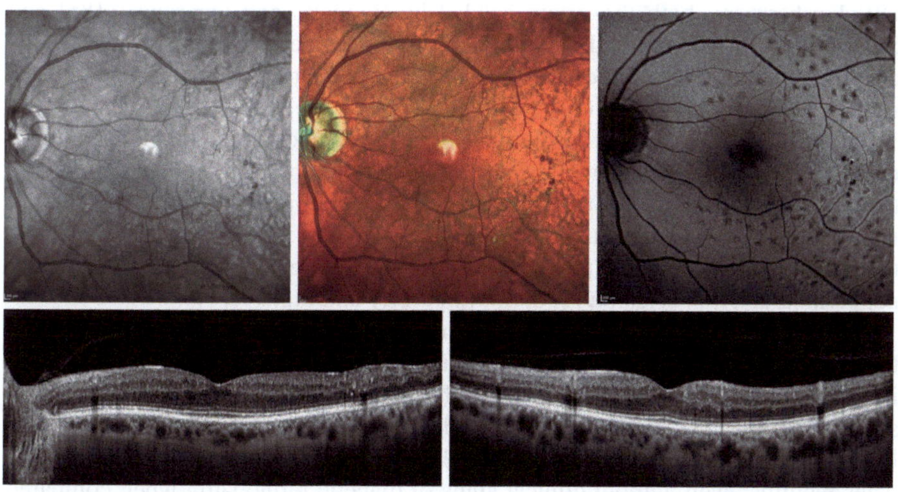

Fig. 17.8 Infrared reflectance (first raw, first column), multicolor image (first raw, second column), short-wavelength fundus autofluorescence (first raw, third column), and horizontal and vertical structural optical coherence tomography (second raw) of a patient affected by diabetic retinopathy. All images were acquired using Spectralis Heidelberg Retinal Angiograph + OCT (Heidelberg Engineering Inc., Heidelberg, Germany). Courtesy of Prof. Querques G and Dr. Sacconi R, Medical Retinal and Imaging Unit, San Raffaele Hospital, Milan, Italy

Table 17.1 New imaging modalities (OCT-A, ultrawide field imaging): the combination of different imaging modalities increase the predictive value of the diagnostic tests in the detection of early retinal pathology

New imaging modalities	Description	Clinical interest	Limitations
OCT-A	A noninvasive dye-free imaging modality provides a highly detailed view of the retinal and choroidal vasculature	The OCT angiography may therefore predict the onset of diabetic retinopathy, and the changes in the radial peripapillary plexus may represent an early subclinical indicator of diabetic microvascular disease (vessel density, retinal capillary plexus) [177–181]	Feasible only in high resource settings
Ultrawide field imaging	Ultrawide field fluorescein angiography enables a simultaneous pole-to-periphery view of the retina. This allows the entire retinal vasculature to be imaged during the dye transit by a noncontact method and increase the rate of diabetic retinopathy detection [182, 183]	The ultrawide field imaging may be useful in diagnosing retinal pathology that may first present in the periphery of the retina, resulting in better patient outcomes and tailored laser treatments to residual peripheral hypoperfusion [4, 6, 8]	Feasible only in high resource settings

remodeling and retinal capillary nonperfusion in T1DM patients without DR. Furthermore, both the group headed by Bandello and Querques [185] and Simonett et al. [186] reported a significantly decreased perfusion density (PD) in the deep retinal vascular complex (DVC) in T1DM patients without evidence of DR signs at fundus examination (Figs. 17.9 and 17.10).

Ultrawide field, ultrahigh-resolution fluorescein angiography enables a simultaneous pole-to-periphery view of the retina. This allows the entire retinal vasculature to be imaged during the dye transit by a noncontact method. This supports ophthalmologists in diagnosing retinal pathology that may first present in the periphery of the retina, resulting in better patient outcomes and tailored laser treatments to residual peripheral hypoperfusion [4, 6, 8] (Table 17.1 and Fig. 17.11).

Recently Stela Vujosevic et al. [177] have evaluated retinal capillary plexus in the most superficial layer (RPC) in the peripapillary region in healthy subjects and in patients with DM without DR and with mild nonproliferative DR using swept-source OCT-A: they found a significant decrease in vessel density, the number of branches. and length in total branches in the peripapillary area in patients with diabetes mellitus, even without clinical signs of diabetic retinopathy when compared with healthy subjects (Figs. 17.12, 17.13, 17.14, 17.15, 17.16, 17.17, and 17.18).

The OCT angiography may therefore predict the onset of diabetic retinopathy, and the changes in the radial peripapillary plexus may represent an early subclinical indicator of diabetic microvascular disease [177–181].

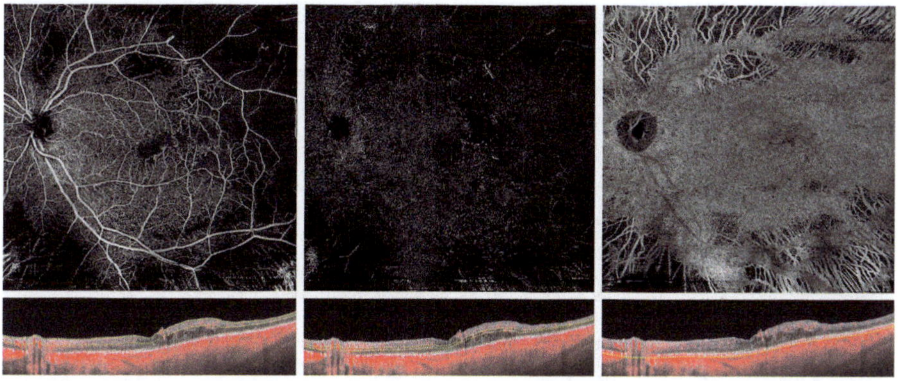

Fig. 17.9 6 × 6 en face optical coherence tomography angiography and corresponding cross-sectional b-scan with flow of superficial capillary plexus (first column), deep capillary plexus (second column), and choriocapillaris (third column) showing the reduction of vessels of a patient affected by diabetic retinopathy and diabetic macular edema. All images were acquired using swept-source OCT-A PLEX® Elite 9000 (Carl Zeiss Meditec Inc., Dublin, CA, USA). Courtesy of Prof. Querques G and Dr. Sacconi R, Medical Retinal and Imaging Unit, San Raffaele Hospital, Milan, Italy

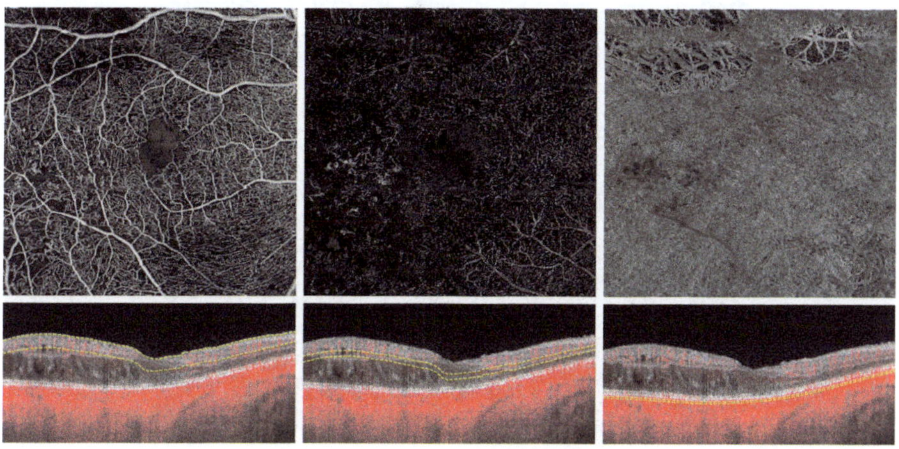

Fig. 17.10 12 × 12 en face optical coherence tomography angiography and corresponding cross-sectional b-scan with flow of superficial capillary plexus (first column), deep capillary plexus (second column), and choriocapillaris (third column) showing the reduction of vessels of a patient affected by diabetic retinopathy and diabetic macular edema. All images were acquired using swept-source OCT-A PLEX® Elite 9000 (Carl Zeiss Meditec Inc., Dublin, CA, USA). Courtesy of Prof. Querques G and Dr. Sacconi R, Medical Retinal and Imaging Unit, San Raffaele Hospital, Milan, Italy

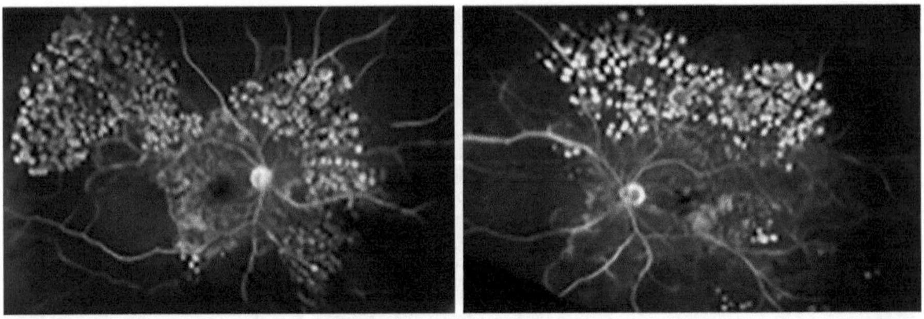

Fig. 17.11 Ultrawide field fluorescein angiography of a patient affected by diabetic retinopathy. All images were acquired using Optos California (Optos PLC, Dunfermline, United Kingdom). Courtesy of Prof. Querques G and Dr. Sacconi R, Medical Retinal and Imaging Unit, San Raffaele Hospital, Milan, Italy

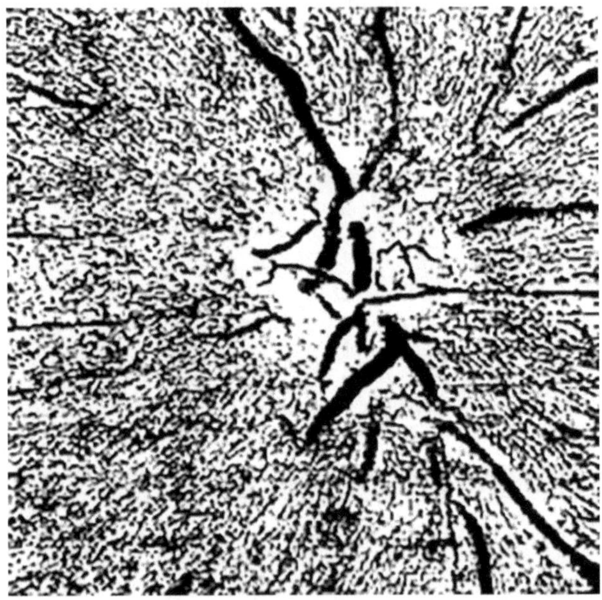

Fig. 17.12 ImageJ analysis of the radial peripapillary capillary plexus (RPC) image. OCT-A images were opened in ImageJ analysis software. All OCT-A images were converted into 8-bit files (320 × 320 pixels; one-pixel macula 9.375 × 9.375 lm^2; one-pixel papilla 14.06 × 14.06 lm^2). All images underwent automatic "default" threshold available in the ImageJ software to neutralize the background noise. The image was then converted into a binarized black-and-white image. RPC slab images were analyzed eliminating the optic disc from the analysis (the region of interest was manually delineated by twp evaluators and confirmed by the expert ophthalmologist) to remove the large vessels of the optic disc. This binary image was used to calculate PD (number of pixels of vessels/total pixels of the analyzed area) [177]. The binarized image was used to create a skeletonized image to measure the statistical length of moving blood column, or VD [(number of pixels of vessels) × (scan width in mm/320) / (area in mm^2)], as previously described [177, 187]. ImageJ binarization. Courtesy of Dr Vujosevic Stela, University Eye Clinic San Giuseppe Hospital (Director Prof. P. Nucci), IRCCS MultiMedica, Milan, Italy

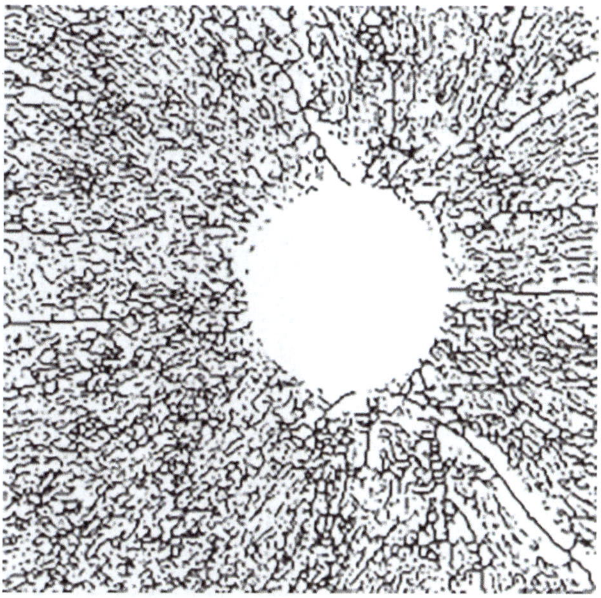

Fig. 17.13 ImageJ analysis of the radial peripapillary capillary plexus (RPC). Image skeletonization. Courtesy of Dr Vujosevic Stela, University Eye Clinic San Giuseppe Hospital (Director Prof. P. Nucci), IRCCS MultiMedica, Milan, Italy

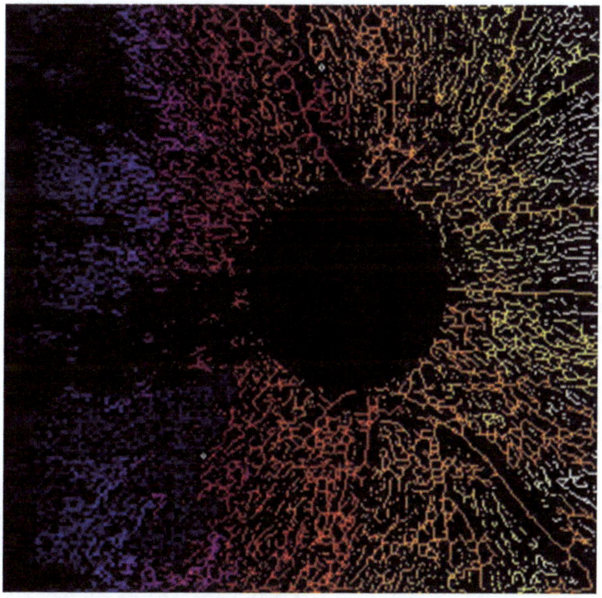

Fig. 17.14 ImageJ-labeled skeletons. AnalyzeSkeleton analysis. Automatic analysis of skeletonized images. From this analysis the number of branches and branch's length can be counted. Courtesy of Dr Vujosevic Stela, University Eye Clinic San Giuseppe Hospital (Director Prof. P. Nucci), IRCCS MultiMedica, Milan, Italy

As shown by the group of Midena and Vujosevic and the group of Wong and Nguyen, there is a coexistence between an early neuronal and microvascular damage in patients with diabetes mellitus without diabetic retinopathy. We can define this interplay as neurovascular coupling: the retina can control local biochemical environment by an interdependent synergy between blood vessels and neural cells

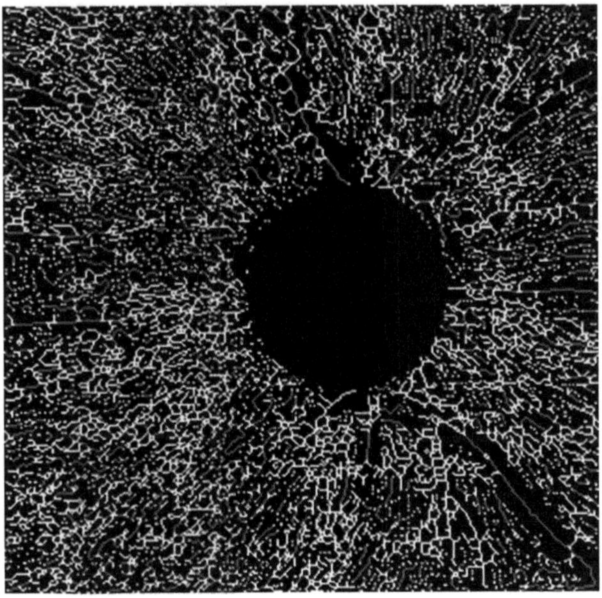

Fig. 17.15 Output image of the shortest (magenta) and the longest (white) path. Courtesy of Dr Vujosevic Stela, University Eye Clinic San Giuseppe Hospital (Director Prof. P. Nucci), IRCCS MultiMedica, Milan, Italy

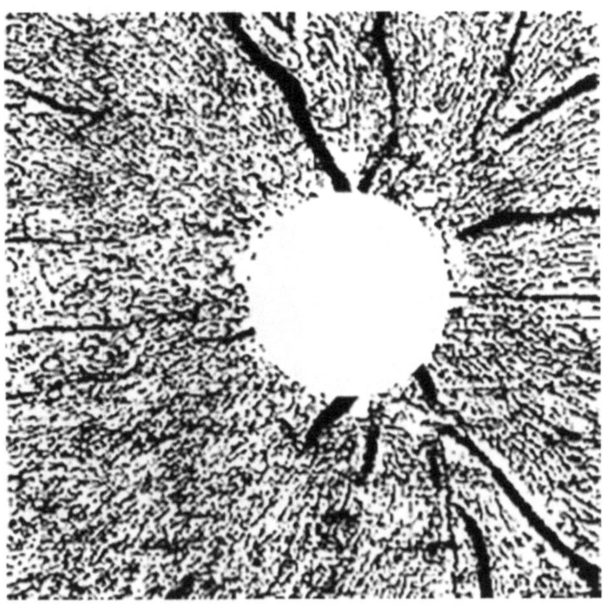

Fig. 17.16 Optic disc manually removed. Skeletonized image with removed optic disc region that was analyzed with plugin AnalyzeSkeleton. Courtesy of Dr Vujosevic Stela, University Eye Clinic San Giuseppe Hospital, IRCCS MultiMedica (Director Prof. P. Nucci), Milan, Italy

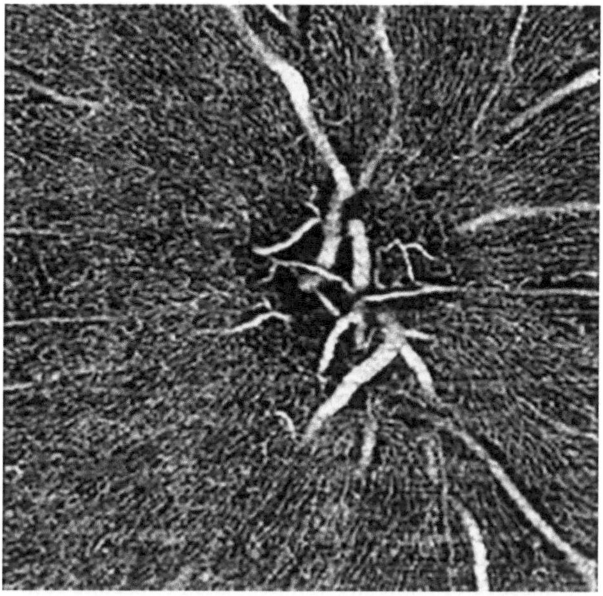

Fig. 17.17 RPC stab image. Courtesy of Dr Vujosevic Stela, University Eye Clinic San Giuseppe Hospital, IRCCS MultiMedica (Director Prof. P. Nucci), Milan, Italy

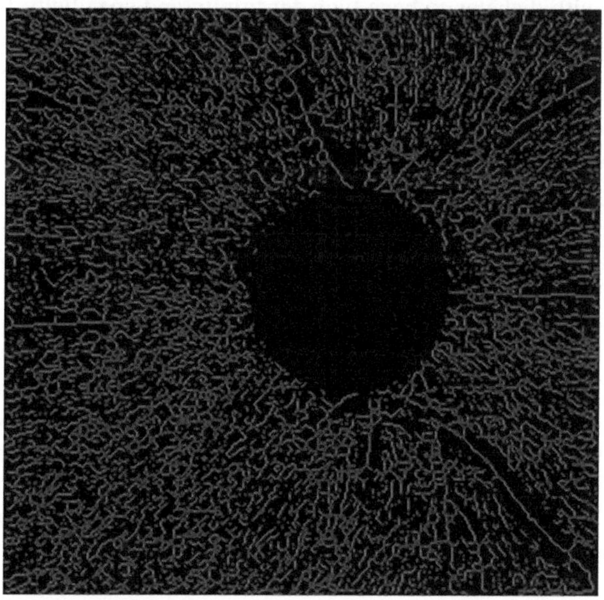

Fig. 17.18 The plugin tagged pixels in the skeleton image (endpoint pixels are displayed in blue, slab pixels in orange, and junction pixels in purple). Courtesy of Dr Vujosevic Stela, University Eye Clinic San Giuseppe Hospital, IRCCS MultiMedica (Director Prof. P. Nucci), Milan, Italy

[27, 52, 54, 78, 132, 188]. The combination of hemodynamic changes secondary to hypertension and metabolic pathways related to diabetes induces maladaptive inflammatory responses that ultimately result in cumulative pathology seen in diabetic and hypertensive retinopathy [28, 56, 132]. The Dynamic Vessel Analyzer

(DVA) was a clinical tool useful to demonstrate the correlation between the microvascular bed and neuronal cells [78, 159–161]. It is becoming increasingly clear that neuronal cells of the retina are also affected by diabetes, resulting in dysfunction and degeneration [174]. As retinal blood flow is coupled with neuronal activity [175], reduced flicker light-induced vasodilation can thus reflect neurodegeneration as well [159, 161, 164, 167]. Therefore in persons with diabetes, reduced flicker light-induced vasodilation may reflect damage to the neural tissues and the microcirculation in diabetes as well as impairment in the myogenic response to posture [132].

The fractal analysis in the eyes with diabetic retinopathy may provide ophthalmologists with new data: retinal vascular geometry measured from fundus photographs may predict the incidence and progression of diabetic retinopathy in adults with diabetes, beyond established risk factors [189–193].

We need to move towards a new paradigm of diabetic retinopathy that integrate also the neuronal damage into classification of diabetic retinal disease: developments of high-resolution structural optical coherence tomography technology have provided ophthalmologists with a reliable tool able to identify and monitor thinning of the inner retinal layers suggesting a gradual loss of neurons may occur, even in the absence of clinically visible signs of vascular retinopathy [3, 4, 169, 194–196].

A deep learning system (DLS) was demonstrated in multiethnic populations with diabetes to have high sensitivity and specificity for identifying diabetic retinopathy and related eye diseases. Current diabetic retinopathy screening programs require manual grading of diabetic retinopathy which is not sustainable in the long run. Therefore there is potential for the use of artificial intelligence (IA) in diabetic retinopathy screening [3]. Further research is needed to understand the clinical applicability of the DLS and to verify the role of the DLS to improve vision outcomes [197–201]. The clinical problem remains to identify diabetic patients int their preclinical asymptomatic phase of the diabetic retinopathy to prevent vision loss [3, 77, 118–127, 132, 159, 164, 181, 196, 202]. In the future, OCT angiography and artificial intelligence could be used to predict the onset of diabetic retinopathy.

The traditional clinical practices operating through a traditional model of "brick-and-mortar" facilities and "face-to-face" patient-physician interaction are not suited for the Covid-19 pandemic and the post-pandemic "new normal." It is important to reduce the non-urgent referrals and not urgent follow-up visits to eye centers. In the current climate of Covid-19, there is a need for digital models of care, such as telemedicine and "virtual clinics" [203–206]. We encourage telemedicine-based approach where digital retinal photographs taken with non-mydriatic cameras in a primary care setting by family physicians or technicians are then transmitted for remote interpretation by ophthalmologists. The peculiarity of ophthalmology is that the ocular examinations are mainly depending on visualization of ocular images (retinal photographs, OCT): in this direction several companies have made available specific softwares to store images in iCloud and ophthalmologists may have access to the images remotely [206]. Mobile device applications may allow teleconsultations and play a role in diabetes education, self-management, and prevention.

Retinal photograph-based artificial intelligence algorithms will help physicians to appropriately differentiate urgent cases from non-urgent cases, medical from surgical cases ("triaging").

An effective alliance between family physicians, endocrinologists, community-based services, and eye centers is warranted. On the other hand, information technology infrastructure, Internet connectivity, and cybersecurity are key factors for these new digital solutions. The European Commission has proposed an ambitious program called the "Next Generation Internet Initiative" to implement an interoperable platform ecosystem between European countries digital-strategy.ec.europa.eu.

Acknowledgments Dr. Tan Nguyen for his true friendship during the months in Melbourne and the original data.

Prof. Franco Veglio who supported me in writing the medical thesis and important publications and helped me to have a wider wisdom not only about ophthalmology.

Prof. Mauro Fioretto who recognized my human characteristics and encouraged me in finding my career path as an ophthalmologist.

To my colleagues for sharing their knowledge and for their patience which has made this chapter possible.

Dedication To my father Pier Carlo who trusted me and encouraged me to do research but not separated from the clinical daily activity ("primum vivere, deinde philosophari"), for his strong support, his true commitment, and presence.

To Tien Yin Wong whom I have met in 2000, my mentor during the clinical research fellowship in Melbourne: I have learned how to do clinical research and the importance of epidemiology and I was involved in the first steps of the artificial intelligence applied to retinal vascular diseases. For his collaboration and for sharing with me his views and comments about ophthalmology and medicine.

To Roberta, my wife, my sweetheart, during the last year at the Turin Eye Hospital, for her lovely assistance and for her kindness. I am deeply indebted to her for the patience and understanding during the time spent in doing research: she never made me miss her presence, support, criticisms, advices, and encouragement.

References

1. Yau JWY, Rogers SL, Kawasaki R, Lamoureux EL, Kowalski JW, Bek T, et al. Global prevalence and major risk factors of diabetic retinopathy. Diabetes Care. 2012;35:556–64.
2. Ting DS, Cheung GC, Wong TY. Diabetic retinopathy: global prevalence, major risk factors, screening practices and public health challenges: a review. Clin Exp Ophthalmol. 2016;44(4):260–77.
3. Wong TY, Sabanayagam C. Euretina lecture: strategies to tackle the global burden of diabetic retinopathy from epidemiology to artificial intelligence. Ophthalmologica. 2020;243(1):9–20.
4. Bandello F, Cicinelli MV. 19th EURETINA congress keynote lecture: diabetic retinopathy today. Ophthalmologica. 2020;243(3):163–71.
5. Wong TY, Sabanayagam C. The war on diabetic retinopathy: where are we now? Asia Pac J Ophthalmol (Phila). 2019;8(6):448–56.
6. Cunha-Vaz J, Ribeiro L, Lobo C. Phenotypes and biomarkers of diabetic retinopathy. Prog Retin Eye Res. 2014;41:90–111.

7. Sabanayagam C, Banu R, Chee ML, Lee R, Wang YX, Tan G, et al. Incidence and progression of diabetic retinopathy: a systematic review. Lancet Diabetes Endocrinol. 2019;7(2):140–9.
8. Lanzetta P, Sarao V, Scanlon PH, Barratt J, Porta M, Bandello F, et al. Vision Academy. Fundamental principles of an effective diabetic retinopathy screening program. Acta Diabetol. 2020;57(7):785–98.
9. Wong TY, Sun J, Kawasaki R, Ruamviboonsuk P, Gupta N, Lansingh VC, et al. Guidelines on diabetic eye care: the international council of ophthalmology recommendations for screening, follow-up, referral, and treatment based on resource settings. Ophthalmology. 2018;125(10):1608–22.
10. Wong TY, Bressler N. Artificial intelligence with deep learning technology looks into diabetic retinopathy screening. JAMA. 2016;316(22):2366–7.
11. Sun JK, Keenan HA, Cavallerano JD, Asztalos BF, Schaefer EJ, Sell DR, et al. Protection from retinopathy and other complications in patients with type 1 diabetes of extreme duration: the joslin 50-year medalist study. Diabetes Care. 2011;34(4):968–74.
12. Sacconi R, Lamanna F, Borrelli E, Mulinacci G, Casaluci M, Gelormini F, et al. Morphofunctional analysis of the retina in patients with type 1 diabetes without complications after 30 years of disease. Sci Rep. 2020;10(1):206.
13. West KM, Erdreich LJ, Stober JA. A detailed study of risk factors for retinopathy and nephropathy in diabetes. Diabetes. 1980;29:501–8.
14. Knowler WC, Bennet PA, Ballantine EJ. Increased incidence of retinopathy in diabetics with elevated elevated blood pressure. A six-year follow-up study in Pima Indians. N Engl J Med. 1980;302:645–50.
15. Klein R, Klein BE, Moss SE. A population-based study of diabetic retinopathy in insulin-using patients diagnosed before 30 years of age. Diabetes Care. 1985;8(Suppl 1):71–6.
16. Rand LI, Krolewesky AS, Aiello LM, Warram JH, Baker RS, Maki T. Multiple factors in prediction of risk of proliferative diabetic retinopathy. N Eng J Med. 1985;3131:1433–8.
17. Holman RR, Paul SK, Bethel MA, Neil HA, Matthews DR. Long-term follow-up after tight control of blood pressure in type 2 diabetes. N Engl J Med. 2008;359(15):1565–76.
18. Matthews DR, Stratton IM, Aldington SJ, Holman RR, Kohner EM, UK Prospective Diabetes Study Group. Risks of progression of retinopathy and vision loss related to tight blood pressure control in type 2 diabetes mellitus: UKPDS 69. Arch Ophthalmol. 2004;122(11):1631–40.
19. Orchard T. Diabetes: a time for excitement-and concern. Hopeful signs exist that the ravages of diabetes can be tamed. BMJ. 1998;317(7160):691–2.
20. UK Prospective Diabetes Study Group. Tight blood pressure control and risk of macrovascular and microvascular complications in type 2 diabetes: UKPDS 38. UK Prospective Diabetes Study Group. BMJ. 1998;317(7160):703–13.
21. Chaturvedi N, Sjolie AK, Stephenson JM, Abrahamian H, Keipes M, Castellarin A, et al. Effect of lisinopril on progression of retinopathy in normotensive people with type 1 diabetes. The EUCLID Study Group. EURODIAB Controlled Trial of Lisinopril in Insulin-Dependent Diabetes Mellitus. Lancet. 1998;351(9095):28–31.
22. Chaturvedi N, Porta M, Klein R, Orchard T, Fuller J, Parving HH, et al. DIRECT Programme Study Group. Effect of candesartan on prevention (DIRECT-Prevent 1) and progression (DIRECT-Protect 1) of retinopathy in type 1 diabetes: randomised, placebo-controlled trials. Lancet. 2008;372(9647):1394–402.
23. Grosso A. Detection and management of vascular hypertension. Compr Ophthalmol Updat. 2007;8(3):145–51; discussion 153–4.
24. Chao JR, Lai MY, Azen SP, Klein R, Varma R. Retinopathy in persons without diabetes: the Los Angeles Latino Eye Study. Invest Ophthalmol Vis Sci. 2007;48:4019–25.
25. Wong TY, McIntosh R. Hypertensive retinopathy signs as risk indicators of cardiovascular morbidity and mortality. Br Med Bull. 2005;7:57–70.
26. Cheung N, Wong TY. Obesity and eye diseases. Surv Ophthalmol. 2007;52:180–95.
27. Wong TY, Mitchell P. Hypertensive retinopathy. N Engl J Med. 2004;351(22):2310–7.
28. Grosso A, Cheung N, Veglio F, Wong TY. Similarities and differences in early retinal phenotypes in hypertension and diabetes. J Hypertens. 2011;29(9):1667–75.

29. Ojaimi E, Nguyen TT, Klein R, Islam FM, Cotch MF, Klein BE, et al. Retinopathy signs in people without diabetes: the multi-ethnic study of atherosclerosis. Ophthalmology. 2011;118(4):656–62.
30. Klein R, Klein BE, Moss SE, Wang Q. Hypertension and retinopathy, arteriolar narrowing, and arteriovenous nicking in a population. Arch Ophthalmol. 1994;112:92–8.
31. Sharrett AR, Hubbard LD, Cooper LS, Sorlie PD, Brothers RJ, Nieto FJ, et al. Retinal arteriolar diameters and elevated blood pressure: the atherosclerosis risk in communities study. Am Epidemiol. 1999;150:263–70.
32. Wong TY, Hubbard LD, Klein R, Marino EK, Kronmal R, Sharrett AR, et al. Retinal microvascular abnormalities and blood pressure in older people: the cardiovascular health study. Br J Ophthalmol. 2002;86:1007–13.
33. Yang C, Kwak L, Ballew SH, Jaar BG, Deal JA, Folsom AR, et al. Retinal microvascular findings and risk of incident peripheral artery disease: an analysis from the atherosclerosis risk in communities (ARIC) study. Atherosclerosis. 2020;294:62–71.
34. Bhargava M, Ikram MK, Wong TY. How does hypertension affect your eyes? J Hum Hypertens. 2012;26(2):71–83.
35. Avery CL, Kucharska-Newton A, Monda KL, Sharrett AR, Mosley TH, Klein BE, et al. Impact of long-term measures of glucose and blood pressure on the retinal microvasculature. Atherosclerosis. 2012;225(2):412–7.
36. Wong TY, Klein R, Sharrett AR, Manolio TA, Hubbard LD, Marino EK, et al. The prevalence and risk factors of retinal microvascular abnormalities in older persons: the cardiovascular health study. Ophthalmology. 2003;110(4):658–66.
37. Tso MO, Jampol LM. Pathophysiology of hypertensive retinopathy. Ophthalmology. 1982;89:1132–45.
38. Buchi ER, Kurosawa A, Tso MO. Retinopathy in diabetic hypertensive monkeys: a pathologic study. Graefes Arch Clin Exp Ophthalmol. 1996;234:388–98.
39. Hayreh SS. Classification of hypertensive fundus changes and their order of appearance. Ophthalmologica. 1989;198:247–60.
40. McLeod D. Why cotton wool spots should not be regarded as regarded as retinal nerve fibre layer infarcts. Br J Ophthalmol. 2005;89:229–37.
41. Ikram MK, Witteman JC, Vingerling JR, Breteler MM, Hofman A, de Jong PT. Retinal vessel diameters and risk of hypertension: the Rotterdam Study. Hypertension. 2006;47:189–94.
42. Nguyen TT, Wong TY. Retinal vascular manifestations of metabolic disorders. Trends Endocrinol Metab. 2006;17:262–8.
43. Klein R, Klein BEK, Moss SE. The relation of systemic hypertension to changes in the retinal vasculature: the Beaver Dam Eye Study. Trans Am Ophthalmol Soc. 1997;95:329–48.
44. Kristinsson JK, Gottfredsdottir MS, Stefansson E. Retinal vessel dilatation and elongation precedes diabetic macular oedema. Br J Ophthalmol. 1997;81:274–8.
45. Gottfredsdottir MS, Stefansson E, Jonasson F, Gislason I. Retinal vasoconstriction after laser treatment for diabetic macular edema. Am J Ophthalmol. 1993;115:64–7.
46. Pappuru RKR, Ribeiro L, Lobo C, Alves D, Cunha-Vaz J. Microaneurysm turnover is a predictor of diabetic retinopathy progression. Br J Ophthalmol. 2019;103(2):222–6.
47. Parravano M, De Geronimo D, Scarinci F, Virgili G, Querques L, Varano M, et al. Progression of diabetic microaneurysms according to the internal reflectivity on structural optical coherence tomography and visibility on optical coherence tomography angiography. Am J Ophthalmol. 2019;198:8–16.
48. Ehlers JP, Jiang AC, Boss JD, Hu M, Figueiredo N, Babiuch A, et al. Quantitative ultra-widefield angiography and diabetic retinopathy severity: an assessment of panretinal leakage index, ischemic index and microaneurysm count. Ophthalmology. 2019;126(11):1527–32.
49. Venkatramani J, Mitchell P. Ocular and systemic causes of retinopathy in patients without diabetes mellitus. BMJ. 2004;328:625–9.
50. Díaz-Coránguez M, Ramos C, Antonetti DA. The inner blood-retinal barrier: cellular basis and development. Vis Res. 2017;139:123–37.

51. Delles C, Michelson G, Harazny J, Oehmer S, Hilgers KF, Schmieder RE. Impaired endothelial function of the retinal vasculature in hypertensive patients. Stroke. 2004;35:1289–93.
52. Gardner TW, Antonetti DA, Barber AJ, LaNoue KF, Levison SW. Diabetic retinopathy: more than meets the eye. Surv Ophthalmol. 2002;47:S253–62.
53. Harhaj NS, Felinski EA, Wolpert EB, Sundstrom JM, Gardner TW, Antonetti DA. VEGF activation of protein kinase C stimulates occludin phosphorylation and contributes to endothelial permeability. Invest Ophthalmol Vis Sci. 2006;47(11):5106–15.
54. Cheung N, Mitchell P, Wong TY. Diabetic retinopathy. Lancet. 2010;376(9735):124–36.
55. Joussen AM, Poulaki V, Le ML, Koizumi K, Esser C, Janicki H, et al. A central role for inflammation in the pathogenesis of diabetic retinopathy. FASEB J. 2004;18:1450–2.
56. Adamis AP. Is diabetic retinopathy an inflammatory disease? Br J Ophthalmol. 2002;86:363–5.
57. Lieth E, Gardner TW, Barber AJ, Antonetti DA, Penn State Retina Research Group. Retinal neurodegeneration: early pathology in diabetes. Clin Exp Ophthalmol. 2000;28(1):3–8.
58. Spaide RF. Retinal vascular cystoid macular edema. Retina. 2016;36:1823–42.
59. Barber AJ, Lieth E, Khin SA, Antonetti DA, Buchanan AG, Gardner TW. Neural apoptosis in the retina during experimental and human diabetes. Early onset and effect of insulin. J Clin Invest. 1998;102:783–91.
60. Kim JH, Kim JH, Jun HO, Yu YS, Kim KW. Inhibition of protein kinase C delta attenuates blood-retinal barrier breakdown in diabetic retinopathy. Am J Pathol. 2010;176(3):1517–24.
61. Dahlof B, Herlitz H, Aurell M, Hansson L. Reversal of cardiovascular structural changes when treating essential hypertension. The importance of the renin-angiotensin-aldosterone system. Am J Hypertens. 1992;5:900–11.
62. Bock KD. Regression of retinal vascular changes by antihypertensive therapy. Hypertension. 1984;6 (6Pt2):III158–62.
63. Chalmers J, Cooper ME. UKPDS and the legacy effect. N Engl J Med. 2008;359(15):1618–20.
64. Engerman RL, Kern TS. Progression of incipient diabetic retinopathy during good glycemic control. Diabetes. 1987;36:808–12.
65. Kowluru RA, Zhong Q, Kanwar M. Metabolic memory and diabetic retinopathy: role of inflammatory mediators in retinal pericytes. Exp Eye Res. 2010;90:617–62.
66. Roy S, Sala R, Cagliero E, Lorenzi M. Overexpression of fibronectin induced by diabetes or high glucose: phenomenon with a memory. Proc Natl Acad Sci U S A. 1990;87(1):404–8.
67. Miller RG, Orchard TJ. Understanding metabolic memory: a tale of two studies. Diabetes. 2020;69(3):291–9.
68. White NH, Sun W, Cleary PA, Tamborlane WV, Danis RP, Hainsworth DP, DCCT-EDIC Research Group. et al; Effect of prior intensive therapy in type 1 diabetes on 10-year progression of retinopathy in the DCCT/EDIC: comparison of adults and adolescents. Diabetes 2010; 59:1244–1253.
69. Lund SS, Rossing P, Vaag AA. Follow-up of intensive glucose control in type 2 diabetes. N Engl J Med. 2009;360(4):416. author reply 418
70. Liu Y, Li J, Ma J, Tong N. The threshold of the severity of diabetic retinopathy below which intensive glycemic control is beneficial in diabetic patients: estimation using data from large randomized clinical trials. J Diabetes Res. 2020;2020:5498528. eCollection 2020. https://doi.org/10.1155/2020/5498528.
71. The Diabetes Control and Complications Trial Research Group. The effect of intensive treatment of diabetes on the development and progression of long-term complications in insulin-dependent diabetes mellitus. N Engl J Med. 1993;329(14):977–86.
72. UK Prospective Diabetes Study (UKPDS) Group. Intensive blood-glucose control with sulphonylureas or insulin com- pared with conventional treatment and risk of complications in patients with type 2 diabetes (UKPDS 33). Lancet. 1998;352(9131):837–53.
73. Kowluru R, Ghulam M. Epigenetics and mitochondrial stability in the metabolic memory phenomenon associated with continued progression of diabetic retinopathy. Sci Rep. 2020;10(1):6655.
74. Reddy MA, Zhang E, Natarajan R. Epigenetic mechanisms in diabetic complications and metabolic memory. Diabetologia. 2015;58(3):443–55.

75. Friedrichs P, Schlotterer A, Sticht C, Kolibabka M, Wohlfart P, Dietrich A, et al. Hyperglycaemic memory affects the neurovascular unit of the retina in a diabetic mouse model. Diabetologia. 2017;60(7):1354–8.
76. Chan PS, Kanwar M, Kowluru RA. Resistance of retinal inflammatory mediators to suppress after reinstitution of good glycemic control: novel mechanism for metabolic memory. J Diabetes Complicat. 2010;24(1):55–63.
77. Liew G, Wang JJ, Mitchell P, Wong TY. Retinal vascular imaging: a new tool in microvascular disease research. Circ Cardiovasc Imaging. 2008;2:156–61.
78. Nguyen TT, Kawasaki R, Wang JJ, Kreis AJ, Shaw J, Vilser W, et al. Flicker light-induced retinal vasodilation in diabetes and diabetic retinopathy. Diabetes Care. 2009;32:2075–80.
79. Lim HB, Lee MW, Park JH, Kim K, Jo YJ, Kim JY. Changes in ganglion cell-inner plexiform layer thickness and retinal microvasculature in hypertension: an optical coherence tomography angiography study. Am J Ophthalmol. 2019;199:167–76.
80. Sjølie AK, Klein R, Porta M, Orchard T, Fuller J, Parving HH, et al; DIRECT Programme Study Group. Effect of candesartan on progression and regression of retinopathy in type 2 diabetes (DIRECT-Protect 2): a randomised placebo-controlled trial. Lancet. 2008;18:1385–93.
81. Antonio PR, Marta PS, Luís DD, Antonio DP, Manuel ST, Rafael MS, et al. Factors associated with changes in retinal microcirculation after antihypertensive treatment. J Hum Hypertens. 2014;28(5):310–5.
82. Rubino F, Kaplan LM, Schauer PR, Cummings DE, Diabetes Surgery Summit Delegates. The diabetes surgery summit consensus conference: recommendations for the evaluation and use of gastrointestinal surgery to treat type 2 diabetes mellitus. Ann Surg. 2010;251:399–405.
83. Pontiroli AE, Merlotti C, Ceriani V, Morabito A. About bariatric surgery and diabetic retinopathy; the debate continues. Eye (Lond). 2018;32(3):652.
84. Chen Y, Laybourne JP, Sandinha MT, de Alwis NM, Avery P, Steel DH, et al. Does bariatric surgery prevent progression of diabetic retinopathy? Eye. 2017;31:1131–9.
85. Cheung D, Switzer NJ, Ehmann D, Rudnisky C, Shi X, Karmali S. The impact of bariatric surgery on diabetic retinopathy: a systematic review and meta-analysis. Obes Surg. 2015;25:1604–9.
86. Pontiroli AE, Ceriani V. Does bariatric surgery influence diabetic retinopathy? Obes Surg. 2015;25:1066–7.
87. Coleman KJ, Haneuse S, Johnson E, Bogart A, Fisher D, O'Connor PJ, et al. Long-term microvascular disease outcomes in patients with type 2 diabetes after bariatric surgery: evidence for the legacy effect of surgery. Diabetes Care. 2016;39:1400–7.
88. Mineo D, Pileggi A, Alejandro R, Ricordi C. Point: steady progress and current challenges in clinical islet transplantation. Diabetes Care. 2009;32:1563–9.
89. Lee TC, Barshes NR, O'Mahony CA, Nguyen L, Brunicardi FC, Ricordi C, et al. The effect of pancreatic islet transplantation on progression of diabetic retinopathy and neuropathy. Transplant Proc. 2005;37(5):2263–5.
90. Merlotti C, Ceriani V, Morabito A, Pontiroli AE. Bariatric surgery and diabetic retinopathy: a systematic review and meta-analysis of controlled clinical studies. Obes Rev. 2017;18:309–16.
91. Bertuzzi F, De Carlis L, Marazzi M, Rampoldi AG, Bonomo M, Antonioli B, et al. Long-term effect of islet transplantation on glycemic variability. Cell Transplant. 2018;27(5):840–6.
92. Thompson DM, Begg IS, Harris C, Ao Z, Fung MA, Meloche RM, et al. Reduced progression of diabetic retinopathy after islet cell transplantation compared with intensive medical therapy. Transplantation. 2008;85(10):1400–5.
93. Robertson PR. Islet transplantation a decade later and strategies for filling a half-full glass. Diabetes. 2010;59(6):1285–91.
94. Parver LM. Temperature modulating action of choroidal blood flow. Eye (Lond). 1991;5(Pt 2):181–5.
95. Nickla DL, Wallman J. The multifunctional choroid. Prog Retin Eye Res. 2010;29(2):144–68.
96. Weinberger D, Kramer M, Priel E, Gaton DD, Axer-Siegel R, Yassur Y. Indocyanine green angiographic findings in nonproliferative diabetic retinopathy. Am J Ophthalmol. 1998;126(2):238–47.

97. Hua R, Liu L, Wang X, Chen L. Imaging evidence of diabetic choroidopathy in vivo: angiographic pathoanatomy and choroidal-enhanced depth imaging. PLoS One. 2013;8(12):e83494.
98. Brancato R, Trabucchi G. Fluorescein and indocyanine green angiography in vascular chorioretinal diseases. Semin Ophthalmol. 1998;13(4):189–98.
99. Mori K, Yoshida S, Kobayashi Y, Ishikawa K, Nakao S, Hisatomi T, et al. Decrease in the number of microaneurysms in diabetic macular edema after anti-vascular endothelial growth factor therapy: implications for indocyanine green angiography-guided detection of refractory microaneurysms. Graefes Arch Clin Exp Ophthalmol. 2020;258(4):735–41.
100. Ferrara D, Waheed NK, Duker JS. Investigating the choriocapillaris and choroidal vasculature with new optical coherence tomography technologies. Prog Retin Eye Res. 2016;52:130–55.
101. Choi W, Waheed NK, Moult EM, Adhi M, Lee B, De Carlo T, et al. Ultra speed swept source optical coherence tomography angiography of retinal and choriocapillaris alterations in diabetic patients with and without retinopathy. Retina. 2017;37(1):11–21.
102. Murakami T, Uji A, Suzuma K, Dodo Y, Yoshitake S, Ghashut R, et al. In vivo choroidal vascular lesions in diabetes on swept-source optical coherence tomography. PLoS One. 2016;11(8):e0160317.
103. Adhi M, Brewer E, Waheed NK, Duker JS. Analysis of morphological features and vascular layers of choroid in diabetic retinopathy using spectral-domain optical coherence tomography. JAMA Ophthalmol. 2013;131(10):1267–74.
104. Hidayat AA, Fine BS. Diabetic choroidopathy. Light and electron microscopic observations of seven cases. Ophthalmology. 1985;92(4):512–22.
105. Cao J, McLeod S, Merges CA, Lutty GA. Choriocapillaris degeneration and related pathologic changes in human diabetic eyes. Arch Ophthalmol. 1998;116(5):589–97.
106. Fryczkowski AW, Sato SE, Hodes BL. Changes in the diabetic choroidal vasculature: scanning electron microscopy findings. Ann Ophthalmol. 1988;20(8):299–305.
107. Lutty GA. Diabetic choroidopathy. Vis Res. 2017;139:161–7.
108. Nagaoka T, Kitaya N, Sugawara R, Yokota H, Mori F, Hikichi T, et al. Alteration of choroidal circulation in the foveal region in patients with type 2 diabetes. Br J Ophthalmol. 2004;88(8):1060–3.
109. Coscas G, Lupidi M, Coscas F, Chhablani J, Cagini C. Optical coherence tomography angiography in healthy subjects and diabetic patients. Ophthalmologica. 2018;239(2–3):61–73.
110. Campos A, Campos EJ, Martins J, Ambrósio AF, Silva R. Viewing the choroid: where we stand, challenges and contradictions in diabetic retinopathy and diabetic macular oedema. Acta Ophthalmol. 2017;95(5):446–59.
111. Pichi F, Aggarwal K, Neri P, Salvetti P, Lembo A, Nucci P, et al. Choroidal biomarkers. Indian J Ophthalmol. 2018;66(12):1716–26.
112. Velazquez-Villoria D, Marti Rodrigo P, DeNicola ML, Zapata Vitori MA, Segura García A, García-Arumí J. Swept source optical coherence tomography evaluation of chorioretinal changes in hypertensive choroidopathy related to HELLP syndrome. Retin Cases Brief Rep. 2019;13(1):30–3.
113. Ugarte M, Horgan S, Rassam S, Leong T, Kon CH. Hypertensive choroidopathy: recognizing clinically significant end-organ damage. Acta Ophthalmol. 2008;86(2):227–8.
114. Rezkallah A, Kodjikian L, Abukhashabah A, Denis P, Mathis T. Hypertensive choroidopathy: Multimodal imaging and the contribution of wide-field swept-source oct-angiography. Am J Ophthalmol Case Rep. 2019;13:131–5.
115. Nakanishi M, Grebe R, Bhutto IA, Edwards M, McLeod DS, Lutty GA. Albumen transport to Bruch's membrane and RPE by choriocapillaris caveolae. Invest Ophthalmol Vis Sci. 2016;57(4):2213–24.
116. Lutty GA, Cao J, McLeod DS. Relationship of polymorphonuclear leukocytes to capillary dropout in the human diabetic choroid. Am J Pathol. 1997;151(3):707–14.
117. Endo H, Kase S, Saito M, Yokoi M, Takahashi M, Ishida S, et al. Choroidal thickness in diabetic patients without diabetic retinopathy: a meta-analysis. Am J Ophthalmol. 2020;218:68–77.
118. Nguyen TT, Wang JJ, Wong TY. Retinal vascular changes in pre-diabetes and prehypertension: new findings and their research and clinical implications. Diabetes Care. 2007;30(10):2708–15.

119. Nguyen TT, Wang JJ, Islam FM, Paul Mitchell P, Tapp RJ, Zimmet PZ, et al. Retinal arteriolar narrowing predicts incidence of diabetes: the Australian diabetes, obesity and lifestyle (AusDiab) study. Diabetes. 2008;57(3):536–9.
120. Wong TY, Klein R, Sharrett AR, Schmidt MI, Pankow JS, Couper DJ, et al. Retinal arteriolar narrowing and risk of diabetes mellitus in middle-aged persons. JAMA. 2002;287(19):2528–33.
121. Wong TY, Shankar A, Klein R, Klein BE, Hubbard LD. Retinal arteriolar narrowing, hypertension, and subsequent risk of diabetes mellitus. Arch Intern Med. 2005;165(9):1060–5.
122. Moss SE, Klein R, Klein BE, Wong TY. Retinal vascular changes and 20-year incidence of lower extremity amputations in a cohort with diabetes. Arch Intern Med. 2003;163(20):2505–10.
123. Cheung N, Rogers SL, Donaghue KC, Jenkins AJ, Tikellis G, Wong TY. Retinal arteriolar dilation predicts retinopathy in adolescents with type 1 diabetes. Diabetes Care. 2008;31(9):1842–6.
124. Rogers SL, Tikellis G, Cheung N, Tapp R, Shaw J, Zimmet PZ, et al. Retinal arteriolar caliber predicts incident retinopathy: the Australian diabetes, obesity and lifestyle (AusDiab) study. Diabetes Care. 2008;31(4):761–3.
125. Alibrahim E, Donaghue KC, Rogers S, Hing S, Jenkins AJ, Chan A, et al. Retinal vascular caliber and risk of retinopathy in young patients with type 1 diabetes. Ophthalmology. 2006;113(9):1499–503.
126. Klein R, Klein BE, Moss SE, Wong TY. Retinal vessel caliber and microvascular and macrovascular disease in type 2 diabetes: XXI: the Wisconsin epidemiologic study of diabetic retinopathy. Ophthalmology. 2007;114(10):1884–92.
127. Wong TY, Shankar A, Klein R, Klein BE. Retinal vessel diameters and the incidence of gross proteinuria and renal insufficiency in people with type 1 diabetes. Diabetes. 2004;53(1):179–84.
128. Stefansson E, Landers MB 3rd, Wolbarsht M. Retinal vessel caliber and diabetic retinopathy. Arch Ophthalmol. 2005;123(5):709.
129. Klein R, Moss SE, Klein BE. Author reply. Ophthalmology. 2007;114(11):2099.
130. Meigs JB, Hu FB, Rifai N, Manson JE. Biomarkers of endothelial dysfunction and risk of type 2 diabetes mellitus. JAMA. 2004;291:1978–86.
131. Stehouwer CD, Lambert J, Donker AJ, van Hinsbergh VW. Endothelial dysfunction and pathogenesis of diabetic angiopathy. Cardiovasc Res. 1997;34:55–68.
132. Tecilazich F, Feke TG, Mazzantini S, Sobrin L, Lorenzi M. Defective myogenic response of retinal vessels is associated with accelerated onset of retinopathy in type 1 diabetic individuals. Invest Ophthalmol Vis Sci. 2016;57:1523–9.
133. Lim LS, Tai ES, Mitchell P, Wang JJ, Tay WT, Lamoureux E, et al. C-reactive protein, body mass index, and diabetic retinopathy. Invest Ophthalmol Vis Sci. 2010;51:4458–63.
134. van Hecke MV, Dekker JM, Nijpels G, Moll AC, Heine RJ, Bouter LM, et al. Inflammation and endothelial dysfunction are associated with retinopathy: the Hoorn Study. Diabetologia. 2005;48:1300–6.
135. Matsumoto K, Sera Y, Ueki Y, Inukai G, Niiro E, Miyake S. Comparison of serum concentrations of soluble adhesion molecules in diabetic microangiopathy and macroangiopathy. Diabet Med. 2002;19:822–6.
136. Siemianowicz K, Francuz T, Gminski J, Telega A, Syzdól M. Endothelium dysfunction markers in patients with diabetic retinopathy. Int J Mol Med. 2005;15:459–62.
137. Spijkerman AM, Gall MA, Tarnow L, et al. Endothelial dysfunction and low-grade inflammation and the progression of retinopathy in type 2 diabetes. Diabet Med. 2007;24:969–76.
138. Boulbou MS, Koukoulis GN, Petinaki EA, Germenis A, Gourgoulianis KI. Soluble adhesion molecules are not involved in the development of retinopathy in type 2 diabetic patients. Acta Diabetol. 2004;41:118–22.
139. Koga M, Otsuki M, Kubo M, Hashimoto J, Kasayama S. Relationship between circulating vascular cell adhesion molecule-1 and microvascular complications in type 2 diabetes mellitus. Diabet Med. 1998;15:661–7.

140. Malecki MT, Osmenda G, Walus-Miarka M, Skupien J, Cyganek K, Mirkiewicz-Sieradzka B, et al. Retinopathy in type 2 diabetes mellitus is associated with increased intima-media thickness and endothelial dysfunction. Eur J Clin Investig. 2008;38:925–30.
141. Suetsugu M, Takebayashi K, Aso Y. Association between diabetic microangiopathy and vascular endothelial function evaluated by flow-mediated vasodilatation in patients with type 2 diabetes. Int J Clin Pract. 2007;61:920–6.
142. Nair BM, Viswanathan V, Snehalatha C, Mohan RS, Ramachandran A. Flow mediated dilatation and carotid intimal media thickness in South Indian type 2 diabetic subjects. Diabetes Res Clin Pract. 2004;65:13–9.
143. Porta M. Endothelium: the main actor in the remodelling of the retinal microvasculature in diabetes. Diabetologia. 1996;39:739–44.
144. Rim TH, Teo AWJ, Yang HHS, Cheung CY, Wong TY. Retinal vascular signs and cerebrovascular diseases. J Neuroophthalmol. 2020;40(1):44–59.
145. Liao D, Wong TY, Klein R, Jones D, Hubbard L, Sharrett AR. Relationship between carotid artery stiffness and retinal arteriolar narrowing in healthy middle-aged persons. Stroke. 2004;35(4):837–42.
146. Yau JW, Xie J, Kawasaki R, Kramer H, Shlipak M, Klein R, et al. Retinal arteriolar narrowing and subsequent development of CKD stage 3: the multi-ethnic study of atherosclerosis (MESA). Am J Kidney Dis. 2011;58(1):39–46.
147. Gishti O, Jaddoe VW, Hofman A, Wong TY, Ikram MK, Gaillard R. Body fat distribution, metabolic and inflammatory markers and retinal microvasculature in school-age children. The Generation R Study. Int J Obes. 2015;39(10):1482–7.
148. Liu M, Wake M, Wong TY, He M, Xiao Y, Burgner DP, et al. Associations of retinal microvascular caliber with intermediate phenotypes of large arterial function and structure: a systematic review and meta-analysis. Microcirculation. 2019;26(7):e12557.
149. Nagel E, Vilser W, Lanzl I. Age, blood pressure, and vessel diameter as factors influencing the arterial retinal flicker response. Invest Ophthalmol Vis Sci. 2004;45:1486–92.
150. Buerk DG, Riva CE, Cranstoun SD. Nitric oxide has a vasodilatory role in cat optic nerve head during flicker stimuli. Microvasc Res. 1996;52:13–26.
151. Kondo M, Wang L, Bill A. The role of nitric oxide in hyperaemic response to flicker in the retina and optic nerve in cats. Acta Ophthalmol Scand. 1997;75:232–5.
152. Buerk DG, Riva CE, Cranstoun SD. Frequency and luminance-dependent blood flow and K+ ion changes during flicker stimuli in cat optic nerve head. Invest Ophthalmol Vis Sci. 1995;36(11):2216–27.
153. Dorner GT, Garhofer G, Kiss B, Polska E, Polak K, Riva CE, et al. Nitric oxide regulates retinal vascular tone in humans. Am J Physiol Heart Circ Physiol. 2003;285(2):H631–6.
154. Polak K, Schmetterer L, Riva CE. Influence of flicker frequency on flicker-induced changes of retinal vessel diameter. Invest Ophthalmol Vis Sci. 2002;43(8):2721–6.
155. Hughes AD, Stanton AV, Jabbar AS, Chapman N, Martinez-Perez ME, McG Thom SA. Effect of antihypertensive treatment on retinal microvascular changes in hypertension. J Hypertens. 2008;26(8):1703–7.
156. Nagaoka T, Takahashi A, Sato E, Yokota H, Izumi N, Yoshida A. Effect of systemic administration of valsartan, an angiotensin II type 1 receptor blocker, on retinal circulation in healthy humans. Eye (Lond). 2009;23(6):1491–2.
157. Horio N, Clermont AC, Abiko A, Abiko T, Shoelson BD, Bursell S-E, et al. Angiotensin AT(1) receptor antagonism normalizes retinal blood flow and acetylcholine-induced vasodilatation in normotensive diabetic rats. Diabetologia. 2004;47(1):113–23.
158. Mandecka A, Dawczynski J, Blum M, Muller N, Kloos C, Wolf G, et al. Influence of flickering light on the retinal vessels in diabetic patients. Diabetes Care. 2007;30:3048–52.
159. Nian S, Lo ACY, Mi Y, Ren K, Yang D. Neurovascular unit in diabetic retinopathy: pathophysiological roles and potential therapeutical targets. Eye Vis (Lond). 2021;8(1):15.
160. Lott MEJ, Slocomb J, Shivkumar V, Smith B, Quillen D, Gabbay RA, et al. Impaired retinal vasodilator responses in prediabetes and type 2 diabetes. Acta Ophthalmol. 2013;91(6):e462–9.

161. Pemp B, Garhofer G, Weigert G, Karl K, Resch H, Wolzt M, et al. Reduced retinal vessel response to flicker stimulation but not to exogenous nitric oxide in type 1 diabetes. Invest Ophthalmol Vis Sci. 2009;50:4029–32.
162. Turner J, Belch JJ, Khan F. Current concepts in assessment of microvascular endothelial function using laser Doppler imaging and iontophoresis. Trends Cardiovasc Med. 2008;18:109–16.
163. Debbabi H, Bonnin P, Ducluzeau PH, Lefthériotis G, Levy BI. Noninvasive assessment of endothelial function in the skin microcirculation. Am J Hypertens. 2010;23:541–6.
164. Nguyen TT, Shaw JE, Robinson C, Kawasaki R, Wang JJ, Kreis AJ, et al. Diabetic retinopathy is related to both endothelium-dependent and -independent responses of skin microvascular flow. Diabetes Care. 2011;34(6):1389–93.
165. Cheung N, Tikellis G, Wang JJ. Diabetic retinopathy. Ophthalmology. 2007;114(11):2098–9.
166. Wong TY. Retinal vessel diameter as a clinical predictor of diabetic retinopathy progression: time to take out the measuring tape. Arch Ophthalmol. 2011;129:95–6.
167. Nguyen TT, Kawasaki R, Kreis AJ, Wang JJ, Shaw J, Vilser W, et al. Correlation of light-flicker-induced retinal vasodilation and retinal vascular caliber measurements in diabetes. Invest Ophthalmol Vis Sci. 2009;50:5609–13.
168. Joussen AM, Poulaki V, Qin W, Kirchhof B, Mitsiades N, Wiegand SJ, et al. Retinal vascular endothelial growth factor induces intercellular adhesion molecule-1 and endothelial nitric oxide synthase expression and initiates early diabetic retinal leukocyte adhesion in vivo. Am J Pathol. 2002;160:501–9.
169. Tang Z, Chan MY, Leung WY, Wong HY, Ng CM, Chan VTT, et al. Assessment of retinal neurodegeneration with spectral-domain optical coherence tomography: a systematic review and meta-analysis. Eye (Lond). 2021;35(5):1317–25.
170. Lecleire-Collet A, Tessier LH, Massin P, Forster V, Brasseur G, Sahel JA, et al. Advanced glycation end products can induce glial reaction and neuronal degeneration in retinal explants. Br J Ophthalmol. 2005;89:1631–3.
171. Antonetti DA, Barber AJ, Bronson SK, Freeman WM, Gardner TW, Jefferson LS, et al; JDRF Diabetic Retinopathy Center Group. Diabetic retinopathy: seeing beyond glucose-induced microvascular disease. Diabetes. 2006;55:2401–11.
172. Vujosevic S, Micera A, Bini S, Berton M, Esposito G, Midena E. Aqueous humor biomarkers of muller cell activation in diabetic eyes. Invest Ophthalmol Vis Sci. 2015;56:3913–8.
173. Vujosevic S, Micera A, Bini S, Berton M, Esposito G, Midena E. Proteome analysis of retinal glia cells-related inflammatory cytokines in the aqueous humour of diabetic patients. Acta Ophthalmol. 2016;94:56–64.
174. Kern TS, Barber AJ. Retinal ganglion cells in diabetes. J Physiol. 2008;586(Pt 18):4401–8.
175. Mulligan SJ, MacVicar BA. Calcium transients in astrocyte endfeet cause cerebrovascular constrictions. Nature. 2004;431(7005):195–9.
176. Vujosevic S, Midena E. Retinal layers changes in human preclinical and early clinical diabetic retinopathy support early retinal neuronal and Müller cells alterations. J Diabetes Res. 2013;2013:905058.
177. Vujosevic S, Muraca A, Gatti V, Masoero L, Brambilla M, Cannillo B, et al. Peripapillary microvascular and neural changes in diabetes mellitus: an OCT-angiography study. Invest Ophthalmol Vis Sci. 2018;59(12):5074–81.
178. Zheng Y, Cheung N, Aung T, Mitchell P, He M, Wong TY. Relationship of retinal vascular caliber with retinal nerve fiber layer thickness: the Singapore Malay Eye Study. Invest Ophthalmol Vis Sci. 2009;50:4091–6.
179. Yu PK, Cringle SJ, Yu DY. Correlation between the radial peripapillary capillaries and the retinal nerve fibre layer in the normal human retina. Exp Eye Res. 2014;129:83–92.
180. Pierro L, Iuliano L, Cicinelli MV, Casalino G, Bandello F. Retinal neurovascular changes appear earlier in type 2 diabetic patients. Eur J Ophthalmol. 2017;27:346–51.
181. Barber AJ, Gardner TW, Abcouwer SF. The significance of vascular and neural apoptosis to the pathology of diabetic retinopathy. Invest Ophthalmol Vis Sci. 2011;52(2):1156–63.

182. Silva PS, Cavallerano JD, Haddad NM, Kwak H, Dyer KH, Omar AF, et al. Peripheral lesions identified on ultrawide field imaging predict increased risk of diabetic retinopathy progression over 4 years. Ophthalmology. 2015;122(5):949–56.
183. Reif R, Qin J, An L, Zhi Z, Dziennis S, Wang R. Quantifying optical microangiography images obtained from a spectral domain optical coherence tomography system. Int J Biomed Imaging. 2012;2012:509783.
184. De Carlo TE, Chin AT, Bonini Filho MA, Adhi M, Branchini L, Salz DA, et al. Detection of microvascular changes in eyes of patients with diabetes but not clinical diabetic retinopathy using optical coherence tomography angiography. Retina. 2015;35:2364–70.
185. Carnevali A, Sacconi R, Corbelli E, Tomasso L, Querques L, Zerbini G, et al. Optical coherence tomography angiography analysis of retinal vascular plexuses and choriocapillaris in patients with type 1 diabetes without diabetic retinopathy. Acta Diabetol. 2017;54:695–702.
186. Simonett JM, Scarinci F, Picconi F, Giorno P, De Geronimo D, Di Renzo A, et al. Early microvascular retinal changes in optical coherence tomography angiography in patients with type 1 diabetes mellitus. Acta Ophthalmol. 2017;95:e751–5.
187. Arganda-Carreras I, Fernández-González R, Muñoz-Barrutia A, Ortiz-De-Solorzano C. 3D reconstruction of histological sections: application to mammary gland tissue. Microsc Res Tech. 2010;73:1019–29.
188. Simó R, Stitt AW, Gardner TW. Neurodegeneration in diabetic retinopathy: does it really matter? Diabetologia. 2018;61(9):1902–12.
189. Cheung CY, Sabanayagam C, Law AK, Kumari N, Ting DS, Tan G, et al. Retinal vascular geometry and 6 year incidence and progression of diabetic retinopathy. Diabetologia. 2017;60(9):1770–81.
190. Zahid S, Dolz-Marco R, Freund KB, Balaratnasingam C, Dansingani K, Gilani F, et al. Fractal dimensional analysis of optical coherence tomography angiography in eyes with diabetic retinopathy. Invest Ophthalmol Vis Sci. 2016;57(11):4940–7.
191. Grauslund J, Green A, Kawasaki R, Hodgson L, Sjolie AK, Wong TY. Retinal vascular fractals and microvascular and macrovascular complications in type 1 diabetes. Ophthalmology. 2010;117:1400–5.
192. Cheung N, Donaghue KC, Liew G, Rogers SL, Wang JJ, Lim S-W, et al. Quantitative assessment of early diabetic retinopathy using fractal analysis. Diabetes Care. 2009;32:106–10.
193. Borrelli E, Sacconi R, Querques L, Battista M, Bandello F, Querques G. Quantification of diabetic macular ischemia using novel three-dimensional optical coherence tomography angiography metrics. J Biophotonics. 2020;13(10):e202000152.
194. Vujosevic S, Muraca A, Alkabes M, Villani E, Cavarzeran F, Rossetti L, et al. Early microvascular and neural changes in patients with type 1 and type 2 diabetes mellitus without clinical signs of diabetic retinopathy. Retina. 2019;39(3):435–45.
195. Abramoff MD, Fort PE, Han IC, Jayasundera KT, Sohn EH, Gardner TW. Approach for a clinically useful comprehensive classification of vascular and neural aspects of diabetic retinal disease. Invest Ophthalmol Vis Sci. 2018;59(1):519–27.
196. Sacconi R, Casaluci M, Borrelli E, Mulinacci G, Lamanna F, Gelormini F, et al. Multimodal imaging assessment of vascular and neurodegenerative retinal alterations in Type 1 diabetic patients without fundoscopic signs of diabetic retinopathy. J Clin Med. 2019;8(9):1409.
197. Ting DSW, Cheung CY, Lim G, Tan GSW, Quang ND, Gan A, et al. Development and validation of a deep learning system for diabetic retinopathy and related eye diseases using retinal images from multiethnic populations with diabetes. JAMA. 2017;318(22):2211–23.
198. Ting DSW, Pasquale LR, Peng L, Campbell JP, Lee AY, Raman R, et al. Artificial intelligence and deep learning in ophthalmology. Br J Ophthalmol. 2019;103(2):167–75.
199. Ting DSW, Peng L, Varadarajan AV, Keane PA, Burlina PM, Chiang MF, et al. Deep learning in ophthalmology: The technical and clinical considerations. Prog Retin Eye Res. 2019;72:100759.
200. Gunasekeran DV, Ting DSW, Tan GSW, Wong TY. Artificial intelligence for diabetic retinopathy screening, prediction and management. Curr Opin Ophthalmol. 2020;31(5):357–65.

201. Cheung CY, Xu D, Cheng CY, Sabanayagam C, Tham YC, Yu M, et al. A deep-learning system for the assessment of cardiovascular disease risk via the measurement of retinal-vessel calibre. Nat Biomed Eng. 2021;5:498–508.
202. Lorenzi M, Feke TG, Pitler L, Berisha F, Kolodjaschna J, McMeel W. Defective myogenic response to posture change in retinal vessels of well-controlled type 1 diabetic patients with no retinopathy. Invest Vis Sci. 2010;51:6770–5.
203. Li JO, Liu H, Ting DSJ, Jeon S, Chan RVP, Kim JE, et al. Digital technology, tele-medicine and artificial intelligence in ophthalmology: a global perspective. Prog Retin Eye Res. 2021;82:100900.
204. Tham YC, Husain R, Teo KYC, Tan ACS, Chew ACY, Ting DS, et al. New digital models of care in ophthalmology, during and beyond the COVID-19 pandemic. Br J Ophthalmol. 2022;106(4):452–7.
205. Gunasekeran DV, Tham YC, Ting DSW, Tan GSW, Wong TY. Digital health during COVID-19: lessons from operationalising new models of care in ophthalmology. Lancet Digit Health. 2021;3(2):e124–34.
206. Grosso A, Rigoli R, Formentini S, Di Perri G, Scotton P, Dapavo G, et al. Suppression of Covid-19 outbreak among healthcare workers at the Treviso Regional Hospital, Italy and lessons for ophthalmologists. Eur J Ophthalmol. 2021;31(6):2901–9.

Part VI

Diabetes and Benefit of Blood Pressure Lowering Treatment

Blood Pressure-Lowering Treatment and Macrovascular Events

18

Costas Thomopoulos

18.1 Stating the Problem

Type 2 diabetes mellitus (DM) is associated with an increased risk of hypertension [1] and cardiovascular and renal disease [2, 3]. In addition, DM and hypertension are comorbid clinical conditions that interact to create an adverse vascular environment, increasing macrovascular disease risk [4]. In the late 1990s, the Hypertension Optimal Treatment trial [5], and subsequently the UK Prospective Diabetes Study (UKPDS) [6], showed that more intensive blood pressure (BP)-lowering treatment reduced fatal and non-fatal cardiovascular events in patients with DM. After that, most DM and hypertension guidelines published in the first decade of the current century recommended that antihypertensive treatment be initiated at a lower systolic BP threshold (i.e., 130 mmHg) in patients with, rather than without, DM (i.e., 140 mmHg). Moreover, lower systolic BP targets should be attained by BP-lowering treatment in patients with DM compared to no-DM counterparts, i.e., less than 130 mmHg vs less than 140 mmHg, respectively [7–10]. However, a critical reappraisal of the evidence [11] called attention to the fact that no direct trial evidence was available to support lower thresholds and targets for patients with DM. Therefore, all subsequent guidelines did not recommend a differential BP-lowering management of hypertensive individuals by DM status [12–19]. The latest guidelines issued by the European Society of Cardiology and the European Society of Hypertension [17] recommend drug treatment initiation by any of the five classes in all hypertensive patients with or without DM. However, in patients with DM starting antihypertensive treatment with a renin-angiotensin system blocker may be reasonable because of specific protective effects on albuminuria and renal function [12–14, 17].

C. Thomopoulos (✉)
Department of Cardiology, Helena Venizelou Hospital, Athens, Greece
e-mail: thokos@otenet.gr

A. E. Berbari, G. Mancia (eds.), *Blood Pressure Disorders in Diabetes Mellitus*, Updates in Hypertension and Cardiovascular Protection,
https://doi.org/10.1007/978-3-031-13009-0_18

In this chapter, we will focus on some relevant clinical questions about the effect of BP-lowering treatment on cardiovascular and renal outcomes in patients with DM by using data from previous specific outcome meta-analyses in the field [20, 21], which have excluded (1) heart failure trials with reduced ejection fraction, (2) trials after acute coronary syndrome, (3) trials in hemodialysis patients, and (4) trials with type 1 diabetes mellitus patients. The clinical questions to address are the following: (1) Is BP-lowering treatment accompanied by favorable effects on fatal and non-fatal outcomes in patients with DM? (2) Are the effects of BP-lowering treatment different between patients with or without DM? (3) Should BP thresholds for treatment initiation and BP targets to achieve during BP-lowering treatment be different between patients with or without DM? (4) Are different classes of BP-lowering drugs differéntly effective on the risk of cardiovascular and renal outcomes in hypertensive patients with and without DM? Finally, (5) Is there any effect modification of BP-lowering treatment at higher levels of baseline cardiovascular risk in patients with DM?

18.2 BP-Lowering Treatment and Macrovascular Outcomes in DM

To date, the BP-lowering treatment effect on various outcomes was reported in 17 entire trials and 24 subgroups of trials [5, 6, 22–60], including patients with DM (Table 18.1), for a total of 61,772 patients [20]. As shown in Fig. 18.1, BP-lowering treatment produced an averaged systolic/diastolic BP reduction of 5.8/2.6 mmHg, which was associated with a significant reduction of most outcomes except for cardiovascular mortality. Notably, the extent of outcome reduction was similar for coronary heart disease (CHD) and stroke, while total mortality was reduced by 10% (95% confidence interval [CI], 4–16%). Furthermore, in an extensive meta-analysis of BP-lowering treatment, including trials or subgroups of trials in patients with DM, Edmin et al. reported the standardized risk estimates to a 10-mmHg systolic BP difference [61]. However, in the Edmin et al. analysis [61] and in another one by Brunström and Carlberg [62], DM patients after an acute coronary syndrome or systolic heart failure were not excluded, making inappropriate the comparability with meta-analyses limited to stable DM patients [20, 21].

Table 18.1 BP-lowering and head-to-head treatment trials repor ting separate data for patients with and without DM

BP-lowering treatment trials			Head-to-head (comparison) treatment trials		
Trial acronym (Ref.)	Treatment	DM/no-DM	Trial acronym (Ref.)	Treatment	DM/no-DM
AASK [63]	More vs less	–/1094	ACCOMPLISH [79]	D vs other	3468 vs 3478/2293 vs 2266
ABCD-H [22]	More vs less	470/–	ALLHAT (vs CCB) [80]		5994 vs 3597/8419 vs 4958
ACCORD [23]	More vs less	4733/–	ALLHAT (vs ACEi) [80]		5994 vs 3510/8419 vs 5034
ACTION [24]	CCB vs placebo	1113/6652	ANBP-2 [81]		212 vs 229/2827 vs 2815
ADVANCE [25]	ACEi+D vs placebo	1140/–	Berglund [100]		–/53 vs 53
Australian mild [77]	D vs placebo	–/3427	COLM [82]		678 vs 684/1895 vs 1884
BENEDICT [26]	ACEI and/or CCB vs placebo	1204/–	HAPPHY [101]		–/3272 vs 3297
CAMELOT [27]	CCB or ACEi vs placebo	363/1628	INSIGHT [83]		653 vs 649/2511 vs 2508
CARDIO-SIS [64]	More vs less	–/1111	MRC-mild [69]		–/4297 vs 4403
DEMAND [28]	ACEi or ACEi+CCB vs placebo	380/–	MRC-old [70]		–/1081 vs 1102
DIABHYCAR [29]	ACEi vs placebo	4912/–	NESTOR [84]		283 vs 286/–
DIRECT protect 2 [30]	ARB vs placebo	1905/–	NICS-EH [102]		–/210 vs 204
DREAM [65]	ACEi vs placebo	–/5269	VA-COOP [103]		–/177 vs 125
EUROPA [31]	ACEi vs placebo	1502/10716	AASK (vs CCB) [63]	BB vs other	–/441 vs 217
EWPHE [32]	D vs placebo	111/729	AASK (vs ACEi) [63]		–/441 vs 436
FEVER [33]	CCB vs placebo	1241/8470	ASCOT [85]		2572 vs 2565/7046 vs 7074
Fogari [34]	CCB + ACEi vs CCB or ACEi	309/–	Berglund [99]		–/53 vs 53
HDPF [35]	D vs little treatment	772/10168	HAPPHY [101]		–/3297 vs 3272
HEP [66]	BB vs no treatment	–/884	INVEST [86]		3231 vs 3169/8078 vs 8098
HOPE [36]	ACEi vs placebo	3577/5720	LIFE [87]		609 vs 586/3979 vs 4019
HOPE-3H [67]	ARB + D vs placebo	–/4240	MRC-mild [69]		–/4403 vs 4297
HOT [5]	More vs less	1501/17289	MRC-old [70]		–/1102 vs 1081
HSCG [37]	Central+D vs placebo	162/290	UKPDS-39 [88]		358 vs 400/–
Hunan Province [68]	CCB vs no treatment	–/2080	VA-COOP [103]		–/125 vs 177

(continued)

Table 18.1 (continued)

BP-lowering treatment trials			Head-to-head (comparison) treatment trials		
Trial acronym (Ref.)	Treatment	DM/no-DM	Trial acronym (Ref.)	Treatment	DM/no-DM
IDNT [38]	ARB or CCB vs placebo	1715/–	AASK (vs BB) [63]	CCB vs other	–/217 vs 441
I-PRESERVE [39]	ARB vs placebo	1134/2991	AASK (vs ACEi) [63]		–/217 vs 436
IRMA-2 [40]	ARB vs placebo	590/–	ABCD-H [22]		235 vs 235/–
JATOS [41]	More vs less	521/3897	ACCOMPLISH [79]		3478 vs 3468/2266 vs 2293
MRC-mild [69]	D or BB vs placebo	–/17354	ALLHAT (vs D) [80]		3597 vs 5994/4958 vs 8419
MRC-old [70]	D or D vs placebo	–/4396	ALLHAT (vs ACEi) [80]		3510 vs 5994/5034 vs 8419
NAVIGATOR [71]	ARB vs placebo	–/9306	ASCOT [85]		2565 vs 2572/7074 vs 7046
NICOLE [42]	CCB vs placebo	85/741	BENEDICT [26]		303 vs 301/–
ORIENT [43]	ARB vs placebo	566/–	CAMELOT [27]		115 vs 118/548 vs 555
OSLO [72]	D vs no treatment	–/785	CASE-J [89]		1007 vs 1011/1342 vs 1343
PEACE [44]	ACEi vs placebo	1384/6906	COLM [82]		684 vs 678/1884 vs 1895
PROFESS [45]	ARB vs placebo	5743/14589	CONVINCE [90]		1616 vs 1623/6563 vs 6674
PROGRESS [46]	ACEi or ACEi-D vs placebo	761/5344	FACET [91]		191 vs 189/–
REIN-2 [73]	More vs less	–/335	Fogari [34]		103 vs 102/–
RENAAL [47]	ARB vs placebo	1513/–	IDNT [38]		567 vs 579/–
ROADMAP [48]	ARB vs placebo	4447/–	INSIGHT [83]		649 vs 653/2508 vs 2511
SANDS [49]	More vs less	499/–	INVEST [86]		3169 vs 3231/8098 vs 8078
SCOPE [50]	ARB vs placebo	599/4338	JMIC-B [92]		199 vs 173/629 vs 649
SHEP [51]	D vs placebo	583/4149	JMIND [93]		228 vs 208/–
SPRINT [74]	More vs less	–/9361	NICS-EH [102]		–/204 vs 210
SPS-3 [52]	More vs less	1106/1914	NORDIL [94]		351 vs 376/5375 vs 5095
STOP [53]	D/BB or ACEi or CCB vs placebo	142/1485	STOP-2 (vs D/BB) [95]		231 vs 253/1964 vs 1960
Syst-China [54]	CCB vs placebo	98/2296	STOP-2 (vs ACEi) [95]		231 vs 235/1964 vs 1970
Syst-Eur [55]	CCB vs placebo	492/4203	VALUE [96]		2428 vs 2395/5168 vs 5254

BP-lowering treatment trials			Head-to-head (comparison) treatment trials		
Trial acronym (Ref.)	Treatment	DM/no-DM	Trial acronym (Ref.)	Treatment	DM/no-DM
TOMHS [75]	Active vs placebo	–/902	AASK (vs BB) [63]	ACEi vs other	–/436 vs 441
TRANSCEND [56]	ARB vs placebo	2118/3808	AASK (vs CCB) [63]		–436 vs 217
UKPDS-38 [6]	More (ACEi or BB) vs less	1148/–	ABCD-H [22]		235 vs 235/–
USPHS [76]	Central+D vs placebo	–/389	ALLHAT (vs D) [80]		3510 vs 3597/5034 vs 8419
VALISH [57]	More vs less	399/2861	ALLHAT (vs CCB) [80]		3510 vs 3597/5034 vs 4958
ABCD-N [58]	More vs less	480/–	ANBP-2 [81]		229 vs 2012/2815 vs 2827
ABCD-2 V [59]	More vs less	129/–	BENEDICT [26]		301 vs 303/–
HOPE-3 N [67]	ARB + D vs placebo	–/8463	CAMELOT [27]		118 vs 115/555 vs 548
PHARAO [60]	ACEi vs no treatment	135/873	CAPPP [97]		309 vs 263/5183 vs 5230
Head-to-head (comparison) treatment trials			DETAIL [98]		130 vs 120/–
			FACET [91]		189 vs 191/–
			Fogari [34]		102 vs 103/–
			JMIC-B [92]		173 vs 199/649 vs 629
CASE-J [89]	ARB vs other	1011 vs 1007/1343 vs 1342	JMIND [93]		208 vs 222/–
DETAIL [98]		120 vs 130/–	NESTOR [84]		286 vs 283/–
IDNT [38]		579 vs 567/–	ONTARGET [99]		3453 vs 3550/5122 vs 4992
E-COST [107]		–/1053 vs 995	REIN-str 1 [104]		–/99 vs 87
E-COST R [108]		–/69 vs 72	REIN-str 2 [105]		–/78 vs 88
LIFE [87]		586 vs 609/4019 vs 3979	ROAD [106]		–/180 vs 180
ONTARGET [99]		3550 vs 3453/4992 vs 5122	STOP-2 (vs D/BB) [95]		235 vs 253/1970 vs 1960
ROAD [106]		–/180 vs 180	STOP-2 (vs CCB) [95]		235 vs 231/1970 vs 1964
VALUE [96]		2395 vs 2428/5254 vs 5168	UKPDS-39 [88]		400 vs 358/–

ACEi angiotensin-converting enzyme inhibitors, *ARB* angiotensin receptor blockers, *BB* beta-blockers, *BP* blood pressure, *CCB* calcium channel blockers, *D* diuretics, *DM* type 2 diabetes mellitus, *Ref.* reference, *vs* versus

Modified from Thomopoulos et al. [20], by courtesy of *Journal of Hypertension*

Outcome	Trials (n)	Difference SBP/DBP (mmHg)	Events (n/patients) Treated	Controls	RR (95% CI)	RR (95% CI)	I-squared (Heterogeneity)
Stroke	30	-5.8/-2.6	1184/25989	1342/25716	0.84 (0.77-0.92)		15%
CHD	27	-5.8/-2.6	1146/22547	1292/22138	0.83 (0.76-0.89)		0%
HF	19	-6.2/-2.7	866/19377	901/18501	0.85 (0.77-0.95)		0%
Stroke + CHD	30	-5.7/-2.6	2180/24687	2469/23709	0.82 (0.77-0.87)		0%
Stroke + CHD + HF	26	-5.9/-2.6	3761/23588	4012/22738	0.86 (0.81-0.90)		29%
CV Death	26	-5.7/-2.6	1020/23483	1097/22463	0.87 (0.74-1.01)		50%
All-cause Death	31	-5.7/-2.6	2074/24843	2139/24277	0.90 (0.84-0.96)		15%

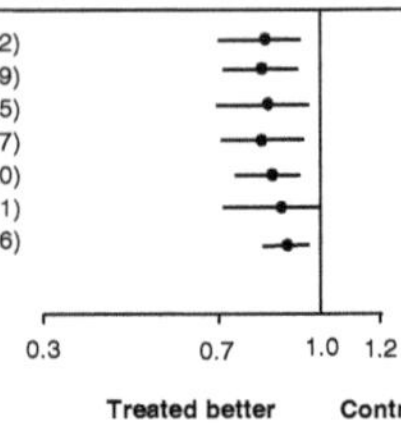

Fig. 18.1 Effects of blood pressure lowering in trials or subgroup of trials in patients with type 2 diabetes mellitus. *CHD* coronary heart disease, *CI* confidence interval, *CV* cardiovascular, *DBP* diastolic blood pressure, *HF* heart failure, *n* number, *RR* risk ratio, *SBP* systolic blood pressure. Modified from Thomopoulos et al. [20], by courtesy of *Journal of Hypertension*

18.3 Macrovascular Outcomes Following BP-Lowering Treatment in Patients With or Without DM

The same meta-analysis [20] compared the 41 trials (or subgroups of trials) [5, 6, 22–60] of stable DM patients ($n = 61{,}772$) with 40 trials (or subgroups of trials) [5, 24, 27, 31–33, 35–37, 39, 41, 43–46, 50–57, 63–77] of patients without DM ($n = 191{,}772$) (Table 18.1). At variance with DM patients, in patients without DM, all outcomes were reduced, including cardiovascular mortality. For a standard systolic/diastolic BP reduction of 10/5 mmHg in patients with DM compared to those without DM, the relative risk reduction was significantly larger for CHD events and all-cause death; however, it was significantly smaller for heart failure (Fig. 18.2). In addition, absolute risk reductions of CHD events, the composite of major cardiovascular outcomes, cardiovascular death, and all-cause death were significantly higher in patients with than without DM.

The difference between the effects of BP-lowering in patients with and without DM could not be observed in two previous sets of meta-analyses that compared responses in the presence and absence of DM. The more recent analysis by Ettehad et al. [78] included 23 trials in patients with DM and 19 trials in patients without DM. A somewhat smaller reduction of major cardiovascular events in the presence than the absence of DM was shown; however, the more detailed data presented in the manuscript supplement [78] indicate that interaction did not attain significance for all other outcomes.

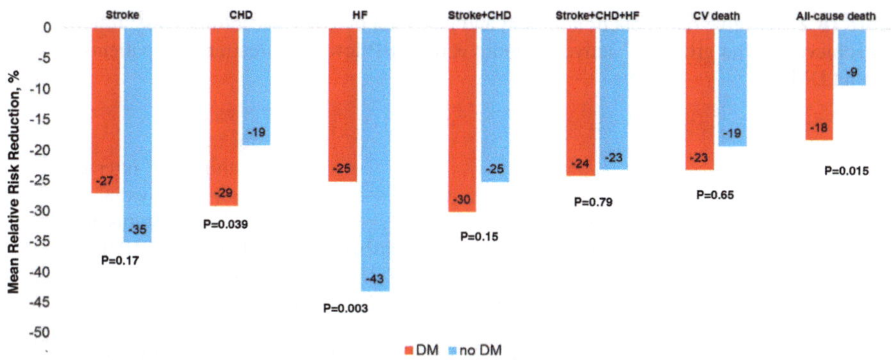

Fig. 18.2 Relative risk reduction of various outcomes in patients with or without type 2 diabetes mellitus. *CHD* coronary heart disease, *CV* cardiovascular, *HF* heart failure. Modified from Thomopoulos et al. [20], by courtesy of *Journal of Hypertension*

18.4 BP Thresholds and Macrovascular Outcomes in Patients with DM

The limited evidence in DM and pre-hypertension or grade 1 or grade 3 hypertension denies any reliable comparative evaluation between different BP threshold categories [20]. However, in ten trials ($n = 6905$ patients) of patients with DM belonging to grade 2 hypertension – without or with a very-low baseline antihypertensive treatment – the relative risk reduction, following systolic/diastolic BP-lowering treatment of −7/−3.5 mmHg on average, was 1) 37% (95% CI, 14–54%) for major cardiovascular events, 2) 42% (95% CI, 21–57%) for stroke, 3) 29% (95% CI, 10–45%) for CHD events, 4) 51% (95% CI, 10–73%) for cardiovascular death, and 5) 21% (95% CI, 5–35%) for all-cause death. For all outcomes, the test for interaction between grade 2 hypertension trials of patients with (ten trials, 6905 patients) or without DM (11 trials, 67,748 individuals) never attained statistical significance, suggesting that treatment initiation at grade 2 hypertension was not different between DM and no-DM strata.

18.5 Systolic BP Targets and Macrovascular Outcomes in Patients with DM

Among trials providing data on hypertensive patients with DM [20], there were (1) 13 trials in which systolic BP in the active or more actively treated group was lowered to values no less than 140 mmHg (average value 143.9 mmHg), (2) 19 trials in which systolic BP was lowered between 130 and 140 mmHg (average value 135.2 mmHg), and (3) six trials in which systolic BP was reduced to less than 130 mmHg (average value 123.3 mmHg). The relative risk reduction by a standardized systolic/diastolic BP difference of 10/5 mmHg was progressively smaller, the lower was the systolic BP achieved on treatment, with a significant trend for CHD events, heart failure, composite events, and cardiovascular death (Table 18.2). A

Table 18.2 Relative risk reduction of fatal and non-fatal outcomes according to systolic BP values achieved in the groups of active (or more active) BP-lowering treatment in patients with or without DM

Outcomes	Diabetes status[a]	Achieved SBP treated group (mmHg)	Trials (*n*)	Standardized RR (95% CI)	*P*-value for trend within each diabetes status group	*P*-interaction by diabetes status at each SBP treated group
Stroke	DM	≥140	11	0.52 (0.29–0.96)		SBP ≥140,
		130–140	13	0.76 (0.80–0.98)	0.13	0.14
		<130	4	0.74 (0.59–0.92)		SBP 130–140,
	No-DM	≥140	9	0.68 (0.60–0.78)		0.071
		130–140	13	0.62 (0.53–0.74)	0.37	SBP <130, 0.73
		<130	6	0.78 (0.55–1.14)		
CHD	DM	≥140	10	0.41 (0.27–0.64)		SBP ≥140,
		130–140	12	0.72 (0.58–0.89)	0.007	0.001
		<130	3	0.86 (0.72–1.02)		SBP 130–140,
	No-DM	≥140	6	0.84 (0.75–0.94)		0.11
		130–140	13	0.88 (0.73–0.94)	0.055	SBP <130, 0.13
		<130	6	0.66 (0.50–0.90)		
HF	DM	≥140	6	0.45 (0.24–0.81)		SBP ≥140,
		130–140	9	0.77 (0.58–1.02)	0.010	0.068
		<130	3	0.92 (0.75–1.14)		SBP 130–140,
	No-DM	≥140	3	0.77 (0.59–0.99)		0.088
		130–140	9	0.60 (0.45–0.79)	0.28	SBP <130, 0.11
		<130	5	0.50 (0.34–0.77)		
Stroke + CHD	DM	≥140	10	0.44 (0.32–0.71)		SBP ≥140,
		130–140	15	0.72 (0.61–0.83)	0.001	<0.001
		<130	3	0.81 (0.70–0.94)		SBP 130–140,
	No-DM	≥140	7	0.79 (0.73–0.86)		0.83
		130–140	13	0.73 (0.68–0.80)	0.36	SBP <130, 0.31
		<130	5	0.70 (0.56–0.90)		
Stroke + CHD + HF	DM	≥140	8	0.49 (0.32–0.71)		SBP ≥140,
		130–140	13	0.77 (0.65–0.91)	0.003	<0.001
		<130	3	0.86 (0.75–0.99)		SBP 130–140,
	No-DM	≥140	6	0.82 (0.74–0.91)		0.85
		130–140	13	0.76 (0.68–0.85)	0.54	SBP <130, 0.29
		<130	6	0.74 (0.58–0.96)		
CV death	DM	≥140	8	0.56 (0.26–1.21)		SBP ≥140,
		130–140	13	0.67 (0.41–1.070	0.008	0.057
		<130	4	1.28 (0.87–1.89)		SBP 130–140,
	No-DM	≥140	5	0.85 (0.75–0.96)		0.035
		130–140	10	0.94 (0.78–1.14)	0.45	SBP <130,
		<130	7	0.56 (0.37–0.89)		0.002

Table 18.2 (continued)

Outcomes	Diabetes status[a]	Achieved SBP treated group (mmHg)	Trials (*n*)	Standardized RR (95% CI)	*P*-value for trend within each diabetes status group	*P*-interaction by diabetes status at each SBP treated group
All-cause death	DM	≥140	10	0.79 (0.58–1.21)		SBP ≥140, 0.022
		130–140	15	0.71 (0.58–0.88)	0.090	
		<130	4	1.08 (0.86–1.23)		SBP 130–140, <0.001
	No-DM	≥140	7	0.95 (0.88–1.02)		
		130–140	13	0.93 (0.85–1.01)	0.030	SBP <130, 0.005
		<130	7	0.71 (0.57–0.88)		

BP blood pressure, *CHD* coronary heart disease, *CI* confidence interval, *CV* cardiovascular, *DM* type 2 diabetes mellitus, *HF* heart failure, *n* number, *RR* risk ratio, *SBP* systolic blood pressure
Modified from Thomopoulos et al. [20] by courtesy of *Journal of Hypertension*
[a]Trials (or subgroups of trials) in patients with DM in which SBP in the active or more active group was lowered to values: no less than 140 mmHg (*n* = 13, 13,566 patients), between 130 and 140 mmHg (*n* = 19, 34,940 patients), and less than 130 mmHg (*n* = 6, 12,532 patients). Trials (or subgroups of trials) in patients without diabetes mellitus: no less than 140 mmHg (*n* = 10, 24,850 patients), between 130 and 140 mmHg (*n* = 17, 11,487 patients), and less than 130 mmHg (*n* = 10, 38,866 patients)

similar trend was not observed for patients without DM (stratum systolic BP 140 mmHg or more, ten trials, average value, 148.8 mmHg; stratum 130–140 mmHg, 17 trials, average value 135.6 mmHg; stratum less than 130 mmHg ten trials, average value 126.2 mmHg). However, as illustrated in Table 18.2, in patients without DM, the risk of most outcomes was significantly reduced even at achieved systolic BP levels below 130 mmHg without a trend for the relative risk reduction to become smaller at lower systolic BP targets. Interaction analyses of risk reductions in patients with and without DM at different levels of achieved systolic BP indicated that (1) at achieved systolic BP no less than 140 mmHg, the relative risk reductions of most outcomes were greater in patients with DM, (2) at achieved systolic BP between 130 and 140 mmHg the relative risk reductions were mostly similar in DM and no-DM, and (3) at achieved systolic BP levels below 130 mmHg, the effects of BP-lowering treatment reversed with greater relative risk reductions of some outcomes in patients without DM (Table 18.2). Although DM is often associated with high or very-high cardiovascular risk, among trials providing data on hypertensive patients with DM, only 29 trials or subgroups of trials, including 52,350 patients, had 10-year cardiovascular mortality of at least 5% (average 14.3%). The effects of stratification by achieved systolic BP levels in patients with DM at high or very-high cardiovascular risk (i.e., 10-year fatal cardiovascular event rate of 5% or more) are reported in Table 18.3. For most outcomes, especially for deaths, a standard systolic/diastolic BP reduction of 10/5 mmHg was accompanied by a significantly smaller risk ratio reduction at lower levels of attained systolic BP.

Table 18.3 Relative risk of various cardiovascular outcomes and death according to systolic BP values achieved in the groups with active (or more active) BP-lowering treatment in patients with DM at high or very-high baseline cardiovascular risk

Outcome	Achieved SBP (mmHg)	Trials, *n*	SBP/DBP difference (mmHg)	Follow-up (years)	Outcome risk, %	RR (95% CI)	Standardized RR (95% CI)	*P*-value trend	*P*-value between targets
Stroke	≥140	10	−3.9/−1.9	3.5	5.5	0.89 (0.74–1.07)	0.62 (0.29–1.32)	0.62	0.48
	130–139	11	−5.2/−2.3	4.1	6.1	0.85 (0.75–0.96)	0.70 (0.54–0.92)		0.90
	<130	2	−13.6/−6.1	4.5	4.5	0.66 (0.49–0.88)	0.72 (0.57–0.90)		
CHD	≥140	9	3.4/−1.7	3.5	4.8	0.72 (0.60–0.85)	0.28 (0.13–0.53)	—	<0.001
	130–139	10	−5.6/−2.3	4.5	7.4	0.86 (0.78–0.94)	0.72 (0.58–0.87)		
	<130	1	—	—	—	—	—		
HF	≥140	5	−3.0/−1.4	3.5	7.4	0.86 (0.70–1.05)	0.54 (0.23–1.22)	0.17	0.45
	130–139	8	−5.7/−2.4	4.5	4.3	0.82 (0.69–0.97)	0.70 (0.52–0.95)		0.53
	<130	2	−11.3/−5.2	4.7	3.7	0.89 (0.65–1.23)	0.85 (0.55–1.33)		
Stroke + CHD	≥140	9	3.6/−1.7	3.6	10.4	0.80 (0.71–0.90)	0.40 (0.25–0.65)	—	<0.001
	130–139	11	−5.5/−2.3	4.5	12.6	0.85 (0.78–0.91)	0.71 (0.59–0.82)		
	<130	1	—	—	—	—	—		
Stroke + CHD + HF	≥140	7	−3.4/−1.6	3.4	18.4	0.85 (0.74–0.97)	0.53 (0.31–1.65)	—	<0.001
	130–139	12	−5.2/−2.3	4.1	18.8	0.87 (0.80–0.94)	0.74 (0.62–0.87)		
	<130	1	—	—	—	—	—		
CV death	≥140	10	3.2/−1.7	3.5	6.6	0.92 (0.75–1.13)	0.71 (0.31–1.65)	0.46	0.45
	130–139	7	−5.6/−2.3	4.5	6.0	0.79 (0.67–0.93)	0.61 (0.43–0.860		0.008
	<130	2	−11.3/−5.2	4.7	2.5	1.12 (0.77–1.63)	1.10 (0.80–1.50)		
All-cause death	≥140	9	−3.4/−1.7	3.5	12.8	0.98 (0.89–1.07)	0.91 (0.59–1.36)	0.35	0.002
	130–139	11	−5.7/−2.5	4.5	9.8	0.85 (0.78–0.92)	0.71 (0.59–0.84)		0.007
	<130	2	−11.3/−5.2	4.7	6.3	1.00 (0.82–1.21)	1.00 (0.85–1.17)		

BP blood pressure, *CHD* coronary heart disease, *CI* confidence interval, *CV* cardiovascular, *DM* type 2 diabetes mellitus, *HF* heart failure, *n* number, *RR* risk ratio, *SBP* systolic blood pressure

P-values between targets refer to differences between standardized risk ratios of two adjacent SBP targets

Modified from Thomopoulos et al. [21], by courtesy of *Journal of Hypertension*

18.6 Blood Pressure-Lowering Treatment and Renal Failure in Patients With or Without DM

In trials or subgroups of trials reporting data for incident end-stage renal disease in patients with DM (14 trials, 33,313 patients), BP-lowering treatment was associated with an attained systolic/diastolic BP reduction −6.1/−2.5 mmHg [20]. In such a case, the renal outcome was reduced by 12% (95% CI, 3–21%). However, in patients without DM (ten trials, 36,599 patients), BP-lowering treatment (attained systolic/diastolic BP reduction −8.6/3.2 mmHg) was not accompanied by a risk reduction of end-stage renal disease (risk ratio 1.01, 95% CI, 0.85–1.19). For a standardized systolic/diastolic BP reduction of 10/5 mmHg, the relative risk reduction of end-stage renal disease was 21% (95% CI, 5–34%) in patients with DM, while no risk reduction was observed in patients without DM (risk ratio 1.01, 95% CI 0.82–1.24). Thus, for a standard BP reduction, the incidence of end-stage renal disease significantly differed between patients with or without DM (*P* for interaction, 0.031).

Focusing on DM patients, at different targets of attained systolic BP, the effect of BP-lowering treatment on the end-stage renal disease was significantly different for a standard systolic/diastolic BP reduction of 10/5 mmHg (Fig. 18.3). Although a significant trend favoring more conservative BP targets ($P = 0.015$) occurred, point estimates in the lower attained systolic BP strata did not suggest an increased risk with more intense BP-lowering treatment.

Outcome: End-stage renal disease	Trials (n)	Difference SBP/DBP (mmHg)	Events (n/patients) Treated	Events (n/patients) Controls	Standardized RR (95% CI)	P-value Interaction
Achieved SBP (mmHg)						
≥ 140	5	-3.5/-1.7	354/5153	318/4246	0.56 (0.37–0.83)	
130-140	6	-6.7/-2.8	117/9375	121/9308	0.93 (0.56–1.57)	0.015
<130	3	-13.2/-5.9	61/2667	60/2564	1.01 (0.78–1.30)	

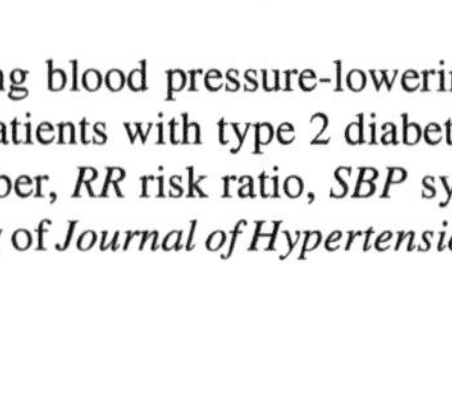

Fig. 18.3 Relative risk reduction of end-stage renal disease following blood pressure-lowering treatment across different systolic blood pressure targets in trials of patients with type 2 diabetes mellitus. *CI* confidence interval, *DBP* diastolic blood pressure, *n* number, *RR* risk ratio, *SBP* systolic blood pressure. Modified from Thomopoulos et al. [20], by courtesy of *Journal of Hypertension*

18.7 BP-Lowering Treatment and Macrovascular Outcomes by Different Drug Classes in Patients With DM

The effect of BP-lowering treatment by separate drug classes is usually investigated by confronting each drug class with a placebo or no treatment [20]. The effects on composite outcomes or end-stage renal disease of different drug classes from trials or subgroups of trials of patients with DM are presented in Table 18.4. The effect of BP-lowering treatment on major cardiovascular events by diuretics and beta-blockers was rather scarce. On the other hand, angiotensin-converting enzyme inhibitors, calcium channel blockers, and renin-angiotensin system blockers (i.e., angiotensin-converting enzyme inhibitors and angiotensin receptor blockers considered together) significantly reduced major cardiovascular events on average by 20%, 19%, and 17%, respectively (Table 18.4). Notably, angiotensin receptor blockers were not associated with a reduction of the composite endpoint of cardiovascular events.

Table 18.4 Effect of BP-lowering treatment by different drug classes (vs placebo) on major cardiovascular events or end-stage renal disease in patients with DM

Drug class	Outcome	Trials, *n*	SBP/DBP, mmHg	Events (*n*/patients) Active drug	placebo	RR (95% CI)
Diuretics	Stroke + CHD	2	−10.8/−2.7	47/338	75/356	0.66 (0.47–0.92)
BB	Stroke + CHD	1	–	–	–	–
CCB	Stroke + CHD + HF	6	−5.2/−2.8	312/2026	382/2189	0.81 (0.66–0.98)
ACEi	Stroke + CHD	7	−3.5/−1.2	622/6077	775/6115	0.80 (0.73–0.89)
	ESRD	3	−3.4/−1.0	25/4651	30/4628	0.83 (0.49–1.40)
ARB	Stroke + CHD + HF	6	−3.8/−2.0	1371/6081	1481/6141	0.92 (0.84–1.01)
	ESRD	4	−3.9/−1.7	308/2674	382/2674	0.81 (0.71–0.93)
RASb	Stroke + CHD	13	−3.6/−1.5	1057/11293	1264/11290	0.83 (0.77–0.90)
	ESRD	7	−3.6/−1.3	333/7322	412/7302	0.81 (0.71–0.92)

ACEi angiotensin-converting enzyme inhibitors, *ARB* angiotensin receptor blockers, *BB* beta-blockers, *BP* blood pressure, *CCB* calcium channel blockers, *CHD* coronary heart disease, *CI* confidence interval, *DBP* diastolic blood pressure, *DM* type 2 diabetes mellitus, *ESRD* end-stage renal disease, *HF* heart failure, *n* number, *RAS* renin-angiotensin system blockers (i.e., ACEi and ARB considered together), *RR* risk ratio, *SBP* systolic blood pressure

Modified from Thomopoulos et al. [20], by courtesy of *Journal of Hypertension*

Regarding the effect of BP-lowering treatment on end-stage renal disease, the available data for angiotensin-converting enzyme inhibitors were quite limited. At the same time, a significant reduction was revealed by angiotensin receptor blockers or renin-angiotensin system blockers (Table 18.4). Overall, renin-angiotensin receptor blockers might be considered an integrated class of agents yielding cardiovascular and renal protection in patients with DM.

18.8 BP-Lowering Independent Effects of Different Drug Classes on Major Cardiovascular Events in Patients With DM

Among 50 randomized controlled trials comparing different drug classes for the same (or almost the same) attained BP reduction [20], trials (or trial subgroups) with DM patients were identified. The comparison vs any other drug class of (1) diuretics (seven comparisons, 23,721 patients) [79–84], (2) beta-blockers (four comparisons, 13,490 patients) [85–88], (3) calcium channel blockers (21 comparisons, 49,620 patients) [22, 26, 27, 34, 38, 79, 80, 82, 83, 85, 86, 89–96], (4) angiotensin-converting enzyme inhibitors (17 comparisons, 26,113 patients) [22, 26, 27, 34, 80, 81, 84, 88, 91–93, 95, 97–99], and (5) angiotensin receptor blockers (six comparisons, 16,435 patients) [38, 87, 89, 96, 98, 99] yielded similar effects for the composite outcome of major cardiovascular events in all comparisons. However, when renin-angiotensin system blockers (i.e., angiotensin-converting enzyme inhibitors and angiotensin receptor blockers) were considered together against all other drug classes, a relative risk reduction of 13% (3–21%) for major cardiovascular events was produced (Fig. 18.4). In the seven comparisons between renin-angiotensin system blockers and other drug classes, the end-stage renal disease incidence was not different (risk ratio, 0.90; 95% CI, 0.66–1.23).

Comparison	Trials (n)	Difference SBP/DBP (mmHg)	Events (n/patients) Treated	Events (n/patients) Controls	RR (95% CI)	RR (95% CI)	I-squared (Heterogeneity)
Outcome: fatal and non-fatal stroke, CHD and HF events							
Diuretics vs other	5	-1.03/0.44	1811/10327	2144/11463	0.97 (0.93-1.02)		56%
BB vs other	3	2.40/1.16	591/3539	524/ 3551	1.11 (0.90-1.36)		68%
CCB vs other	14	-1.02/-1.21	2256/14643	3720/20769	1.06 (0.97-1.15)		60%
ACEi vs other	13	1.60/0.74	1916/9000	3655/15355	0.91 (0.82-1.01)		64%
ARB vs other	5	-0.05/0.22	1326/7230	1387/7187	0.91 (0.78-1.06)		72%
RASb vs other	14	1.57/0.88	1763/8977	3563/15289	0.87 (0.79-0.97)		69%

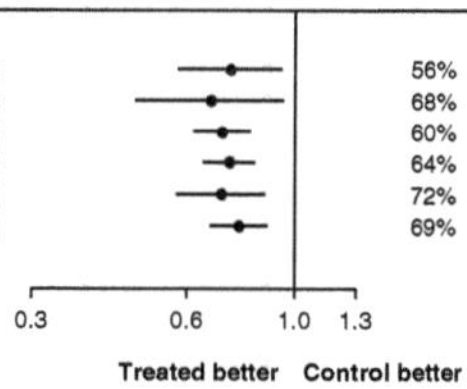

Fig. 18.4 Relative risk reduction of major cardiovascular events in head-to-head (comparison) trials of each drug class compared to any other drug class in patients with type 2 diabetes mellitus. *ACEi* angiotensin-converting enzyme inhibitors, *ARB* angiotensin receptor blockers, *BB* beta-blockers, *CCB* calcium channel blockers, *CI* confidence interval, *DBP* diastolic blood pressure, *n* number, *RASb* renin-angiotensin system blockers, *RR* risk ratio, *SBP* systolic blood pressure. Modified from Thomopoulos et al. [20], by courtesy of *Journal of Hypertension*

18.9 Are the Independent BP-Lowering Effects of Various Drug Classes Different Between Patients With and Without DM?

From the same analysis [20], we also identified trials (or subgroups of trials) in patients without DM. The comparison vs any other drug class of (1) diuretics (12 comparisons, 55,684 patients) [69, 70, 80–83, 100–103], (2) beta-blockers (ten comparisons, 57,248 patients) [63, 69, 70, 85–87, 99, 101, 103], (3) calcium channel blockers (18 comparisons, 108,561 patients) [27, 63, 79, 80, 82, 83, 85, 86, 89, 90, 92, 94, 96, 102], (4) angiotensin-converting enzyme inhibitors (14 comparisons, 54,661 patients) [27, 63, 80, 81, 92, 95, 97, 104–106], and (5) angiotensin receptor blockers (seven comparisons, 33,768 patients) [87, 89, 96, 99, 106–108] yielded similar effects for the composite outcome of major cardiovascular events in all comparisons except for beta-blockers where a 15% increase in relative risk was shown (95% CI, 5–26%). In addition, the end-stage renal disease incidence was not different in the seven comparisons between renin-angiotensin system blockers and other classes (risk ratio, 1.19; 95% CI, 0.90–1.58). Figure 18.5 illustrates the relative risk of major cardiovascular events in head-to-head trials of one drug class with all other classes in patients with or without DM. No significant interaction was observed by DM status in all drug comparisons (Fig. 18.5) for the relative risk of major

Comparison	DM status	Trials (n)	Events (n/patients) Drug	Events (n/patients) Others	RR (95% CI)	RR (95% CI)	P-value for interaction
Diuretics vs others	DM	5	1811/10327	2144/11463	0.97 (0.93-1.02)	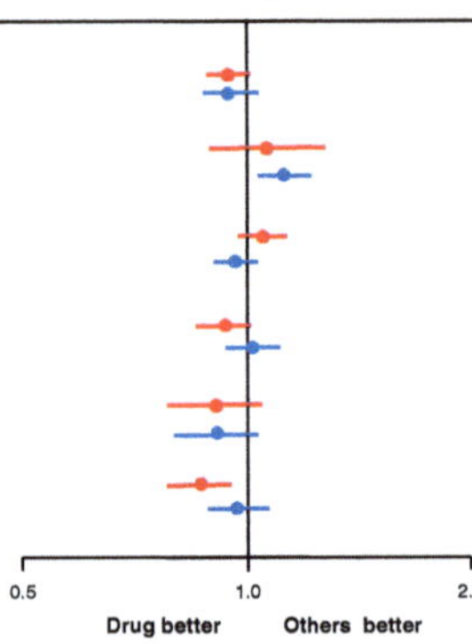	0.91
	No-DM	9	2305/24910	2671/26587	0.96 (0.87-1.06)		
BB vs other	DM	3	591/ 3539	524/ 3551	1.11 (0.90-1.36)		0.79
	No-DM	5	1695/19827	1469/19743	1.15 (1.05-1.26)		
CCB vs other	DM	14	2256/14643	3720/20769	1.06 (0.97-1.15)		0.18
	No-DM	12	2995/30694	4956/40996	0.96 (0.89-1.04)		
ACEi vs other	DM	13	1916/ 9000	3655/15355	0.91 (0.82-1.01)		0.082
	No-DM	10	2812/21508	4486/31707	1.01 (0.94-1.10)		
ARB vs other	DM	5	1326/ 7230	1387/ 7187	0.91 (0.78-1.06)		0.87
	No-DM	6	1742/15567	1815/15516	0.91 (0.79-1.04)		
RASb vs other	DM	10	1763/ 8977	3563/15289	0.87 (0.79-0.97)		0.087
	No-DM	10	3137/26601	4884/36749	0.97 (0.89-1.06)		

Fig. 18.5 Relative risk of major cardiovascular events in head-to-head (comparison) trials of one drug class vs all other classes in patients with or without type 2 diabetes mellitus. *ACEi* angiotensin-converting enzyme inhibitors, *ARB* angiotensin receptor blockers, *BB* beta-blockers, *CCB* calcium channel blockers, *CI* confidence interval, *DM* type 2 diabetes mellitus, *n* number, RASb renin-angiotensin system blockers, *RR* risk ratio. Modified from Thomopoulos et al. [20], by courtesy of *Journal of Hypertension*

cardiovascular events. This finding was extended to end-stage renal disease for the comparison between renin-angiotensin system blocker and other drug classes ($P = 0.17$).

18.10 Conclusions

- BP-lowering treatment in patients with DM is associated with a relative risk reduction of all outcomes except for cardiovascular mortality. Notably, outcome reduction is almost identical for stroke and CHD events.
- Relative risk reductions of CHD events and all-cause mortality are greater in patients with than without DM.
- End-stage renal disease is the only outcome that BP-lowering treatment appears to reduce only in the presence of DM.
- In DM patients with at least a high baseline cardiovascular risk, a significantly smaller outcome benefit of a standardized systolic/diastolic BP reduction of 10/5 mmHg was observed at lower attained BP targets.
- The effects of BP-lowering treatment differ between hypertensive patients with or without DM when trials are stratified according to the attained systolic BP. For attained systolic BP of more than 140 mmHg, reductions of most outcomes are significantly greater for patients with than without DM, whereas for achieved BP lower than 130 mmHg, the difference between the effects in patients with and without DM disappears or even reverses. A systolic BP target below 130 mmHg in patients with DM is associated with no additional benefit, although it never indicates significant harm.
- Calcium channel and renin-angiotensin system blockers are protective for fatal and non-fatal major cardiovascular events in patients with DM, as shown in the BP-lowering treatment trials against placebo. In addition, renin-angiotensin system blockers, particularly angiotensin receptor blockers, are protective for end-stage renal disease.
- Head-to-head (i.e., comparison) trials aiming to investigate the BP-independent effects of different drug classes demonstrated no significant outcome differences in patients with or without DM. However, in patients with DM, renin-angiotensin system blockers appear more effective than all other drug classes in preventing major fatal and non-fatal cardiovascular events. Furthermore, for the same BP reduction obtained in head-to-head trials on DM, the prevention of end-stage renal disease of renin-angiotensin system blockers was similar to all other drugs.

The conclusions above from a comprehensive overview of randomized trials in patients with and without DM may give support to the following clinical recommendations: (1) BP-lowering treatment is indicated to reduce the macrovascular risk of hypertensive patients with or without DM; (2) systolic BP targets may be less aggressive in patients with than without DM; although systolic BP reduction to less than 130 mmHg in patients with DM does not add further benefit, it does not increase cardiovascular risk also; (3) BP-lowering treatment in patients with DM reduces the risk of end-stage renal disease, whereas most of the benefit occurs at a relatively high attained systolic BP; and (4) renin-angiotensin system blockers are more protective for cardiovascular events in patients with than without DM.

Acknowledgments The data, concepts, and figures reported in this chapter are largely taken from two original articles published by the author in the *Journal of Hypertension* [20, 21]. Wolters Kluwer Health Inc. is thanked for permission.

References

1. Hypertension in Diabetes Study (HDS). Prevalence of hypertension in newly presenting type 2 diabetic patients and the association with risk factors for cardiovascular and diabetic complications. J Hypertens. 1993;11:309–17.
2. Woodward M, Zhang X, Barzi F, Pan W, Ueshima H, Rodgers A, et al. The effects of diabetes on the risks of major cardiovascular diseases and death in the Asia-Pacific region. Diabetes Care. 2003;26:360–6.
3. Jha V, Garcia-Garcia G, Iseki K, Li Z, Naicker S, Plattner B, et al. Chronic kidney disease: global dimension and perspectives. Lancet. 2013;382:260–72.
4. Stratton IM, Cull CA, Adler AI, Matthews DR, Neil HA, Holman RR. Additive effects of glycaemia and blood pressure exposure on risk of complications in type 2 diabetes: a prospective observational study (UKPDS 75). Diabetologia. 2006;49:1761–9.
5. Hansson L, Zanchetti A, Carruthers SG, Dahlof B, Elmfeldt D, Julius S, et al. Effects of intensive blood pressure lowering and low-dose aspirin in patients with hypertension: principal results of the Hypertension Optimal Treatment (HOT) randomised trial. HOT Study Group. Lancet. 1998;351:1755–62.
6. UK Prospective Diabetes Study Group. Tight blood pressure control and risk of macrovascular and microvascular complications in type 2 diabetes: UKPDS 38. BMJ. 1998;317:703–13.
7. Chobanian AV, Bakris GL, Black HR, Cushman WC, Green LA, Izzo JL Jr, et al. National Heart, Lung, Blood Institute Joint National Committee on Prevention, Detection, Evaluation, and Treatment of High Blood Pressure. National High Blood Pressure Education Program Coordinating Committee. The seventh report of the joint national committee on prevention, detection, evaluation, and treatment of high blood pressure: the JNC 7 report. JAMA. 2003;289:2560–72.
8. European Society of Hypertension-European Society of Cardiology Guidelines Committee. 2003 European Society of Hypertension- European Society of Cardiology guidelines for the management of arterial hypertension. J Hypertens. 2003;2003(21):1011–53.
9. Mancia G, De Backer G, Dominiczak A, Cifkova R, Fagard R, Germano G, et al. The task force for the management of arterial hypertension of the European Society of Hypertension. The task force for the management of arterial hypertension of the European Society of Cardiology. 2007 Guidelines for the management of arterial hypertension: The task force for the management of arterial hypertension of the European Society of Hypertension (ESH) and of the European Society of Cardiology (ESC). Eur Heart J. 2007;28:1462–536.
10. Buse JB, Ginsberg HN, Bakris GL, Clark NG, Costa F, Eckel R, et al; American Heart Association; American Diabetes Association. Primary prevention of cardiovascular diseases in people with diabetes mellitus: a scientific statement from the American Heart Association and the American Diabetes Association. Circulation. 2007;115:114–26.
11. Zanchetti A, Grassi G, Mancia G. When should antihypertensive drug treatment be initiated and to what levels should systolic blood pressure be lowered? A critical reappraisal. J Hypertens. 2009;27:923–34.
12. Mancia G, Fagard R, Narkiewicz K, Redon J, Zanchetti A, Bohm M, et al. The Task Force for the management of arterial hypertension of the European Society of Hypertension (ESH), of

the European Society of Cardiology (ESC). 2013 ESH/ESC Guidelines for the management of arterial hypertension. J Hypertens. 2013;31:1281–357.
13. Ryden L, Grant PJ, Anker SD, Berne C, Cosentino F, Danchin N, et al. ESC Guidelines on diabetes, prediabetes, and cardiovascular diseases developed in collaboration with the EASD: the Task Force on diabetes, prediabetes, and cardiovascular diseases of the European Society of Cardiology (ESC) and developed in collaboration with the European Association for the Study of Diabetes (EASD). Eur Heart J. 2013;34:3035–87.
14. Weber MA, Schiffrin EL, White WB, Mann S, Lindholm LH, Kenerson JG, et al. Clinical practice guidelines for the management of hypertension in the community. A statement by the American Society of Hypertension and the International Society of Hypertension. J Hypertens. 2014;32:3–15.
15. James PA, Oparil S, Carter BL, Cushman WC, Dennison-Himmelfarb C, Handler J, et al. 2014 evidence-based guideline for the management of high blood pressure in adults: report from the panel members appointed to the Eighth Joint National Committee (JNC 8). JAMA. 2014;311:507–20.
16. American Diabetes Association. Standards of medical care in diabetes- 2015: summary of revisions. Diabetes Care. 2015;38:S4.
17. Williams B, Mancia G, Spiering W, Agabiti Rosei E, Azizi M, Burnier M, et al; Authors/Task Force Members. 2018 ESC/ESH Guidelines for the management of arterial hypertension: The Task Force for the management of arterial hypertension of the European Society of Cardiology and the European Society of Hypertension: The Task Force for the management of arterial hypertension of the European Society of Cardiology and the European Society of Hypertension. J Hypertens. 2018;36:1953–2041.
18. Whelton PK, Carey RM, Aronow WS, Casey DE Jr, Collins KJ, Dennison Himmelfarb C, et al. 2017 ACC/AHA/AAPA/ABC/ACPM/AGS/APhA/ASH/ASPC/NMA/PCNA Guideline for the Prevention, Detection, Evaluation, and Management of High Blood Pressure in Adults: A Report of the American College of Cardiology/American Heart Association Task Force on Clinical Practice Guidelines. Circulation. 2018;138:e484–594.
19. Unger T, Borghi C, Charchar F, Khan NA, Poulter NR, Prabhakaran D, et al. 2020 International Society of Hypertension global hypertension practice guidelines. J Hypertens. 2020;38:982–1004.
20. Thomopoulos C, Parati G, Zanchetti A. Effects of blood-pressure-lowering treatment on outcome incidence in hypertension: 10 - Should blood pressure management differ in hypertensive patients with and without diabetes mellitus? Overview and meta-analyses of randomized trials. J Hypertens. 2017;35:922–44.
21. Thomopoulos C, Parati G, Zanchetti A. Effects of blood-pressure-lowering treatment on outcome incidence in hypertension. 11. Effects of total cardiovascular risk and achieved blood pressure: overview and meta-analyses of randomized trials. J Hypertens. 2017;35:2138–49.
22. Estacio RO, Jeffers BW, Gifford N, Schrier RW. Effect of blood pressure control on diabetic microvascular complications in patients with hypertension and type 2 diabetes. Diabetes Care. 2000;23:B54–64.
23. The ACCORD Study Group. Effects of intensive blood-pressure control in type 2 diabetes mellitus. N Engl J Med. 2010;362:1575–85.
24. Poole-Wilson PA, Lubsen J, Kirwan BA, van Dalen FJ, Wagener G, Danchin N, et al. Effect of long-acting nifedipine on mortality and cardiovascular morbidity in patients with stable angina requiring treatment (ACTION trial): randomised controlled trial. Lancet. 2004;364:849–57.
25. ADVANCE Collaborative Group. Effects of a fixed combination of perindopril and indapamide on macrovascular and microvascular outcomes in patients with type 2 diabetes mellitus (the ADVANCE trial): a randomised controlled trial. Lancet. 2007;37:829–40.
26. Ruggenenti P, Fassi A, Ilieva AP, Bruno S, Iliev IP, Brusegan V, et al. Bergamo Nephrologic Diabetes Complications Trial (BENEDICT) Investigators. Preventing microalbuminuria in type 2 diabetes. N Engl J Med. 2004;351:1941–51.

27. Nissen SE, Tuzcu EM, Libby P, Thompson PD, Ghali M, Garza D, et al. Effect of antihypertensive agents on cardiovascular events in patients with coronary disease and normal blood pressure: the CAMELOT study: a randomized controlled trial. JAMA. 2004;292:2217–25.
28. Ruggenenti P, Lauria G, Iliev IP, Fassi A, Ilieva AP, Rota S, et al. DEMAND Study Investigators. Effects of manidipine and delapril in hypertensive patients with type 2 diabetes mellitus: The Delapril and Manidipine for Nephroprotection in Diabetes (DEMAND) randomized clinical trial. Hypertension. 2011;58:776–83.
29. Marre M, Lievre M, Chatellier G, Mann JF, Passa P, Me'nard J, DIABHYCAR Study Investigators. Effects of low dose ramipril on cardiovascular and renal outcomes in patients with type 2 diabetes and raised excretion of urinary albumin: randomised, double blind, placebo controlled trial (the DIABHYCAR study). BMJ. 2004;328:495.
30. Tillin T, Orchard T, Malm A, Fuller J, Chaturvedi N. The role of antihypertensive therapy in reducing vascular complications of type 2 diabetes. Findings from the DIabetic REtinopathy Candesartan Trials Protect 2 study. J Hypertens. 2011;29:1457–62.
31. Fox KM. Efficacy of perindopril in reduction of cardiovascular events among patients with stable coronary artery disease: randomised, double-blind, placebo-controlled, multicentre trial (the EUROPA study). Lancet. 2003;362:782–8.
32. Amery A, Brixko P, Clement D, De Schaepdryver A, Fagard R, Forte J, et al. Mortality and morbidity results from the European Working Party on High Blood Pressure in the Elderly trial. Lancet. 1985;325:1349–54.
33. Liu L, Zhang Y, Liu G, Li W, Zhang X, Zanchetti A. The Felodipine Event Reduction (FEVER) Study: a randomized long-term placebo controlled trial in Chinese hypertensive patients. J Hypertens. 2005;23:2157–72.
34. Fogari R, Preti P, Zoppi A, Rinaldi A, Corradi L, Pasotti C, et al. Effects of amlodipine fosinopril combination on microalbuminuria in hypertensive type 2 diabetic patients. Am J Hypertens. 2002;15:1042–9.
35. The Hypertension Detection, Follow-up Program Cooperative Research Group. Mortality findings for stepped-care and referred care participants in the hypertension detection and follow-up program, stratified by other risk factors. Prev Med. 1985;14:312–35.
36. The Heart Outcomes Prevention Evaluation Study Investigators. Effects of an angiotensin-converting-enzyme inhibitor, ramipril, on cardiovascular events in high-risk patients. N Engl J Med. 2000;342:145–53.
37. Hypertension-Stroke Cooperative Study Group. Effect of antihypertensive treatment on stroke recurrence. JAMA. 1974;229:409–18.
38. Lewis EJ, Hunsicker LG, Clarke WR, Berl T, Pohl MA, Lewis JB, et al. Renoprotective effect of the angiotensin-receptor antagonist irbesartan in patients with nephropathy due to type 2 diabetes. N Engl J Med. 2001;345:851–60.
39. Massie BM, Carson PE, McMurray JJ, Komajda M, McKelvie R, Zile MR, et al. Irbesartan in patients with heart failure and preserved ejection fraction. N Engl J Med. 2008;359:2456–67.
40. Parving HH, Lehnert H, Bröchner-Mortensen J, Gomis R, Andersen S, Arner P, Irbesartan in Patients with Type 2 Diabetes Microalbuminuria Study Group. The effect of irbesartan on the development of diabetic nephropathy in patients with type 2 diabetes. N Engl J Med. 2001;345:870–8.
41. JATOS Study Group. Principal results of the Japanese Trial to assess Optimal Systolic blood pressure in elderly hypertensive patients (JATOS). Hypertens Res. 2008;31:2115–27.
42. Dens JA, Desmet WJ, Coussement P, De Scheerder IK, Kostopoulos K, Kerdsinchai P, et al. Long term effects of nisoldipine on the progression of coronary atherosclerosis and the occurrence of clinical events: the NICOLE study. Heart. 2003;89:887–92.
43. Imai E, Chan JC, Ito S, Yamasaki T, Kobayashi F, Haneda M, et al. ORIENT Study Investigators. Effects of olmesartan on renal and cardiovascular outcomes in type 2 diabetes with overt nephropathy: a multicentre, randomised, placebo-controlled study. Diabetologia. 2011;54:2978–86.
44. The PEACE Trial Investigators. Angiotensin-converting-enzyme inhibition in stable coronary artery disease. N Engl J Med. 2004;351:2058–68.

45. Yusuf S, Diener HC, Sacco RL, Cotton D, Ounpuu S, Lawton WA, et al. Telmisartan to prevent recurrent stroke and cardiovascular events. N Engl J Med. 2008;359:1225–37.
46. PROGRESS Collaborative Group. Randomised trial of a perindopril based blood-pressure-lowering regimen among 6105 individuals with previous stroke or transient ischaemic attack. Lancet. 2001;358:1033–41.
47. Brenner BM, Cooper ME, de Zeeuw D, Keane WF, Mitch WE, Parving HH, et al. Effects of losartan on renal and cardiovascular outcomes in patients with type 2 diabetes and nephropathy. N Engl J Med. 2001;345:861–9.
48. Haller H, Ito S, Izzo JL Jr, Januszewicz A, Katayama S, Menne J, et al. ROADMAP Trial Investigators. Olmesartan for the delay or prevention of microalbuminuria in type 2 diabetes. N Engl J Med. 2011;364:907–17.
49. Howard BV, Roman MJ, Devereux RB, Fleg JL, Galloway JM, Henderson JA, et al. Effect of lower targets for blood pressure and LDL cholesterol on atherosclerosis in diabetes: the SANDS randomized trial. JAMA. 2008;299:1678–89.
50. Lithell H, Hansson L, Skoog I, Elmfeldt D, Hofman A, Olofsson B, et al. The Study on Cognition and Prognosis in the Elderly (SCOPE): principal results of a randomized double-blind intervention trial. J Hypertens. 2003;21:875–86.
51. SHEP Co-operative Research Group. Prevention of stroke by antihypertensive drug treatment in older persons with isolated systolic hypertension. Final results of the Systolic Hypertension in the Elderly Program (SHEP). JAMA. 1991;265:3255–64.
52. SPS3 Study Group; Benavente OR, Coffey CS, Conwit R, Hart RG, McClure LA, Pearce LA, et al. Blood-pressure targets in patients with recent lacunar stroke: the SPS3 randomised trial. Lancet. 2013;382:507–15.
53. Dahlof B, Lindholm LH, Hansson L, Schersten B, Ekbom T, Wester PO. Morbidity and mortality in the Swedish Trial in Old Patients with Hypertension (STOP-Hypertension). Lancet. 1991;338:1281–5.
54. Liu L, Wang JG, Gong L, Liu G, Staessen JA. Comparison of active treatment and placebo in older Chinese patients with isolated systolic hypertension. Systolic Hypertension in China (Syst-China) Collaborative Group. J Hypertens. 1998;16:1823–9.
55. Staessen JA, Fagard R, Thijs L, Celis H, Arabidze GG, Birkenhager WH, et al. Randomised double-blind comparison of placebo and active treatment for older patients with isolated systolic hypertension. The Systolic Hypertension in Europe (Syst-Eur) Trial Investigators. Lancet. 1997;350:757–64.
56. Telmisartan Randomized Assessment Study in ACE Intolerant Subjects with Cardiovascular Disease (TRANSCEND) Investigators. Effects of the angiotensin-receptor blocker telmisartan on cardiovascular events in high-risk patients intolerant to angiotensin-converting enzyme inhibitors: a randomised controlled trial. Lancet. 2008;372:1174–83.
57. Ogihara T, Saruta T, Rakugi H, Matsuoka H, Shimamoto K, Shimada K, et al. Target blood pressure for treatment of isolated systolic hypertension in the elderly: valsartan in elderly isolated systolic hypertension study. Hypertension. 2010;56:196–202.
58. Schrier RW, Estacio RO, Esler A, Mehler P. Effects of aggressive blood pressure control in normotensive type 2 diabetic patients on albuminuria, retinopathy and strokes. Kidney Int. 2002;61:1086–97.
59. Estacio RO, Coll JR, Tran ZV, Schrier RW. Effect of intensive blood pressure control with valsartan on urinary albumin excretion in normotensive patients with type 2 diabetes. Am J Hypertens. 2006;19:1241–8.
60. Luders S, Schrader J, Berger J, Unger T, Zidek W, Böhmet M, et al. PHARAO Study Group. The PHARAO study: prevention of hypertension with the angiotensin converting enzyme inhibitor ramipril in patients with high-normal blood pressure: a prospective, randomized, controlled prevention trial of the German Hypertension League. J Hypertens. 2008;26:1487–96.
61. Emdin CA, Rahimi K, Neal B, Callender T, Perkovic V, Patel A. Blood pressure lowering in type 2 diabetes. A systematic review and metaanalysis. JAMA. 2015;313:603–15.

62. Brunstrom M, Carlberg B. Effect of antihypertensive treatment at different blood pressure levels in patients with diabetes mellitus: systematic review and meta-analyses. BMJ. 2016;352(i717):63–76.
63. Appel LJ, Wright JT Jr, Greene T, Agodoa LY, Astor BC, Bakris GL, et al. Intensive blood-pressure control in hypertensive chronic kidney disease. N Engl J Med. 2010;363:918–29.
64. Verdecchia P, Staessen JA, Angeli F, De Simone G, Achilli A, Ganau A, et al. Usual vs. tight control of systolic blood pressure in nondiabetic patients with hypertension (Cardio-Sis): an open-label randomized trial. Lancet. 2009;374:525–33.
65. DREAM Trial Investigators, Dagenais GR, Gerstein HC, Holman R, Budaj A, Escalante A, Hedner T, et al. Effects of ramipril and rosiglitazone on cardiovascular and renal outcomes in people with impaired glucose tolerance or impaired fasting glucose: results of the Diabetes REduction Assessment with ramipril and rosiglitazone Medication (DREAM) trial. Diabetes Care. 2008;31:1007–14.
66. Coope J, Warrender TS. Randomised trial of treatment of hypertension in elderly patients in primary care. BMJ. 1986;293:1145–51.
67. Lonn EM, Bosch J, Lopez-Jaramillo P, Zhu J, Liu L, Pais P, et al. Blood pressure lowering in intermediate-risk persons without cardiovascular disease. N Engl J Med. 2016;374:2009–20.
68. Sun M, Zhou H, Jia Z. Prevention and treatment of stroke after hypertension for ten years in Hunan Province. Zhonghua Nei Ke Za Zhi. 1997;36:312–4.
69. Medical Research Council Working Party. MRC trial on treatment of mild hypertension: principal results. BMJ. 1985;291:97–104.
70. MRC Working Party. Medical Research Council trial of treatment of hypertension in older adults: principal results. BMJ. 1992;304:405–12.
71. The NAVIGATOR Study Group. Effect of valsartan on the incidence of diabetes and cardiovascular events. N Engl J Med. 2010;362:1477–90.
72. Helgeland A. Treatment of mild hypertension: a five year controlled drug trial. The Oslo study. Am J Med. 1980;69:725–32.
73. Ruggenenti P, Perna A, Loriga G, Ganeva M, Ene-Iordache B, Turturro M, et al. Blood-pressure control for renoprotection in patients with nondiabetic chronic renal disease (REIN-2): multicentre, randomized controlled trial. Lancet. 2005;365:939–46.
74. The SPRINT Research Group. A randomized trial of intensive versus standard blood-pressure control. N Engl J Med. 2015;373:2103–16.
75. Neaton JD, Grimm RH Jr, Prineas RJ, Stamler J, Grandits GA, Elmer PJ, et al. Treatment of Mild Hypertension Study. Final results. Treatment of mild hypertension study research group. JAMA. 1993;270:713–24.
76. Smith WM. Treatment of mild hypertension: results of a ten-year intervention trial. Circ Res. 1977;40:I98–105.
77. Management Committee. The Australian therapeutic trial in mild hypertension. Lancet. 1980;315:1261–7.
78. Ettehad D, Emdin CA, Kiran A, Anderson SG, Callender T, Emberson J, et al. Blood pressure lowering for prevention of cardiovascular disease and death: a systematic review and meta-analysis. Lancet. 2016;387:957–67.
79. Jamerson K, Weber MA, Bakris GL, Dahlof B, Pitt B, Shi V, et al. Benazepril plus amlodipine or hydrochlorothiazide for hypertension in high-risk patients. N Engl J Med. 2008;359:2417–28.
80. ALLHAT Officers, Coordinators for the ALLHAT Collaborative Research Group. Major outcomes in high-risk hypertensive patients randomized to angiotensin-converting enzyme inhibitor or calcium channel blocker vs. diuretic: the Antihypertensive and Lipid-Lowering Treatment to Prevent Heart Attack Trial (ALLHAT). JAMA. 2002;288:2981–97.
81. Wing LM, Reid CM, Ryan P, Beilin LJ, Brown MA, Jennings GL, et al. A comparison of outcomes with angiotensin-converting enzyme inhibitors and diuretics for hypertension in the elderly. N Engl J Med. 2003;348:583–92.
82. Ogihara T, Saruta T, Rakugi H, Saito I, Shimamoto K, Matsuoka H, et al. COLM Investigators. Combinations of olmesartan and a calcium channel blocker or a diuretic in elderly hypertensive patients: a randomized, controlled trial. J Hypertens. 2014;32:2054–63.

83. Brown MJ, Palmer CR, Castaigne A, de Leeuw PW, Mancia G, Rosenthal T, et al. Morbidity and mortality in patients randomized to double-blind treatment with a long-acting calcium-channel blocker or diuretic in the International Nifedipine GITS study: Intervention as a Goal in Hypertension Treatment (INSIGHT). Lancet. 2000;356:366–72.
84. Marre M, Puig JG, Kokot F, Fernandez M, Jermendy G, Opie L, et al. Equivalence of indapamide SR and enalapril on microalbuminuria reduction in hypertensive patients with type 2 diabetes: the NESTOR Study. J Hypertens. 2004;22:1613–22.
85. Dahlof B, Sever PS, Poulter NR, Wedel H, Beevers DG, Caulfield M, et al. Prevention of cardiovascular events with an antihypertensive regimen of amlodipine adding perindopril as required versus atenolol adding bendroflumethiazide as required, in the Anglo-Scandinavian Cardiac Outcomes Trial-Blood Pressure Lowering Arm(ASCOT-BPLA): a multicentre randomised controlled trial. Lancet. 2005;366:895–906.
86. Pepine CJ, Handberg EM, Cooper-DeHoff RM, Marks RG, Kowey P, Messerli FH, et al. A calcium antagonist vs. a noncalcium antagonist hypertension treatment strategy for patients with coronary artery disease. The International Verapamil-Trandolapril Study (INVEST): a randomized controlled trial. JAMA. 2003;290:2805–16.
87. Dahlof B, Devereux RB, Kjeldsen SE, Julius S, Beevers G, de Faire U, et al. Cardiovascular morbidity and mortality in the Losartan Intervention. For Endpoint reduction in hypertension study (LIFE): a randomised trial against atenolol. Lancet. 2002;359:995–1003.
88. UK Prospective Diabetes Study Group. Efficacy of atenolol and captopril in reducing risk of macrovascular and microvascular complications in type 2 diabetes: UKPDS 39. UK Prospective Diabetes Study Group. BMJ. 1998;317:713–20.
89. Ogihara T, Nakao K, Fukui T, Fukiyama K, Ueshima K, Oba K, et al. Effects of candesartan compared with amlodipine in hypertensive patients with high cardiovascular risks: candesartan antihypertensive survival evaluation in Japan trial. Hypertension. 2008;51:393–8.
90. Black HR, Elliott WJ, Grandits G, Grambsch P, Lucente T, White WB, et al. Principal results of the Controlled Onset Verapamil Investigation of Cardiovascular End Points (CONVINCE) trial. JAMA. 2003;289:2073–82.
91. Tatti P, Pahor M, Byington RP, Di Mauro P, Guarisco R, Strollo G, et al. Outcome results of the Fosinopril Versus Amlodipine Cardiovascular Events Randomized Trial (FACET) in patients with hypertension and NIDDM. Diabetes Care. 1998;21:597–603.
92. Yui Y, Sumiyoshi T, Kodama K, Hirayama A, Nonogi H, Kanmatsuse K, et al. Comparison of nifedipine retard with angiotensin converting enzyme inhibitors in Japanese hypertensive patients with coronary artery disease: the Japan Multicenter Investigation for Cardiovascular Diseases-B (JMIC-B) randomized trial. Hypertens Res. 2004;27:181–91.
93. Baba S, J-MIND Study Group. Nifedipine and enalapril equally reduce the progression of nephropathy in hypertensive type 2 diabetics. Diabetes Res Clin Pract. 2001;54:191–201.
94. Hansson L, Hedner T, Lund-Johansen P, Kjeldsen SE, Lindholm LH, Syvertsen JO, et al. Randomised trial of effects of calcium antagonists compared with diuretics and beta-blockers on cardiovascular morbidity and mortality in hypertension: the Nordic Diltiazem (NORDIL) study. Lancet. 2000;356:359–65.
95. Hansson L, Lindholm LH, Ekbom T, Dahlöf B, Lanke J, Scherstén B, et al. Randomised trial of old and new antihypertensive drugs in elderly patients: cardiovascular mortality and morbidity. The Swedish Trial in Old Patients with Hypertension-2 study. Lancet. 1999;354:1751–6.
96. Julius S, Kjeldsen SE, Weber M, Brunner HR, Ekman S, Hansson L, et al. Outcomes in hypertensive patients at high cardiovascular risk treated with regimens based on valsartan or amlodipine: the VALUE randomised trial. Lancet. 2004;363:2022–31.
97. Hansson L, Lindholm LH, Niskanen L, Lanke J, Hedner T, Niklason A, et al. Effect of angiotensin-converting-enzyme inhibition compared with conventional therapy on cardiovascular morbidity and mortality in hypertension: the Captopril Prevention Project (CAPPP) randomized trial. Lancet. 1999;353:611–6.
98. Barnett AH, Bain SC, Bouter P, Karlberg B, Madsbad S, Jervell J, et al. Angiotensin-receptor blockade versus converting-enzyme inhibition in type 2 diabetes and nephropathy. N Engl J Med. 2004;351:1952–61.

99. ONTARGET., Investigators. Telmisartan, ramipril, or both in patients at high risk for vascular events. N Eng J Med. 2008;358:1547–59.
100. Berglund G, Andersson O, Widgren B. Low-dose antihypertensive treatment with a thiazide diuretic is not diabetogenic. A 10-year controlled trial with bendroflumethiazide. Acta Med Scand. 1986;220:419–21.
101. Wilhelmsen L, Berglund G, Elmfeldt D, Fitzsimons T, Holzgreve H, Hosie J, et al. Beta-blockers versus diuretics in hypertensive men: main results from the HAPPHY trial. J Hypertens. 1987;5:561–72.
102. National Intervention Cooperative Study in Elderly Hypertensives Study Group. Randomized double-blind comparison of a calcium antagonist and a diuretic in elderly hypertensives. Hypertension. 1999;34:1129–33.
103. Veterans Administration Cooperative Study Group on Antihypertensive Agents. Comparison of propranolol and hydrochlorothiazide for the initial treatment of hypertension. II. Results of long-term therapy. JAMA. 1982;248:2004–11.
104. Ruggenenti P, Perna A, Gherardi G, Garini G, Zoccali C, Salvadori M, et al. Renoprotective properties of ACE-inhibition in non-diabetic nephropathies with non-nephrotic proteinuria. Lancet. 1999;354:359–64.
105. The GISEN Group (Gruppo Italiano di Studi Epidemiologici in Nefrologia). Randomised placebo-controlled trial of effect of ramipril on decline in glomerular filtration rate and risk of terminal renal failure in proteinuric, nondiabetic nephropathy. Lancet. 1997;349:1857–63.
106. Hou FF, Xie D, Zhang X, Chen PY, Zhang WR, Liang M, et al. Renoprotection of Optimal Antiproteinuric Doses (ROAD) Study: a randomized controlled study of benazepril and losartan in chronic renal insufficiency. J Am Soc Nephrol. 2007;18:1889–98.
107. Suzuki H, Kanno Y, Efficacy of Candesartan on Outcome in Saitama Trial (E-COST) Group. Effects of candesartan on cardiovascular outcomes in Japanese hypertensive patients. Hypertens Res. 2005;28:307–14.
108. Nakamura T, Kanno Y, Takenaka T, Suzuki H, Efficacy of Candesartan on Outcome in Saitama Trial Group. An angiotensin receptor blocker reduces the risk of congestive heart failure in elderly hypertensive patients with renal insufficiency. Hypertens Res. 2005;28:415–23.

Blood Pressure Lowering and Microvascular Complications of Diabetes

19

Scott D. Cohen and Charles Faselis

19.1 Introduction

There is a worldwide epidemic of diabetes mellitus (DM). Four hundred sixty-three million adults have been diagnosed with diabetes around the world as of 2019 [1]. An estimated 700 million adults worldwide will have diabetes by 2045 [2]. Diabetes is associated with devastating macrovascular and microvascular complications including diabetic nephropathy, retinopathy, and neuropathy. Diabetic kidney disease is the number one cause of end-stage kidney disease (ESKD) leading to dialysis and transplantation [3]. The physical and economic burden of diabetes and its complications is extensive [4–6]. Diabetics have two times the rate of hypertension compared with nondiabetics [7–9]. The role of intensive blood pressure control to treat the microvascular complications of diabetes has been well studied [10, 11]. In the general population, there is a continuous risk of BP elevations greater than 115/70 and adverse outcomes [12, 13]. Similar risk has been reported in patients with type 2 diabetes. There is a debate on the optimal target blood pressure in patients with diabetes with some guidelines recommending <140/90 and others <130/80. The results of the Systolic Blood Pressure Intervention Trial (SPRINT) in nondiabetics have moved recent consensus guidelines toward lower BP targets [7, 14].

S. D. Cohen (✉) · C. Faselis
Department of Veterans Affairs, Washington, DC, USA

Department of Medicine, George Washington University School of Medicine, Washington, DC, USA
e-mail: Scott.cohen@va.gov

A. E. Berbari, G. Mancia (eds.), *Blood Pressure Disorders in Diabetes Mellitus*, Updates in Hypertension and Cardiovascular Protection,
https://doi.org/10.1007/978-3-031-13009-0_19

19.2 Diabetic Neuropathy

Peripheral and autonomic neuropathies are the most common types of diabetic neuropathy, and they typically coexist [15]. There is at least a 50% incidence of peripheral neuropathy among type 2 diabetes [16]. Hypertension and hyperglycemia can predispose to the development of a sensory peripheral neuropathy. Multiple studies support the association between hypertension and the development of diabetic neuropathy. Hypertension was found to be associated with a 60% greater chance of sensory neuropathy in a cross-sectional study [17]. Jarmuzeska et al. [18] also found a strong link between hypertension and sensorimotor peripheral neuropathy in type 2 diabetes. In a prospective cohort study, Forrest et al. [19] found hypertension was strongly associated with the onset of a distal sensory polyneuropathy in 463 children with type 1 diabetes.

The mechanisms linking diabetic neuropathy with hypertension are unclear. Hypertensive rat models show a decrease in motor and sensory nerve conduction velocities and myelinated fiber density [20]. Reduction of blood flow and oxygen delivery to peripheral nerves may play an important role in leading to nerve injury [21]. Ischemia can lead to oxidative stress injury to nerves. Antihypertensive medications may help to increase blood flow to peripheral nerves and oxygenation [21]. In human studies, antihypertensive medications increased nerve conduction velocities and sensation to temperature and vibration [20]. The target blood pressure to prevent diabetic neuropathy is uncertain, but control to at least 130/80 or less is likely to be beneficial. It is unclear if there is a specific beneficial effect of one class of antihypertensive medication over another as there is for the development of diabetic nephropathy.

Didangelos et al. [15] evaluated the effect of quinapril on autonomic and peripheral neuropathy in 63 patients with DM (36 with type 2 DM and 27 with type 1 DM). Quinapril 20 mg daily was given for 2 years, and the incidence of diabetic cardiovascular autonomic neuropathy and peripheral neuropathy was evaluated. Quinapril was found to improve diabetic cardiovascular autonomic neuropathy but had no impact on the indices of peripheral neuropathy. Additional studies are needed to determine the effect of RAAS blockade on the incidence and progression of diabetic neuropathy.

19.3 Diabetic Retinopathy

Diabetic retinopathy is associated with significant morbidity in patients with diabetes and is the number one cause of blindness for diabetics between the ages of 30–70 years old [22]. Diabetic retinopathy occurs from endothelial cell injury from hyperglycemia, breakdown of the blood-retina barrier, and hyperperfusion damage to the eyes [23]. It progresses from the mild nonproliferative phase to severe proliferative forms. Treatment to slow progression of diabetic retinopathy includes glycemic control. The results of the Diabetes Control and Complications Trial (DCCT) [24] and the United Kingdom Prospective Diabetes Study (UKPDS) [25] both showed the benefit of tight glycemic control to reduce the incidence of diabetic retinopathy [26]. Intensive blood pressure control can also prevent the development of diabetic retinopathy. Hypertension can lead to macroaneurysms and vascular occlusion of the retina leading to ischemic optic neuropathy. It is possible that the hypertensive effects on blood vessels will lead to retinopathy. However, there are mixed results on the impact of tight blood pressure control on the development of diabetic retinopathy. The UKPDS data demonstrated that higher systolic blood pressure lead to increased rates of retinopathy [25]. Patients in the baseline SBP range above 140 mm Hg had a 2.8 times higher likelihood to develop retinopathy as compared with patients in the lowest tertile range of SBP < 125 mm Hg [26]. Diastolic blood pressure predicted onset of proliferative diabetic retinopathy in type 1 diabetes over a 14-year period in the Wisconsin Epidemiologic Study of Diabetic Retinopathy (WESDR) [26, 27]. However, systolic and diastolic blood pressure did not predict progression of retinopathy in type 2 diabetic patients. The Action to Control Cardiovascular Risk in Diabetes (ACCORD) study [28] found that tight blood pressure reduction did not ameliorate the rate of diabetic retinopathy in subjects with type 2 diabetes.

In a meta-analysis of eight trials randomizing almost 7000 patients, intensive blood pressure control was associated with a 17% reduction in the incidence of diabetic retinopathy [29]. In another meta-analysis of 15 randomized controlled clinical trials that included 4157 type 1 and 9512 type 2 diabetes, there was a 12% decrease in risk of progression of diabetic retinopathy over 4–5 years with tighter blood pressure control among subjects with baseline retinopathy but no benefit among normotensive type 1 diabetes [30]. These meta-analyses should be interpreted with caution as they have inherent limitations including the heterogeneity of the clinical trials with different blood pressure targets, hba1c level, and the definition of diabetic retinopathy.

It is unclear if specific classes of antihypertensive agents will help to slow progression of diabetic retinopathy. Mauer et al. [31] evaluated 285 normotensive type 1 diabetic patients without albuminuria and randomly assigned them to receive Losartan 100 mg daily, Enalapril 20 mg daily, or placebo with 5 years of follow-up. The risk of progressive diabetic retinopathy decreased by 65% in the Enalapril arm and 70% in the losartan group compared with the placebo arm. The effect of other antihypertensive medications on progressive diabetic retinopathy was not assessed in this study. Lin et al. [32] evaluated type 2 diabetic patients with concomitant hypertension in the Longitudinal Health Insurance Database in 2005. Patients on beta blockers and calcium channel blockers (CCBs) had a lower risk of diabetic retinopathy compared with those taking ACEIs or ARBs. The reason for the disparate results is unclear, but other confounders including blood pressure and glycemic control in the groups may have played a role.

The EUCLID study [33] evaluated the effect of lisinopril to reduce the rate of the development of diabetic retinopathy in normotensive patients. Patients taking lisinopril had a 50% decreased rate of progression of retinopathy over a 2-year period compared with patients not taking this medication. Proliferative retinopathy incidence was decreased by 82% in those taking lisinopril compared with placebo. The mechanism by which ACEI can prevent diabetic retinopathy is uncertain but may include favorable hemodynamic effects and increased nitric oxide levels. It is also possible that the antihypertensive effect of lisinopril may be beneficial at preventing onset of diabetic retinopathy even in patients that would otherwise be considered normotensive [26].

The degree of blood pressure control needed to prevent retinopathy is unclear. In the UKPDS trial [25], 1048 patients with hypertension received either "tight control" of blood pressure defined as <150/85 or more "liberalized control" of <180/105 using atenolol or captopril. Patients randomized to blood pressure of less than 150/85 had a 35% decrease rate of retinal photocoagulation. Over a 7.5 year follow-up period, there was a decrease in progression of retinopathy of approximately one-third, and almost 50 pct decrease in the decline in visual acuity. Atenolol and captopril were equivalent in decreasing risk of diabetic retinopathy. It should be noted that the definition of "tight" blood pressure control in this study would not meet the standard of care for hypertension management in 2021 where values of <130/80 are considered goal readings.

Another study evaluated the impact of diastolic blood pressure to a goal of 75 mm Hg or 80–89 mm Hg on patients with hypertension and type 2 DM in the Appropriate Blood Pressure Control in Diabetes (ABCD) trial [34]. Patients received nisoldipine, enalapril, or placebo. Mean blood pressure was 132/78 in the DBP goal 75 mm Hg arm and 138/86 in the DBP goal 80–89 mm Hg arm. In this study, there was no difference in the progression to diabetic retinopathy over a 5-year follow-up. The reasons for the disparate results may be related to the lower overall blood pressures in the ABCD trial compared with the UKPDS trial. Based on the results of the UKPDS and ABCD trials, blood pressure control to at least 140/90 or less is essential.

19.4 Diabetic Nephropathy

There is a debate on the target blood pressure to prevent progression to diabetic nephropathy. Several clinical trials support the role of "tight" blood pressure control. In the MDRD study of 840 patients randomized to a mean arterial pressure of 107 vs 92 mm Hg over a 2.2 year treatment duration, the group of patients with proteinuria above 1 g per day had a significant benefit to BP lowering to 126/77 compared 134/80 in the standard arm [35]. In the African American Study of Kidney Disease and Hypertension (AASK) [36], 1094 African Americans without diabetes with hypertensive kidney disease and GFR between 20 and 65 were randomized to a mean arterial pressure of 102 mm Hg vs 107 mm Hg over a 3–6.4 year treatment follow-up; there was no differences between the two groups over the follow-up period. In follow-up over 8.8–12.2 years, patients in the tight BP control arm had a decrease in the number of renal events if they had a higher degree of proteinuria at baseline.

The ADVANCE trial [37] studied 11,140 type 2 diabetes and randomized patients to perindopril and indapamide or placebo to achieve a SBP of <135 mm Hg or approximately 140 mm Hg. Patients in the SBP < 135 mm Hg arm had significantly lower rates of moderate albuminuria, dialysis, or need for kidney transplant. Patients with baseline CKD in this study also had improved outcomes with tighter BP control [38]. Patients with CKD and SBP < 135 mm Hg had a trend toward decreased incidence of cardiovascular events compared with patients who maintained SBP > 140 mm Hg while receiving antihypertensive medication [37].

The Irbesartan Diabetic Nephropathy Trial (IDNT) [39] studied 1590 type 2 diabetic patients with hypertension and diabetic nephropathy (mean serum creatinine of 1.7 mg/dl and 24 h urine protein of 1.9 g/day) to treatment with irbesartan vs amlodipine. In those patients with a systolic blood pressure above 149 mm Hg, there was a 2.2-fold higher risk of doubling of serum creatinine or ESKD compared with those patients with a systolic blood pressure of less than 134 mm Hg. The IDNT also showed that a decrease of >20 mm Hg in SBP was associated with an almost 50% decrease in the doubling of serum creatinine or development of ESKD [39].

The ONTARGET trial [40] showed that decreased SBP from 154 to 125 mm Hg led to a lower degree of proteinuria and higher rate of regression to normoalbuminuria. In the Appropriate Blood Pressure Control in Diabetes-Part 2 with Valsartan (ABCD-2 V) trial [41], a blood pressure of 118/75 (intensive arm) in the group with baseline microalbuminuria led to greater proteinuria lowering from 54.2 to 5.5 μg/min. However, the microalbuminuria group randomized to (moderate control) a blood pressure of 124/80 saw an increase in proteinuria from 70.4 to 121.7 μg/min. Decreased blood pressures also led to a reduction in incident development of microalbuminuria and reduced risk of CVA although the number of CVA and microalbuminuria events were small leading to concerns that the study was under powered to assess this outcome. Reduction of proteinuria is strongly correlated with risk of developing ESKD and therefore is a crucial surrogate measure of outcomes in these clinical trials. In diabetic patients, there was a more pronounced effect of proteinuria reduction compared with blood pressure reduction on the risk of progressive CKD [42, 43].

In meta-analyses, decreased BP has been shown to slow progression of CKD [44]. In one meta-analysis, an SBP < 120 mm Hg was associated with the lowest rate of CKD progression. In patients with diabetic kidney disease, a mean arterial pressure of 89 mm Hg or BP 120/75 was associated with the slowest rate of progressive CKD [45]. Multiple clinical trials have also shown that there is a decreased risk of developing albuminuria in diabetic and nondiabetic patients with lower BPs especially to SBP < 120 mm Hg [46].

Not all studies support the beneficial effect of intensive blood pressure control to reduce diabetic nephropathy. The studies showing an improvement in outcomes were based on post hoc analyses and not from prospective randomized controlled trials. In the MDRD study [35], those randomized to a BP 126/77 vs 134/80 did not have a decrease in progression of CKD. There was also no difference in CKD progression in the AASK trial in those randomized to a BP 128/78 vs 141/85 [36]. In the ACCORD trial [28], progression of CKD to ESKD and cardiovascular events were not significantly different in patients who were randomized to SBP >130 mm

Hg or <120 mm Hg. Despite this difference, clinical studies consistently show that intensive blood pressure control will prevent development of moderate albuminuria and in many instances will lead to a regression in albuminuria stages.

Intensive blood pressure control is also not without risk. There is a higher risk of orthostatic hypotension in diabetic and elderly patients with autonomic neuropathies [47–49]. Careful attention to postural changes in blood pressure should be monitored prior to further intensification of antihypertensive medication regimens. Hypotension also carries an increased risk for hemodynamically mediated AKI, which is typically reversible once renal autoregulation is restored.

Based on the results of randomized controlled clinical trials and guidelines, the BP goal in patients with severe albuminuria (macroalbuminuria) should be to <130/80 mmHg while balancing the risk of decreased coronary blood flow if BP is too low. There is a debate on the optimal target blood pressure in patients with moderate albuminuria (microalbuminuria). RAAS inhibitors are recommended first line for the treatment of hypertension to prevent further microvascular complications in patients with diabetes.

19.5 Conclusion

Diabetes is associated with multiple complications including macrovascular and microvascular disease. Tight glycemic and blood pressure control may help to alleviate some of these deleterious effects. The exact target blood pressure to prevent microvascular complications is unclear, but control to at least <130/80 mmHg is reasonable for most patients except those with autonomic neuropathies. All patients should be placed on a RAAS inhibitor first line for blood pressure control unless contraindication such as angioedema reaction exists. Newer oral hypoglycemic agents including sodium–glucose cotransporter-2 inhibitors (SGLT2is) have the dual beneficial effect of reducing BP and controlling glucose and should also be considered if no contraindication exists. Further studies are needed to precisely define the appropriate target blood pressure and to identify those patients most at risk for the development of microvascular disease.

References

1. International Diabetes Federation. IDF Diabetes Atlas. 9th edition. 2019.
2. International Diabetes Federation. IDF Diabetes Atlas 10th edition. 2020.
3. USRDS 2020 Annual Report. www.usrds.org, Accessed 1 June 2021.
4. O'Connell JM, Manson SM. Understanding the economic costs of diabetes and prediabetes and what we may learn about reducing the health and economic burden of these conditions. Diabetes Care. 2019;42(9):1609–11.
5. Dall TM, Zhang Y, Chen YJ, Quick WW, Yang WG, Fogli J. The economic burden of diabetes. Health Aff (Millwood). 2010;29(2):297–303.
6. Bommer C, Heesemann E, Sagalova V, Manne-Goehler J, Atun R, Bärnighausenet T, et al. The global economic burden of diabetes in adults aged 20-79 years: a cost-of-illness study. Lancet Diabetes Endocrinol. 2017;5(6):423–30.

7. Sowers JR. Recommendations for special populations: diabetes mellitus and the metabolic syndrome. Am J Hypertens. 2003;16(11 Pt 2):41S–5S.
8. Arauz-Pacheco C, Parrott MA, Raskin P. Hypertension management in adults with diabetes. Diabetes Care. 2004;27(Suppl 1):S65–7.
9. Arauz-Pacheco C, Parrott MA, Raskin P. The treatment of hypertension in adult patients with diabetes. Diabetes Care. 2002;25(1):134–47.
10. Aggarwal R, Steinkamp J, Chiu N, Petrie B, Mirzan H. Intensive blood pressure targets for diabetic and other high-risk populations: a pooled individual patient data analysis. Hypertension. 2018;71(5):833–9.
11. Tsujimoto T, Kajio H. Benefits of intensive blood pressure treatment in patients with type 2 diabetes mellitus receiving standard but not intensive glycemic control. Hypertension. 2018;72(2):323–30.
12. Lewington S, Clarke R, Qizilbash N, Peto R, Collins R. Prospective studies collaboration. Age-specific relevance of usual blood pressure to vascular mortality: a meta-analysis of individual data for one million adults in 61 prospective studies. Lancet. 2002;360(9349):1903–13.
13. Neaton JD, Wentworth D. Serum cholesterol, blood pressure, cigarette smoking, and death from coronary heart disease. Overall findings and differences by age for 316,099 white men. Multiple risk factor intervention trial research group. Arch Intern Med. 1992;152(1):56–64.
14. Wright JT Jr, Williamson JD, Whelton PK, Snyder JK, Sink KM, Rocco MV, et al. A randomized trial of intensive versus standard blood-pressure control. N Engl J Med. 2015;373(22):2103–16.
15. Didangelos T, Tziomalos K, Margaritidis C, Kontoninas Z, Stergiou I, Tsotoulidis S, et al. Efficacy of administration of an angiotensin converting enzyme inhibitor for two years on autonomic and peripheral neuropathy in patients with diabetes mellitus. J Diabetes Res. 2017;2017:6719239.
16. Malik RA. Can diabetic neuropathy be prevented by angiotensin-converting enzyme inhibitors? Ann Med. 2000;32(1):1–5.
17. Harris M, Eastman R, Cowie C. Symptoms of sensory neuropathy in adults with NIDDM in the U.S. population. Diabetes Care. 1993;16(11):1446–52.
18. Jarmuzewska EA, Ghidoni A, Mangoni AA. Hypertension and sensorimotor peripheral neuropathy in type 2 diabetes. Eur Neurol. 2007;57(2):91–5.
19. Forrest KY, Maser RE, Pambianco G, Becker DJ, Orchard TJ. Hypertension as a risk factor for diabetic neuropathy: a prospective study. Diabetes. 1997;46(4):665–70.
20. Ponirakis G, Petropoulos IN, Alam U, Ferdousi M, Asghar O, Marshall A, et al. Hypertension contributes to neuropathy in patients with type 1 diabetes. Am J Hypertens. 2019;32(8):796–803.
21. Østergaard L, Finnerup NB, Terkelsen AJ, Olesen RA, Drasbek KR, Knudsen L, et al. The effects of capillary dysfunction on oxygen and glucose extraction in diabetic neuropathy. Diabetologia. 2015;58(4):666–77.
22. Williams R, Airey M, Baxter H, Forrester J, Kennedy-Martin T, Girach A. Epidemiology of diabetic retinopathy and macular oedema: a systematic review. Eye. 2004;18(10):963–83.
23. Eshaq RS, Aldalati AMZ, Alexander JS, Harris NR. Diabetic retinopathy: breaking the barrier. Pathophysiology. 2017;24(4):229–41.
24. Nathan DM, Genuth S, Lachin J, Cleary P, Crofford O, Davis M, et al. The effect of intensive treatment of diabetes on the development and progression of long-term complications in insulin-dependent diabetes mellitus. N Engl J Med. 1993;329(14):977–86.
25. UK Prospective Diabetes Study Group. Tight blood pressure control and risk of macrovascular and microvascular complications in type 2 diabetes. BMJ. 1998;317:703–13.
26. Klein R, Klein BE. Blood pressure control and diabetic retinopathy. Br J Ophthalmol. 2002;86(4):365–7.
27. Klein R, Klein BE, Moss SE, Davis MD, DeMets DL. The Wisconsin epidemiologic study of diabetic retinopathy. II. Prevalence and risk of diabetic retinopathy when age at diagnosis is less than 30 years. Arch Ophthalmol. 1984;102(4):520–6.
28. Accord Study Group; Cushman WC, Evans GW, Byington RP, Goff DC Jr, Grimm RH Jr, Cutler JA, et al. Effects of intensive blood-pressure control in type 2 diabetes mellitus. N Engl J Med. 2010;362:1575–85.

29. Zhou JB, Song ZH, Bai L, Zhu XR, Li HB, Yang JK. Could intensive blood pressure control really reduce diabetic retinopathy outcomes? Evidence from meta-analysis and trial sequential analysis from randomized controlled trials. Diabetes Ther. 2018;9(5):2015–27.
30. Do DV, Wang X, Vedula SS, Marrone M, Sleilati G, Hawkins BS, et al. Blood pressure control for diabetic retinopathy. Cochrane Database Syst Rev. 2015;1:CD006127.
31. Mauer M, Zinman B, Gardiner R, Suissa S, Sinaiko A, Strand T, et al. Renal and retinal effects of enalapril and losartan in type 1 diabetes. N Engl J Med. 2009;361(1):40–51.
32. Lin JC, Lai MS. Antihypertensive drugs and diabetic retinopathy in patients with type 2 diabetes. Ophthalmologica. 2016;235(2):87–96.
33. Chaturvedi N, Sjolie AK, Stephenson JM, Abrahamian H, Keipes M, Castellarin A, et al. Effect of lisinopril on progression of retinopathy in normotensive people with type 1 diabetes. The EUCLID Study Group. EURODIAB controlled trial of lisinopril in insulin-dependent diabetes mellitus. Lancet. 1998;351(9095):28–31.
34. Estacio RO, Jeffers BW, Gifford N, Schrier RW. Effect of blood pressure control on diabetic microvascular complications in patients with hypertension and type 2 diabetes. Diabetes Care. 2000;23(Suppl 2):B54–64.
35. Klahr S, Levey AS, Beck GJ, Caggiula AW, Hunsicker L, Kusek JW, et al. The effects of dietary protein restriction and blood pressure control on the progression of chronic renal disease. Modification of Diet in Renal Disease Study Group. N Engl J Med. 1994;330:877–84.
36. Wright JT Jr, Bakris G, Greene T, Agodoa LY, Appel LJ, Charleston J, et al. African American Study of Kidney Disease and Hypertension Study Group. Effect of blood pressure lowering and antihypertensive drug class on progression of hypertensive kidney disease: results from the AASK trial. JAMA. 2002;288:2421–31.
37. Patel A. Effects of a fixed combination of perindopril and indapamide on macrovascular and microvascular outcomes in patients with type 2 diabetes mellitus (the ADVANCE trial): a randomised controlled trial. Lancet. 2007;370(9590):829–40.
38. Heerspink HJ, Ninomiya T, Perkovic V, Woodward M, Zoungas S, Casset A, et al. Effects of a fixed combination of perindopril and indapamide in patients with type 2 diabetes and chronic kidney disease. Eur Heart J. 2010;31(23):2888–96.
39. Berl T, Hunsicker LG, Lewis JB, Pfeffer MA, Porush JG, Rouleau JL, et al. Impact of achieved blood pressure on cardiovascular outcomes in the irbesartan diabetic nephropathy trial. J Am Soc Nephrol. 2005;16:2170–9.
40. Mancia G, Schumacher H, Redon J, Verdecchia P, Schmieder R, Jennings G, et al. Blood pressure targets recommended by guidelines and incidence of cardiovascular and renal events in the Ongoing Telmisartan Alone and in Combination With Ramipril Global Endpoint Trial (ONTARGET). Circulation. 2011;124(16):1727–36.
41. Estacio RO, Coll JR, Tran ZV, Schrier RW. Effect of intensive blood pressure control with valsartan on urinary albumin excretion in normotensive patients with type 2 diabetes. Am J Hypertens. 2006;19(12):1241–8.
42. Yusuf S, Teo KK, Pogue J, Dyal L, Copland I, Schumacher H, et al. Telmisartan, ramipril, or both in patients at high risk for vascular events. N Engl J Med. 2008;358(15):1547–59.
43. Schmieder RE, Schutte S, Schumacher H, Böhm M, Mancia G, Weber MA, et al. Mortality and morbidity in relation to changes in albuminuria, glucose status and systolic blood pressure: an analysis of the ONTARGET and TRANSCEND studies. Diabetologia. 2014;57(10):2019–29.
44. Jafar TH, Stark PC, Schmid CH, Landa M, Maschio G, de Jong PE, et al. Progression of chronic kidney disease: the role of blood pressure control, proteinuria, and angiotensin-converting enzyme inhibition: a patient-level meta-analysis. Ann Intern Med. 2003;139(4):244–52.
45. Yamout H, Lazich I, Bakris GL. Blood pressure, hypertension, RAAS blockade, and drug therapy in diabetic kidney disease. Adv Chronic Kidney Dis. 2014;21(3):281–6.
46. Ruilope LM, Segura J. The nephroprotective effect of antihypertensive treatment. In: Mancia G, Grassi G, Redon J, editors. Manual of hypertension of the European Society of Hypertension. 2nd ed. Boca Raton, FL: CRC Press; 2014. p. 291–8.
47. Campese VM. Orthostatic hypotension: idiopathic and uremic. Kidney Int Suppl. 1988;25:S152–5.

48. Savica V, Musolino R, Di Leo R, Santoro D, Vita G, Bellinghieri G. Autonomic dysfunction in uremia. Am J Kidney Dis. 2001;38(4 Suppl 1):S118–21.
49. Grassi G, Bertoli S, Seravalle G. Sympathetic nervous system: role in hypertension and in chronic kidney disease. Curr Opin Nephrol Hypertens. 2012;21(1):46–51.

New Antidiabetic Agents: Relevance to Cardiovascular Outcomes

20

Reinhold Kreutz and Engi Abd El-Hady Algharably

20.1 Sodium Glucose Cotransporter Type 2 (SGLT2) Inhibitors

20.1.1 Physiology of SGLT2 and Its Pharmacological Inhibition

Membrane-associated transport proteins responsible for renal glucose reabsorption include two classes of carrier proteins: the sodium–glucose cotransporters (SGLTs) and the glucose transporters (GLUTs) [1].

SGLTs belong to the human solute carrier family 5 (SLC5) and include, among others, SGLT1 and SGLT2 that are situated at the luminal surface of the proximal tubule epithelium [1].

SGLT2, situated at the S1 segment of the proximal tubule, is a low affinity high-capacity transporter that uses one sodium ion per glucose molecule while SGLT1, a high affinity but low capacity transporter, uses two sodium ions per glucose transport. SGLT2 is selectively expressed in the kidney and accounts for almost all proximal tubular glucose reabsorption (~97%) while the remaining (~2–3%) filtered glucose is reabsorbed via SGLT-1 in the distal segments of the proximal tubules [2]. SGLT1 is also expressed in the small intestine to a greater extent than in the kidney and in the heart [3]. In normoglycemia and with normal renal function, up to 180 g of glucose are filtered and almost fully reabsorbed by the kidney daily. In diabetes, however, an increased tubular glucose load combined with higher expression of SGLT2 [4] enhances renal glucose reabsorption, hence becoming counterproductive and conserve hyperglycemia [5].

R. Kreutz (✉) · E. A. E.-H. Algharably
Institute of Clinical Pharmacology and Toxicology, Charité—Universitätsmedizin Berlin, corporate member of Freie Universität Berlin and Humboldt-Universität zu Berlin, Berlin, Germany
e-mail: reinhold.kreutz@charite.de

A. E. Berbari, G. Mancia (eds.), *Blood Pressure Disorders in Diabetes Mellitus*, Updates in Hypertension and Cardiovascular Protection,
https://doi.org/10.1007/978-3-031-13009-0_20

Table 20.1 Pharmacology characteristics of SGLT2 inhibitors

Drug	Oral bioavailability (%)	Dose range (mg/day)	Half-life (h)	Renal elimination (%)	SGLT2/SGLT1 selectivity
Canagliflozin	65	100–300	11–13	<2	~250-fold
Dapagliflozin	78	5–10	13	<1	~1200-fold
Empagliflozin	90	10–25	13	28.6	~2500-fold
Ertugliflozin	70–90	5, 15	17	50	~2000-fold
Ipragliflozin[a]	90	50–100	15–16	≤2	~250-fold
Luseogliflozin[a]	86	2.5–5	10-12	4	~1770-fold
Sotagliflozin[b]	71	200– 400	21	57	~20-fold
Tofogliflozin [a]	97.5	20	5–6	6.8	~2930-fold

[a] Approved and available in Japan
[b] Approved and available in the European Union

The inhibition of SGLT2 prevents glucose and sodium reabsorption into the blood stream, promotes glucosuria, reduces blood glucose concentrations, and improves subsequently glycosylated hemoglobin (HbA1c) levels through an "insulin-independent" pathway [6]. SGLT1 plays a complementary but still relevant role beside SGLT2 in renal glucose reabsorption [2]. In addition to the kidney, SGLT1 is also abundantly expressed in the brush-border membrane of villi of the upper small intestine, where it takes part in the absorption of postprandial glucose or galactose from the gastrointestinal tract [3]. Therefore, enhanced transport of glucose in kidney and intestine mediated by SGLT1 may weaken the glucose-lowering effect of SGLT2 inhibitors [7]. The role of SGLT1 in both renal and intestinal glucose reabsorption thus provides also a rationale for dual SGLT1/2 inhibitors use by means of achieving better glycemic control and improving cardiovascular (CV) outcomes further as compared with more selective SGLT2 inhibitors in patients with type 2 diabetes mellitus (T2DM). Pharmacology characteristics of SGLT2 inhibitors are shown in Table 20.1.

20.1.2 Effects of SGLT2 Inhibitors on CV Outcomes

The first three landmark CV outcome trials (CVOTs) with SGLT2 inhibitors were the EMPA-REG OUTCOME with empagliflozin [8], the Canagliflozin Cardiovascular Assessment Study (CANVAS) Program with canagliflozin (including in fact two trials, namely, CANVAS [9] and Canagliflozin Cardiovascular Assessment Study-Renal (CANVAS-R) [10]), and the Dapagliflozin Effect on Cardiovascular Events (DECLARE-TIMI 58) with dapagliflozin [11]. These CVOTs yielded impressive positive results in terms of CV protection. All trials were multicentered, randomized, double-blind, and placebo-controlled and included patients with history of long-standing T2DM and established atherosclerotic CV disease (ASCVD) or at high CV risk. In addition, patients received a standard background therapy for T2DM and CV prevention. The primary outcome in EMPA-REG OUTCOME, CANVAS Program, and the DECLARE-TIMI 58 was the composite of three major CV events (three-point MACE) defined as CV death, non-fatal myocardial infarction (MI), or non-fatal stroke. Hospitalization for heart failure (HHF) was a prespecified secondary outcome in all trials and a co-primary composite outcome in the DECLARE-TIMI 58 [11].

The EMPA-REG OUTCOME [8] trial was the first to identify a protective effect to reduce heart failure (HF) events and mortality of empagliflozin in patients with and without HF at baseline, while patients with HHF had a lower risk of death. Results were relatively consistent across the three trials with a risk reduction in the composite primary three-point MACE endpoint in EMPA-REG Outcome and in CANVAS with a 14% risk reduction in both studies compared with placebo [8, 12]. This effect was driven mainly by a 38% reduction in CV death (HR 0.62; 95% CI 0.49–0.77; $p < 0.001$) in case of empagliflozin. Empagliflozin also reduced significantly HHF (HR 0.65; 95% CI 0.50–0.85; $p = 0.002$) and reduced overall mortality (HR 0.68; 95% CI 0.57–0.82; $p < 0.001$). Furthermore, the cardioprotective effects were recognized within the first three months of treatment as shown by the early separation of placebo and empagliflozin curves in Kaplan-Meier analysis [8].

The CANVAS Program [12] combining data from two RCTs (CANVAS and CANVAS-R) reported for canagliflozin comparable results with a 33% reduction in HHF (HR 0.67; 95% CI 0.52–0.87).

The benefit of dapagliflozin with respect to CV death or HHF was revealed by DECLARE-TIMI 58 [11], the largest of the CVOTs 3 trials conducted so far. However, this study included a higher proportion of patients (59%) without evidence of cardiovascular disease (CVD) as compared with EMPA-REG OUTCOME and CANVAS. Although no significant reduction in three-point MACE was found, dapagliflozin reduced the risk of the composite outcome of CV death plus HHF significantly by 17% (HR 0.83; 95% CI 0.73–0.95; $p = 0.005$), which was driven by a 27% lower rate of HHF (HR 0.73; 95% CI 0.61–0.88). Notably, DECLARE-TIMI 58 excluded patients with a creatinine clearance <60 mL/min while EMPA-REG OUTCOME and CANVAS included patients with an estimated glomerular rate (eGFR) above 30 mL/min/1.73 m^2. A meta-analysis of the three CVOTs pooling data from 34,322 patients (60.2% with established ASCVD) indicated a consistent reduction of three-point MACE by 11% in those patients with ASCVD and a reduction in the composite of HHF or CV death by 23% [13]. The latter effect was similar in patients with and without ASCVD and in those with and without a history of HF. SGLT2 inhibitors also reduced progression of kidney disease in either atherosclerotic patients or with a history of HF [13]. The CREDENCE trial with canagliflozin, specifically dedicated to patients with T2DM and chronic kidney disease (CKD) as defined by an eGFR of 30–90 mL/min/1.73 m^2 and albuminuria (urinary albumin-to-creatinine ratio 300–5000 mg/g), confirmed the results of the previous CVOTs by showing a reduction in three-point MACE (HR 0.80; 95% CI 0.67–0.95) and HHF (HR 0.61; 95% CI 0.47–0.80) [14]. This study included only 15% of the patients with a history of HF; however, the results of this study indicate that the cardioprotective benefits of canagliflozin may extend to high-risk patients with T2DM and CKD.

The DAPA-HF was the first dedicated trial to investigate SGLT-2 inhibition exclusively in HF patients with reduced ejection fraction (HFrEF) irrespective of the presence of T2DM at baseline. Dapagliflozin reduced significantly the primary endpoint of CV death or worsening HF (HR 0.74; 95% CI 0.65–0.85) and CV mortality (HR 0.82; 95% CI 0.69–0.98) demonstrating the beneficial role in the treatment of HF independent from the presence of T2DM [15].

Ertugliflozin, another SGLT-2 inhibitor, was subsequently investigated in the VERTIS CV, a similar CVOT study that included patients with T2DM and established CVD [16]. However, ertugliflozin did not significantly reduce the primary endpoint of three-point MACE [16]. Nevertheless, ertugliflozin reduced the risk of HHF especially for those with EF $\leq$ 45% at baseline (HR 0.48;95% CI 0.30–0.76) with greater benefits seen in patients with eGFR<60 mL/min/1.73 m^2, albuminuria, and diuretic use. Furthermore, the events for total HHF and the combined outcome of HHF plus CV death were significantly reduced [17].

More recently, sotagliflozin, a combined SGLT-1 and SGLT-2 inhibitor [18], was evaluated in two trials: the SOLOIST-WHF [19] and the SCORED trials [20], both including T2DM patients and a fraction of patients with HF with preserved ejection fraction (HFpEF). The SOLOIST-WHF was the first to include patients with acute decompensated HF, recently hospitalized, but in stable condition. Sotagliflozin reduced the composite of total CV deaths, HHF, and urgent HF visits by 33%. Those benefits were shown as early as 1 month after therapy and were consistent among HF subgroups with either HF with reduced ejection fraction (HFrEF) or HFpEF [19].

In the SCORED trial, T2DM patients with HF and CKD at baseline were enrolled with a median eGFR of 44 mL/min/1.73 m^2 including 7% of patients with an eGFR<30 mL/min/1.73 m^2. Sotagliflozin exhibited cardioprotective effects and reduced significantly the same composite outcome as in SOLOIST-WHF by 26% [20]. However, both studies lost funding and were terminated early; hence, the studies had a shortened follow-up duration, and statistical power was limited to observe significant reductions in CV death or in kidney outcomes.

Furthermore, EMPEROR-Reduced [21] and EMPEROR-Preserved [22] using empagliflozin targeted specifically patients with HF with either HFrEF or HFpEF and included patients with or without T2DM at baseline.

In EMPEROR-Reduced, empagliflozin reduced the risk of the primary outcome of CV death or HHF in patients with and without diabetes (HR 0.72; 95% CI 0.60–0.87 and 0.78; 95% CI 0.64–0.97, respectively). In EMPEROR-Preserved, the primary endpoint was a composite of CV death or HHF and was significantly reduced by empagliflozin (HR 0.73; 95% CI 0.61–0.88); this benefit was again independent from the presence or absence of diabetes.

20.1.3 Effects of SGLT2 Inhibitors on Renal Outcomes

The potential nephroprotection offered by SGLT-2 inhibition was already indicated by a reduction of albuminuria (on average about 25%) as compared with placebo or other antidiabetic agents in glycemic trials [23, 24]. This effect was enhanced in patients with more severe albuminuria [25]. In those trials, renal outcomes were studied as secondary endpoints, but they were subsequently confirmed by the analyses of renal endpoints that emerged from the large CVOTs including EMPA-REG OUTCOME [26], CANVAS program [12], DECLARE-TIMI 58 [11], and VERTIS CV [16].

In the EMPA-REG OUTCOME trial, T2DM patients treated with empagliflozin showed significantly higher reductions in the composite outcome of progression to macroalbuminuria, doubling of serum creatinine (SCr), initiation of renal replacement therapy (RRT), or death from renal disease (HR 0.61; 95% CI 0.53–0.70) with similar reduction for the individual renal endpoints. Notably, about 26% of the patients had eGFR values <60 mL/min/1.73 m^2 at baseline [26].

Similar benefits were demonstrated by the CANVAS program study where canagliflozin reduced the composite outcome of sustained 40% reduction in eGFR, need for RRT, or death from renal causes compared with placebo (HR 0.60; 95% CI 0.47–0.77). Furthermore, the reduction in renal composite endpoints was consistent in patients with and without CKD and across different eGFR levels (baseline eGFR ≥90, 60 to <90, 45 to <60 and <45 mL/min/1.73 m^2) [27]. However, only 20.1% of participants had an eGFR <60 mL/min/1.73 m^2 at baseline.

In the DECLARE-TIMI 58 trial, dapagliflozin reduced the prespecified renal composite of ≥40% reduction in eGFR, end-stage kidney disease (ESKD), or death due to renal or CV causes (HR 0.76; 95% CI 0.67–0.87) [28]. A meta-analysis of the three trials showed that SGLT-2 inhibitors reduced the risk of worsening of renal function, ESKD or renal death by 45% (HR 0.55; 95% CI 0.48–0.64), with an identical effect in patients with and without ASCVD [13]. However, DECLARE-TIMI-58, EMPA-REG OUTCOME, and CANVAS explored the renal benefits of SGLT2 inhibitors in patients with mostly preserved renal function (eGFR >60 mL/min/1.73 m^2). In the VERTIS CV study, although ertugliflozin exhibited trends for beneficial effect on renal outcomes in T2DM with established CVD, it did not significantly reduce the secondary composite renal endpoint (death from renal causes, RRT, or doubling of SCr levels) (HR 0.81; 95% CI 0.63, $p = 1.04$) [16].

The Canagliflozin and Renal Events in Diabetes with Established Nephropathy Clinical Evaluation (CREDENCE) trial was the first dedicated trial to address patients with moderate to severe CKD as it was designed to explore the effect of SGLT2 inhibition in T2DM with high risk of kidney disease progression [14]. Credence included specifically patients with CKD and eGFR<60 mL/min/1.73 m^2 (60% of the study population) and with albuminuria defined by urinary albumin to creatinine ratio (UACR) of >300–5000 mg/g. Renoprotective effects were observed at all levels of kidney function, including participants with baseline eGFR of 30–45 mL/min/1.73 m^2 (HR 0.75; 95% CI 0.59–0.95) in whom these drugs were originally not approved for use in diabetes [14]. These findings are important given that these patients are at increased risk of rapid progression of CKD. The CREDENCE trial also provided new information supporting the role of SGLT2 inhibitors in advanced CKD. In this respect, the offered renal benefits are not compromised by low GFR since glycemic control resulting from SGLT2 inhibitors depends on GFR and renal glucose excretion. Therefore, despite the lower reductions in HbA1C levels, renal protection persists suggesting that SGLT2 inhibitors should be continued in patients with CKD and that their prescription in diabetic kidney disease should be separated from their use in T2DM with regard to glucose lowering.

In this regard, the more recent DAPA-CKD trial was important as it was the first to investigate the safety and renal outcomes in patients with CKD, both with and without T2DM [29]. The study had a more ambitious target of the composite of sustained decline in the eGFR (at least 50%), ESKD, or death from renal or CV causes. The HR for the primary endpoint was 0.61 (95% CI 0.51–0.72; $p < 0.001$) and was consistent in patients with and without T2DM. Like CREDENCE, DAPA-CKD provides further insight in the role of SGLT2 inhibitors in the progression of CKD and supports their use for the prevention of CV and renal complications among CKD patients including patients with glomerulonephritis [29]. An ongoing trial, the EMPA-KIDNEY (NCT03594110) designed specifically to evaluate the protective effect of empagliflozin on the CV and renal systems in patients with CKD, is yet to reveal more data.

20.1.4 Mechanisms of Cardiorenal Protection of SGLT2 Inhibitors

Being originally developed "only" as glucose lowering, i.e., antihyperglycemic, drugs for the treatment of T2DM, the profound protective cardiorenal effects appeared initially completely unexpected and could not be explained. Hence, the reduction in CV and renal events were not related to either baseline or achieved HbA1c levels in participants with diabetes. In the meantime, a veritable avalanche of experimental and clinical mechanistic studies has been triggered by the data obtained in randomized outcome trials identifying or at least postulating several mechanisms that contribute to cardiorenal protection by SGLT2 inhibition (as recently reviewed in [30, 31] and summarized in Fig. 20.1).

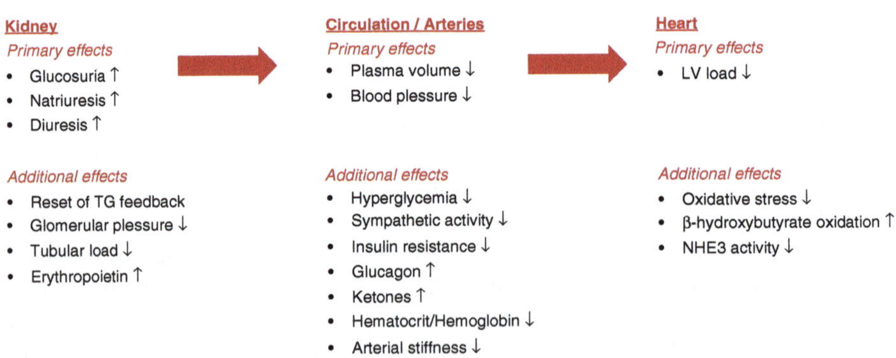

Fig. 20.1 Primary and additional effects of SGLT2 inhibition in the kidney, systemic circulation/arteries, and heart. *LV* left ventricle, *NHE3* sodium-hydrogen exchanger, *TG* tubuloglomerular

20.2 Glucagon-Like Peptide-1 Receptor Agonists (GLP-1RAs)

20.2.1 Physiology of GLP-1 and Pharmacological Activation of GLP-1 Receptors

Glucagon-like peptide-1 (GLP-1) is a natural incretin hormone synthesized and secreted from the neuroendocrine L cells localized in the distal ileum and ascending colon in response to glucose absorption [32]. GLP-1 secretion stimulates insulin release from pancreatic β cells (insulinotropic) in a glucose-dependent manner limiting the risk of hypoglycemia. Simultaneously, GLP-1 suppresses glucagon secretion from pancreatic α-cells, which is inappropriately elevated in T2DM. These effects are primarily responsible for lowering the postprandial blood glucose excursions. In addition, GLP-1 promotes proliferation of β cells and prevents their apoptosis and delays gastric emptying, resulting in regulation of glucose homeostasis [33, 34]. GLP-1 is also a physiological regulator of appetite and food intake by acting on the central GLP-1 receptors enhancing satiety and limiting food intake, thereby contributing to body weight regulation [34]. In diabetes, endogenous GLP-1 effects on insulin secretion are suboptimal [35] compared with healthy individuals. However, they can be to a great extent restored by exogenous GLP-1 administration in supraphysiological doses. Thus, GLP-1 receptor stimulation is a suitable method for reducing blood glucose levels constituting a good therapeutic target for the treatment of T2DM [36].

20.2.2 Characteristics of Available GLP-1RAs

The physiologic rapid proteolytic degradation of GLP-1 by endogenous dipeptidyl-peptidase 4 (DPP4) activity precludes its therapeutic utility. Synthetic GLP-1 analogues have been developed to activate the endogenous GLP-1 receptor, thus mimicking the effects of GLP-1 after subcutaneous application with a longer half-life and duration of action depending on the molecular design of the compound [37]. The currently approved GLP-1RAs include exenatide, liraglutide, lixisenatide, dulaglutide, and semaglutide, while another GLP-1 RA, i.e., albiglutide, was discontinued from global use in 2018. They are all applied by subcutaneous injection and are classified based on their pharmacokinetics and pharmacodynamics into short- or long-acting GLP-1RAs [38]. Short-acting GLP-1RAs have a half-life of 2–4 h mandating once or twice daily administration while long-acting GLP-1RAs have a half-life >12 h up to more than 100 h, thereby allowing once daily or even once weekly dosing [38] (Table 20.2). Of interest, an oral formulation of semaglutide was recently developed.

Table 20.2 Pharmacology characteristics of GLP-1 receptor agonists

Drug	Molecular origin/ backbone	Type	Dosage	Half-life (h)	Protein binding (%)	Elimination
Injectable						
Exenatide	Exendin-4	Short acting	5–10 μg twice daily	2.4	NA	Mainly renal (80%)
Exenatide[a] extended release	Exendin-4	Long acting	2 mg weekly	NA	NA	Mainly renal
Dulaglutide	Human GLP-1	Long acting	0.75–1.5 mg weekly	120	NA	Mainly proteolytic degradation
Liraglutide	Human GLP-1	Long acting	0.6–1.8 mg once daily	13	>98	Mainly proteolytic degradation; renal (very low)
Lixisenatide	Exendin-4	Short acting	10–20 μg once daily	3	55	Mainly renal
Semaglutide	Human GLP-1	Long acting	0.25–1 mg weekly	168	>99	Proteolytic degradation; renal (3%)
Oral						
Oral Semaglutide	Human GLP-1	Long acting	3–14 mg once daily	168	>99%	Mainly proteolytic degradation; renal (3%)

NA not available

Injectable preparations are available as prefilled pens

[a] Encapsulated in a biodegradable polymer of poly(lactic-co-glycolic acid) microspheres

20.2.3 Effects of GLP-1 RAs on CV Outcomes

Lixisenatide, liraglutide, semaglutide, oral semaglutide, exenatide, and dulaglutide have been tested in six CVOTs in patients with T2DM: ELIXA [39], LEADER [40], SUSTAIN-6 [41], PIONEER 6 [42], EXSCEL [43], and REWIND [44], respectively. Albiglutide, a GLP-1RA that has been withdrawn from the market, was tested in the Harmony Outcomes trial [45]. Lixisenatide in the ELIXA trial was non-inferior to placebo, but did not significantly affect a 4-point MACE (the three-point MACE plus hospitalization for unstable angina) in patients with T2DM post-acute coronary syndrome [39]. Similarly, in the EXSCEL study, where 73% of participants had experienced a previous CV event, once weekly exenatide showed non-inferiority to placebo. The intention-to-treat analysis revealed a significant reduction in all-cause death by exenatide of 14% ($p = 0.016$) while subgroup analysis for CV disease patients revealed a significant 10% reduction for MACE (HR 0.90; 95% CI 0.816–0.999) [43]. In the LEADER trial, however, with 81% of patients having previous CVD, positive results were shown as liraglutide significantly reduced the three-point MACE by 13% and CV death and total death by 22% and 15%, respectively [40].

Semaglutide, in SUSTAIN-6, which had similar inclusion criteria as LEADER including patients with high CV risk, reduced the three-point MACE by 26% mainly driven by a 39% significant reduction of nonfatal stroke [41]. The PIONEER-6 trial confirmed non-inferiority for CV safety of oral semaglutide compared with placebo with a significantly reduced risk for CV death (HR 0.49, $p = 0.03$) and all cause death (HR 0.51; $p = 0.008$) [42]. Once weekly albiglutide in the Harmony Outcomes trial significantly reduced three-point MACE by 22% and myocardial infarction by 25% compared with placebo [45]. The REWIND, with the longest median follow-up of 5.4 years among these trials, showed a significant reduction of three-point MACE by once weekly dulaglutide vs. placebo (HR 0.88; 95% CI 0.79–0.99; $p = 0.026$) [44]. A recent meta-analysis of the seven trials showed that GLP-RAs reduce three-point MACE by 12% (HR 0.88; 95% CI 0.84–0.94; $p < 0.001$], all-cause mortality by 12% (HR 0.88; 95% CI 0.83–0.95; $p = 0.001$) and HHF by 9% (95% CI 0.91–0.99; $p = 0.028$) [46]. Moreover, the favorable effect on MACE was mainly consistent among subgroups stratified by history of CVD, body mass index, age, and kidney function at baseline [46]. Overall, these data underscore the protective CV effects of GLP-1RAs in addition to their positive effects on other CV risk factors, such as body weight and blood pressure (BP).

20.2.4 Effects of GLP-1 RAs on Renal Outcomes

GLP-1RA exhibited also a renoprotective potential, although less substantial as compared with those observed with SGLT2 inhibitors. The corresponding data come from the CVOTs in which renal outcomes were prespecified secondary endpoints [47]. The first trial reporting renal outcomes was the ELIXA trial in which a modest decrease in UACR in favor of lixisenatide was found [39].

In contrast to ELIXA, the LEADER and the SUSTAIN-6 trial had a prespecified renal outcome of new or worsening nephropathy defined as a composite of new-onset persistent macroalbuminuria, persistent doubling of serum creatinine and eGFR≤45 mL/min/1.73 m^2, need for RRT, and renal death [40, 48]. Liraglutide reduced the composite by 22% (HR 0.78; 95% CI; 0.67–0.92; $p = 0.003$) driven by a reduction in persistent macroalbuminuria, with no evident effect on the harder renal outcomes. Notably, LEADER also reported a 2% slower decline in renal function (eGFR) with liraglutide versus placebo, which was stronger in patients with moderate or severe renal impairment at baseline [48]. Semaglutide in SUSTAIN-6 reduced the renal composite outcome (HR 0.64; 95% CI 0.46–0.88; $p = 0.005$) [41], mainly caused by lower risk of albuminuria progression. Analysis of renal data from the EXCEL trial revealed that lixisenatide use caused a significant reduction in UACR (−39.18%, 95% CI −68.53 to −9.84; $p = 0.007$) in patients with macroalbuminuria compared with placebo and reduced new onset macroalbuminuria by 20% (HR 0.808; 95% CI 0.660–0.991; $p = 0.0404$) when adjusted for baseline HbA1c and other renal risk factors [49]. In REWIND, dulaglutide reduced the composite outcome of first occurrence of new macroalbuminuria (UACR >33.9 mg/mmol), a sustained decline in eGFR of ≥30% from baseline, or chronic RRT (HR 0.85; 95% CI 0.77–0.93; $p = 0.0004$) with a more evident effect for macroalbuminuria (HR 0.77; 95% CI 0.68–0.87; $p < 0.0001$). Meta-analyses of trials with GLP-1 RA agents indicated a statistically significant 17% reduction in the composite renal endpoint of new-onset macroalbuminuria, decline in eGFR, progression to ESKD, or death attributable to kidney causes (HR 0.83; 95% CI 0.78–0.89; $p < 0.0001$) with macroalbuminuria acting as the main driver for renal outcome [46]. The most pertinent data for kidney protection beyond reducing risk of albuminuria come from the AWARD-7 trial. This trial compared once weekly dulaglutide in two doses to insulin glargine including patients with moderate-to-severe CKD (mean eGFR: 38 mL/min/1.73 m^2) in which the secondary outcomes were eGFR and UACR [50]. Dulaglutide demonstrated a smaller decline in eGFR compared with glargine; the protective effect was greater in patients with baseline macroalbuminuria, who also had the greatest reduction in UACR [50]. Another trial with liraglutide conducted in patients with eGFR between 30 and 59 mL/min1.73 m^2 demonstrated no significant changes on renal function with liraglutide use with only a numerical 17% reduction in UACR (HR 0.83; 95% CI 0.62–1.10; $p = 0.1856$) [51].

20.2.5 Potential Mechanisms of CV Protection

The mechanism by which GLP-1 RAs may reduce primarily CV atherosclerotic events is not yet clear. These benefits might be related to glycemic control, weight loss, small reductions in BP mainly systolic BP and arterial stiffness, and improvement of lipid profiles, in addition to favorable effects on the kidney [52]. Their efficacy in lowering blood glucose, therefore reducing exposure to other antidiabetic agents such as insulin or sulfonylureas with less benefits, besides, lower rates of hypoglycemia associated with GLP-1RAs use, might also contribute to their protective effects [53]. Direct vascular or cardiac effects of GLP-1RAs such as favorable effects on cardiac function, cardiac ischemia, and on inflammatory markers, resulting in the prevention or delay of the atherosclerotic processes, may contribute to the CV favorable outcomes [33]. Regarding renoprotection, the effects offered by GLP-1RA comprise mainly a reduction in the emergence and progression of albuminuria/proteinuria, with a marginal effect on eGFR decline and neutral effects on hard renal endpoints, e.g., need for RRT [47].

References

1. Wright EM, Loo DD, Hirayama BA. Biology of human sodium glucose transporters. Physiol Rev. 2011;91(2):733–94.
2. Vallon V, Platt KA, Cunard R, Schroth J, Whaley J, Thomson SC, et al. SGLT2 mediates glucose reabsorption in the early proximal tubule. J Am Soc Nephrol. 2011;22(1):104–12.
3. Drozdowski LA, Thomson AB. Intestinal sugar transport. World J Gastroenterol. 2006;12(11):1657–70.
4. Rahmoune H, Thompson PW, Ward JM, Smith CD, Hong G, Brown J. Glucose transporters in human renal proximal tubular cells isolated from the urine of patients with non–insulin-dependent diabetes. Diabetes. 2005;54(12):3427–34.
5. Vallon V. Glucose transporters in the kidney in health and disease. Pflügers Arch. 2020;472:1345–70.

6. Vasilakou D, Karagiannis T, Athanasiadou E, Mainou M, Liakos A, Bekiari E, et al. Sodium–glucose cotransporter 2 inhibitors for type 2 diabetes: a systematic review and meta-analysis. Ann Intern Med. 2013;159(4):262–74.
7. Abdul-Ghani MA, DeFronzo RA, Norton L. Novel hypothesis to explain why SGLT2 inhibitors inhibit only 30–50% of filtered glucose load in humans. Diabetes. 2013;62(10):3324–8.
8. Zinman B, Wanner C, Lachin JM, Fitchett D, Bluhmki E, Hantel S, et al. Empagliflozin, cardiovascular outcomes, and mortality in type 2 diabetes. N Engl J Med. 2015;373(22):2117–28.
9. Neal B, Perkovic V, de Zeeuw D, Mahaffey KW, Fulcher G, Stein P, et al. Rationale, design, and baseline characteristics of the Canagliflozin Cardiovascular Assessment Study (CANVAS)—a randomized placebo-controlled trial. Am Heart J. 2013;166(2):217–23.e11.
10. Neal B, Perkovic V, Matthews DR, Mahaffey KW, Fulcher G, Meininger G, et al. Rationale, design and baseline characteristics of the CANagliflozin cardioVascular assessment study-renal (CANVAS-R): a randomized, placebo-controlled trial. Diabetes Obes Metab. 2017;19(3):387–93.
11. Wiviott SD, Raz I, Bonaca MP, Mosenzon O, Kato ET, Cahn A, et al. Dapagliflozin and cardiovascular outcomes in type 2 diabetes. N Engl J Med. 2019;380(4):347–57.
12. Neal B, Perkovic V, Mahaffey KW, de Zeeuw D, Fulcher G, Erondu N, et al. Canagliflozin and cardiovascular and renal events in type 2 diabetes. N Engl J Med. 2017;377(7):644–57.
13. Zelniker TA, Wiviott SD, Raz I, Im K, Goodrich EL, Bonaca MP, et al. SGLT2 inhibitors for primary and secondary prevention of cardiovascular and renal outcomes in type 2 diabetes: a systematic review and meta-analysis of cardiovascular outcome trials. Lancet. 2019;393(10166):31–9.
14. Perkovic V, Jardine MJ, Neal B, Bompoint S, Heerspink HJL, Charytan DM, et al. Canagliflozin and renal outcomes in type 2 diabetes and nephropathy. N Engl J Med. 2019;380(24):2295–306.
15. McMurray JJV, DeMets DL, Inzucchi SE, Køber L, Kosiborod MN, Langkilde AM, et al. A trial to evaluate the effect of the sodium-glucose co-transporter 2 inhibitor dapagliflozin on morbidity and mortality in patients with heart failure and reduced left ventricular ejection fraction (DAPA-HF). Eur J Heart Fail. 2019;21(5):665–75.
16. Cannon CP, Pratley R, Dagogo-Jack S, Mancuso J, Huyck S, Masiukiewicz U, et al. Cardiovascular outcomes with ertugliflozin in type 2 diabetes. N Engl J Med. 2020;383(15):1425–35.
17. Cosentino F, Cannon CP, Cherney DZI, Masiukiewicz U, Pratley R, Dagogo-Jack S, et al. Efficacy of ertugliflozin on heart failure-related events in patients with type 2 diabetes mellitus and established atherosclerotic cardiovascular disease: results of the VERTIS CV trial. Circulation. 2020;142(23):2205–15.
18. Rendell MS. Sotagliflozin: a combined SGLT1/SGLT2 inhibitor to treat diabetes. Expert Rev Endocrinol Metab. 2018;13(6):333–9.
19. Bhatt DL, Szarek M, Steg PG, Cannon CP, Leiter LA, McGuire DK, et al. Sotagliflozin in patients with diabetes and recent worsening heart failure. N Engl J Med. 2021;384(2):117–28.
20. Bhatt DL, Szarek M, Pitt B, Cannon CP, Leiter LA, McGuire DK, et al. Sotagliflozin in patients with diabetes and chronic kidney disease. N Engl J Med. 2021;384(2):129–39.
21. Packer M, Anker SD, Butler J, Filippatos G, Pocock SJ, Carson P, et al. Cardiovascular and renal outcomes with empagliflozin in heart failure. N Engl J Med. 2020;383(15):1413–24.
22. Anker SD, Butler J, Filippatos GS, Jamal W, Salsali A, Schnee J, et al. Evaluation of the effects of sodium-glucose co-transporter 2 inhibition with empagliflozin on morbidity and mortality in patients with chronic heart failure and a preserved ejection fraction: rationale for and design of the EMPEROR-preserved trial. Eur J Heart Fail. 2019;21(10):1279–87.
23. Ridderstråle M, Andersen KR, Zeller C, Kim G, Woerle HJ, Broedl UC. Comparison of empagliflozin and glimepiride as add-on to metformin in patients with type 2 diabetes: a 104-week randomised, active-controlled, double-blind, phase 3 trial. Lancet Diabetes Endocrinol. 2014;2(9):691–700.
24. Roden M, Weng J, Eilbracht J, Delafont B, Kim G, Woerle HJ, et al. Empagliflozin monotherapy with sitagliptin as an active comparator in patients with type 2 diabetes: a randomised, double-blind, placebo-controlled, phase 3 trial. Lancet Diabetes Endocrinol. 2013;1(3):208–19.

25. Piperidou A, Sarafidis P, Boutou A, Thomopoulos C, Loutradis C, Alexandrou ME, et al. The effect of SGLT-2 inhibitors on albuminuria and proteinuria in diabetes mellitus: a systematic review and meta-analysis of randomized controlled trials. J Hypertens. 2019;37(7):1334–43.
26. Wanner C, Inzucchi SE, Lachin JM, Fitchett D, von Eynatten M, Mattheus M, et al. Empagliflozin and progression of kidney disease in type 2 diabetes. N Engl J Med. 2016;375(4):323–34.
27. Neuen BL, Ohkuma T, Neal B, Matthews DR, de Zeeuw D, Mahaffey KW, et al. Cardiovascular and renal outcomes with canagliflozin according to baseline kidney function. Circulation. 2018;138(15):1537–50.
28. Mosenzon O, Wiviott SD, Cahn A, Rozenberg A, Yanuv I, Goodrich EL, et al. Effects of dapagliflozin on development and progression of kidney disease in patients with type 2 diabetes: an analysis from the DECLARE-TIMI 58 randomised trial. Lancet Diabetes Endocrinol. 2019;7(8):606–17.
29. Heerspink HJL, Stefánsson BV, Correa-Rotter R, Chertow GM, Greene T, Hou FF, et al. Dapagliflozin in patients with chronic kidney disease. N Engl J Med. 2020;383(15):1436–46.
30. Tuttle KR, Brosius FC 3rd, Cavender MA, Fioretto P, Fowler KJ, Heerspink HJL, et al. SGLT2 inhibition for CKD and cardiovascular disease in type 2 diabetes: report of a scientific workshop sponsored by the national kidney foundation. Am J Kidney Dis. 2021;77(1):94–109.
31. Mohebi R, Januzzi JL. Cardiovascular benefit of SGLT2 inhibitors. Crit Rev Clin Lab Sci. 2021:1–14.
32. Girard J. The incretins: from the concept to their use in the treatment of type 2 diabetes. Part A: incretins: concept and physiological functions. Diabetes Metab. 2008;34(6):550–9.
33. Drucker DJ. The biology of incretin hormones. Cell Metab. 2006;3(3):153–65.
34. Kim W, Egan JM. The role of incretins in glucose homeostasis and diabetes treatment. Pharmacol Rev. 2008;60(4):470–512.
35. Muscelli E, Mari A, Casolaro A, Camastra S, Seghieri G, Gastaldelli A, et al. Separate impact of obesity and glucose tolerance on the incretin effect in normal subjects and type 2 diabetic patients. Diabetes. 2008;57(5):1340–8.
36. Heuvelman VD, Van Raalte DH, Smits MM. Cardiovascular effects of glucagon-like peptide 1 receptor agonists: from mechanistic studies in humans to clinical outcomes. Cardiovasc Res. 2020;116(5):916–30.
37. Gilbert MP, Pratley RE. GLP-1 analogs and DPP-4 inhibitors in type 2 diabetes therapy: review of head-to-head clinical trials. Front Endocrinol (Lausanne). 2020;11:178.
38. Nauck MA, Quast DR, Wefers J, Meier JJ. GLP-1 receptor agonists in the treatment of type 2 diabetes–state-of-the-art. Mol Metab. 2021;46:101102.
39. Pfeffer MA, Claggett B, Diaz R, Dickstein K, Gerstein HC, Køber LV, et al. Lixisenatide in patients with type 2 diabetes and acute coronary syndrome. N Engl J Med. 2015;373(23):2247–57.
40. Marso SP, Daniels GH, Brown-Frandsen K, Kristensen P, Mann JF, Nauck MA, et al. Liraglutide and cardiovascular outcomes in type 2 diabetes. N Engl J Med. 2016;375(4):311–22.
41. Marso SP, Bain SC, Consoli A, Eliaschewitz FG, Jódar E, Leiter LA, et al. Semaglutide and cardiovascular outcomes in patients with type 2 diabetes. N Engl J Med. 2016;375:1834–44.
42. Husain M, Birkenfeld AL, Donsmark M, Dungan K, Eliaschewitz FG, Franco DR, et al. Oral semaglutide and cardiovascular outcomes in patients with type 2 diabetes. N Engl J Med. 2019;381(9):841–51.
43. Holman RR, Bethel MA, Mentz RJ, Thompson VP, Lokhnygina Y, Buse JB, et al. Effects of once-weekly exenatide on cardiovascular outcomes in type 2 diabetes. N Engl J Med. 2017;377(13):1228–39.
44. Gerstein HC, Colhoun HM, Dagenais GR, Diaz R, Lakshmanan M, Pais P, et al. Dulaglutide and cardiovascular outcomes in type 2 diabetes (REWIND): a double-blind, randomised placebo-controlled trial. Lancet. 2019;394(10193):121–30.
45. Hernandez AF, Green JB, Janmohamed S, D'Agostino RB Sr, Granger CB, Jones NP, et al. Albiglutide and cardiovascular outcomes in patients with type 2 diabetes and cardiovascular disease (harmony outcomes): a double-blind, randomised placebo-controlled trial. Lancet. 2018;392(10157):1519–29.

46. Kristensen SL, Rørth R, Jhund PS, Docherty KF, Sattar N, Preiss D, et al. Cardiovascular, mortality, and kidney outcomes with GLP-1 receptor agonists in patients with type 2 diabetes: a systematic review and meta-analysis of cardiovascular outcome trials. Lancet Diabetes Endocrinol. 2019;7(10):776–85.
47. Yin WL, Bain SC, Min T. The effect of glucagon-like peptide-1 receptor agonists on renal outcomes in type 2 diabetes. Diabetes Ther. 2020;11(4):835–44.
48. Mann JF, Ørsted DD, Brown-Frandsen K, Marso SP, Poulter NR, Rasmussen S, et al. Liraglutide and renal outcomes in type 2 diabetes. N Engl J Med. 2017;377(9):839–48.
49. Muskiet MHA, Tonneijck L, Huang Y, Liu M, Saremi A, Heerspink HJL, et al. Lixisenatide and renal outcomes in patients with type 2 diabetes and acute coronary syndrome: an exploratory analysis of the ELIXA randomised, placebo-controlled trial. Lancet Diabetes Endocrinol. 2018;6(11):859–69.
50. Tuttle KR, Lakshmanan MC, Rayner B, Busch RS, Zimmermann AG, Woodward DB, et al. Dulaglutide versus insulin glargine in patients with type 2 diabetes and moderate-to-severe chronic kidney disease (AWARD-7): a multicentre, open-label, randomised trial. Lancet Diabetes Endocrinol. 2018;6(8):605–17.
51. Davies MJ, Bain SC, Atkin SL, Rossing P, Scott D, Shamkhalova MS, et al. Efficacy and safety of liraglutide versus placebo as add-on to glucose-lowering therapy in patients with type 2 diabetes and moderate renal impairment (LIRA-RENAL): a randomized clinical trial. Diabetes Care. 2016;39(2):222–30.
52. Nauck MA, Meier JJ, Cavender MA. Abd El Aziz M, Drucker DJ. Cardiovascular actions and clinical outcomes with glucagon-like peptide-1 receptor agonists and dipeptidyl peptidase-4 inhibitors. Circulation. 2017;136(9):849–70.
53. Sattar N, Petrie MC, Zinman B, Januzzi JL. Novel diabetes drugs and the cardiovascular specialist. J Am Coll Cardiol. 2017;69(21):2646–56.

Advances on Long-Term Antihypertensive Treatment and Diabetes

21

John Chalmers and Nelson Wang

21.1 Establishing Personalized Goals in the Treatment of Hypertension

There is strong evidence from randomized controlled trials that lowering systolic blood pressure (SBP) to <140 mmHg and diastolic blood pressure (DBP) to <90 mmHg in patients with diabetes reduces the risk of all-cause mortality, stroke, coronary artery disease, kidney disease, and retinopathy [1]. Stricter blood pressure targets with either treatment among patients with baseline SBP <140 mmHg or target SBP ≤130 mmHg, reduces the risk of stroke but not other diabetic complications [1, 2].

The 2017 American College of Cardiology/American Heart Association (ACC/AHA) guidelines have the most positive treatment strategy, recommending the use of blood pressure-lowering medications for secondary prevention in all patients with clinical atherosclerotic cardiovascular disease (ASCVD) and blood pressure ≥ 130/80 mmHg and for primary prevention in adults with blood pressures ≥130/80 mmHg and estimated 10-year ASCVD risk ≥10% [3]. These guidelines go on to outline that patients with diabetes fit within the high-risk category of 10-year ASCVD risk ≥10%, placing them in the group requiring initiation of antihypertensive therapy when blood pressure is ≥130/80 mmHg. The 2018 European Society of Cardiology (ESC)/European Society of Hypertension (ESH) guidelines recommend initiation of antihypertensives in patients with diabetes and blood pressure ≥140/90 mmHg and to treat toward a target SBP of 130 mmHg or <130 mmHg if tolerated [4].

J. Chalmers (✉) · N. Wang
The George Institute for Global Health, University of New South Wales, Sydney, NSW, Australia

The Royal Prince Alfred Hospital, Sydney, NSW, Australia
e-mail: chalmers@georgeinstitute.org.au

A. E. Berbari, G. Mancia (eds.), *Blood Pressure Disorders in Diabetes Mellitus*, Updates in Hypertension and Cardiovascular Protection,
https://doi.org/10.1007/978-3-031-13009-0_21

However, the cardiovascular risk in patients with diabetes spans a continuum – from moderate risk in individuals with few additional risk factors to very high risk in patients with recurrent major macrovascular and microvascular disease. Clinicians should engage with patients in a shared decision-making process to determine individualized blood pressure targets, with the acknowledgement that the benefits and risks of intensive blood pressure targets are uncertain and may vary across patients. Factors that may influence treatment targets include comorbidities, tolerance of lower blood pressures, patient motivation, preferences, resources, and support systems. Specific factors to consider are the individual's absolute risk of cardiovascular events, risk of progressive kidney disease as reflected by albuminuria and estimated glomerular filtration rate (eGFR), adverse effects from antihypertensives, age, and overall treatment burden. For example, patients at high risk of cardiovascular and renal events and who can tolerate intensive blood pressure control may be best suited to more intensive blood pressure targets. In contrast, patients with conditions more common in older adults, such as functional limitations, multimorbidity, and polypharmacy, may be best suited to less stringent blood pressure targets.

Treatment decisions should consider the absolute benefits and harms of a particular treatment and not the relative benefits and harms. Several risk calculators including the ACC/AHA ASCVD risk are available and can be applied to patients with diabetes [5]. Components of the ASCVD risk calculator include age, sex, race, blood pressure, cholesterol levels, the presence or absence of diabetes, history of smoking, and concurrent antihypertensive, statin, or aspirin use. All patients with diabetes are classified as at least moderate ASCVD risk (10-year risk 7.5–20%). Those individuals with an estimated ASCVD risk (≥20%) are at high risk. Individuals with diabetes and hypertension are automatically considered at very high risk if they have either recurrent ASCVD or 1 major ASCVD event and one other high-risk condition(s) (age ≥ 65 years, heterozygous familial hypercholesterolemia, chronic kidney disease, current smoking, and low-density lipoprotein cholesterol (LDL-C) ≥ 2.6 mmol/L despite maximal therapy and history of congestive heart failure) [6].

The European guidelines reserve the use of the SCORE risk predictor for only those persons with type 1 diabetes without hypertension-mediated organ damage (HMOD). All other individuals with diabetes are risk-stratified accordingly: Individuals with type 2 diabetes and ASCVD or type 2 diabetes with HMOD (including proteinuria, estimated GFR <30 mL/min/1.73 m^2) are at very high risk (10-year risk of cardiovascular death >10%). Patients with three or more major risk factors or with diabetes duration >20 years are also at very high risk. Most others with diabetes are at high risk (10-year risk of cardiovascular death 5–10%), with exception of those at moderate risk including young patients (aged <35 years) with type 1 diabetes of short duration (<10 years) and patients with type 2 diabetes aged <50 years with a duration of diabetes of <10 years and without major risk factors [7].

Once the absolute risk of ASCVD has been established, treatment goals should be tailored based on the patient's priorities, adverse effects of blood pressure lowering, and the physical, psychological, and financial burden of treatment. These factors can be identified through discussion with the patient and family, with particular emphasis on the individual's risk tolerance and personal preferences. Individuals susceptible to the adverse effects of antihypertensives may include those with prior serious adverse effects to blood pressure-lowering or older individuals in whom the consequences of adverse effects may be particularly harmful (e.g., fall secondary to orthostatic hypotension resulting in head trauma or fracture). Once a blood pressure target has been established through shared decision-making, clinicians should remain adaptable and frequently revisit targets during subsequent physician–patient encounters.

21.1.1 Building Antihypertensive Therapies with Single-Pill Combinations (SPC) for People with Diabetes

Although all major antihypertensive classes (angiotensin-converting enzyme (ACE) inhibitors, angiotensin receptor blockers (ARB), calcium channel blockers (CCB), and diuretics) have proven efficacy in the reduction of incident cardiovascular events in diabetes [1, 4], treatment regimens for patients with diabetes should specifically incorporate an ACE inhibitor or ARB when tolerated because of the proven reduction in progressive kidney disease in patients with macroalbuminuria or chronic kidney disease [8]. If an ACE inhibitor is not tolerated, then substitution with an ARB is recommended. ACE inhibitors should not be combined with ARBs because the combination is accompanied by an excess of renal adverse events [9].

CCBs appear to be the most appropriate second-line therapy to be used in combination with an ACE inhibitor/ARB. A large randomized trial of 11,506 patients, of whom 60% had diabetes, found that the combination of an ACE inhibitor with a CCB was superior to an ACE inhibitor and a thiazide diuretic [10]. Combining an ARB with a CCB is also associated with improved insulin sensitivity compared with an ARB and a diuretic [11]. In patients requiring triple therapy, thiazide or thiazide-like diuretics should be added to the combination of an ACE inhibitor (or ARB) and CCB, unless there is a compelling indication for the use of a different class of drug such as heart failure or ischemic heart disease requiring beta-blockers or benign prostatic hyperplasia requiring alpha-blockers. The beta-blocker/diuretic combination favors the development of diabetes and should be avoided in prediabetes, unless required for other reasons. Among beta-blockers, nebivolol has been shown not to worsen insulin sensitivity in patients with metabolic syndrome [12].

Blood pressure control is more difficult to achieve in patients with than in those without diabetes, and most patients with diabetes require multiple antihypertensive agents to achieve blood pressure targets. When available, a combination of two or more drugs at fixed doses in a single-pill combination (SPC) should be used as the first-line blood pressure-lowering drug. Evidence supporting the use of dual combination antihypertensives in individuals with diabetes comes from the Action in Diabetes and Vascular Disease: PreterAx and DiamicroN MR Controlled Evaluation–Blood Pressure (ADVANCE blood pressure) trial, which compared a SPC containing perindopril 4 mg and indapamide 1.25 mg with placebo in 11,140 participants with type 2 diabetes and found that the combination antihypertensive reduced the composite of macrovascular and microvascular events by 9%, cardiovascular mortality by 18%, and all-cause mortality by 14% [13].

Therapeutic inertia, defined as failure to intensify blood pressure-lowering therapy in individuals with inadequately controlled blood pressure, remains one of the biggest challenges in hypertension management. Large observational studies have reported that only 17% of primary care visits with documented blood pressures exceeding blood pressure targets resulted in treatment intensification. In a clinical trial setting, only 36% of patients with uncontrolled blood pressures receive treatment intensification [14]. There is some concern that SPCs may be associated with more therapeutic inertia. In a recent polypill-based blood pressure trial in the United States, there was a significant improvement in blood pressure control in participants randomized to the polypill, although individuals receiving the polypill were less likely to have other blood pressure medications added or increased [15]. Early treatment intensification with SPCs provides large reductions in blood pressure, which may lead to greater reluctance to uptitrate blood pressure therapy, particularly when blood pressures are only modestly above the target. However, SPCs will provide better blood pressure control earlier, such that fewer patients will require further uptitration of medications in the first place. Even if the use of FDC pills increases therapeutic inertia, the negative outcome may be offset by the substantial upfront advantage in blood pressure control. Nevertheless, strategies to address therapeutic inertia are needed. Implementation of SPCs into clinical practice should be part of longitudinal care pathways, with reassessment of blood pressures over time and algorithms to uptitrate therapy for those whose blood pressure remains above the target value. It is important to provide multiple dosing options for SPC, to allow clinicians greater prescribing flexibility without losing the simplicity of a combination pill.

21.1.2 Moving Toward the Use of Low-Dose SPC for Lowering Blood Pressure

In general, all patients with diabetes and hypertension should begin first-line blood pressure-lowering treatment with an SPC containing two or three antihypertensive classes. Initiation of dual combination antihypertensive therapy, particularly at low-to-standard doses is more effective than standard-dose monotherapy, without an associated increase in adverse events [16]. Several observations suggest triple low-dose combination therapy may produce even greater blood pressure control without increasing adverse effects compared with dual combination therapy. A meta-analysis of 14 randomized controlled trials enrolling 11,457 participants found that triple therapy reduced SBP/DBP by 5.4/3.2 mmHg and improved the percentage of people achieving blood pressure control by 58% in triple therapy vs. 45% in dual therapy [relative risk (RR) 1.33 (95% CI 1.25–1.41)] [17]. There was no increase in the incidence of withdrawals because of adverse events in the triple therapy group compared to dual therapy.

SPCs provide better blood pressure lowering not only partly because they reduce the "pill burden" for the patient and the risk of nonadherence but also partly because most of the blood pressure-lowering effects can be obtained with a fraction of the full dose of a single antihypertensive drug. Compared with a standard dose, quarter dose antihypertensives produce 50–60% of the blood pressure-lowering effect, and half-dose antihypertensives achieve 70–80% [18, 19]. At quarter or half the standard dose, there are little or no drug-specific adverse effects, and drug-specific adverse effects generally rise steeply and steadily as the dose increases [18, 19]. Given the blood pressure-lowering effects across drug classes are additive, SPC antihypertensives can provide potent blood pressure reduction while minimizing adverse effects.

The Triple Pill vs. Usual Care Management for Patients with Mild-to-Moderate Hypertension (TRIUMPH) trial randomized 700 patients with mild-to-moderate hypertension to either usual care or triple SPC therapy consisting of telmisartan 20 mg, amlodipine 2.5 mg, and chlorthalidone 12.5 mg [14]. The trial included 220 (29%) patients with diabetes. The trial found that significantly more patients on the triple pill reached the blood pressure targets of less than 140/90 mmHg (less than 130/80 mmHg in patients with diabetes) at 6 months compared with usual care (70% in triple pill vs. 55% in usual care). There was no significant heterogeneity in the effect of the triple pill compared with usual care when stratified by the presence of diabetes.

A low-dose triple-pill combination containing half standard doses of an ARB, CCB, and thiazide or thiazide-like diuretic has several advantages in comparison with monotherapy. Firstly, it provides more potent therapy without an increase in adverse effects. Secondly, the use of SPC therapies improve adherence [20]. Thirdly, the combination of an ARB and thiazide diuretic offsets the incidence of peripheral edema associated with a CCB [21]. The addition of an ARB reduces the incidence of hypokalemia associated with thiazide diuretics [22]. When available, low-dose dual or triple combination antihypertensives should be used as the first-line treatment in all patients with diabetes and hypertension.

Figure 21.1 outlines an approach toward the use of SPC antihypertensive therapy for patients with diabetes. Patients with SBP 130–159 mmHg may start treatment with a dual combination antihypertensive at half standard dose, while patients with higher levels of blood pressure should begin treatment with a triple combination antihypertensive at half standard dose. If blood pressure control is not achieved with initiation of a fixed-dose double or triple antihypertensive, uptitration of blood pressure therapy is warranted from low-dose double to low-dose triple or from low-dose to standard dose, as the case may be.

One major issue that must be addressed is that many of our recommendations would be difficult to implement in parts of the world where individuals experience economic disadvantage and poverty, which has been exacerbated by the current shock of the coronavirus pandemic, particularly in Africa, India, and South/Latin America. In many countries in these regions, standard dose antihypertensive drugs are often not available or affordable, and half dose or even lower dose drug formulations are not even on the horizon!

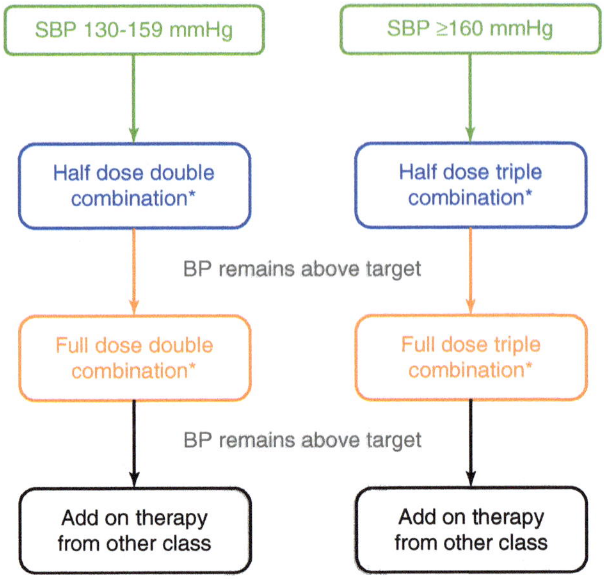

Fig. 21.1 Approach for the use of SPC antihypertensives in patients with diabetes. Initiation of pharmacological therapy should begin with half standard dose double or triple antihypertensive SPC. If blood pressure remains above target, uptitration of therapy should include increasing to full dose double or triple SPC. *Patients with albuminuria and chronic kidney disease should use a combination containing an ACE inhibitor or ARB

21.1.3 Management of Multiple Risk Factors and Potential for Combination Hypertension-Diabetes Polypill

Besides elevated blood pressure, there are multiple risk factors that contribute toward organ damage in patients with diabetes including elevated blood glucose, deranged lipid metabolism, hyperuricemia, and lifestyle factors including overweight and obesity, smoking, alcohol, dietary habits, and sedentary lifestyle. Multifaceted management plans that target all relevant risk factors are needed.

Adequate glucose control is of fundamental importance for minimizing disease progression and also because the deleterious effects of hypertension and hyperglycemia appear to be additive. The United Kingdom Prospective Diabetes Study (UKPDS) trial showed that for each 1% decrease in HbA1c and each 10 mmHg decrease in blood pressure, there was a 21% and an 11% decrease in diabetes-related endpoints, respectively [23]. Tests for interaction confirmed that the effects of glucose control and blood pressure-lowering were additive. Similar trends were seen for diabetes-related deaths with glucose control and all-cause mortality with blood pressure lowering. There were significantly fewer diabetes-related endpoints among those patients who were randomized to both intensive glucose control and intensive blood pressure management compared with those individuals who were randomized to either intervention alone. Similarly, the Action in Diabetes and Vascular Disease: PreterAx and DiamicroN Controlled Evaluation (ADVANCE) trial reported the combined effects of routine blood pressure lowering and intensive glucose control on macrovascular and microvascular events in 11,140 patients with type 2 diabetes [24]. The trial showed that there was no interaction between these two interventions for any of the clinical outcomes. The combined effects of blood pressure lowering and intensive glucose control reduced all-cause mortality by 18% and nephropathy by 33% [24]. It is important to note that ADVANCE was conducted in the twenty-first century, a decade later than the UKPDS. Patients who entered the ADVANCE trial had much better controlled baseline blood pressures and blood glucose (mean SBP/DBP 145/81 vs. 160/94 mmHg in ADVANCE vs. UKPDS, respectively), and HbA1c reduced from 7.5% to 6.5% in the intensively treated arm vs. an achieved 7.3% in the standard treatment group, compared with HbA1c levels achieved 10 years earlier, in the UKPDS, of 7.0% in the intensive group and 7.9% in the conventional treatment group. The Steno-2 study demonstrated the efficacy of multifactorial risk factor management including behavioral modification, ACE inhibitor therapy, intensive glucose control, and statins as required, which reduced the risk of major cardiovascular disease (hazard ratio 0.47 [95% CI 0.24–0.73]), nephropathy (hazard ratio 0.39 [95% CI 0.17–0.87]), and retinopathy (hazard ratio, 0.42 [95% CI 0.21–0.86]) by >50% over a 7.8 year follow-up period [25].

An analysis of 271,174 patients with type 2 diabetes in the Swedish National Diabetes Register found that those patients with adequate control of five major risk factors (elevated glycated hemoglobin, elevated LDL-C, albuminuria, smoking, and elevated blood pressure) appeared to have a similar risk of death, myocardial infarction, and stroke compared with the matched general population without diabetes [26]. Therefore, it may be possible to almost entirely mitigate the cardiovascular risk associated with type 2 diabetes through intensive management of multiple risk factors.

One strategy to target multiple risk factors simultaneously is through the use of fixed-dose combinations of cholesterol and blood pressure-lowering drugs as a SPC or polypill. A prior meta-analysis of 13 trials including 9059 patients with prior ASCVD or cardiovascular risk factors including hypertension, hypercholesterolemia, and/or diabetes showed that a polypill strategy for primary and secondary prevention of ASCVD led to improvements in adherence, LDL-C levels, and blood pressure among patients with appropriate indications for therapy [27]. Adverse events, such as cough, myalgias, or dyspepsia, were higher among patients randomized to prescribed polypills compared with control (31% vs. 27%), although these were largely expected adverse effects from greater exposure to cholesterol and blood pressure-lowering drugs.

The PolyIran trial randomized 6838 participants (15% had pre-existing diabetes) to a four-component polypill containing hydrochlorothiazide 12.5 mg, aspirin 81 mg, atorvastatin 20 mg, and enalapril 5 mg compared with usual care in a largely primary prevention setting [28]. Compared with usual care, the polypill was associated with a 2.9% absolute risk reduction in ASCVD events over 5 years (adjusted hazard ratio = 0.66 [95% CI, 0.55–0.80]). The primary prevention Southern Community Cohort Study polypill trial [15] enrolled 303 participants (13% with diabetes) across federally qualified health centers in the United States and demonstrated greater reductions in LDL-C and blood pressure in the polypill group compared with usual care (15 mg/dL reduction in LDL-C in polypill vs. 4 mg/dL reduction in LDL-C in usual care; 9 mmHg reduction in SBP in polypill vs. 2 mmHg reduction in SBP in usual care), with no between-group difference in frequency of serious adverse events. Several trials have also demonstrated the efficacy and safety of polypills that do not include aspirin, which is relevant because aspirin has recently been shown to increase the risk of major bleeding with only a modest reduction in cardiovascular events in a primary prevention setting [29, 30]. For primary prevention, aspirin is only recommended in patients with diabetes at high or very high cardiovascular risk.

Given patients with type 2 diabetes frequently use the components of a polypill, there is potential for the development of a "diabetic polypill" that would include additional oral hypoglycemic drugs in addition to a statin and two blood pressure-lowering drugs. Metformin remains the most prescribed first-line oral hypoglycemic in type 2 diabetes and would be a suitable inclusion in a diabetic polypill. Dipeptidyl peptidase-4 (DPP4) inhibitors and sulfonylureas are other commonly used oral hypoglycemic drugs that could be included in a polypill.

More recently, the sodium-dependent glucose cotransporter 2 (SGLT2) inhibitors have proven to be remarkably effective in reducing the risk of ASCVD, heart failure hospitalizations, and progression of diabetic kidney disease [31, 32]. Although the exact mechanisms driving these benefits remain uncertain, the benefits of SGLT2 inhibitors extend beyond their glucose-lowering effects. SGLT2 inhibitors are increasingly used as first-line therapy, either as an add-on to metformin or in drug naïve patients, particularly in those patients with prior history of ASCVD, heart failure, or at high cardiovascular risk. Considering most diabetic patients with prior ASCVD or at high cardiovascular risk require treatment with antihypertensive agents and statins, there is potential for the inclusion of SGLT2 inhibitors in a diabetic polypill. However, practical implications regarding the suspension of SGLT2 inhibitors before major surgery or other medical conditions that predispose to diabetic ketoacidosis need to be considered.

Along with SGLT2 inhibitors, glucagon-like peptide-1 receptor agonists (GLP1-RAs) have also been effective in reducing the risk of cardiovascular events in patients with type 2 diabetes. The PIONEER trials have demonstrated the efficacy of oral semaglutide, an oral GLP1-RA that is administered as a once-daily pill and would be suitable for inclusion in a diabetic polypill [33]. The remaining GLP1-RAs are administered subcutaneously and would not be suitable in a polypill design (instead they would be used as add on therapy). Although SGLT2 inhibitors and GLP1-RAs are not used for their blood pressure lowering effects, both drug classes have small but significant reductions in blood pressure, which should be recognized.

It is important to remember that population-based and individual risk-based strategies are not mutually exclusive. Polypills should be incorporated as part of a longitudinal treatment strategy, where it will likely serve as a foundational therapy for patients with diabetes, with the option of add on medications for those patients with good adherence who remain at elevated risk. Polypills should not preclude or minimize the importance of other interventions, such as diet, exercise, and smoking cessation. It is worth emphasizing that polypills may not be readily accessible in low- and middle-income countries, areas where they appear to be most effective [15].

21.1.4 Long-Term Blood Pressure and Glucose Control, with a Focus on Treatment Adherence

Prevention of microvascular and macrovascular complications should focus on the long-term control of elevated blood pressures and glucose levels, rather than isolated blood pressure or glucose readings at a single time point. Several longitudinal cohort studies have shown that blood pressure levels in middle age and young adulthood are predictors of future cardiovascular risk independent of current or later adult exposures [34, 35]. Post-trial analyses suggest that blood pressure lowering over a period of time appears to have sustained benefits lasting many years afterward. In the ADVANCE post-trial analyses of 11,140 diabetic participants, there was a clear persistence in the reduction of all-cause (9% risk reduction) and cardiovascular mortality (12% risk reduction) 6 years after cessation of treatment and convergence of blood pressure levels between the randomized groups [36]. The UKPDS post-trial monitoring of 1148 patients assigned to 4 years of intensive or standard blood pressure control found nonsignificant trends for lower all-cause mortality, myocardial infarction, microvascular disease, and any diabetes-related complications over a 10-year post interventional follow-up period [37].

Similar concepts apply for glycemic control in the prevention of diabetic complications. Data from post-trial follow-up analyses in patients with type 1 and type 2 diabetes have revealed the benefits of intensive glucose control on major cardiovascular disease that were not evident during the initial trial period [38, 39]. In the Diabetes Control and Complications Trial, the Epidemiology of Diabetes Interventions and Complications Group found that intensive glucose control reduced the risk of cardiovascular death, nonfatal myocardial infarction, and stroke by 57% compared with conventional therapy [38] during a mean follow-up of 17 years (mean treatment/randomization period of 6.5 years). In the UKPDS, 10 years of post-trial monitoring found that intensive glucose control resulted in a continued reduction in microvascular risk and emergent risk reductions for myocardial infarction and death despite the early loss of glycemic differences [39].

Recent Mendelian randomization studies have challenged traditional perceptions about the benefits of blood pressure lowering, suggesting a 10 mmHg SBP difference sustained over a lifetime will reduce coronary artery disease by almost 50% [40]. It has been hypothesized that the benefits of exposure to lower SBP may accumulate over time. Unfortunately, evaluating the impact of long-term blood pressure treatment in young asymptomatic people over decades within the context of a clinical trial may be impractical. However, these studies suggest that the cumulative exposure to elevated SBP (defined as an integration of the magnitude and duration of exposure) may be an important risk factor for lifetime risk of cardiovascular disease. Given trajectories of blood pressure can vary between individuals, further research is needed to quantify more precisely the cumulative lifetime exposure to blood pressure that incorporates differing individual trajectories over the life course. A similar concept for glycemic control has also been hypothesized from Mendelian randomization. One study demonstrated that lifetime exposure to glucose-lowering alleles is associated with significant reductions in coronary heart disease, a relationship that is not fully appreciated in randomized controlled trials with relatively short-term follow-up (<7 years) [41].

To achieve sustained and long-term risk factor control, greater emphasis on medication adherence is needed. Nonadherence to antihypertensive therapy correlates with a higher risk of cardiovascular events [42, 43]. After 6 months and after 1 year, more than one-third and about one-half of patients may stop their initial treatment [44]. Adherence measured by the detection of antihypertensive medications in urine has shown that poor adherence affects up to 50% of patients with apparently resistant hypertension and that the number of prescribed pills is strongly correlated with worse adherence [45]. Other barriers to adherence are related to health care system factors, physician factors, therapy-related factors, and patient factors.

Adherence to blood pressure therapy can be improved by several interventions. The most useful interventions are those that link drug intake with habits [46], provide feedback to patients, self-monitoring of blood pressure [47], use of pillboxes and other special packaging, motivational interviewing, and multidisciplinary involvement from pharmacists and nurses. SPC antihypertensives can improve adherence by simplifying the medication regimen and decreasing the pill burden. In a secondary analysis of TRIUMPH, a triple fixed-dose combination antihypertensive was able to substantially simplify treatment regimens (23 unique antihypertensive treatment regimens per 100 treated patients in triple pill vs. 54 unique treatment regimens per 100 treated patients in usual care) while improving blood pressure control [48]. Similar concepts can also be applied to adherence to statins and glucose-lowering therapies. Currently available polypills that contain a statin and two or more antihypertensive medications are an attractive option to decrease pill burden and improve medication adherence. The development of a diabetic polypill, as discussed in the prior section, will also become a potentially important advance in improving adherence.

21.2 Conclusions

Hypertension is a strong, modifiable risk factor for macrovascular and microvascular complications of diabetes. Evidence from clinical trials and meta-analyses strongly support the need to lower blood pressure in individuals with diabetes to 130/80 mmHg, or even lower in high-risk patients. Individualized targets should be established through a shared decision-making process between the clinician and the individual that considers the patient's absolute risk of macrovascular and microvascular disease, treatment burden, available resources, risk of adverse drug effects, and personal preference. Blood pressure management should include the use of a double or triple low-dose combination antihypertensive as a single pill in the first instance because they are associated with greater blood pressure reductions and improved medication adherence, without increase in adverse effects. A multifactorial approach that targets all macrovascular and microvascular risk factors including but not limited to elevated blood pressure, hyperglycemia, cholesterol, sedentary lifestyle, and obesity is needed, with special emphasis on sustainable strategies that can provide long-term control. SPCs, both full dose and low dose, that contain antihypertensives, statins, and potentially glucose-lowering drugs, will become an attractive treatment option for patients with diabetes because they are able to address multiple risk factors simultaneously, reduce adverse effects, improve medication adherence, and hence prevent the major long-term complications of both hypertension and diabetes.

References

1. Emdin CA, Rahimi K, Neal B, Callender T, Perkovic V, Patel A. Blood pressure lowering in type 2 diabetes: a systematic review and meta-analysis. JAMA. 2015;313:603–15.
2. Bangalore S, Kumar S, Lobach I, Messerli FH. Blood pressure targets in subjects with type 2 diabetes mellitus/impaired fasting glucose: observations from traditional and bayesian random-effects meta-analyses of randomized trials. Circulation. 2011;123:2799–810.
3. Whelton PK, Carey RM, Aronow WS, Casey DE, Collins KJ, Himmelfarb CD, et al. 2017 ACC/AHA/AAPA/ABC/ACPM/AGS/APhA/ASH/ASPC/NMA/PCNA guideline for the prevention, detection, evaluation, and management of high blood pressure in adults: a report of the American College of Cardiology/American Heart Association Task Force on Clinical Practice Guidelines. J Am Coll Cardiol. 2018;71:e127–248.
4. Williams B, Mancia G, Spiering W, Agabiti Rosei E, Azizi M, Burnier M, et al. 2018 ESC/ESH Guidelines for the management of arterial hypertension: The Task Force for the management of arterial hypertension of the European Society of Cardiology and the European Society of Hypertension. J Hypertens. 2018;36:1953–2041.
5. Goff DC, Lloyd-Jones DM, Bennett G, Coady S, D'agostino RB, Gibbons R, et al. 2013 ACC/AHA guideline on the assessment of cardiovascular risk: a report of the American College of Cardiology/American Heart Association Task Force on Practice Guidelines. J Am Coll Cardiol. 2014;63:2935–59.
6. Grundy SM, Stone NJ, Bailey AL, Beam C, Birtcher KK, Blumenthal RS, et al. 2018 AHA/ACC/AACVPR/AAPA/ABC/ACPM/ADA/AGS/APhA/ASPC/NLA/PCNA Guideline on the Management of Blood Cholesterol: A Report of the American College of Cardiology/American Heart Association Task Force on Clinical Practice Guidelines. Circulation. 2019;139:e1082–143.
7. Cosentino F, Grant PJ, Aboyans V, Bailey CJ, Ceriello A, Delgado V, et al. 2019 ESC guidelines on diabetes, pre-diabetes, and cardiovascular diseases developed in collaboration with the EASD: the task force for diabetes, pre-diabetes, and cardiovascular diseases of the European Society of Cardiology (ESC) and the European Association for the Study of Diabetes (EASD). Eur Heart J. 2020;41:255–323.
8. Thomopoulos C, Parati G, Zanchetti A. Effects of blood-pressure-lowering treatment on outcome incidence. 12. Effects in individuals with high-normal and normal blood pressure: overview and meta-analyses of randomized trials. J Hypertens. 2017;35:2150–60.
9. Fried LF, Emanuele N, Zhang JH, Brophy M, Conner TA, Duckworth W, et al. Combined angiotensin inhibition for the treatment of diabetic nephropathy. N Engl J Med. 2013;369:1892–903.
10. Jamerson K, Weber MA, Bakris GL, Dahlöf B, Pitt B, Shi V, et al. Benazepril plus amlodipine or hydrochlorothiazide for hypertension in high-risk patients. N Engl J Med. 2008;359:2417–28.
11. Derosa G, Querci F, Franzetti I, Dario Ragonesi P, D'Angelo A, Maffioli P. Comparison of the effects of barnidipine+losartan compared with telmisartan+hydrochlorothiazide on several

parameters of insulin sensitivity in patients with hypertension and type 2 diabetes mellitus. Hypertens Res. 2015;38:690–4.
12. Ayers K, Byrne LM, DeMatteo A, Brown NJ. Differential effects of nebivolol and metoprolol on insulin sensitivity and plasminogen activator inhibitor in the metabolic syndrome. Hypertension. 2012;59:893–8.
13. Bakris GL, Weir MR, Study of Hypertension and the Efficacy of Lotrel in Diabetes (SHIELD) Investigators. Achieving goal blood pressure in patients with type 2 diabetes: conventional versus fixed-dose combination approaches. J Clin Hypertens (Greenwich). 2003;5:202–9.
14. Webster R, Salam A, de Silva HA, Selak V, Stepien S, Rajapakse S, et al. Fixed low-dose triple combination antihypertensive medication vs usual care for blood pressure control in patients with mild to moderate hypertension in Sri Lanka: a randomized clinical trial. JAMA. 2018;320:566–79.
15. Muñoz D, Uzoije P, Reynolds C, Miller R, Walkley D, Pappalardo S, et al. Polypill for cardiovascular disease prevention in an underserved population. N Engl J Med. 2019;381:1114–23.
16. Salam A, Kanukula R, Atkins E, Wang X, Islam S, Kishore SP, et al. Efficacy and safety of dual combination therapy of blood pressure-lowering drugs as initial treatment for hypertension: a systematic review and meta-analysis of randomized controlled trials. J Hypertens. 2019;37:1768–74.
17. Salam A, Atkins ER, Hsu B, Webster R, Patel A, Rodgers A. Efficacy and safety of triple versus dual combination blood pressure-lowering drug therapy: a systematic review and meta-analysis of randomized controlled trials. J Hypertens. 2019;37:1567–73.
18. Bennett A, Chow CK, Chou M, Dehbi HM, Webster R, Salam A, et al. Efficacy and safety of quarter-dose blood pressure-lowering agents: a systematic review and meta-analysis of randomized controlled trials. Hypertension. 2017;70:85–93.
19. Law MR, Wald NJ, Morris JK, Jordan RE. Value of low dose combination treatment with blood pressure lowering drugs: analysis of 354 randomised trials. BMJ. 2003;326:1427.
20. Corrao G, Parodi A, Nicotra F, Zambon A, Merlino L, Cesana G, et al. Better compliance to antihypertensive medications reduces cardiovascular risk. J Hypertens. 2011;29:610–8.
21. Jadhav U, Hiremath J, Namjoshi DJ, Gujral VK, Tripathi KK, Siraj M, et al. Blood pressure control with a single-pill combination of indapamide sustained-release and amlodipine in patients with hypertension: the EFFICIENT study. PLoS One. 2014;9:e92955.
22. Lindholm LH, Persson M, Alaupovic P, Carlberg B, Svensson A, Samuelsson O. Metabolic outcome during 1 year in newly detected hypertensives: results of the antihypertensive treatment and lipid profile in a north of Sweden efficacy evaluation (ALPINE study). J Hypertens. 2003;21:1563–74.
23. Stratton I, Cull C, Adler A, Matthews D, Neil H, Holman R. Additive effects of glycaemia and blood pressure exposure on risk of complications in type 2 diabetes: a prospective observational study (UKPDS 75). Diabetologia. 2006;49:1761–9.
24. Zoungas S, De Galan BE, Ninomiya T, Grobbee D, Hamet P, Heller S, et al. Combined effects of routine blood pressure lowering and intensive glucose control on macrovascular and microvascular outcomes in patients with type 2 diabetes: new results from the ADVANCE trial. Diabetes Care. 2009;32:2068–74.
25. Gæde P, Vedel P, Larsen N, Jensen GVH, Parving H-H, Pedersen O. Multifactorial intervention and cardiovascular disease in patients with type 2 diabetes. N Engl J Med. 2003;348:383–93.
26. Rawshani A, Rawshani A, Franzén S, Sattar N, Eliasson B, Svensson A-M, et al. Risk factors, mortality, and cardiovascular outcomes in patients with type 2 diabetes. N Engl J Med. 2019;379:633–44.
27. Bahiru E, de Cates AN, Farr MR, Jarvis MC, Palla M, Rees K, et al. Fixed-dose combination therapy for the prevention of atherosclerotic cardiovascular diseases. Cochrane Database Syst Rev. 2017;3:Cd009868.
28. Roshandel G, Khoshnia M, Poustchi H, Hemming K, Kamangar F, Gharavi A, et al. Effectiveness of polypill for primary and secondary prevention of cardiovascular diseases (PolyIran): a pragmatic, cluster-randomised trial. Lancet. 2019;394:672–83.

29. Saito Y, Okada S, Ogawa H, Soejima H, Sakuma M, Nakayama M, et al. Low-dose aspirin for primary prevention of cardiovascular events in patients with type 2 diabetes mellitus: 10-year follow-up of a randomized controlled trial. Circulation. 2017;135:659–70.
30. Bowman L, Mafham M, Wallendszus K, Stevens W, Buck G, Barton J, et al. Effects of aspirin for primary prevention in persons with diabetes mellitus. N Engl J Med. 2018;379:1529–39.
31. Neal B, Perkovic V, Mahaffey KW, De Zeeuw D, Fulcher G, Erondu N, et al. Canagliflozin and cardiovascular and renal events in type 2 diabetes. N Engl J Med. 2017;377:644–57.
32. Perkovic V, Jardine MJ, Neal B, Bompoint S, Heerspink HJL, Charytan DM, et al. Canagliflozin and renal outcomes in type 2 diabetes and nephropathy. N Engl J Med. 2019;380:2295–306.
33. Husain M, Birkenfeld AL, Donsmark M, Dungan K, Eliaschewitz FG, Franco DR, et al. Oral semaglutide and cardiovascular outcomes in patients with type 2 diabetes. N Engl J Med. 2019;381:841–51.
34. Zhang Y, Vittinghoff E, Pletcher MJ, Allen NB, Zeki Al Hazzouri A, Yaffe K, et al. Associations of blood pressure and cholesterol levels during young adulthood with later cardiovascular events. J Am Coll Cardiol. 2019;74:330–41.
35. Bonifonte A, Ayer T, Veledar E, Clark A, Wilson PW. Antecedent blood pressure as a predictor of cardiovascular disease. J Am Soc Hypertens. 2015;9:690–6.e1.
36. Zoungas S, Chalmers J, Neal B, Billot L, Li Q, Hirakawa Y, et al. Follow-up of blood-pressure lowering and glucose control in type 2 diabetes. N Engl J Med. 2014;371:1392–406.
37. Holman RR, Paul SK, Bethel MA, Neil HAW, Matthews DR. Long-term follow-up after tight control of blood pressure in type 2 diabetes. N Engl J Med. 2008;359:1565–76.
38. Nathan DM, Cleary PA, Backlund JY, Genuth SM, Lachin JM, Orchard TJ, et al. Intensive diabetes treatment and cardiovascular disease in patients with type 1 diabetes. N Engl J Med. 2005;353:2643–53.
39. Holman RR, Paul SK, Bethel MA, Matthews DR, Neil HA. 10-year follow-up of intensive glucose control in type 2 diabetes. N Engl J Med. 2008;359:1577–89.
40. Ference BA, Bhatt DL, Catapano AL, Packard CJ, Graham I, Kaptoge S, et al. Association of genetic variants related to combined exposure to lower low-density lipoproteins and lower systolic blood pressure with lifetime risk of cardiovascular disease. JAMA. 2019;322:1381–91.
41. Ahmad OS, Morris JA, Mujammami M, Forgetta V, Leong A, Li R, et al. A Mendelian randomization study of the effect of type-2 diabetes on coronary heart disease. Nat Commun. 2015;6:7060.
42. Wang YR, Alexander GC, Stafford RS. Outpatient hypertension treatment, treatment intensification, and control in Western Europe and the United States. Arch Int Med. 2007;167:141–7.
43. Burnier M, Wuerzner G, Struijker-Boudier H, Urquhart J. Measuring, analyzing, and managing drug adherence in resistant hypertension. Hypertension. 2013;62:218–25.
44. Naderi SH, Bestwick JP, Wald DS. Adherence to drugs that prevent cardiovascular disease: meta-analysis on 376,162 patients. Am J Med. 2012;125(882–7):e1.
45. Jung O, Gechter JL, Wunder C, Paulke A, Bartel C, Geiger H, et al. Resistant hypertension? Assessment of adherence by toxicological urine analysis. J Hypertens. 2013;31:766–74.
46. Conn VS, Ruppar TM, Chase J-AD, Enriquez M, Cooper PS. Interventions to improve medication adherence in hypertensive patients: systematic review and meta-analysis. Curr Hypertens Rep. 2015;17:94.
47. Parati G, Omboni S. Role of home blood pressure telemonitoring in hypertension management: an update. Blood Press Monit. 2010;15:285–95.
48. Wang N, Salam A, Webster R, de Silva A, Guggilla R, Stepien S, et al. Association of low-dose triple combination therapy with therapeutic inertia and prescribing patterns in patients with hypertension: a secondary analysis of the TRIUMPH trial. JAMA Cardiol. 2020;5(11):1219–26.

Part VII

Strategies for Blood Pressure Control

Lifestyle Modifications 22

Renata Cífková

22.1 Introduction

Most of the lifestyle modifications recommended to diabetic patients also reduce blood pressure (BP). Although the benefits of lifestyle changes are undisputed, few patients are able to achieve blood pressure control with these interventions alone [1]. Lifestyle modification is an important part of hypertension management because it lowers blood pressure, increases the effectiveness of some antihypertensive drugs, and may improve a number of metabolic parameters.

Lifestyle management of a diabetic patient with hypertension should include the reduction of excess body weight through caloric restriction, restriction of sodium intake, increased consumption of fruits and vegetables and low-fat dairy products, avoiding excessive alcohol consumption, and increased physical activity. In addition, counseling should include smoking cessation in tobacco users and e-cigarette smokers.

The Da Qing Diabetes Prevention Outcome Study found that lifestyle intervention in individuals with impaired glucose tolerance delayed the onset of type 2 diabetes and reduced the incidence of macrovascular events and microvascular changes and decreased cardiovascular and all-cause mortality in the longer term [2]. Systolic and diastolic BP was lower in the intervention group (143.9/74.2 vs. 148.1/77.6 mm Hg) after 30 years.

Lifestyle measures in diabetic patients with elevated blood pressure should be implemented by behavioral changes to be included in diabetes self-management education and support, nutrition therapy, physical activity, smoking cessation counseling, and psychosocial care [3]. There is a need to evaluate diabetes

R. Cífková (✉)
First Faculty of Medicine and Thomayer University Hospital, Center for Cardiovascular Prevention, Charles University in Prague, Prague, Czech Republic
e-mail: renata.cifkova@ftn.cz

A. E. Berbari, G. Mancia (eds.), *Blood Pressure Disorders in Diabetes Mellitus*, Updates in Hypertension and Cardiovascular Protection,
https://doi.org/10.1007/978-3-031-13009-0_22

self-management education at the time of diagnosis, annually and/or when not meeting treatment targets and when changes in life and care occur.

22.2 Weight Reduction

Weight reduction is recommended to any overweight or obese diabetic patient using dietary changes, increased physical activity, and behavioral therapy to achieve and maintain ≥5% weight loss. Modest and sustained weight loss improves glycemic control and lipid profile and reduces BP and, potentially, the need for drugs to control these risk factors. Although these interventions are generally recommended to obese and overweight hypertensive patients, the average weight loss is rather small, and most of the patients will increase their body weight within a few months or years [4]. Most of the data regarding the BP decrease and weight loss were obtained from short-term studies. Indeed, the beneficial effects of weight loss on neurohormonal activity can be most noticeable within a relatively short time-period and may be attenuated when body weight is stabilized.

The Look AHEAD (Action for Health in Diabetes) trial showed a greater BP reduction in the intensive lifestyle intervention arm, compared with diabetes support and education serving as the control group (– 5.33 vs. –2.97 mm Hg for systolic BP, $p < 0.001$; – 2.92 vs. –2.48 mm Hg for diastolic BP, $p < 0.01$) over a period of 4 years in a large cohort of obese type 2 diabetic patients [5]. This was the first study providing evidence that lifestyle interventions can induce long-term weight loss, improvement in fitness, and cardiovascular disease (CVD) risk factors.

In the Diabetes Remission Clinical Trial (DiRECT), intensive lifestyle changes with a low-calorie diet and mean weight loss of 10 kg induced remission of type 2 diabetes in 46% of the intervention group at 1 year and in 36% after 2 years [6, 7]. Mean systolic BP at 24 months had decreased by 1.4 mm Hg in the control group and by 4.3 mm Hg in the intervention group.

22.2.1 Caloric Restrictions

Significant weight loss can be attained with lifestyle programs achieving a 500–750 kcal/day energy deficit. Some clinical benefits may start with 3–5% weight loss [8, 9] and will increase with more intensive weight reduction. Dietary interventions should take into consideration a patient's health status and preferences, including food availability and affordability [10]. Meal replacement prescribed by nutritionists/dieticians with close monitoring can be beneficial. Interventions can be provided in either individual or group sessions [4].

Intensive dietary intervention such as structured, very low-calorie diets (800–1000 kcal/day), utilizing high-protein foods and meal replacement products, may be prescribed to selected patients, e.g., requiring weight loss prior to surgery or needing greater weight loss and improvement in glycemic control.

22.3 Increased Physical Activity

Physical activity in general includes all movement that increases energy use, thus becoming an important part of hypertension management in diabetes, whereas exercise is a more specific form of physical activity designed to improve physical fitness. Exercise has been shown to improve blood glucose control, reduce CV risk factors, facilitate a decrease in body weight, and promote overall well-being.

Physical activity can be characterized either by absolute or relative intensity. Absolute intensity is the amount of energy expended per minute of activity, evaluated by oxygen uptake per unit of time (ml/min or L/min) or by metabolic equivalent of task (MET). Classification of physical activity and examples are provided in Table 22.1 [11].

Physical activity is associated with an acute rise in BP, particularly systolic BP, followed by a decline possibly lasting for several hours [12]. A meta-analysis of randomized clinical trials based on self-reported exercise has shown that aerobic endurance training, dynamic resistance training, and isometric training reduce resting systolic and diastolic BP by 3.5/3.5, 1.8/3.2, and 10.9/6.2 mm Hg, respectively, in the general population [13]. There is evidence that endurance training, but no other types of training, induces a greater BP reduction in hypertensive individuals (8.3/5.2 mm Hg). Physical activity of lower intensity and duration performed on a regular basis not only is associated with a smaller BP reduction than with

Table 22.1 Classification of physical activity[a]

Absolute intensity			Relative intensity		
Intensity	MET	Examples	$\%HR_{max}$	RPE (Borg scale score)	Talk test
Light	1.1–2.9	Walking <4.7 km/h, light household work	57–63	10–11	
Moderate	3–5.9	Walking with moderate or brisk pace (4.1–6.5 km/h), slow cycling (15 km/h), painting/decorating, vacuuming, gardening (mowing lawn), golf (pulling clubs in trolley), tennis (doubles), ballroom dancing, water aerobics	64–76	12–13	Breathing is faster but compatible with speaking full sentences
Vigorous	≥6	Race-walking, jogging or running, cycling >15 km/h, heavy gardening (continuous digging or hoeing), swimming laps, tennis (single)	77–95	14–17	Breathing very hard, incompatible with carrying on a conversation comfortably

%HRmax percentage of measured or estimated maximum heart rate (220-age), *MET* metabolic equivalent, O_2 oxygen, *PA* physical activity, *RPE* rating of perceived exertion (Borg scale 6–20), *VO2* oxygen consumption

MET is estimated as the energy cost of a given activity divided by resting energy expenditure: 1 MET = 3.5 ml O_2 kg^{-1} min^{-1} VO_2

[a]Modified from Howley [11]

moderate- or high-intensity training but also is associated with a substantial decrease in mortality [14, 15]. The 2018 ESC/ESH guidelines recommend at least 30 min of moderate intensity dynamic aerobic exercise (walking, jogging, cycling, or swimming) 5–7 days per week [16].

The American Diabetes Association (ADA) guidelines suggest that most adults with type 1 and type 2 diabetes should engage in 150 min or more of physical activity of moderate to vigorous intensity spread over at least 3 days per week, with no more than two consecutive days without activity. Younger and more physically fit individuals may have exercise sessions of more vigorous intensity or interval training with a minimum duration of 75 min per week [3].

Both sets of guidelines suggest two to three sessions per week of resistance exercise on nonconsecutive days.

A careful assessment of patient history, focusing on CV risk factors, should be performed prior to initiating physical activity in diabetic patients. Following the ADA consensus report, "Screening for Coronary Artery Disease in Patients with Diabetes" [17], routine testing is not needed. However, physicians should be aware of possible atypical presentation of coronary artery disease such as a decrease in exercise tolerance.

There is rather new evidence that all individuals including those with diabetes should be advised to reduce sedentary activities such as sitting at a computer or watching TV, or at least disrupt these practices every 30 min by standing up, walking, or performing light physical activities (e.g., stretching) [18, 19]. The avoidance of extended sedentary periods may improve glycemic control or prevent type 2 diabetes in at risk individuals.

22.4 Sodium Intake Reduction

Dietary sodium restriction has been shown to have a BP lowering effect. A meta-analysis of trials showed that a reduction of ~1.75 g sodium per day (4.4 g salt/day) was associated with a mean BP reduction of 4.2/2.1 mm Hg, more pronounced in hypertensive individuals [20]. The beneficial effect of reduced sodium intake on BP tends to diminish with time, partly due to poor adherence to a low-sodium diet. There is a greater BP lowering effect of sodium restriction in individuals of Afro-Caribbean descent, in the elderly, and in patients with diabetes, metabolic syndrome, or chronic kidney disease [21]. In drug-treated hypertensive patients, sodium restriction may reduce the number of drugs and improve BP control [22, 23].

There are huge differences in sodium intake between countries and even within countries ranging from 3.5 to 5.5 g/day, corresponding to 9–12 g of salt/day. The ADA guidelines recommend a ˂2300 mg/day sodium intake for diabetic patients with hypertension, which is the same as for the general population [24]. The 2018 European guidelines on hypertension are stricter, recommending a sodium intake of less than 2 g/day (the equivalent of 5 g of salt/day) [16]. Sodium restriction below 1500 g is not recommended [25–27]. It should be emphasized that 80% of salt consumption is in processed foods; therefore, the sodium restriction can only be achieved by a joint effort between the food industry, governments, and the public. Indeed, high-sodium foods and using additional salt should be avoided.

22.5 Increased Consumption of Fruits and Vegetables

The ADA guidelines suggest an increased consumption of fruit and vegetables (8–10 servings per day) [3]. This can be achieved by a Dietary Approaches to Stop Hypertension (DASH), style eating pattern [28], which has been shown to decrease BP in nondiabetic hypertensive patients [29]. While rich in fruits, vegetables, and lean proteins, it restricts red meat, salt, added sugars, and fat. In the original landmark clinical trial, a "combination diet" rich in fruits, vegetables, and low-fat dairy products and with reduced saturated and total fat induced a greater BP reduction than the diet rich only in fruits and vegetables (5.5/3.0 vs. 2.8/1.1 mm Hg) [29].

Despite the number of studies using the DASH eating plan in diabetes being limited [30–33], all show a significant BP reduction. In a well-designed crossover clinical trial in 31 type 2 diabetic patients, the DASH diet, in addition to decreasing BP, improved lipids and hemoglobin A1C (Hb A1c) [31]. Further research evaluating the effects of the DASH diet in diabetes is needed [34].

Some examples of daily and weekly servings of the DASH eating plan are given in Table 22.2.

Table 22.2 Examples of daily/weekly servings meeting DASH targets for a 2000 calorie eating plan

Food group	Daily/weekly recommended servings	Serving size definition
Grains and grain products	7–8	1 slice bread 1 cup (240 ml) ready-to-eat cereal 1/2 cup (120 ml) cooked rice, pasta, or cereal
Lean meats, poultry, and fish	≤2	3 oz (85 g) cooked lean meat, skinless poultry, or fish
Vegetables	4–5	1 cup (240 ml) raw leafy vegetable 1/2 cup (120 ml) cooked vegetable 6 oz (177 ml) vegetable juice
Fruit	4–5	1 medium piece of fruit 1/4 cup (60 ml) dried fruit 1/2 cup (120 ml) fresh, frozen, or canned fruit 6 oz (177 ml) fruit juice
Low-fat or fat-free dairy foods	2–3	8 oz (237 ml) milk 1 cup (240 ml) yogurt 1 1/2 oz (42 g) cheese
Nuts, seeds, and dry beans	4–5 per week	1/3 cup (80 ml) or 1 1/2 oz (42 g) nuts 1 Tbsp. or 1/2 oz (14 g) seeds 1/2 cup (120 ml) cooked dry beans
Fats and oils†	2–3	1 tsp. soft margarine 1 tsp. low-fat mayonnaise 1 Tbsp. regular salad dressing 2 Tbsp. light salad dressing 1 tsp. vegetable oil
Sweets	≤5 per week	1 Tbsp. sugar 1 Tbsp. jelly or jam 1/2 oz (14 g) jelly beans 8 oz (237 ml) lemonade
Sodium	<2300 mg	Total from prepared/packaged foods and added during cooking or at the table

Tbsp. tablespoon, *tsp.* teaspoon
Adapted from Ref. [32]

22.6 Avoiding Excessive Alcohol Consumption

There is a well-established linear association between alcohol consumption, BP, the prevalence of hypertension, and CVD risk [35]. Binge drinking has a strong BP increasing effect. Mendelian randomization studies do not support the previously believed beneficial effect of moderate alcohol consumption, suggesting that the lowest CVD risk is in nondrinkers [36, 37]. Alcohol consumption also increases BMI and glycemia, particularly in those consuming excessive amounts [38].

Alcohol consumption may also induce hypoglycemia, particularly in those treated with insulin or insulin secretagogue therapies [39].

The Prevention and Treatment of Hypertension Study (PATHS) examined the effects of alcohol reduction on BP, finding a small BP decrease (1.2/0.7 mm Hg) in the intervention group after 6 months [40].

Diabetic patients with hypertension should reduce their alcohol consumption to 14 units per week for men and eight units for women, with some alcohol-free days during the week and the avoidance of binge drinking [16].

22.7 Smoking Cessation

Smoking cessation is probably the single most effective lifestyle measure in the prevention of CVD, with a substantial reduction of recurrent myocardial infarction or death [41, 42]. For heavy smokers (≥20 cigarettes/day), stopping tobacco use is associated with significant CVD risk reduction within 5 years; however, it remains higher than in nonsmokers [42]. Ambulatory BP monitoring studies have shown that hypertensive smokers have higher daily BP values than nonsmokers [43]. However, no chronic effect of smoking has been found for office BP, as most smokers don't smoke 30–60 min prior to visiting a doctor, thus ameliorating the BP increasing effect of smoking [44].

The history of tobacco use should be reviewed at each patient visit. Nicotine dependence, which is associated with difficulty in quitting and relapse, should also be assessed [45]. Brief advice from a physician has a small but significant effect on increasing smoking cessation rates [46]. This could be further enhanced by nicotine replacement therapy. Pharmacotherapy (varenicline or bupropion), combined with behavioral support, may substantially increase the chance of successfully quitting smoking [47]. There are no convincing studies demonstrating that e-cigarettes are a healthier alternative to smoking or that they can assist in smoking cessation [48–50]. Recent evidence indicates that e-cigarettes are likely to be more effective than nicotine replacement therapy in quitting smoking [51–53], however, e-cigarettes are addictive.

Voulgari et al. found in smokers with newly diagnosed type 2 diabetes that smoking cessation was associated with an improvement of metabolic parameters, a reduction of BP, and urinary albumin excretion after 1 year [54].

Regardless of any possible minor weight gain following smoking cessation, the overall beneficial effect is well demonstrated [55].

22.8 Conclusions

Lifestyle changes should be recommended to any diabetic patient with high-normal BP (130–139/85–89 mm Hg) or hypertension. The American guidelines suggest initiating lifestyle modification in individuals with BP > 120/80 mm Hg [24]. Both the American and European guidelines agree on initiating drug treatment in diabetic patients with BP ≥ 140/90 mm Hg, meaning antihypertensive medication should not be delayed when lifestyle measures are ineffective.

The 1998 National Health Interview Survey showed that in diabetic patients with hypertension, physicians´ advice to lose weight, and to take antihypertension medication is effective in modifying hypertension-related lifestyle, regardless of sex or ethnicity [56]. Advice to increase physical activity seemed to be less effective.

References

1. Konzem SL, Devore VS, Bauer DW. Controlling hypertension in patients with diabetes. Am Fam Physician. 2002;66(7):1209–14.
2. Gong Q, Zhang P, Wang J, Ma J, An Y, Chen Y, et al. Morbidity and mortality after lifestyle intervention for people with impaired glucose tolerance: 30-year results of the Da Qing diabetes prevention outcome study. Lancet Diabetes Endocrinol. 2019;7(6):452–61.
3. American Diabetes Association. 5. Facilitating behavior change and well-being to improve health outcomes: standards of medical care in diabetes-2021. Diabetes Care. 2021;44(Suppl 1):S53–72.
4. Stevens VJ, Obarzanek E, Cook NR, Lee IM, Appel LJ, Smith West D, et al. Long-term weight loss and changes in blood pressure: results of the trials of hypertension prevention, phase II. Ann Intern Med. 2001;134(1):1–11.
5. Wing RR. Long-term effects of a lifestyle intervention on weight and cardiovascular risk factors in individuals with type 2 diabetes mellitus: four-year results of the look AHEAD trial. Arch Intern Med. 2010;170(17):1566–75.
6. Lean ME, Leslie WS, Barnes AC, Brosnahan N, Thom G, McCombie L, et al. Primary care-led weight management for remission of type 2 diabetes (DiRECT): an open-label, cluster-randomised trial. Lancet. 2018;391(10120):541–51.
7. Lean MEJ, Leslie WS, Barnes AC, Brosnahan N, Thom G, McCombie L, et al. Durability of a primary care-led weight-management intervention for remission of type 2 diabetes: 2-year results of the DiRECT open-label, cluster-randomised trial. Lancet Diabetes Endocrinol. 2019;7(5):344–55.
8. Jensen MD, Ryan DH, Apovian CM, Ard JD, Comuzzie AG, Donato KA, et al. 2013 AHA/ACC/TOS guideline for the management of overweight and obesity in adults: a report of the American College of Cardiology/American Heart Association Task Force on Practice Guidelines and The Obesity Society. J Am Coll Cardiol. 2014;63(25 Pt B):2985–3023.
9. Franz MJ, Boucher JL, Rutten-Ramos S, VanWormer JJ. Lifestyle weight-loss intervention outcomes in overweight and obese adults with type 2 diabetes: a systematic review and meta-analysis of randomized clinical trials. J Acad Nutr Diet. 2015;115(9):1447–63.
10. Leung CW, Epel ES, Ritchie LD, Crawford PB, Laraia BA. Food insecurity is inversely associated with diet quality of lower-income adults. J Acad Nutr Diet. 2014;114(12):1943–53.e2.
11. Howley ET. Type of activity: resistance, aerobic and leisure versus occupational physical activity. Med Sci Sports Exerc. 2001;33(6 Suppl):S364–9; discussion S419–20.
12. Pescatello LS, Franklin BA, Fagard R, Farquhar WB, Kelley GA, Ray CA. American college of sports medicine position stand. Exercise and hypertension. Med Sci Sports Exerc. 2004;36(3):533–53.

13. Cornelissen VA, Smart NA. Exercise training for blood pressure: a systematic review and meta-analysis. J Am Heart Assoc. 2013;2(1):e004473.
14. Leitzmann MF, Park Y, Blair A, Ballard-Barbash R, Mouw T, Hollenbeck AR, et al. Physical activity recommendations and decreased risk of mortality. Arch Intern Med. 2007;167(22):2453–60.
15. Rossi A, Dikareva A, Bacon SL, Daskalopoulou SS. The impact of physical activity on mortality in patients with high blood pressure: a systematic review. J Hypertens. 2012;30(7):1277–88.
16. Williams B, Mancia G, Spiering W, Agabiti Rosei E, Azizi M, Burnier M, et al. 2018 ESC/ESH Guidelines for the management of arterial hypertension: The Task Force for the management of arterial hypertension of the European Society of Cardiology and the European Society of Hypertension: The Task Force for the management of arterial hypertension of the European Society of Cardiology and the European Society of Hypertension. J Hypertens. 2018;36(10):1953–2041.
17. Bax JJ, Young LH, Frye RL, Bonow RO, Steinberg HO, Barrett EJ. Screening for coronary artery disease in patients with diabetes. Diabetes Care. 2007;30(10):2729–36.
18. Katzmarzyk PT, Church TS, Craig CL, Bouchard C. Sitting time and mortality from all causes, cardiovascular disease, and cancer. Med Sci Sports Exerc. 2009;41(5):998–1005.
19. Dempsey PC, Larsen RN, Sethi P, Sacre JW, Straznicky NE, Cohen ND, et al. Benefits for type 2 diabetes of interrupting prolonged sitting with brief bouts of light walking or simple resistance activities. Diabetes Care. 2016;39(6):964–72.
20. He FJ, Li J, Macgregor GA. Effect of longer-term modest salt reduction on blood pressure. Cochrane Database Syst Rev. 2013;(4):Cd004937.
21. Suckling RJ, He FJ, Markandu ND, MacGregor GA. Modest salt reduction lowers blood pressure and albumin excretion in impaired glucose tolerance and type 2 diabetes mellitus: a randomized double-blind trial. Hypertension. 2016;67(6):1189–95.
22. Graudal NA, Hubeck-Graudal T, Jürgens G. Effects of low-sodium diet vs. high-sodium diet on blood pressure, renin, aldosterone, catecholamines, cholesterol, and triglyceride (Cochrane review). Am J Hypertens. 2012;25(1):1–15.
23. He FJ, MacGregor GA. How far should salt intake be reduced? Hypertension. 2003;42(6):1093–9.
24. American Diabetes Association. 10. Cardiovascular disease and risk management: standards of medical care in diabetes-2021. Diabetes Care. 2021;44(Suppl 1):S125–50.
25. Thomas MC, Moran J, Forsblom C, Harjutsalo V, Thorn L, Ahola A, et al. The association between dietary sodium intake, ESRD, and all-cause mortality in patients with type 1 diabetes. Diabetes Care. 2011;34(4):861–6.
26. Ekinci EI, Clarke S, Thomas MC, Moran JL, Cheong K, MacIsaac RJ, et al. Dietary salt intake and mortality in patients with type 2 diabetes. Diabetes Care. 2011;34(3):703–9.
27. Lennon SL, DellaValle DM, Rodder SG, Prest M, Sinley RC, Hoy MK, et al. 2015 evidence analysis library evidence-based nutrition practice guideline for the management of hypertension in adults. J Acad Nutr Diet. 2017;117(9):1445–58.e17.
28. Campbell AP. DASH eating plan: an eating pattern for diabetes management. Diabetes Spectr. 2017;30(2):76–81.
29. Appel LJ, Moore TJ, Obarzanek E, Vollmer WM, Svetkey LP, Sacks FM, et al. A clinical trial of the effects of dietary patterns on blood pressure. DASH collaborative research group. N Engl J Med. 1997;336(16):1117–24.
30. Paula TP, Viana LV, Neto AT, Leitão CB, Gross JL, Azevedo MJ. Effects of the DASH diet and walking on blood pressure in patients with type 2 diabetes and uncontrolled hypertension: a randomized controlled trial. J Clin Hypertens (Greenwich). 2015;17(11):895–901.
31. Azadbakht L, Fard NR, Karimi M, Baghaei MH, Surkan PJ, Rahimi M, et al. Effects of the dietary approaches to stop hypertension (DASH) eating plan on cardiovascular risks among type 2 diabetic patients: a randomized crossover clinical trial. Diabetes Care. 2011;34(1):55–7.
32. de Paula TP, Steemburgo T, de Almeida JC, Dall'Alba V, Gross JL, de Azevedo MJ. The role of dietary approaches to stop hypertension (DASH) diet food groups in blood pressure in type 2 diabetes. Br J Nutr. 2012;108(1):155–62.

33. Hashemi R, Rahimlou M, Baghdadian S, Manafi M. Investigating the effect of DASH diet on blood pressure of patients with type 2 diabetes and prehypertension: randomized clinical trial. Diabetes Metab Syndr. 2019;13(1):1–4.
34. Tseng E, Appel LJ, Yeh HC, Pilla SJ, Miller ER, Juraschek SP, et al. Effects of the dietary approaches to stop hypertension diet and sodium reduction on blood pressure in persons with diabetes. Hypertension. 2021;77(2):265–74.
35. Wood AM, Kaptoge S, Butterworth AS, Willeit P, Warnakula S, Bolton T, et al. Risk thresholds for alcohol consumption: combined analysis of individual-participant data for 599 912 current drinkers in 83 prospective studies. Lancet. 2018;391(10129):1513–23.
36. Millwood IY, Walters RG, Mei XW, Guo Y, Yang L, Bian Z, et al. Conventional and genetic evidence on alcohol and vascular disease aetiology: a prospective study of 500 000 men and women in China. Lancet. 2019;393(10183):1831–42.
37. Holmes MV, Dale CE, Zuccolo L, Silverwood RJ, Guo Y, Ye Z, et al. Association between alcohol and cardiovascular disease: Mendelian randomisation analysis based on individual participant data. BMJ. 2014;349:g4164.
38. Mozaffarian D. Dietary and policy priorities for cardiovascular disease, diabetes, and obesity: a comprehensive review. Circulation. 2016;133(2):187–225.
39. Evert AB, Dennison M, Gardner CD, Garvey WT, Lau KHK, MacLeod J, et al. Nutrition therapy for adults with diabetes or prediabetes: a consensus report. Diabetes Care. 2019;42(5):731–54.
40. Cushman WC, Cutler JA, Hanna E, Bingham SF, Follmann D, Harford T, et al. Prevention and treatment of hypertension study (PATHS): effects of an alcohol treatment program on blood pressure. Arch Intern Med. 1998;158(11):1197–207.
41. Critchley JA, Capewell S. Mortality risk reduction associated with smoking cessation in patients with coronary heart disease: a systematic review. JAMA. 2003;290(1):86–97.
42. Anthonisen NR, Skeans MA, Wise RA, Manfreda J, Kanner RE, Connett JE. The effects of a smoking cessation intervention on 14.5-year mortality: a randomized clinical trial. Ann Intern Med. 2005;142(4):233–9.
43. Groppelli A, Giorgi DM, Omboni S, Parati G, Mancia G. Persistent blood pressure increase induced by heavy smoking. J Hypertens. 1992;10(5):495–9.
44. Primatesta P, Falaschetti E, Gupta S, Marmot MG, Poulter NR. Association between smoking and blood pressure: evidence from the health survey for England. Hypertension. 2001;37(2):187–93.
45. Ranney L, Melvin C, Lux L, McClain E, Lohr KN. Systematic review: smoking cessation intervention strategies for adults and adults in special populations. Ann Intern Med. 2006;145(11):845–56.
46. Stead LF, Buitrago D, Preciado N, Sanchez G, Hartmann-Boyce J, Lancaster T. Physician advice for smoking cessation. Cochrane Database Syst Rev. 2013;2013(5):Cd000165.
47. Stead LF, Koilpillai P, Fanshawe TR, Lancaster T. Combined pharmacotherapy and behavioural interventions for smoking cessation. Cochrane Database Syst Rev. 2016;3:Cd008286.
48. Bam TS, Bellew W, Berezhnova I, Jackson-Morris A, Jones A, Latif E, et al. Position statement on electronic cigarettes or electronic nicotine delivery systems. Int J Tuberc Lung Dis. 2014;18(1):5–7.
49. Bhatnagar A, Whitsel LP, Ribisl KM, Bullen C, Chaloupka F, Piano MR, et al. Electronic cigarettes: a policy statement from the American Heart Association. Circulation. 2014;130(16):1418–36.
50. Young-Hyman D, de Groot M, Hill-Briggs F, Gonzalez JS, Hood K, Peyrot M. Psychosocial care for people with diabetes: a position statement of the American Diabetes Association. Diabetes Care. 2016;39(12):2126–40.
51. Hartmann-Boyce J, McRobbie H, Lindson N, Bullen C, Begh R, Theodoulou A, et al. Electronic cigarettes for smoking cessation. Cochrane Database Syst Rev. 2020;10:Cd010216.
52. Hajek P, Phillips-Waller A, Przulj D, Pesola F, Myers Smith K, Bisal N, et al. A randomized trial of E-cigarettes versus nicotine-replacement therapy. N Engl J Med. 2019;380(7):629–37.

53. Li J, Hajek P, Pesola F, Wu Q, Phillips-Waller A, Przulj D, et al. Cost-effectiveness of e-cigarettes compared with nicotine replacement therapy in stop smoking services in England (TEC study): a randomized controlled trial. Addiction. 2020;115(3):507–17.
54. Voulgari C, Katsilambros N, Tentolouris N. Smoking cessation predicts amelioration of microalbuminuria in newly diagnosed type 2 diabetes mellitus: a 1-year prospective study. Metabolism. 2011;60(10):1456–64.
55. Clair C, Rigotti NA, Porneala B, Fox CS, D'Agostino RB, Pencina MJ, et al. Association of smoking cessation and weight change with cardiovascular disease among adults with and without diabetes. JAMA. 2013;309(10):1014–21.
56. Egede LE. Lifestyle modification to improve blood pressure control in individuals with diabetes: is physician advice effective? Diabetes Care. 2003;26(3):602–7.

Blood Pressure Thresholds for Initiation of Drug Treatment: Blood Pressure Targets in Diabetes

23

Omar Al Dhaybi and George L. Bakris

23.1 Introduction

Despite advancing therapeutics, diabetes mellitus (DM) continues to be an increasing global health problem. Its prevalence is increasing worldwide due to population aging, obesity epidemic, physical inactivity, and changing lifestyle/food consumption patterns in the setting of rapid urbanization [1, 2]. DM remains the leading cause of chronic kidney disease (CKD) and End-Stage Renal Disease (ESRD) in the Western Hemisphere [3]. Conversely, hypertension is the single most important modifiable risk factor that leads to renal failure and cardiovascular (CV) disease in patients with type 2 diabetes [4–7].

The pathophysiology of hypertension in diabetes is complicated, with multiple intricate and intersecting pathways. In brief, the two paramount factors are increased arterial stiffness leading, in turn, to reduced nitric oxide release and increased sympathetic tone and interstitial volume expansion. Furthermore, in persons with diabetes, the glomerulus is especially susceptible to barotrauma inflicted by systemic arterial hypertension due to its portal nature [8]. The UKPDS trial was the first to establish the benefits of lowering blood pressure (BP) on microvascular and macrovascular outcomes in diabetic patients [9]. How low should we go poses much less controversy today than it did in previous years? This chapter discusses the thresholds for BP treatment initiation and focuses on the range of BP to achieve to reduce both renal and CV risk.

O. Al Dhaybi · G. L. Bakris (✉)
Department of Medicine, Am. Heart Assoc. Comprehensive Hypertension Center, University of Chicago Medicine, Chicago, IL, USA
e-mail: gbakris@uchicago.edu

A. E. Berbari, G. Mancia (eds.), *Blood Pressure Disorders in Diabetes Mellitus*, Updates in Hypertension and Cardiovascular Protection,
https://doi.org/10.1007/978-3-031-13009-0_23

23.2 Review of Data on Blood Pressure Targets

Hypertension in all adults was redefined in 2017 by the American College of Cardiology/American Heart Association (ACC/AHA) Blood Pressure Guidelines to >130/80 mm Hg for all adults with >10% CV risk [10]. This change in the definition of hypertension has raised the estimated prevalence of hypertension from 39.1%, as per the Seventh Report of the Joint National Committee (JNC7), to 43.6%, which is the equivalent of 103 million adults in the United States (US), or roughly 1.8 billion persons worldwide with hypertension [11]. No other guidelines worldwide followed this guidance except for the Canadian guidelines, which stressed that those at higher CV risk, such as those with diabetes, start treatment when BP is >130/80 mmHg [12].

The European, Latin American, and Canadian guidelines did not follow the American lead. Still, they stress the importance of the lower threshold of 130/80 mm Hg in individuals at higher CV risk, including those with diabetes [5, 13–15]. In short, all hypertension guidelines from around the world, including the American Diabetes Association, recommend a BP goal <130/80 mm Hg for all those with diabetes; however, pharmacologic treatment by most guidelines is recommended to start at 140/90 mmHg.

Data for these recommendations date back to the UKPDS and subsequent trials [6, 9], along with observational data, and is incorporated in the most recent American Diabetes Association Guidelines of 2021 [16]. In concert with this, a review of treatment guidelines integrating all this information and data from nonpharmacological trials offers an approach similar to what is put forth by the American Diabetes Association [17].

In contrast, there have only been three prospective randomized controlled trials to date. All failed to demonstrate a benefit of a lower BP on their primary analysis, which was reduced CV events with intensive BP reduction (Table 23.1). The oldest of the three is the UKPDS study, which evaluated the effect of different BP levels on CV outcomes in patients with Type 2 DM [9]. This landmark trial demonstrated that BP control below 150/85 mmHg with captopril or atenolol was associated with a 34% risk reduction in risk of developing macrovascular disease (myocardial infarction (MI), sudden death, and stroke) and, additionally, a 37% risk reduction in the risk of microvascular disease (retinopathy and microalbuminuria). Intensive BP control did not reduce the incidence of MI, nor all-cause mortality, albeit it did

Table 23.1 Achieved BP values in prospective diabetes outcome clinical trials after 2000. Two of the three did NOT show significant reduction in combined CV events in intensive group when below 140 mmHg systolic

Clinical outcome trial	Achieved level of systolic BP (mmHg)
ACCORD (primary)	119 (intensive); 133 (conventional)
UKPDS (primary)	144 (intensive); 154 (conventional)
J-DOIT 3 (primary)	122 (intensive); 129 (conventional)

improve many outcomes related to diabetes. It is noteworthy that the level of BP achieved in the intensive group far exceeded the currently established society guidances. The UKPDS study confirmed the benefits of BP control in DM and demonstrated that it is as necessary as glucose control in preventing complications from diabetes [9].

The Action to Control Cardiovascular Risk in Diabetes (ACCORD) trial was a landmark trial that evaluated the effects of intensive BP reduction on CV outcomes in its BP trial component in a randomized prospective fashion. It is the largest long-term follow-up study evaluating the effects of BP reduction on CV outcomes in diabetes [18]. There were 4733 high risk CV patients (10-year CV > 15%) with type 2 DM randomized to intensive BP control (systolic BP (SBP) < 120 mm Hg) versus standard control (SBP < 140 mm Hg). Patients in the intensive BP control arm achieved an SBP of 119 mm Hg, compared with 133 mm Hg in the standard control group. After an average of 4.7 years of follow-up, there were no differences in CV events' primary composite outcome (nonfatal MI, nonfatal stroke, and death from CV causes), HR = 0.88 (95% CI: 0.73–1.06, $p = 0.2$) between the two groups.

Furthermore, CV mortality and all-cause mortality were similar in both groups. The incidence of strokes was significantly reduced with intensive therapy (HR = 0.59, 95% CI:0.39–0.89, $p = 0.01$). However, serious adverse events such as hypotension, syncope, bradycardia/arrhythmias, or hyperkalemia occurred at higher rates with intensive therapy (3.3% versus 1.3%, $p < 0.001$). Moreover, kidney function deterioration was significantly more frequent with intensive treatment ($p < 0.001$) [18]. Hence, at first sight, the ACCORD-BP trial indicated that intensive BP control in people with type 2 diabetes was associated with a more significant nephropathy progression in the medium term.

One should consider the fact that patients were randomized in a 2 by 2 factorial design to intensive versus standard glycemic control; this is important because the premature termination of the ACCORD glycemia study (due to the higher mortality in the intensive glucose control arm) may have led to a loss of power in the original well-powered target BP assessment group, thus complicating the primary BP outcome analyses. Also, the target of SBP < 120 mm Hg in the intensive treatment group was a step further than what existing guidelines recommend (SBP target < 130 mm Hg). Finally, the achieved BP of 133 mm Hg in the standard group was close to clinicians' BPs in the real world. However, outside of the controlled settings of trials, nonadherence, and dietary indiscretions are the norm. Those with blood pressures in the 130 s systolic may have dissipated any tangible between-group differences in outcomes.

Most outcomes in ACCORD are tilted toward the intensive group, despite not achieving statistical significance. Having a high event rate could have tipped the results in favor of the intensive study group. Henceforth, one cannot objectively say that ACCORD BP provided any definitive answers to the BP target question. This observation is further exemplified in a post hoc analysis of people randomized in ACCORD, by Buckley et al. called "ACCORDION" [19]. In this analysis, ACCORD-BP patients from the standard glycemic arm and who had CKD established CV disease or high CV risk (≥ 15% 10-year risk) or who were older than 74 years were followed for an average of 9 years. The composite outcome of CV mortality, nonfatal MI/strokes, decreased by 25% in the intensive BP control arm (HR = 0.75, 95% CI: 0.60–0.95, $p = 0.02$). Lower rates of nonfatal MI mainly drove this.

Finally, the Intensified Multifactorial Intervention on Cardiovascular Outcomes and Mortality in type 2 Diabetes (J-DOIT 3) also failed to demonstrate tangible benefits with intensive BP reduction in diabetics [20]. The study randomized 2540 patients with type 2 diabetes to intensive versus standard BP reduction. BP achieved in the intensive group was 123/71 mm Hg, whereas that achieved in the standard group was 129/74 mm Hg, which was below 130 mm Hg and which may have hindered the analyses results since the study did not show a reduction of the composite of MI, stroke, revascularization, and all-cause mortality with intensive BP reduction. Nonetheless, the secondary endpoint of the composite of MI, stroke, and all-cause mortality approached statistical significance, with a risk reduction of 26% with intensive therapy (HR = 0.74, 95% CI: 0.54–1.01, $p = 0.055$) [20].

Despite these negative prospective studies, three recent meta-analyses show clear benefit on CV events with aggressive BP reduction to <130 mm Hg systolic compared with the standard range above 130 mmHg [21–23]. The meta-analysis by Ettehad et al. revealed a 13% decline in mortality and significant CV benefits for each 10 mm Hg BP reduction in pooled data from 123 studies with ≥600,000 patients, even at levels <130 mm Hg [22].

23.3 Nuanced Approach to BP Management: In Search of the "Sweet Spot"

The RENAAL and IDNT trials, while not blood pressure trials, were landmark studies that ushered a new era in the management of diabetic nephropathy in the twenty-first century. In RENAAL, patients with diabetic nephropathy (albumin/creatinine ratio ≥ 300 mg/g) were randomized to losartan versus placebo and followed for a mean of 3.4 years [24, 25]. In RENAAL, losartan therapy reduced the risk of the primary composite outcome of doubling serum creatinine, ESRD, or death by 16% when compared with placebo ($p = 0.02$). Losartan reduced the incidence of doubling of serum creatinine by 25% ($p = 0.006$) and ESRD by 28% ($p = 0.002$), results extrapolating to a 2-year delay in dialysis initiation. While BP was reduced by about 3 mm Hg systolic over placebo, the benefits were independent of the magnitude of BP reduction, as ascertained by dedicated analyses. BP achieved at the end of the study was 140/74 mm Hg in the losartan group, as compared with 142/74 mm Hg in the placebo group [26].

The IDNT trial went a step further when it compared the effect of Irbesartan on renal outcomes with those of amlodipine, giving the results further validation when it comes to the independence from BP lowering effects [25]. The risk of doubling of serum creatinine was 37% lower in the Irbesartan group ($p < 0.001$), and Irbesartan therapy reduced the risk of the composite primary outcome of doubling serum

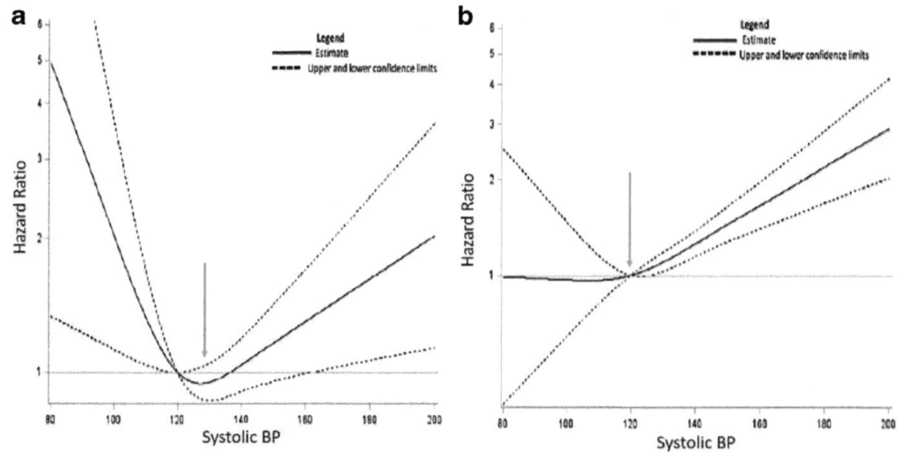

Fig. 23.1 Achieved BP values in prospective diabetes outcome clinical trials after 2000. These are randomized prospective outcome trials evaluating different levels of blood pressure on cardiovascular and to a much lesser extent renal outcomes in diabetes. Two of the three did NOT show significant reduction in combined CV events in intensive group when below 140 mmHg systolic. Due to issues with recruitment a post hoc analysis of the BP data from ACCORD did show a reduced CV event rate in the group randomized to lower BP [45] (**a**) Increment of risk to develop Acute Myocardial Infarction, Stroke, Peripheral Vascular Disease and All-cause mortality events and all-cause mortality in presence of HTN (gray light) as compared with T2DM without HTN (gray dark) (see text). (**b**) Increment of risk to develop Chronic Kidney Disease, Atrial fibrillation and Heart Failure in presence of HTN (gray light) as compared with T2DM without HTN (gray dark) (see text)

creatinine, ESRD, or death by 23% compared with amlodipine ($p = 0.006$). Again, those benefits were independent of BP reduction. Mean BP achieved in the Irbesartan arm was 140/77 mm Hg, compared with 141/77 mm Hg in the amlodipine group [27], both above any current or previous guideline goals.

A post hoc analysis of IDNT showed that the best renal outcomes were attained in patients who achieved an SBP < 134 mm Hg, as only 17% of those reached renal endpoints at the end of follow-up (compared with 32.6% in the Irbesartan group who reached the primary renal outcome in IDNT). The effects of Irbesartan and BP-lowering were independent and synergistic ($p = 0.61$ for interaction). Patients who achieved SBP < 120 mm Hg conversely had increased mortality and a greater risk of renal disease progression [28]. The signal that emanates from these studies is that a SBP target <134 mm Hg seems optimal, given it is tolerated, and SBP remains >120 mm Hg. Those findings were reinforced in an analysis of NHANES III/DHS patient cohorts. Investigators demonstrated that CV mortality and SBP had a U-shaped association in type 2 diabetes patients. The mortality nadir occurred at a BP of 120–135 mm Hg, and the mortality rate increased exponentially at an SBP < 120 mm Hg and linearly at an SBP > 135 mm Hg (Fig. 23.1). Conversely, CV mortality and SBP had J-shaped relationship in nondiabetics, with the lowest CV risk extending down to 110 mm Hg systolic [29].

23.4 Diastolic Blood Pressure: Is It Important?

Diastolic BP (DBP) has been somewhat in the "background" ever since the Franklin analyses, which showed that SBP mainly determines CV outcomes in individuals older than 50 years [30]. In the post hoc IDNT analysis, DBP lowering was not associated with improved renal outcomes, even when DBP exceeded 100 mm Hg at baseline [28]. Extrapolating from the studies mentioned earlier, the J-curve phenomenon, where intensive SBP lowering can lead to worse CV outcomes due to excessive DBP lowering, holds truth in diabetic patients, but not as much in nondiabetics. In the overall scheme of things, we know that DBP lowering below 60 mm Hg can lead to cardiac ischemia in patients with disturbed coronary autoregulatory flow reserves in the setting of advanced atherosclerotic disease and marked vascular stiffness.

A DBP < 60 mm Hg at baseline was independently associated with progressive myocardial ischemia in patients from the Atherosclerosis Risk in Communities (ARiC) cohort of 11,565 adults followed over 6 years. Also, a DBP < 60 mm Hg was independently associated with incident coronary disease and mortality compared with a DBP of 80–89 mm Hg, but not with stroke [31]. Patients with DM, especially those with concomitant diabetic nephropathy and CKD, have increased arterial stiffness, which only worsens as they get older. Henceforth, those who have DBP < 60 mm Hg have more advanced atherosclerosis and are at greater risk of cardiovascular events with more aggressive BP lowering, especially when the concomitant pulse pressure is increased [32].

In a post hoc analysis of 4731 ACCORD BP patients, Ilkun and colleagues showed that baseline DBP did not influence the effect of intensive SBP control on cardiovascular outcomes. Nonetheless, despite robust analytical methods, the authors chose a DBP of 70 mm Hg as cutoff, both in linear and categorical modeling, which exceeds the 60 mm Hg cutoff believed to trigger nefarious cardiac outcomes [33].

Another post hoc analysis of the Systolic Blood Pressure Intervention Trial (SPRINT) showed that the effect of intensive SBP reduction on CV outcomes was not affected by baseline DBP, albeit there was a discernible U-shaped association between the risk of primary CV outcomes and baseline DBP [34].

Thus, the available evidence regarding CV outcomes and the J/U curves is derived from observational studies and post analyses of outcome trials. These analyses are typically not powered to detect the studied primary effect post hoc. Those observations are of great practical interest. However, they cannot define BP goals for patients with diabetes without confirmation from randomized trials.

23.5 Barriers to Achieving the Desired Blood Pressure Targets

Many barriers hinder the ability to reduce BP to the desired levels. One modifiable factor is the infrequent use of combination pills, which is proven to improve medication adherence and outcomes. The average number of antihypertensive medications in a patient with diabetic kidney disease and controlled BP is 2.7 medications

[35, 36]. This average increases to 3.3 medicines in patients with stage 3 or greater CKD [37]. Using single combined pills improves patient compliance and lowers the number of daily pills [38]. The RAS blocker/CCB combination is superior in reducing CV and renal events in high-risk patients in the ACCOMPLISH trial and can be a good starting point [39, 40].

A significant hindrance to using single-pill combinations remains the widespread reflex among physicians to hold or stop RAS blockers at the advent of serum creatinine increases, which is a common occurrence. Creatinine increases in patients with diabetic kidney disease, and uncontrolled hypertension is a given once their BP is under control and associated with improved long-term renal outcomes [41–43]. The creatinine bump mentioned earlier is mostly hemodynamic in >90% of cases, as ascertained by analyses from SPRINT [44]. GFR decreases of up to 46% in the acute setting were not associated with adverse long-term outcomes in post hoc analyses of ACCORD and SPRINT, strongly validating the accepted 30% threshold for creatinine elevation with RAS blockade and even allowing more leniency in the acute setting approach, unless confirmed ischemic renal injury/hyperkalemia occurs [45].

Hyperkalemia by itself remains an impediment to achieving the desired BP targets because many patients with diabetic nephropathy have underlying type IV renal tubular acidosis, making them susceptible to hyperkalemia with any RAS blockade. Tackling this problem with dietary interventions is not straightforward because most foods low in potassium are high in sodium, and vice versa, making pharmacologic therapy indispensable for the long-term continuation of RAS inhibitors [46, 47]. The risk of hyperkalemia with RAS blockade depends on several factors; the most important of which is the baseline level of kidney function and baseline potassium levels [48]. RAS blockade is advocated for in hypertensive CKD by both the ACC/AHA guidelines and the ADA, as defined by an albumin/creatinine ratio ≥ 300 mg/day and an eGFR <60 mL/min/1.73m^2. When hyperkalemia becomes a barrier to using RAS blockers, then the newer potassium binding agents becomes an effective strategy for keeping those patients on RAS blockers [49], as demonstrated by the AMBER trial, which allowed the continued usage of spironolactone in patients with resistant HTN, needing an add-on agent to the already maximized RAS blockade [50].

23.6 Conclusion

The BP lowering targets in people with diabetes have been a source of controversy over the past two decades. Randomized well-powered prospective controlled trials did not demonstrate a clear benefit on CV risk reduction with intensive BP lowering, albeit secondary analyses of those studies did show benefits with BP reduction to the 125–130 mm Hg range. Recent meta-analyses and systematic reviews also pointed in that direction. The negative results from prospective trials most likely come from the fact that too aggressive BP lowering was pursued, negating the benefits seen when BP is reduced to 125–130 mm Hg range, which is suggested by more pertinent and targeted analyses as the most befitting target for HTN in DM patients with high CV risk, if well tolerated and devoid of signs or symptoms of CV and/or adverse kidney effects. Indeed, this 125–130 mm Hg seems like the "sweet spot," the optimal BP level that is associated with the largest reduction in CV events, beyond which CV events are increased and slowed the progression of CKD [16, 51].

Furthermore, it is clinically relevant to determine whether this lower BP target is appropriate for all patients with DM or that different targets should be applied according to underlying patient characteristics (baseline CV risk, age, race, renal function, history of cerebrovascular accident, etc.). This observation warrants further evaluation. The addition of SGLT2 inhibitors to our arsenal in the management of diabetic nephropathy will help achieve BP targets by providing an additional 3.5 mmHg BP reduction on average, independent of glycemic control or reduction [52]. Moreover, they improve primary renal outcomes [53].

References

1. Al-Rubeaan K, Youssef AM, Subhani SN, Ahmad NA, Al-Sharqawi AH, Al-Mutlaq HM, et al. Diabetic nephropathy and its risk factors in a society with a type 2 diabetes epidemic: a Saudi National Diabetes Registry-based study. PLoS One. 2014;9(2):e88956. https://doi.org/10.1371/journal.pone.0088956.
2. Bhupathiraju SN, Hu FB. Epidemiology of obesity and diabetes and their cardiovascular complications. Circ Res. 2016;118(11):1723–35. https://doi.org/10.1161/CIRCRESAHA.115.306825.
3. Umanath K, Lewis JB. Update on diabetic nephropathy: core curriculum 2018. Am J Kidney Dis. 2018;71(6):884–95. https://doi.org/10.1053/j.ajkd.2017.10.026.
4. Ali W, Bakris G. The management of hypertension in 2018: what should the targets be? Curr Hypertens Rep. 2019;21(6):41. https://doi.org/10.1007/s11906-019-0946-7.
5. Antza C, Doundoulakis I, Stabouli S, Kotsis V. Comparison among recommendations for the management of arterial hypertension issued by last US, Canadian, British and European Guidelines. High Blood Press Cardiovasc Prev. 2018;25(1):9–16. https://doi.org/10.1007/s40292-017-0236-x.
6. de Boer IH, Bangalore S, Benetos A, Davis AM, Michos ED, Muntner P, et al. Diabetes and hypertension: a position statement by the american diabetes association. Diabetes Care. 2017;40(9):1273–84. https://doi.org/10.2337/dci17-0026.
7. de Boer IH, Bakris G, Cannon CP. Individualizing blood pressure targets for people with diabetes and hypertension: comparing the ADA and the ACC/AHA recommendations. JAMA. 2018;319(13):1319–20. https://doi.org/10.1001/jama.2018.0642.
8. Zatz R, Dunn BR, Meyer TW, Anderson S, Rennke HG, Brenner BM. Prevention of diabetic glomerulopathy by pharmacological amelioration of glomerular capillary hypertension. J Clin Invest. 1986;77(6):1925–30. https://doi.org/10.1172/JCI112521.
9. UK Prospective Diabetes Study Group. Tight blood pressure control and risk of macrovascular and microvascular complications in type 2 diabetes: UKPDS 38. UK Prospective Diabetes Study Group. BMJ. 1998;317(7160):703–13.
10. Whelton PK, Carey RM, Aronow WS, Casey DE Jr, Collins KJ, Himmelfarb CD, et al. 2017 ACC/AHA/AAPA/ABC/ACPM/AGS/APhA/ASH/ASPC/NMA/PCNA Guideline for the Prevention, Detection, Evaluation, and Management of High Blood Pressure in Adults: Executive Summary: A Report of the American College of Cardiology/American Heart Association Task Force on Clinical Practice Guidelines. Hypertension. 2018;71(6):1269–324. https://doi.org/10.1161/HYP.0000000000000066.

11. Muntner P, Carey RM, Gidding S, Jones DW, Taler SJ, Wright JT Jr, et al. Potential US population impact of the 2017 ACC/AHA high blood pressure guideline. Circulation. 2018;137(2):109–18. https://doi.org/10.1161/CIRCULATIONAHA.117.032582.
12. Rabi DM, McBrien KA, Sapir-Pichhadze R, Nakhla M, Ahmed SB, Dumanski SM, et al. Hypertension Canada's 2020 comprehensive guidelines for the prevention, diagnosis, risk assessment, and treatment of hypertension in adults and children. Can J Cardiol. 2020;36(5):596–624. https://doi.org/10.1016/j.cjca.2020.02.086.
13. Williams B, Mancia G, Spiering W, Agabiti Rosei E, Azizi M, Burnier M, et al. 2018 ESC/ESH guidelines for the management of arterial hypertension: the task force for the management of arterial hypertension of the European Society of Cardiology (ESC) and the European Society of Hypertension (ESH). Eur Heart J. 2018;39(33):3021–104. https://doi.org/10.1093/eurheartj/ehy339.
14. Bakris G. Similarities and differences between the ACC/AHA and ESH/ESC guidelines for the prevention, detection, evaluation, and management of high blood pressure in adults. Circ Res. 2019;124(7):969–71. https://doi.org/10.1161/CIRCRESAHA.118.314664.
15. Task Force of the Latin American Society of Hypertension. Guidelines on the management of arterial hypertension and related comorbidities in Latin America. J Hypertens. 2017;35(8):1529–45. https://doi.org/10.1097/HJH.0000000000001418.
16. American Diabetes Association Professional Practice Committee. 10. Cardiovascular Disease and Risk Management: Standards of Medical Care in Diabetes-2022. Diabetes Care. 2022; 45(Suppl 1):S144–74. https://diabetesjournals.org/care/article/45/Supplement_1/S144/138910/10-Cardiovascular-Disease-and-Risk-Management.
17. American Diabetes Association. 10. Cardiovascular Disease and Risk Management: Standards of Medical Care in Diabetes-2020. Diabetes Care. 2020;43(Suppl 1):S111–34. https://doi.org/10.2337/dc20-S010.
18. ACCORD Study Group; Cushman WC, Evans GW, Byington RP, Goff DC Jr, Grimm RH Jr, Cutler JA, et al. Effects of intensive blood-pressure control in type 2 diabetes mellitus. N Engl J Med. 2010;362(17):1575–85. https://doi.org/10.1056/NEJMoa1001286.
19. Buckley LF, Dixon DL, Wohlford GF, Wijesinghe DS, Baker WL, Van Tassell BW. Effect of intensive blood pressure control in patients with type 2 diabetes mellitus over 9 years of follow-up: a subgroup analysis of high-risk ACCORDION trial participants. Diabetes Obes Metab. 2018;20(6):1499–502. https://doi.org/10.1111/dom.13248.
20. Ueki K, Sasako T, Okazaki Y, Kato M, Okahata S, Katsuyama H, et al. Effect of an intensified multifactorial intervention on cardiovascular outcomes and mortality in type 2 diabetes (J-DOIT3): an open-label, randomised controlled trial. Lancet Diabetes Endocrinol. 2017;5(12):951–64. https://doi.org/10.1016/S2213-8587(17)30327-3.
21. Emdin CA, Rahimi K, Neal B, Callender T, Perkovic V, Patel A. Blood pressure lowering in type 2 diabetes: a systematic review and meta-analysis. JAMA. 2015;313(6):603–15. https://doi.org/10.1001/jama.2014.18574.
22. Ettehad D, Emdin CA, Kiran A, Anderson SG, Callender T, Emberson J, et al. Blood pressure lowering for prevention of cardiovascular disease and death: a systematic review and meta-analysis. Lancet. 2016;387(10022):957–67. https://doi.org/10.1016/S0140-6736(15)01225-8.
23. Thomopoulos C, Parati G, Zanchetti A. Effects of blood-pressure-lowering treatment on outcome incidence. 12. Effects in individuals with high-normal and normal blood pressure: overview and meta-analyses of randomized trials. J Hypertens. 2017;35(11):2150–60. https://doi.org/10.1097/HJH.0000000000001547.
24. Brenner BM, Cooper ME, de Zeeuw D, Keane WF, Mitch WE, Parving HH, et al. Effects of losartan on renal and cardiovascular outcomes in patients with type 2 diabetes and nephropathy. N Engl J Med. 2001;345(12):861–9. https://doi.org/10.1056/NEJMoa011161.
25. Lewis EJ, Hunsicker LG, Rodby RA, Collaborative Study Group. A clinical trial in type 2 diabetic nephropathy. Am J Kidney Dis. 2001;38(4 Suppl 1):S191–4. https://doi.org/10.1053/ajkd.2001.27442.

26. Bakris GL, Weir MR, Shanifar S, Zhang Z, Douglas J, van Dijket DJ, et al. Effects of blood pressure level on progression of diabetic nephropathy: results from the RENAAL study. Arch Intern Med. 2003;163(13):1555–65. https://doi.org/10.1001/archinte.163.13.1555.
27. Lewis EJ, Hunsicker LG, Clarke WR, Berl T, Pohl MA, Lewis JB, et al. Renoprotective effect of the angiotensin-receptor antagonist irbesartan in patients with nephropathy due to type 2 diabetes. N Engl J Med. 2001;345(12):851–60. https://doi.org/10.1056/NEJMoa011303.
28. Pohl MA, Blumenthal S, Cordonnier DJ, De Alvaro F, Deferrari G, Eisner G, et al. Independent and additive impact of blood pressure control and angiotensin II receptor blockade on renal outcomes in the irbesartan diabetic nephropathy trial: clinical implications and limitations. J Am Soc Nephrol. 2005;16(10):3027–37. https://doi.org/10.1681/ASN.2004110919.
29. Gomadam P, Shah A, Qureshi W, Yeboah PN, Freedman BI, Bowden D, et al. Blood pressure indices and cardiovascular disease mortality in persons with or without diabetes mellitus. J Hypertens. 2018;36(1):85–92. https://doi.org/10.1097/HJH.0000000000001509.
30. Franklin SS. Cardiovascular risks related to increased diastolic, systolic and pulse pressure. An epidemiologist's point of view. Pathol Biol (Paris). 1999;47(6):594–603.
31. McEvoy JW, Chen Y, Rawlings A, Hoogeveen RC, Ballantyne CM, Blumenthal RS, et al. Diastolic blood pressure, subclinical myocardial damage, and cardiac events: implications for blood pressure control. J Am Coll Cardiol. 2016;68(16):1713–22. https://doi.org/10.1016/j.jacc.2016.07.754.
32. Kannel WB, Wilson PW, Nam BH, D'Agostino RB, Li J. A likely explanation for the J-curve of blood pressure cardiovascular risk. Am J Cardiol. 2004;94(3):380–4. https://doi.org/10.1016/j.amjcard.2004.04.043.
33. Ilkun OL, Greene T, Cheung AK, Whelton PK, Wei G, Boucher RE, et al. The influence of baseline diastolic blood pressure on the effects of intensive blood pressure lowering on cardiovascular outcomes and all-cause mortality in type 2 diabetes. Diabetes Care. 2020;43(8):1878–84. https://doi.org/10.2337/dc19-2047.
34. Beddhu S, Chertow GM, Cheung AK, Cushman WC, Rahman M, Greene T, et al. Influence of baseline diastolic blood pressure on effects of intensive compared with standard blood pressure control. Circulation. 2018;137(2):134–43. https://doi.org/10.1161/CIRCULATIONAHA.117.030848.
35. Omboni S, Kario K, Bakris G, Parati G. Effect of antihypertensive treatment on 24-h blood pressure variability: pooled individual data analysis of ambulatory blood pressure monitoring studies based on olmesartan mono or combination treatment. J Hypertens. 2018;36(4):720–33. https://doi.org/10.1097/HJH.0000000000001608.
36. Al Dhabyi O, Bakris GL. Initial single-pill blood pressure-lowering therapy: should it be for most people? J Am Heart Assoc. 2017;6(11):e007760. https://doi.org/10.1161/JAHA.117.007760.
37. Sarafidis PA, Khosla N, Bakris GL. Antihypertensive therapy in the presence of proteinuria. Am J Kidney Dis. 2007;49(1):12–26. https://doi.org/10.1053/j.ajkd.2006.10.014.
38. Gradman AH, Basile JN, Carter BL, Bakris GL, American Society of Hypertension Writing Group. Combination therapy in hypertension. J Clin Hypertens (Greenwich). 2011;13(3):146–54. https://doi.org/10.1111/j.1751-7176.2010.00397.x.
39. Bakris GL, Sarafidis PA, Weir MR, Dahlöf B, Pitt B, Jamersonet K, et al. Renal outcomes with different fixed-dose combination therapies in patients with hypertension at high risk for cardiovascular events (ACCOMPLISH): a prespecified secondary analysis of a randomised controlled trial. Lancet. 2010;375(9721):1173–81. https://doi.org/10.1016/S0140-6736(09)62100-0.
40. Jamerson K, Weber MA, Bakris GL, Dahlöf B, Pitt B, Shi V, et al. Benazepril plus amlodipine or hydrochlorothiazide for hypertension in high-risk patients. N Engl J Med. 2008;359(23):2417–28. https://doi.org/10.1056/NEJMoa0806182.
41. Bakris GL, Weir MR. Angiotensin-converting enzyme inhibitor-associated elevations in serum creatinine: is this a cause for concern? Arch Intern Med. 2000;160(5):685–93.
42. Bakris GL, Agarwal R. Creatinine bump following antihypertensive therapy. Hypertension. 2018;72(6):1274–6. https://doi.org/10.1161/HYPERTENSIONAHA.118.12051.

43. Malhotra R, Craven T, Ambrosius WT, Killeen AA, Haley WE, Cheung AK, et al. Effects of intensive blood pressure lowering on kidney tubule injury in CKD: a longitudinal subgroup analysis in SPRINT. Am J Kidney Dis. 2019;73(1):21–30. https://doi.org/10.1001/jamainternmed.2020.0193.
44. Malhotra R, Craven T, Ambrosius WT, Killeen AA, Haley WE, Cheung AK, et al. Effects of intensive blood pressure lowering on kidney tubule injury in ckd: a longitudinal subgroup analysis in SPRINT. Am J Kidney Dis. 2019;73(1):21–30. https://doi.org/10.1053/j.ajkd.2018.07.015.
45. Collard D, Brouwer TF, Olde Engberink RHG, Zwinderman AH, Vogt L, van den Born BH. Initial estimated glomerular filtration rate decline and long-term renal function during intensive antihypertensive therapy: a post hoc analysis of the SPRINT and ACCORD-BP randomized controlled trials. Hypertension. 2020;75(5):1205–12. https://doi.org/10.1161/HYPERTENSIONAHA.119.14659.
46. Palmer BF. Potassium binders for hyperkalemia in chronic kidney disease-diet, renin-angiotensin-aldosterone system inhibitor therapy, and hemodialysis. Mayo Clin Proc. 2020;95(2):339–54. https://doi.org/10.1016/j.mayocp.2019.05.019.
47. Ai Dhaybi O, Bakris GL. Renal targeted therapies of antihypertensive and cardiovascular drugs for patients with stages 3 through 5d kidney disease. Clin Pharmacol Ther. 2017;102(3):450–8. https://doi.org/10.1002/cpt.758.
48. Lazich I, Bakris GL. Prediction and management of hyperkalemia across the spectrum of chronic kidney disease. Semin Nephrol. 2014;34(3):333–9. https://doi.org/10.1016/j.semnephrol.2014.04.008.
49. Pitt B, Bakris GL. New potassium binders for the treatment of hyperkalemia: current data and opportunities for the future. Hypertension. 2015;66(4):731–8. https://doi.org/10.1161/HYPERTENSIONAHA.115.04889.
50. Agarwal R, Rossignol P, Romero A, Garza D, Mayo MR, Warrenet S, et al. Patiromer versus placebo to enable spironolactone use in patients with resistant hypertension and chronic kidney disease (AMBER): a phase 2, randomised, double-blind, placebo-controlled trial. Lancet. 2019;394(10208):1540–50. https://doi.org/10.1016/S0140-6736(19)32135-X.
51. Flynn C, Bakris GL. Blood pressure targets for patients with diabetes or kidney disease. Curr Hypertens Rep. 2011;13(6):452–5. https://doi.org/10.1007/s11906-011-0228-5.
52. Sternlicht H, Bakris GL. Blood pressure lowering and sodium-glucose co-transporter 2 inhibitors (SGLT2is): more than osmotic diuresis. Curr Hypertens Rep. 2019;21(2):12. https://doi.org/10.1007/s11906-019-0920-4.
53. Briasoulis A, Al Dhaybi O, Bakris GL. SGLT2 inhibitors and mechanisms of hypertension. Curr Cardiol Rep. 2018;20(1):1. https://doi.org/10.1007/s11886-018-0943-5.

24 Choice of Antihypertensive Drugs and Antihypertensive Drug Combination in Diabetes

Alexander A. Leung

24.1 Introduction

Diabetes mellitus is a highly prevalent medical condition that commonly coexists with hypertension [1]. People with diabetes and hypertension have a greatly increased risk of coronary heart disease, heart failure, stroke, chronic kidney disease, and cardiovascular death [2–4]. Compelling evidence from randomized controlled trials demonstrates that blood pressure (BP) reduction effectively prevents major cardiovascular events and death [5–8]. While efforts to prevent cardiovascular morbidity and mortality for patients with diabetes have traditionally focused on blood glucose management [9–11], there is a growing awareness of the importance of BP control for these individuals. In fact, the benefits of BP lowering may even exceed those of glycemic control for the prevention of cardiovascular complications [9, 12].

24.2 Initial Therapy

24.2.1 Approach to Treatment

All patients with high BP should be advised on healthy behaviors, including maintaining healthy weight; consuming a diet that emphasizes fruit, vegetables, and whole grain foods; limiting dietary sodium to 2 g per day; avoiding excessive alcohol consumption; and engaging in at least 150 min of moderate to vigorous physical activity per week [13–15]. In addition to healthy lifestyle and behaviors, patients

A. A. Leung (✉)
Division of Endocrinology and Metabolism, Departments of Medicine and Community Health Sciences, Cumming School of Medicine, University of Calgary, Calgary, AB, Canada
e-mail: aacleung@ucalgary.ca

A. E. Berbari, G. Mancia (eds.), *Blood Pressure Disorders in Diabetes Mellitus*, Updates in Hypertension and Cardiovascular Protection,
https://doi.org/10.1007/978-3-031-13009-0_24

with diabetes and hypertension commonly require drug therapy to achieve target BP control.

The choice of initial drug therapy is partly based on the severity of hypertension. At conventional doses, most major antihypertensive drugs lower systolic BP by approximately 5–10 mmHg and diastolic BP by 5 mmHg when used as monotherapy [16, 17]. As such, while treatment with a single drug may occasionally be sufficient, there is growing consensus that initial combination therapy with two antihypertensive agents should be considered as first-line treatment [18–21], acknowledging that the majority of patients will eventually require more than one agent to achieve long-term BP control (vide infra) [22, 23]. Moreover, on the whole, antihypertensive medications from multiple major drug classes (i.e., angiotensin-converting enzyme [ACE] inhibitors, angiotensin II receptor blockers [ARBs], non-dihydropyridine calcium channel blockers [CCBs], thiazide or thiazide-like diuretics, and beta-blockers) appear broadly similar in their ability to reduce cardiovascular disease [24–27], end-stage renal disease [25, 28], and mortality [29, 30]. Many of the purported differences in effectiveness between drug classes in clinical trials can be accounted for by adjusting for the magnitude of BP reduction achieved [26–29], though there may still be some small residual differences in selected clinical outcomes between agents [25, 27, 30, 31].

The selection of a specific antihypertensive drug should be chiefly informed by the tolerability of the medication, the presence of other medical conditions, and patient preference. Accordingly, a summary of the main antihypertensive drugs used in diabetes along with the evidence base that support their use is presented in the succeeding text.

24.2.2 Renin-Angiotensin System Blockers

Overall, ACE inhibitors and ARBs (collectively referred to as renin-angiotensin system [RAS] blockers) appear to have similar (or even interchangeable) clinical benefits with strong evidence from randomized trials proving their effectiveness in reducing myocardial infarction, stroke, hospitalizations for heart failure, progression to end-stage renal disease, and death compared with placebo [32–35]. Moreover, in patients with type 1 diabetes, there is some evidence to suggest that RAS inhibitors may lower the risk of diabetic retinopathy compared with other antihypertensive drugs [36].

Most clinical practice guidelines recommend RAS blockers as initial therapy for the treatment of hypertension in patients with diabetes and chronic kidney disease, especially among those with albuminuria (e.g., albumin ≥300 mg/day or albumin-to-creatinine ratio ≥ 30 mg/g), to reduce the risk of progression to end-stage renal disease [18–20, 37]. It is popularly held that RAS blockers have renoprotective properties that are independent of their BP-lowering effect [38], but these inferences are largely drawn from placebo-controlled trials [39–43] with few head-to-head studies with other active drug comparators [44]. While some meta-analyses have presented data to support the hypothesis that RAS blockers may have pleotropic effects [33], others have been able to attribute their renoprotective benefits entirely to BP lowering [28, 45]. Even so, amidst the controversy, ACE inhibitors and ARBs are still admittedly the only drugs with strong trial-based evidence available to prove their effectiveness in reducing the progression of diabetic nephropathy, albeit in comparison with placebo, but direct evidence of their superiority over other antihypertensive drug classes is weak [31, 46].

In the absence of albuminuria or retinopathy, however, there is little to no evidence to support the use of ACE inhibitors or ARBs preferentially over other common antihypertensive agents. In a methodologically rigorous meta-analysis of 19 randomized controlled trials comprising 25,414 participants with diabetes and high BP (excluding placebo-controlled trials so as to mitigate against between-arm BP differences), treatment with RAS blockers was not associated with any significant differences in myocardial infarction, stroke, revascularization, end-stage renal disease, or cardiovascular death when compared with other common BP-lowering drugs, such as beta-blockers, CCBs, or thiazide diuretics [25]. These findings are consistent with other comprehensive systematic reviews and meta-analyses showing similar cardiovascular and renoprotective effects across all major drug classes for patients with diabetes [27, 28, 47].

Overall, ACE inhibitors and ARBs are generally safe and well-tolerated [48]. The most common side effect unique to ACE inhibitors is the development of a dry cough, which may affect up to 30% of patients [49–51]. ACE inhibitors are also associated with the rare, but potentially life-threatening, side effect of angioedema with an estimated incidence of 0.1–0.2% per year [51, 52]. The use of either RAS blocker may occasionally be limited by hyperkalemia, particularly in patients with chronic kidney disease. In such cases, measures to control high potassium (e.g., dietary changes and the use of gastrointestinal cation exchangers) may be helpful [37]. Finally, the combination of an ACE inhibitor and an ARB, which was once recommended for the management of diabetic nephropathy, is no longer advisable. Several large trials comparing dual RAS blockade with monotherapy failed to show any significant differences in the rates of progression in chronic kidney disease, the occurrence of major cardiovascular events, or mortality, but rather reported higher rates of adverse treatment-related effects, including hyperkalemia, acute kidney injury, and hypotension [53, 54]. In light of the generally unfavorable risk-to-benefit ratio, the simultaneous use of an ACE inhibitor and an ARB is not recommended [18–20, 37].

24.2.3 Calcium Channel Blockers

Several randomized controlled trials have shown that long-acting CCBs are safe and effective for reducing cardiovascular events in patients with diabetes [55–58]. In the Antihypertensive and Lipid-Lowering Treatment to Prevent Heart Attack Trial (ALLHAT), a subgroup of 13,101 patients with diabetes were randomized to receive either amlodipine, lisinopril, or chlorthalidone for hypertension [55]. Although the achieved systolic BP was notably higher among participants who received amlodipine or lisinopril compared with chlorthalidone, there were no significant differences in the primary composite outcome of nonfatal myocardial infarction and fatal coronary heart disease after a mean follow-up of 4.9 years for patients receiving amlodipine (relative risk [RR], 0.97; 95% confidence interval [CI], 0.86–1.10) or lisinopril (RR, 0.97; 95% CI, 0.85–1.10) compared with chlorthalidone. The risk of other secondary cardiovascular outcomes and all-cause mortality were generally similar as well, but the study was underpowered to detect differences in the risk of progression to end-stage renal disease. Correspondingly, these findings were important in establishing CCBs as potential first-line drugs for patients with diabetes in the absence of albuminuria [55].

Additional data supporting the use of CCBs, particularly in combination with RAS blockers, derives from the Avoiding Cardiovascular Events through Combination Therapy in Patients Living with Systolic Hypertension (ACCOMPLISH) trial, which randomized 11,506 adults at high cardiovascular risk to either a combination of benazepril plus amlodipine or benazepril plus hydrochlorothiazide [48]. Notably, this trial was prematurely terminated after a mean follow-up of 36 months because of a significant reduction in the composite outcome of major adverse cardiovascular events or cardiovascular death with benazepril plus amlodipine compared with benazepril plus hydrochlorothiazide. In the prespecified analysis of a subgroup of 6946 participants with diabetes, the combination of benazepril plus amlodipine compared with benazepril plus hydrochlorothiazide resulted in a lower risk of the composite outcome (8.8% vs. 11.0%; hazard ratio [HR], 0.79; 95% CI, 0.68–0.92), corresponding to a number needed to treat of 46 people over 30 months to prevent one event [59]. Altogether, the results of the ACCOMPLISH trial informed the use of a CCB in combination with a RAS blocker for patients with diabetes and chronic kidney disease [59].

While CCBs are generally well tolerated, the most frequent side effect is the occurrence of peripheral edema [60], which can lead to medication discontinuation [61]. This adverse effect is dose-dependent and is believed to arise from preferential arteriolar dilatation, resulting in a high-pressure gradient in the capillaries, leading to extravasation of intravascular fluid [62, 63]. The risk of edema is lessened when a CCB is combined with a RAS blocker because the latter effectively decreases postcapillary resistance [62]. Accordingly, combination therapy is associated with 38% lower rates of peripheral edema (RR, 0.62; 95% CI, 0.53–0.74) and 62% lower rates of medication discontinuation (RR, 0.38; 95% CI, 0.22–0.66) [63].

24.2.4 Thiazide and Thiazide-Like Diuretics

Multiple randomized controlled trials have jointly proved the safety and effectiveness of diuretics in people with diabetes [55, 64–68]. In the Systolic Hypertension in the Elderly Program (SHEP) trial, the use of low-dose chlorthalidone compared with placebo resulted in 34% relative risk reduction in major cardiovascular events (RR, 0.66; 95% CI, 0.46–0.94) for patients with diabetes with little to no evidence of adverse treatment effects [64]. Among those with diabetes, the number needed to treat was ten to prevent one major cardiovascular event over 5 years. Moreover, in ALLHAT, chlorthalidone, lisinopril, and amlodipine were compared with no significant differences seen between the three agents in the primary outcome of nonfatal and fatal coronary heart disease (even among the 36% of patients with diabetes), though participants randomized to chlorthalidone had a lower risk of heart failure [55, 65, 67]. Based on these collective findings, thiazide and thiazide-like diuretics have found their place as a potential first-line agent for patients with diabetes and high BP, especially given their overall safety, effectiveness, and low cost.

Accumulating evidence suggests that longer-acting, thiazide-like diuretics (e.g., chlorthalidone and indapamide) are preferable to thiazide diuretics (e.g., hydrochlorothiazide) for controlling BP and reducing cardiovascular events [69, 70]. In a meta-analysis of 14 randomized controlled trials, the use of indapamide or chlorthalidone resulted in greater BP reduction compared with hydrochlorothiazide without any detectable differences in drug side effects [71]. Moreover, in a meta-analysis of 21 randomized controlled trials, the use of thiazide-like diuretics compared with thiazides led to an additional 12% risk reduction in cardiovascular events and 21% risk reduction in heart failure, after accounting for differences in BP achieved [72]. Both types of diuretics reduced the risk of cardiovascular events, stroke, and heart failure compared with placebo, but only thiazide-like diuretics reduced the risk of coronary events and death.

While there are a number of known adverse metabolic effects associated with thiazide and thiazide-like diuretics (e.g., hypokalemia, hyponatremia, hyperglycemia, hyperlipidemia, and hyperglycemia), these risks are generally small, particularly when lower doses are used [17, 65, 73], and they probably do not outweigh the benefits of treatment if BP can be controlled. Alternative antihypertensive agents should be considered for patients with significant renal impairment (e.g., estimated glomerular filtration rate less than 30 mL/min/1.73 m^2), as thiazide and thiazide-like diuretics are less likely to be effective.

24.2.5 Beta-Blockers

Beta-blockers reduce the risk of myocardial infarction and stroke compared with placebo [24], and they appear similarly effective as other antihypertensive agents when prescribed as monotherapy for preventing cardiovascular death in patients with diabetes [29], though direct head-to-head comparisons between active agents are admittedly limited [25, 26, 30]. Once widely recommended as a possible option for first-line treatment of uncomplicated hypertension, beta-blockers now feature less prominently in most guidelines in the absence of heart failure or ischemic heart disease [19, 20]. Enthusiasm for this particular drug class was dampened over a decade ago following the release of a widely publicized meta-analysis of 13 randomized controlled trials incorporating 105,951 participants, which reported an increased risk of stroke among patients treated with beta-blockers compared with other drug classes [74]. Subsequent analyses have not only confirmed this general finding but also noted that the signal of excess risk of stroke largely derives from trials enrolling older patients (i.e., 60 years and higher) [75, 76]. Indeed, the efficacy of beta-blockers may go down with age, owing to differences in the pathophysiology of hypertension in younger vs. older patients [77, 78]. Correspondingly, studies that have stratified according to age groups have consistently shown that beta-blockers perform well in preventing major cardiovascular events in patients under 60 years of age [75, 76], a finding that is obscured when age is not been taken into account [44, 74, 79].

Like all antihypertensive drugs, there are potential adverse effects with beta-blockers. However, historical concerns about hyperglycemia and dyslipidemia from treatment are less significant with newer beta-blockers [80, 81]. Moreover, the absolute risks of depression, fatigue, and sexual dysfunction are generally small [82]. Although beta-blockers may theoretically contribute to impaired perception of hypoglycemia in some patients with diabetes (i.e., due to blunted adrenergic symptoms), this is unlikely to be a common problem in practice [83, 84]. In the UK Prospective Diabetes Study (UKPDS) 39, a randomized controlled trial comparing atenolol with captopril in 758 patients with type 2 diabetes and hypertension (among whom 6.5% were taking insulin and 26.4% a sulfonylurea), there were no differences between treatment arms for either the number or severity of hypoglycemic episodes over a follow-up period of 9 years [85]. Still, these agents should be used cautiously in patients with a known history of frequent hypoglycemia or hypoglycemic unawareness.

Given the global evidence related to their effectiveness and overall safety, beta-blockers remain a reasonable choice for young and middle-aged patients (i.e., under 60 years) or individuals of any age with heart failure or symptomatic ischemic heart disease. They are not recommended as first-line in the elderly, but may be considered as "add-on" treatment.

24.2.6 Mineralocorticoid Receptor Antagonists

Treatment-resistant hypertension is common in patients with diabetes [86–88], yet evidence informing optimal drug selection in this setting is sparse. To date, the strongest data come from the Prevention And Treatment of Hypertension With Algorithm-based therapy (PATHWAY)-2 trial, which was a crossover trial that randomly assigned 335 participants (14% with diabetes) with uncontrolled BP to spironolactone, doxazosin, bisoprolol, and placebo (each for 12 weeks) in addition to standard three-drug therapy (i.e., an ACE inhibitor or ARB, amlodipine, and indapamide) [89]. Spironolactone was associated with the greatest reductions in systolic BP compared with the other active treatments and placebo. Overall, target BP control was achieved in 58% of people with spironolactone vs. 44% with bisoprolol vs. 42% with doxazosin vs. 24% with placebo. In a subsequent open-label substudy, some participants received an additional 12 weeks of amiloride and had similar BP reductions as those seen with spironolactone [90]. The major limitation of this study was the lack of data on cardiovascular outcomes or mortality. Still, these results are important as they indicate that resistant hypertension is frequently volume-mediated and therefore highly responsive to mineralocorticoid receptor blockade. This is consistent with other systematic reviews and meta-analyses, which support the addition of spironolactone, compared with other antihypertensive agents, for the treatment of resistant hypertension [91–94]. Finally, apart from being highly effective for controlling BP in most patients with resistant hypertension, mineralocorticoid receptor antagonists have also been shown to help reduce albuminuria in patients with diabetic nephropathy [95–99].

Common to all mineralocorticoid receptor antagonists, there is a two-fold increased risk of hyperkalemia [100, 101], which may be even higher in individuals with diabetes, chronic kidney disease, and concurrent users of ACE inhibitors or ARBs [102]. Exposure to spironolactone may also lead to antiandrogenic side effects in men, such as gynecomastia or decreased libido, or progestin-like side effects in women, including mastodynia and menstrual irregularities [103, 104]. The risks may potentially increase with prolonged exposure and limit treatment in some patients [105]. Newer mineralocorticoid receptor antagonists (e.g., eplerenone and finerenone) not only are less likely to cause antiandrogen- and progestin-like effects [104, 106, 107], but also are more costly. Amiloride can also be considered as an alternative with fewer side effects [90].

24.2.7 Antihypertensive Drug Combinations

In a sense, debates over which drug class is best for initial treatment may be largely irrelevant, as most patients with high BP require multiple antihypertensive drugs to achieve adequate control. Indeed, the majority of people who have participated in large hypertension trials, such as ALLHAT [55, 67, 108], the UKPDS 38 [12], the Hypertension Optimal Treatment (HOT) trial [56], the Anglo-Scandinavian Cardiac Outcomes Trial (ASCOT) [109], and the Valsartan Antihypertensive Long-term Use Evaluation (VALUE) trial [110] required at least two to three agents to achieve target BP levels.

Correspondingly, major clinical practice guidelines increasingly recommend the use of an antihypertensive drug combination for initial treatment in most patients and preferably prescribed as a single-pill combination (i.e., one pill with multiple active ingredients in a fixed-dose combination) [18–21]. Specifically, the use of single-pill combinations have been shown to lower the risk of cardiovascular events [111–113], improve rates of BP control [22, 23, 48, 111, 112, 114], promote medication adherence [47, 115, 116], and reduce the frequency of treatment-related side effects [17].

The therapeutic efficacy of single-pill combinations was demonstrated in the Heart Outcomes Prevention Evaluation (HOPE)-3 trial, which randomized 12,705 individuals at intermediate risk of cardiovascular disease (among whom 5.8% had diabetes and 12.7% had prediabetes) to receive a fixed-dose combination of candesartan and hydrochlorothiazide or placebo [114]. Among the subgroup of patients with hypertension (i.e., baseline systolic BP >143.5 mmHg), fixed-dose combination therapy reduced the risk of the composite outcome of cardiovascular death, nonfatal myocardial infarction, or nonfatal stroke (4.8% vs. 6.5% for placebo; HR, 0.73; 95% CI, 0.56–0.94) after 5.6 years of follow-up. Moreover, the safety of using a single-pill combination for initial treatment was demonstrated in the Action in Diabetes and Vascular disease: Preterax and Diamicron-MR Controlled Evaluation (ADVANCE) trial [117]. Here, 11,140 patients with type 2 diabetes were randomly assigned to receive a fixed-dose combination of perindopril and indapamide vs. placebo, irrespective of baseline BP level. Recipients of active treatment had greater reductions in major macrovascular and microvascular complications (15.5% vs. 16.8%; HR, 0.91; 95% CI, 0.30–1.00) and death (7.3% vs. 8.5%; HR, 0.86; 95% CI, 0.75–0.98), compared with those who received placebo, with corresponding numbers needed to treat of 66 and 79 to prevent one event over 5 years, respectively. Importantly, there were no detectable differences in treatment effects according to initial BP level, or whether patients received other BP-lowering therapy at baseline or not. Serious adverse event rates were identical between the two arms.

The cardinal advantage to combining drugs together that act through different mechanisms is the ability to achieve lower BP while at the same time reducing the frequency of medication-related side effects, which are often dose-dependent [16, 17]. Several "synergistic" combinations are particularly appealing where one drug may antagonize the potential adverse effects of another. Namely, combining a RAS blocker with a thiazide or thiazide-like diuretic may help to mitigate the risk of potassium disorders, while the combination of a RAS blocker with a CCB has been shown to reduce the frequency of peripheral edema (vide supra) [63, 118]. Notably, the clinical efficacy of the combinations of an ACE inhibitor with a CCB [22, 59, 60], an ACE inhibitor with a diuretic [23, 117], and an ARB with a diuretic [23, 114], in particular, is proven in multiple clinical trials. Consistent with these findings, "real-world" observational studies have also shown that initial treatment with a combination of antihypertensive drugs compared with monotherapy is associated with improved cardiovascular outcomes, shorter time to achieve BP control, and reduced healthcare utilization [111, 112].

24.3 Summary

Clinicians should recognize that there may not be a single overriding treatment that is appropriate for all patients. The selection of an antihypertensive drug needs to be personalized based on side-effect profile, coexisting conditions, and personal preferences. Reassuringly, current evidence suggests that the benefits of treatment mainly derive from BP reduction itself with minimal differences (if any) between most major drug classes. In general, it is reasonable to consider any effective and tolerated antihypertensive agent, acknowledging that many patients may require combination therapy. Accordingly, the use of single-pill combinations reduces the risk of adverse cardiovascular outcomes, improve medication adherence, and help to minimize drug side effects. In all of this, it should be remembered that BP control is of paramount importance for everyone with diabetes.

References

1. Kabakov E, Norymberg C, Osher E, Koffler M, Tordjman K, Greenman Y, et al. Prevalence of hypertension in type 2 diabetes mellitus: impact of the tightening definition of high blood pressure and association with confounding risk factors. J Cardiometab Syndr. 2006;1(2):95–101.
2. Haffner SM, Lehto S, Ronnemaa T, Pyorala K, Laakso M. Mortality from coronary heart disease in subjects with type 2 diabetes and in nondiabetic subjects with and without prior myocardial infarction. N Engl J Med. 1998;339(4):229–34.
3. Stamler J, Vaccaro O, Neaton JD, Wentworth D. Diabetes, other risk factors, and 12-yr cardiovascular mortality for men screened in the multiple risk factor intervention trial. Diabetes Care. 1993;16(2):434–44.
4. Adler AI, Stratton IM, Neil HA, Yudkin JS, Matthews DR, Cull CA, et al. Association of systolic blood pressure with macrovascular and microvascular complications of type 2 diabetes (UKPDS 36): prospective observational study. BMJ. 2000;321(7258):412–9.
5. Blood Pressure Lowering Treatment Trialists' Collaboration. Blood pressure-lowering treatment based on cardiovascular risk: a meta-analysis of individual patient data. Lancet. 2014;384(9943):591–8.
6. Ettehad D, Emdin CA, Kiran A, Anderson SG, Callender T, Emberson J, et al. Blood pressure lowering for prevention of cardiovascular disease and death: a systematic review and meta-analysis. Lancet. 2016;387:957–67.
7. Xie X, Atkins E, Lv J, Bennett A, Neal B, Ninomiya T, et al. Effects of intensive blood pressure lowering on cardiovascular and renal outcomes: updated systematic review and meta-analysis. Lancet. 2016;387:435–43.
8. Emdin CA, Rahimi K, Neal B, Callender T, Perkovic V, Patel A. Blood pressure lowering in type 2 diabetes: a systematic review and meta-analysis. JAMA. 2015;313(6):603–15.
9. UK Prospective Diabetes Study (UKPDS) Group. Intensive blood-glucose control with sulphonylureas or insulin compared with conventional treatment and risk of complications in patients with type 2 diabetes (UKPDS 33). Lancet. 1998;352(9131):837–53.
10. Duckworth W, Abraira C, Moritz T, Reda D, Emanuele N, Reaven PD, et al. Glucose control and vascular complications in veterans with type 2 diabetes. N Engl J Med. 2009;360(2):129–39.
11. Patel A, MacMahon S, Chalmers J, Neal B, Billot L, Woodward M, et al. Intensive blood glucose control and vascular outcomes in patients with type 2 diabetes. N Engl J Med. 2008;358(24):2560–72.
12. UK Prospective Diabetes Study (UKPDS) Group. Tight blood pressure control and risk of macrovascular and microvascular complications in type 2 diabetes: UKPDS 38. BMJ. 1998;317(7160):703–13.
13. Appel LJ, Moore TJ, Obarzanek E, Vollmer WM, Svetkey LP, Sacks FM, et al. A clinical trial of the effects of dietary patterns on blood pressure. DASH collaborative research group. N Engl J Med. 1997;336(16):1117–24.
14. Appel LJ, Champagne CM, Harsha DW, Cooper LS, Obarzanek E, Elmer PJ, et al. Effects of comprehensive lifestyle modification on blood pressure control: main results of the PREMIER clinical trial. JAMA. 2003;289(16):2083–93.
15. Whelton SP, Chin A, Xin X, He J. Effect of aerobic exercise on blood pressure: a meta-analysis of randomized, controlled trials. Ann Intern Med. 2002;136(7):493–503.
16. Wald DS, Law M, Morris JK, Bestwick JP, Wald NJ. Combination therapy versus monotherapy in reducing blood pressure: meta-analysis on 11,000 participants from 42 trials. Am J Med. 2009;122(3):290–300.
17. Law MR, Wald NJ, Morris JK, Jordan RE. Value of low dose combination treatment with blood pressure lowering drugs: analysis of 354 randomised trials. BMJ. 2003;326(7404):1427.
18. American Diabetes Association. 10. Cardiovascular disease and risk management: standards of medical care in diabetes-2021. Diabetes Care. 2021;44(Suppl 1):S125–50.

19. Whelton PK, Carey RM, Aronow WS, Casey DE Jr, Collins KJ, Dennison Himmelfarb C, et al. 2017 ACC/AHA/AAPA/ABC/ACPM/AGS/APhA/ASH/ASPC/NMA/PCNA Guideline for the Prevention, Detection, Evaluation, and Management of High Blood Pressure in Adults: A Report of the American College of Cardiology/American Heart Association Task Force on Clinical Practice Guidelines. J Am Coll Cardiol. 2018;71(19):e127–248.
20. Williams B, Mancia G, Spiering W, Agabiti Rosei E, Azizi M, Burnier M, et al. 2018 ESC/ESH guidelines for the management of arterial hypertension. Eur Heart J. 2018;39(33):3021–104.
21. Leung AA, Daskalopoulou SS, Dasgupta K, McBrien K, Butalia S, Zarnke KB, et al. Hypertension Canada's 2017 guidelines for diagnosis, risk assessment, prevention, and treatment of hypertension in adults. Can J Cardiol. 2017;33(5):557–76.
22. Bakris GL, Weir MR; Study of Hypertension and the Efficacy of Lotrel in Diabetes (SHIELD) Investigators. Achieving goal blood pressure in patients with type 2 diabetes: conventional versus fixed-dose combination approaches. J Clin Hypertens (Greenwich). 2003;5(3):202–9.
23. Feldman RD, Zou GY, Vandervoort MK, Wong CJ, Nelson SA, Feagan BG. A simplified approach to the treatment of uncomplicated hypertension: a cluster randomized, controlled trial. Hypertension. 2009;53(4):646–53.
24. Wei J, Galaviz KI, Kowalski AJ, Magee MJ, Haw JS, Narayan KMV, et al. Comparison of cardiovascular events among users of different classes of antihypertension medications: a systematic review and network meta-analysis. JAMA Netw Open. 2020;3(2):e1921618.
25. Bangalore S, Fakheri R, Toklu B, Messerli FH. Diabetes mellitus as a compelling indication for use of renin angiotensin system blockers: systematic review and meta-analysis of randomized trials. BMJ. 2016;352:i438.
26. Turnbull F, Neal B, Algert C, Chalmers J, Chapman N, Cutler J, et al. Effects of different blood pressure-lowering regimens on major cardiovascular events in individuals with and without diabetes mellitus: results of prospectively designed overviews of randomized trials. Arch Intern Med. 2005;165(12):1410–9.
27. Law MR, Morris JK, Wald NJ. Use of blood pressure lowering drugs in the prevention of cardiovascular disease: meta-analysis of 147 randomised trials in the context of expectations from prospective epidemiological studies. BMJ. 2009;338:b1665.
28. Casas JP, Chua W, Loukogeorgakis S, Vallance P, Smeeth L, Hingorani AD, et al. Effect of inhibitors of the renin-angiotensin system and other antihypertensive drugs on renal outcomes: systematic review and meta-analysis. Lancet. 2005;366(9502):2026–33.
29. Remonti LR, Dias S, Leitao CB, Kramer CK, Klassman LP, Welton NJ, et al. Classes of antihypertensive agents and mortality in hypertensive patients with type 2 diabetes-network meta-analysis of randomized trials. J Diabetes Complicat. 2016;30(6):1192–200.
30. Chen YJ, Li LJ, Tang WL, Song JY, Qiu R, Li Q, et al. First-line drugs inhibiting the renin angiotensin system versus other first-line antihypertensive drug classes for hypertension. Cochrane Database Syst Rev. 2018;11:CD008170.
31. Brunstrom M, Eliasson M, Nilsson PM, Carlberg B. Blood pressure treatment levels and choice of antihypertensive agent in people with diabetes mellitus: an overview of systematic reviews. J Hypertens. 2017;35(3):453–62.
32. Catala-Lopez F, Macias Saint-Gerons D, Gonzalez-Bermejo D, Rosano GM, Davis BR, Ridao M, et al. Cardiovascular and renal outcomes of renin-angiotensin system blockade in adult patients with diabetes mellitus: a systematic review with network meta-analyses. PLoS Med. 2016;13(3):e1001971.
33. Palmer SC, Mavridis D, Navarese E, Craig JC, Tonelli M, Salanti G, et al. Comparative efficacy and safety of blood pressure-lowering agents in adults with diabetes and kidney disease: a network meta-analysis. Lancet. 2015;385(9982):2047–56.
34. Barnett AH, Bain SC, Bouter P, Karlberg B, Madsbad S, Jervell J, et al. Angiotensin-receptor blockade versus converting-enzyme inhibition in type 2 diabetes and nephropathy. N Engl J Med. 2004;351(19):1952–61.
35. Strippoli GF, Bonifati C, Craig M, Navaneethan SD, Craig JC. Angiotensin converting enzyme inhibitors and angiotensin II receptor antagonists for preventing the progression of diabetic kidney disease. Cochrane Database Syst Rev. 2006;(4):CD006257.

36. Wang B, Wang F, Zhang Y, Zhao SH, Zhao WJ, Yan SL, et al. Effects of RAS inhibitors on diabetic retinopathy: a systematic review and meta-analysis. Lancet Diabetes Endocrinol. 2015;3(4):263–74.
37. Kidney Disease: Improving Global Outcomes (KDIGO) Diabetes Work Group. KDIGO 2020 clinical practice guideline for diabetes management in chronic kidney disease. Kidney Int. 2020;98(4S):S1–S115.
38. Sleight P, Yusuf S, Pogue J, Tsuyuki R, Diaz R, Probstfield J, et al. Blood-pressure reduction and cardiovascular risk in HOPE study. Lancet. 2001;358(9299):2130–1.
39. Parving HH, Lehnert H, Brochner-Mortensen J, Gomis R, Andersen S, Arner P, et al. The effect of irbesartan on the development of diabetic nephropathy in patients with type 2 diabetes. N Engl J Med. 2001;345(12):870–8.
40. Makino H, Haneda M, Babazono T, Moriya T, Ito S, Iwamoto Y, et al. Prevention of transition from incipient to overt nephropathy with telmisartan in patients with type 2 diabetes. Diabetes Care. 2007;30(6):1577–8.
41. Brenner BM, Cooper ME, de Zeeuw D, Keane WF, Mitch WE, Parving HH, et al. Effects of losartan on renal and cardiovascular outcomes in patients with type 2 diabetes and nephropathy. N Engl J Med. 2001;345(12):861–9.
42. Keane WF, Brenner BM, de Zeeuw D, Grunfeld JP, McGill J, Mitch WE, et al. The risk of developing end-stage renal disease in patients with type 2 diabetes and nephropathy: the RENAAL study. Kidney Int. 2003;63(4):1499–507.
43. Lewis EJ, Hunsicker LG, Clarke WR, Berl T, Pohl MA, Lewis JB, et al. Renoprotective effect of the angiotensin-receptor antagonist irbesartan in patients with nephropathy due to type 2 diabetes. N Engl J Med. 2001;345(12):851–60.
44. Dahlof B, Devereux RB, Kjeldsen SE, Julius S, Beevers G, de Faire U, et al. Cardiovascular morbidity and mortality in the losartan intervention for endpoint reduction in hypertension study (LIFE): a randomised trial against atenolol. Lancet. 2002;359(9311):995–1003.
45. Svensson P, de Faire U, Sleight P, Yusuf S, Ostergren J. Comparative effects of ramipril on ambulatory and office blood pressures: a HOPE substudy. Hypertension. 2001;38(6):E28–32.
46. Thomopoulos C, Parati G, Zanchetti A. Effects of blood-pressure-lowering treatment on outcome incidence in hypertension: 10 - Should blood pressure management differ in hypertensive patients with and without diabetes mellitus? Overview and meta-analyses of randomized trials. J Hypertens. 2017;35(5):922–44.
47. Bangalore S, Kamalakkannan G, Parkar S, Messerli FH. Fixed-dose combinations improve medication compliance: a meta-analysis. Am J Med. 2007;120(8):713–9.
48. Jamerson K, Weber MA, Bakris GL, Dahlof B, Pitt B, Shi V, et al. Benazepril plus amlodipine or hydrochlorothiazide for hypertension in high-risk patients. N Engl J Med. 2008;359(23):2417–28.
49. Bangalore S, Kumar S, Messerli FH. Angiotensin-converting enzyme inhibitor associated cough: deceptive information from the Physicians' desk reference. Am J Med. 2010;123(11):1016–30.
50. Tseng DS, Kwong J, Rezvani F, Coates AO. Angiotensin-converting enzyme-related cough among Chinese-Americans. Am J Med. 2010;123(2):183 e11–5.
51. McDowell SE, Coleman JJ, Ferner RE. Systematic review and meta-analysis of ethnic differences in risks of adverse reactions to drugs used in cardiovascular medicine. BMJ. 2006;332(7551):1177–81.
52. Banerji A, Blumenthal KG, Lai KH, Zhou L. Epidemiology of ACE inhibitor angioedema utilizing a large electronic health record. J Allergy Clin Immunol Pract. 2017;5(3):744–9.
53. Fried LF, Emanuele N, Zhang JH, Brophy M, Conner TA, Duckworth W, et al. Combined angiotensin inhibition for the treatment of diabetic nephropathy. N Engl J Med. 2013;369(20):1892–903.
54. Yusuf S, Teo KK, Pogue J, Dyal L, Copland I, Schumacher H, et al. Telmisartan, ramipril, or both in patients at high risk for vascular events. N Engl J Med. 2008;358(15):1547–59.
55. Whelton PK, Barzilay J, Cushman WC, Davis BR, Iiamathi E, Kostis JB, et al. Clinical outcomes in antihypertensive treatment of type 2 diabetes, impaired fasting glucose

concentration, and normoglycemia: antihypertensive and lipid-lowering treatment to prevent heart attack trial (ALLHAT). Arch Intern Med. 2005;165(12):1401–9.
56. Hansson L, Zanchetti A, Carruthers SG, Dahlof B, Elmfeldt D, Julius S, et al. Effects of intensive blood-pressure lowering and low-dose aspirin in patients with hypertension: principal results of the hypertension optimal treatment (HOT) randomised trial. HOT Study Group. Lancet. 1998;351(9118):1755–62.
57. Tuomilehto J, Rastenyte D, Birkenhager WH, Thijs L, Antikainen R, Bulpitt CJ, et al. Effects of calcium-channel blockade in older patients with diabetes and systolic hypertension. Systolic Hypertension in Europe Trial Investigators. N Engl J Med. 1999;340(9):677–84.
58. Ostergren J, Poulter NR, Sever PS, Dahlof B, Wedel H, Beevers G, et al. The Anglo-Scandinavian cardiac outcomes trial: blood pressure-lowering limb: effects in patients with type II diabetes. J Hypertens. 2008;26(11):2103–11.
59. Weber MA, Bakris GL, Jamerson K, Weir M, Kjeldsen SE, Devereux RB, et al. Cardiovascular events during differing hypertension therapies in patients with diabetes. J Am Coll Cardiol. 2010;56(1):77–85.
60. Elliott WJ. Rationale for a single-pill combination of perindopril arginine and amlodipine besylate. J Am Soc Hypertens. 2015;9(4):257–65.
61. Brown MJ, Palmer CR, Castaigne A, de Leeuw PW, Mancia G, Rosenthal T, et al. Morbidity and mortality in patients randomised to double-blind treatment with a long-acting calcium-channel blocker or diuretic in the international Nifedipine GITS study: intervention as a goal in hypertension treatment (INSIGHT). Lancet. 2000;356(9227):366–72.
62. Messerli FH, Grossman E. Pedal edema--not all dihydropyridine calcium antagonists are created equal. Am J Hypertens. 2002;15(11):1019–20.
63. Makani H, Bangalore S, Romero J, Wever-Pinzon O, Messerli FH. Effect of renin-angiotensin system blockade on calcium channel blocker-associated peripheral edema. Am J Med. 2011;124(2):128–35.
64. Curb JD, Pressel SL, Cutler JA, Savage PJ, Applegate WB, Black H, et al. Effect of diuretic-based antihypertensive treatment on cardiovascular disease risk in older diabetic patients with isolated systolic hypertension. Systolic hypertension in the elderly program cooperative research group. JAMA. 1996;276(23):1886–92.
65. Barzilay JI, Davis BR, Bettencourt J, Margolis KL, Goff DC Jr, Black H, et al. Cardiovascular outcomes using doxazosin vs. chlorthalidone for the treatment of hypertension in older adults with and without glucose disorders: a report from the ALLHAT study. J Clin Hypertens (Greenwich). 2004;6(3):116–25.
66. Hansson L, Lindholm LH, Niskanen L, Lanke J, Hedner T, Niklason A, et al. Effect of angiotensin-converting-enzyme inhibition compared with conventional therapy on cardiovascular morbidity and mortality in hypertension: the captopril prevention project (CAPPP) randomised trial. Lancet. 1999;353(9153):611–6.
67. ALLHAT Officers and Coordinators for the ALLHAT Collaborative Research Group. Major outcomes in high-risk hypertensive patients randomized to angiotensin-converting enzyme inhibitor or calcium channel blocker vs diuretic: the antihypertensive and lipid-lowering treatment to prevent heart attack trial (ALLHAT). JAMA. 2002;288(23):2981–97.
68. Niskanen L, Hedner T, Hansson L, Lanke J, Niklason A, CAPPP Study Group. Reduced cardiovascular morbidity and mortality in hypertensive diabetic patients on first-line therapy with an ACE inhibitor compared with a diuretic/beta-blocker-based treatment regimen: a subanalysis of the captopril prevention project. Diabetes Care. 2001;24(12):2091–6.
69. Pareek AK, Messerli FH, Chandurkar NB, Dharmadhikari SK, Godbole AV, Kshirsagar PP, et al. Efficacy of low-dose chlorthalidone and hydrochlorothiazide as assessed by 24-h ambulatory blood pressure monitoring. J Am Coll Cardiol. 2016;67(4):379–89.
70. Chen P, Chaugai S, Zhao F, Wang DW. Cardioprotective effect of thiazide-like diuretics: a meta-analysis. Am J Hypertens. 2015;28(12):1453–63.
71. Roush GC, Ernst ME, Kostis JB, Tandon S, Sica DA. Head-to-head comparisons of hydrochlorothiazide with indapamide and chlorthalidone: antihypertensive and metabolic effects. Hypertension. 2015;65(5):1041–6.

72. Olde Engberink RH, Frenkel WJ, van den Bogaard B, Brewster LM, Vogt L, van den Born BJ. Effects of thiazide-type and thiazide-like diuretics on cardiovascular events and mortality: systematic review and meta-analysis. Hypertension. 2015;65(5):1033–40.
73. Harper R, Ennis CN, Heaney AP, Sheridan B, Gormley M, Atkinson AB, et al. A comparison of the effects of low- and conventional-dose thiazide diuretic on insulin action in hypertensive patients with NIDDM. Diabetologia. 1995;38(7):853–9.
74. Lindholm LH, Carlberg B, Samuelsson O. Should beta blockers remain first choice in the treatment of primary hypertension? A meta-analysis. Lancet. 2005;366(9496):1545–53.
75. Khan N, McAlister FA. Re-examining the efficacy of beta-blockers for the treatment of hypertension: a meta-analysis. CMAJ. 2006;174(12):1737–42.
76. Kuyper LM, Khan NA. Atenolol vs nonatenolol beta-blockers for the treatment of hypertension: a meta-analysis. Can J Cardiol. 2014;30(5 Suppl):S47–53.
77. Messerli FH, Grossman E, Goldbourt U. Are beta-blockers efficacious as first-line therapy for hypertension in the elderly? A systematic review. JAMA. 1998;279(23):1903–7.
78. Cruickshank JM. The role of beta-blockers in the treatment of hypertension. Adv Exp Med Biol. 2017;956:149–66.
79. Thomopoulos C, Parati G, Zanchetti A. Effects of blood pressure lowering on outcome incidence in hypertension: 4. Effects of various classes of antihypertensive drugs--overview and meta-analyses. J Hypertens. 2015;33(2):195–211.
80. Jacob S, Rett K, Henriksen EJ. Antihypertensive therapy and insulin sensitivity: do we have to redefine the role of beta-blocking agents? Am J Hypertens. 1998;11(10):1258–65.
81. Bakris GL, Fonseca V, Katholi RE, McGill JB, Messerli FH, Phillips RA, et al. Metabolic effects of carvedilol vs metoprolol in patients with type 2 diabetes mellitus and hypertension: a randomized controlled trial. JAMA. 2004;292(18):2227–36.
82. Ko DT, Hebert PR, Coffey CS, Sedrakyan A, Curtis JP, Krumholz HM. Beta-blocker therapy and symptoms of depression, fatigue, and sexual dysfunction. JAMA. 2002;288(3):351–7.
83. Herings RM, de Boer A, Stricker BH, Leufkens HG, Porsius A. Hypoglycaemia associated with use of inhibitors of angiotensin converting enzyme. Lancet. 1995;345(8959):1195–8.
84. Shorr RI, Ray WA, Daugherty JR, Griffin MR. Antihypertensives and the risk of serious hypoglycemia in older persons using insulin or sulfonylureas. JAMA. 1997;278(1):40–3.
85. UK Prospective Diabetes Study (UKPDS) Group. Efficacy of atenolol and captopril in reducing risk of macrovascular and microvascular complications in type 2 diabetes: UKPDS 39. BMJ. 1998;317(7160):713–20.
86. Borghi C, Tubach F, De Backer G, Dallongeville J, Guallar E, Medina J, et al. Lack of control of hypertension in primary cardiovascular disease prevention in Europe: results from the EURIKA study. Int J Cardiol. 2016;218:83–8.
87. Sim JJ, Bhandari SK, Shi J, Liu IL, Calhoun DA, McGlynn EA, et al. Characteristics of resistant hypertension in a large, ethnically diverse hypertension population of an integrated health system. Mayo Clin Proc. 2013;88(10):1099–107.
88. Daugherty SL, Powers JD, Magid DJ, Tavel HM, Masoudi FA, Margolis KL, et al. Incidence and prognosis of resistant hypertension in hypertensive patients. Circulation. 2012;125(13):1635–42.
89. Williams B, MacDonald TM, Morant S, Webb DJ, Sever P, McInnes G, et al. Spironolactone versus placebo, bisoprolol, and doxazosin to determine the optimal treatment for drug-resistant hypertension (PATHWAY-2): a randomised, double-blind, crossover trial. Lancet. 2015;386(10008):2059–68.
90. Williams B, MacDonald TM, Morant SV, Webb DJ, Sever P, McInnes GT, et al. Endocrine and haemodynamic changes in resistant hypertension, and blood pressure responses to spironolactone or amiloride: the PATHWAY-2 mechanisms substudies. Lancet Diabetes Endocrinol. 2018;6(6):464–75.
91. Makai P, IntHout J, Deinum J, Jenniskens K, Wilt GJV. A network meta-analysis of clinical management strategies for treatment-resistant hypertension: making optimal use of the evidence. J Gen Intern Med. 2017;32(8):921–30.

92. Sinnott SJ, Tomlinson LA, Root AA, Mathur R, Mansfield KE, Smeeth L, et al. Comparative effectiveness of fourth-line anti-hypertensive agents in resistant hypertension: a systematic review and meta-analysis. Eur J Prev Cardiol. 2017;24(3):228–38.
93. Tataru AP, Barry AR. A systematic review of add-on pharmacologic therapy in the treatment of resistant hypertension. Am J Cardiovasc Drugs. 2017;17(4):311–8.
94. Zhao D, Liu H, Dong P, Zhao J. A meta-analysis of add-on use of spironolactone in patients with resistant hypertension. Int J Cardiol. 2017;233:113–7.
95. Bakris GL, Agarwal R, Chan JC, Cooper ME, Gansevoort RT, Haller H, et al. Effect of finerenone on albuminuria in patients with diabetic nephropathy: a randomized clinical trial. JAMA. 2015;314(9):884–94.
96. Filippatos G, Anker SD, Bohm M, Gheorghiade M, Kober L, Krum H, et al. A randomized controlled study of finerenone vs. eplerenone in patients with worsening chronic heart failure and diabetes mellitus and/or chronic kidney disease. Eur Heart J. 2016;37(27):2105–14.
97. Mehdi UF, Adams-Huet B, Raskin P, Vega GL, Toto RD. Addition of angiotensin receptor blockade or mineralocorticoid antagonism to maximal angiotensin-converting enzyme inhibition in diabetic nephropathy. J Am Soc Nephrol. 2009;20(12):2641–50.
98. Sato A, Hayashi K, Naruse M, Saruta T. Effectiveness of aldosterone blockade in patients with diabetic nephropathy. Hypertension. 2003;41(1):64–8.
99. Oxlund CS, Henriksen JE, Tarnow L, Schousboe K, Gram J, Jacobsen IA. Low dose spironolactone reduces blood pressure in patients with resistant hypertension and type 2 diabetes mellitus: a double blind randomized clinical trial. J Hypertens. 2013;31(10):2094–102.
100. Vukadinovic D, Lavall D, Vukadinovic AN, Pitt B, Wagenpfeil S, Bohm M. True rate of mineralocorticoid receptor antagonists-related hyperkalemia in placebo-controlled trials: a meta-analysis. Am Heart J. 2017;188:99–108.
101. Chatterjee S, Moeller C, Shah N, Bolorunduro O, Lichstein E, Moskovits N, et al. Eplerenone is not superior to older and less expensive aldosterone antagonists. Am J Med. 2012;125(8):817–25.
102. Kovesdy CP, Matsushita K, Sang Y, Brunskill NJ, Carrero JJ, Chodick G, et al. Serum potassium and adverse outcomes across the range of kidney function: a CKD prognosis consortium meta-analysis. Eur Heart J. 2018;39(17):1535–42.
103. Pitt B, Zannad F, Remme WJ, Cody R, Castaigne A, Perez A, et al. The effect of spironolactone on morbidity and mortality in patients with severe heart failure. Randomized Aldactone Evaluation Study Investigators. N Engl J Med. 1999;341(10):709–17.
104. Parthasarathy HK, Menard J, White WB, Young WF Jr, Williams GH, Williams B, et al. A double-blind, randomized study comparing the antihypertensive effect of eplerenone and spironolactone in patients with hypertension and evidence of primary aldosteronism. J Hypertens. 2011;29(5):980–90.
105. Engbaek M, Hjerrild M, Hallas J, Jacobsen IA. The effect of low-dose spironolactone on resistant hypertension. J Am Soc Hypertens. 2010;4(6):290–4.
106. Garthwaite SM, McMahon EG. The evolution of aldosterone antagonists. Mol Cell Endocrinol. 2004;217(1–2):27–31.
107. Pitt B, Bakris G, Ruilope LM, DiCarlo L, Mukherjee R; EPHESUS Investigators. Serum potassium and clinical outcomes in the eplerenone post-acute myocardial infarction heart failure efficacy and survival study (EPHESUS). Circulation. 2008;118(16):1643–50.
108. Cushman WC, Ford CE, Cutler JA, Margolis KL, Davis BR, Grimm RH, et al. Success and predictors of blood pressure control in diverse north American settings: the antihypertensive and lipid-lowering treatment to prevent heart attack trial (ALLHAT). J Clin Hypertens (Greenwich). 2002;4(6):393–404.
109. Dahlof B, Sever PS, Poulter NR, Wedel H, Beevers DG, Caulfield M, et al. Prevention of cardiovascular events with an antihypertensive regimen of amlodipine adding perindopril as required versus atenolol adding bendroflumethiazide as required, in the Anglo-Scandinavian Cardiac Outcomes Trial-Blood Pressure Lowering Arm (ASCOT-BPLA): a multicentre randomised controlled trial. Lancet. 2005;366(9489):895–906.

110. Julius S, Kjeldsen SE, Weber M, Brunner HR, Ekman S, Hansson L, et al. Outcomes in hypertensive patients at high cardiovascular risk treated with regimens based on valsartan or amlodipine: the VALUE randomised trial. Lancet. 2004;363(9426):2022–31.
111. Corrao G, Nicotra F, Parodi A, Zambon A, Heiman F, Merlino L, et al. Cardiovascular protection by initial and subsequent combination of antihypertensive drugs in daily life practice. Hypertension. 2011;58(4):566–72.
112. Gradman AH, Parise H, Lefebvre P, Falvey H, Lafeuille MH, Duh MS. Initial combination therapy reduces the risk of cardiovascular events in hypertensive patients: a matched cohort study. Hypertension. 2013;61(2):309–18.
113. Yusuf S, Joseph P, Dans A, Gao P, Teo K, Xavier D, et al. Polypill with or without aspirin in persons without cardiovascular disease. N Engl J Med. 2021;384(3):216–28.
114. Lonn EM, Bosch J, Lopez-Jaramillo P, Zhu J, Liu L, Pais P, et al. Blood-pressure lowering in intermediate-risk persons without cardiovascular disease. N Engl J Med. 2016;374(21):2009–20.
115. Sherrill B, Halpern M, Khan S, Zhang J, Panjabi S. Single-pill vs free-equivalent combination therapies for hypertension: a meta-analysis of health care costs and adherence. J Clin Hypertens (Greenwich). 2011;13(12):898–909.
116. Taylor AA, Shoheiber O. Adherence to antihypertensive therapy with fixed-dose amlodipine besylate/benazepril HCl versus comparable component-based therapy. Congest Heart Fail. 2003;9(6):324–32.
117. Patel A, Group AC, MacMahon S, Chalmers J, Neal B, Woodward M, et al. Effects of a fixed combination of perindopril and indapamide on macrovascular and microvascular outcomes in patients with type 2 diabetes mellitus (the ADVANCE trial): a randomised controlled trial. Lancet. 2007;370(9590):829–40.
118. Epstein M, Bakris G. Newer approaches to antihypertensive therapy. Use of fixed-dose combination therapy. Arch Intern Med. 1996;156(17):1969–78.

Part VIII

Antihypertensive Drugs and Diabetes Mellitus: Special Problems

25 Adverse Reactions in Renal Function and Electrolytes Associated with Antihypertensive and Antidiabetic Therapy

Adel E. Berbari, Najla A. Daouk, and Majida M. Daouk

25.1 Introduction

Cardiovascular disorders remain global health burden and major causes of morbidity and mortality worldwide [1]. Hypertension, diabetes mellitus (DM), and chronic kidney disease (CKD) constitute important determinants of the continuum of vascular diseases [2, 3]. It is well established that the renin–angiotensin–aldosterone system (RAAS) plays an important role in the pathogenesis of a wide spectrum of the cardiorenal disorders through hemodynamic, inflammatory, neurohormonal, and humoral mechanisms [2].

Numerous studies have demonstrated that attenuation of the cascade of the renin–angiotensin system (RAS) provides effective blood pressure (BP) control and confers cardiorenal protection in a wide spectrum of cardiovascular diseases [2, 4]. In the light of these findings, this class of antihypertensive medications has been recommended as first-class therapy in subjects with hypertension, diabetes mellitus, and diabetic and nondiabetic CKD [4–7]. However, blockade of RAS therapy may be associated with significant renal functional impairment and/or electrolyte disturbances in a subset of these patients [4, 8–14].

25.2 Adverse Renal Reactions to Renin–Angiotensin–Aldosterone System Blockade

RAAS blockade therapy is used extensively in the management of a wide spectrum of vascular disorders [6, 7]. However, emergence of safety concerns on renal function has evoked a more cautious approach in the use of RAAS inhibitors [8–16].

A. E. Berbari (✉) · N. A. Daouk · M. M. Daouk
Department of Internal Medicine, American University of Beirut Medical Center, Beirut, Lebanon
e-mail: ab01@aub.edu.lb

A. E. Berbari, G. Mancia (eds.), *Blood Pressure Disorders in Diabetes Mellitus*, Updates in Hypertension and Cardiovascular Protection,
https://doi.org/10.1007/978-3-031-13009-0_25

25.2.1 Renin–Angiotensin–Aldosterone System Blockade Associated Decline in Renal Function: General Features

It is well established that initiation of RAAS inhibitors is associated with an acute decline in renal function characterized by an acute increase in baseline serum creatinine levels, decrease in baseline glomerular filtration rate (eGFR), or both [17, 18]. However, the threshold at which changes in these renal functional parameters are considered nonphysiologic remain undetermined [19].

According to experts, an acute increase in baseline serum creatinine levels to less than 30% (<30%) equivalent to a 27% decline in eGFR following ACEI/ARB (angiotensin-converting enzyme inhibitors/angiotensin receptor blockers) treatment is accepted as a physiologic, primarily functional, and potentially reversible phenomenon [19, 20]. This change in renal function is reported to occur within 2 weeks of RAAS blockade treatment, appears to be safe being associated with minimal cardiovascular events, and may even afford long-term renoprotection [9, 19–21]. Several clinical studies provide support to this concept [19]. Review of 12 randomized clinical trials of CKD patients revealed that, following initiation of RAAS blockade therapy, an increase in baseline serum creatinine levels to less than 30% was common, occurred within 2 weeks, and was not associated with any harm [9, 19]. Conversely, higher serum creatinine concentrations were associated with cerebrovascular complications [22]. In a large population-based study of patients on RAS inhibition treatment, elevation of serum creatinine levels to 30% or more was associated with increased rates of cardiorenal complications [22]. Compared with patients with an increased serum creatinine levels of less than 30%, those with serum creatinine elevation of more than 30% (i) were more frequently elderly women (56.1% vs. 46.1%) and (ii) had (a) more severe advanced CKD (stages 3b-4: 8.9% vs. 4.3%) and (b) higher rates of multiple cardiovascular events (52.7% vs. 18.6%) [22]. Further, those patients who displayed an increase of serum creatinine concentrations of 30% or more were often receiving medications that by themselves are associated with adverse renal outcomes, such as loop and K sparing diuretics and nonsteroidal anti-inflammatory drugs [22].

This study reports additional interesting observations: significant renal impairment (increase in serum creatinine ≥30%) associated with start of ACEI/ARB therapy appears to be uncommon in clinical practice. In this very large population-based cohort of over 300,000 patients, only 1.7% exhibited an increase of serum creatinine levels of ≥30% [16]. In contrast, in the Stockholm Creatinine Measurements (SCREAM) project, in a large health care–based observational study, an increase of serum creatinine >30% was reported in 4% subjects on RAS blockade therapy [22]; further, milder degrees of serum creatinine elevations following RAS blockade were not infrequent and not negligible [22]. There was a trend of increasing risk of cardiorenal events associated with increasing baseline serum creatinine levels [22]. Detailed categorization of serum creatinine elevations was associated with dose response and graduated enhanced risk of cardiorenal events [22]. Using serum creatinine increases of less than 10% as reference, incidence rate ratios of end-stage renal disease increased steadily from patients with serum creatinine increases of

10–19% to those with serum creatinine elevations of 40% (1.73 vs. 4.04) [22]. Similarly, increased incidence of rate ratios were noted for cardiovascular outcomes; a reverse relationship between duration of RAS blockade administration and enhanced risk of cardiorenal complications has been observed in patients with significant renal functional impairment (serum creatinine increase >30%) [9, 22]. The incidence rates of CKD decreased from 12.2-fold during the first year to 2.5-fold within 5–10 years [16]. Similarly, the mortality rate ratio declined from a 3.5 increase within the first year and remained 50% less thereafter [16].

Conversely, long-term RAAS blockade therapy also has been reported to be associated with deterioration of renal function and late onset azotemia in a subgroup of high-risk patients [23, 24]. In a cohort of 6102 subjects with long-standing diabetes mellitus treated with various antihypertensive medications were followed up until the development of end-stage renal failure (ESRF) [12]. The rate ratio of ESRF with the use of angiotensin converting enzyme inhibitors (ACEI) was 0.8 during the first 3 years of follow-up but increased to 4.2 after 3 years thereafter [12]. Further relative to thiazide diuretic use, the adjusted risk ratio of ESRF associated with ACEI was 2.5, whereas it was 0.8 for beta-blockers and 0.7 for calcium channel antagonists [12]. A small study reported similar observations [25]. Although the mechanism underlying late onset azotemia with RAAS blockade therapy remains unclear, it has been attributed to microvascular disease as many patients are elderly [16].

25.2.2 Determinants of Impairment of Renal Function Associated with Renin–Angiotensin–Aldosterone System Blockade Therapy

It is well established that, in most patients, initiation of RAAS blockade therapy is commonly associated with mild reversible renal functional impairment and affords cardiorenovascular protection in the long term [9, 23]. Conversely, administration of ACEI or ARB drugs may cause significant and progressive renal functional impairment (acute increase in baseline serum creatinine ≥30%, equivalent to acute reduction in baseline eGFR ≥27) in one or more of the following settings: (i) patients with comorbidities (diabetes mellitus, CKD, and cardiovascular disease); (ii) altered extracellular fluid volumes and/or systemic parameters (severe dehydration, excessive diuresis, and low BP/hypotension); (iii) the use of concurrent drugs that are by themselves associated with adverse renal outcomes (diuretics, nonsteroidal anti-inflammatory drugs, and cyclosporine) [16, 23].

25.2.3 Role of Renin–Angiotensin–Aldosterone System in Pathogenesis of Chronic Kidney Disease

Overaction of the RAAS plays an important role in the initiation and progression of chronic kidney disease [8, 23]. Both circulating and renally expressed RAAS enhances the vascular tone of systemic and glomerular precapillary resistance vessels, leading to increased systemic BP and glomerular hydraulic pressure, damage to glomerular filtration barrier, and increased ultrafiltration of plasma proteins, an additional damaging process [8, 23]. In addition, non-hemodynamic factors, through enhanced aldosterone secretion and stimulation of inflammatory processes, contribute to the glomerulotubular and target organ disease, predisposing to the development of cardiorenal events [23].

25.2.4 Initiation/Withdrawal of Renin–Angiotensin–Aldosterone System Blockade Therapy in Advanced Stages of Chronic Kidney Disease

Numerous clinical studies support the benefits for initiating RAS blockade therapy in the earlier stages of CKD for the prevention of CKD progression, especially among patients with proteinuria [8, 23, 26]. However, fewer studies have evaluated the renal benefits of RAS inhibition in the setting of advanced stages of CKD (eGFR ≤30 ml/min/1.73m^2 and/or serum creatinine levels ≥2 mg/dl), whether these agents, when already prescribed, should be continued or withdrawn in those groups of patients.

25.2.4.1 De Novo Initiation of Renin–Angiotensin–Aldosterone System Blockade Therapy in Advanced Stages of Chronic Kidney Disease

The renal benefits offered by RAS blockade therapy in advanced stages of CKD remain unclear.

Among the few studies that reported beneficial renal effects, a clinical trial conducted in China evaluated the renal benefits of ACE inhibitors in two groups of untreated nondiabetic advanced stages of CKD (group 1: baseline serum creatinine levels: 1.5–3.0 mg/dl vs. group 2: baseline serum creatinine levels: 3.1–5.0 mg/dl) [8, 27]. Compared with placebo, administration of benazepril, an ACE inhibitor, delayed further progression of CKD (as evidenced by composite outcome of doubling serum creatinine levels, end-stage renal disease (ESRD)), or death in both groups [8, 27]. However, more participants in group 2 (baseline serum creatinine: 3.1–5.0 mg/dl) receiving benazepril treatment reached the composite endpoint compared with those with serum creatinine levels of <3 mg/dl (group 1) [27]. According to the investigators, these findings suggest that ACE inhibition may be maximized if used in earlier stages of advanced CKD [9, 12].

Other trials have reported similar observations. Both Ramipril Efficacy in Nephrology (REIN) and African American Study of Kidney Disease and Hypertension (AASK) demonstrated that RAS inhibition treatment reduced the risk of progression of advanced stages of CKD, in both proteinuric and non-proteinuric patients [9, 19].

In contrast, other investigations indicate that RAS inhibition treatment worsens the course of advanced stages of CKD. In a prior nested case–control study in a cohort of diabetic patients, reported that the risk of ESRD was fourfold higher among those who were receiving ACE inhibition treatment during long-term follow-up [12].

25.2.4.2 Indication for Continuation/Cessation of Renin–Angiotensin–Aldosterone System Blockade Therapy in Advanced Chronic Kidney Disease

There are limited studies that address the question of continuation versus withdrawal of RAS inhibition therapy in advanced stages of CKD [28]. Further, these studies have reported conflicting observations [28].

Some studies support the benefit and recommend continuation of ACEI/ARB treatment in advanced stages of CKD [28]. In a randomized double blind clinical trial, the effect of an ACEI was evaluated on the course of advanced nondiabetic CKD patients [27]. Administration of benazepril, an ACE inhibitor (ACEI), to patients with advanced CKD with baseline serum creatinine levels of 3.1–5 mg/dl and persistent proteinuria over a follow-up of 3 years, compared with placebo, revealed a 51% reduction in risk of doubling serum creatinine and 40% reduction on the risk of ESRD [27]. Similar findings were reported in other studies. Post hoc analysis of data of REIN and RENAAL clinical trials revealed that administration of Ramipril and Losartan was associated with a greater reduction in risk of renal failure in lowest tertiles of GFR compared with higher GFR among patients with advanced CKD stages [29, 30].

In contrast to the above studies that support the use of ACEI/ARB administration in advanced CKD, other examinations do not. In a retrospective propensity score matched study that enrolled 3239 patients with stages 4 and 5 CKD, the use of ACEI/ARB was associated with enhanced risk of ESRD and higher rate of hospitalization of hyperkalemia compared with nonusers [26, 31]. Further, in a small observational study of 100 patients with advanced CKD who developed 25% increase in baseline serum creatinine while on ACEI/ARB treatment during follow-up, withdrawal of RAS blockade therapy resulted in improvement in renal function and delay in the need for renal replacement therapy [26, 32]. Other small observations studies reported similar findings [9].

Withdrawal of RAS blockade therapy has been recommended in the following subset of patients with advanced CKD: (i) rapid and significant increase in baseline serum creatinine and/or reduction in baseline eGFR, (ii) persistent hyperkalemia when measures to control serum K fail, (iii) renal artery stenosis, (iv) repeated episodes of acute kidney injury, and v) hypotension [9, 33].

25.3 Hyperkalemia-Antihypertensive Drugs Association

Antihypertensive medications are frequently associated with adverse disturbances in electrolyte homeostasis [13]. Hyperkalemia is one of the most common serum electrolyte abnormalities and represents a very serious adverse drug reaction due to its potential for causing life-threatening arrhythmias [13].

25.3.1 Definition/Frequency

There is no universally agreed definition of hyperkalemia, although most studies use the European Resuscitation Council Definition of serum K as >5.5 mmol/L [34, 35]. However, recent data suggest that, in patients with CKD, the upper limit of serum K levels should not exceed 4.8 mmol/L as mortality increases above this level [36, 37].

Hyperkalemia has been further characterized by the abnormality of serum K as (i) mild (serum K = 5.5–5.9 mnol/L), (ii) moderate (serum K = 6.0–6.4 mmol/L), and (iii) severe (serum K > 6.4 mmol/L) [35, 36].

Incidence and prevalence rates of hyperkalemia are quite variable and depend, to a larger extent on the definition used, the condition studied, the presence of comorbidities, acuteness/chronicity of serum K elevation, and type of medications prescribed [36].

Although not well studied, the incidence and prevalence rates of hyperkalemia appear to be low in the general population [37]. In a large study involving 129,076 hospital admissions among elderly patients (older than 65 years) in Canada, hyperkalemia was reported in 2.6% of emergency room visits and 3.5% hospital admission [38]. Similar findings of low hyperkalemia rates of 3.2% and 2.6%, respectively, were reported in two large studies in US veterans [39, 40].

25.3.2 Predictors of Hyperkalemia

Reduced glomerular filtration rate, diabetes mellitus, and some classes of antihypertensive medications constitute the most important predictors of hyperkalemia [38, 40, 41]. Further, clustering of several of these conditions enhance significantly the risk of an increase in serum K levels [38, 41].

In a large study that included 245, 808 hospitalized US veterans, CKD and the use of RAAS inhibitors were the most important factors associated with hyperkalemia [38, 41, 42].

25.3.2.1 Reduced Glomerular Filtration Rate

Hyperkalemia is very common in patients with CKD [40]. In a study of 1277 US veterans with a mean estimated glomerular filtration rate (eGFR) of 37 ml/min/1.73m^2, the incidence of baseline serum K > 5.3 mmol/L was 7.7% [38]. In another smaller study of 238 patients with eGFR = 14.6 ml/min/1.73m^2, the incidence rates of serum K levels above 5.0 mmol/L and 5.5 mmol/L were 54% and 40%, respectively [38, 43].

Several factors enhance the risk of hyperkalemia in patients with CKD: (i) inappropriate high K intake in relation to the degree of renal functional impairment, (ii) commonly observed extracellular K shift associated with metabolic acidosis of renal failure, and (iii) frequent administration of RAAS inhibitors [40].

Potassium homeostasis is tightly controlled by a fine balance between intake and excretion of K [43]. During the course of progression of CKD, adaptive structural changes occur in the remaining nephrons, which, however, have a very limited capacity to enhance K secretion in response to an exogenous K load, compared with subjects with normal healthy kidneys [44].

As GFR falls, the decrease in urinary K excretion causes an elevation in serum K levels and creates a new K steady state [45, 46]. As a result, kaliuretic mechanisms are stimulated; enhancing kaliuresis and overcoming further increase in serum K levels [40, 46]. However, as GFR falls to 45 ml/min/1.73m^2, these mechanisms are disrupted, enhancing the development of hyperkalemia [40, 47].

25.3.2.2 Diabetes Mellitus

Disturbances in electrolyte homeostasis occur frequently in patients with diabetes mellitus and have been attributed to an altered acid-base status, the presence of comorbid disorders, and/or side effects of pharmacotherapeutic treatment [14].

Patients with diabetes mellitus are at an increased risk of an elevation in serum K levels [48]. Hyperkalemia is common and is a serious electrolyte abnormality in these patients [48].

Occurrence rates of hyperkalemia vary and are dependent upon the patient population evaluated. Whereas estimated at 0.3% in the general population, prevalence rates of hyperkalemia appear to be much higher, with reported rates of 1–10% [49]. In a large study conducted in 68, 601 diabetic Danish subjects that initiated on antidiabetic treatment at baseline, 16% developed hyperkalemia during a follow-up period of 4.1 years [49]. However, many of these patients suffered from comorbid disorders (CKD, cardiovascular disease) and/or were receiving antihypertensive medications [49].

25.3.2.3 Antihypertensive Pharmacotherapy

Among the wide spectrum of antihypertensive medications, RAAS inhibitors represent the most common causes of hyperkalemia in the general population [18, 34].

Renin–Angiotensin–Aldosterone System Inhibitors

Hyperkalemia is commonly reported in patients prescribed with RAAS inhibitors. In a patient-based study of 262, 375 patients from Denmark who were newly prescribed with an ACEI, 16% developed hyperkalemia within time period of 2.2 years [50, 51]. Another study including US veterans reported a similar incidence of 11% hyperkalemia over 1 year of follow-up [50, 52].

In over 50% of hospitalized patients of one study, hyperkalemia was first detected within 15 days following initiation of an ARB, with the highest occurrence rate during the first 24 h [53].

RAAS inhibitors, the most commonly used cardiovascular drugs in the treatment of a wide range of cardiorenal disorders, encompass a large class of drugs including angiotensin converting enzyme inhibitors (ACEI), angiotensin receptor blockers (ARB), angiotensin receptor-neprilysin inhibitors (ARNI), and mineralocorticoid receptor antagonists (MRA) [34, 43, 50]. All these subclasses of RAAS inhibitors enhance the risk of an elevation in serum K [43]. A population-based study from Sweden revealed that ACEI, ARB, and MRA increased the odds for hyperkalemia by 57%, 22%, and 44%, respectively [54]. Some studies, however, suggest that the risk of hyperkalemia appears to be slightly lower with ARB compared with ACEI [55].

RAAS inhibitors are more commonly associated with an adverse elevation in serum K levels than with other BP lowering medications [13, 50]. In a study that included 1094 hypertensive nondiabetic CKD patients who randomly assigned to treatment with an ACEI, beta-blocker, or calcium channel blocker and followed-up for 3–6 years [50, 56], administration of an ACEI was associated with a nearly threefold higher risk of hyperkalemia compared with beta-blockers and a sevenfold higher risk of hyperkalemia with calcium channel blockers [50, 56].

In patients prescribed with RAAS inhibitors, the presence of CKD enhances significantly the risk of hyperkalemia. A prospective analysis of records of 245, 808 US veterans revealed that, among patients receiving RAAS inhibitors, the adjusted rate of hyperkalemia was higher in those with CKD compared with those without CKD, both inpatient (7.67 vs. 2.30 per 100 patients-months) and outpatient (8.22 vs. 1.77 per 100 patients-months) settings [38].

Mineralocorticoid Receptor Antagonists

Mineralocorticoid receptor antagonists (MRAs), also known as K sparing diuretics, represent a steroidal class of cardiovascular compounds that, by antagonizing aldosterone, inhibit the epithelial sodium channel and reduce renal K excretion, increasing the risk of elevation of serum K levels [36, 57]. The MRAs class of steroidal drugs includes the nonselective agent spironolactone, its active metabolite canrenone and the selective eplerenone [36, 57].

Moderate to severe hyperkalemia has been reported in 4–19% of patients prescribed with these medications, particularly in those with CKD and/or also receiving RAAS inhibitors [13, 58–60].

The rate of hyperkalemia appears to be dose dependent. In the Randomized Aldactone Evaluation Study (RALES) trial in patients with heart failure, hyperkalemia occurred in 13%, 20%, and 24% of patients receiving 25 mg, 50 mg, and 75 mg of spironolactone, respectively [36, 61].

Beta-Blockers

Beta-blockers represent another class of antihypertensive drugs that may cause elevation in serum K levels [13]. Hyperkalemia, generally mild, has been reported with older nonselective (propranolol and labetolol) and few selective (atenolol and metoprolol), beta-blocking agents [13, 62]. In addition, a recent case report described hyperkalemia in Nebivolol, a third generation beta-blocking agent [63].

25.3.3 Clinical Manifestations and Outcomes of Hyperkalemia

Hyperkalemia is one of the most serious and graded adverse electrolyte disturbances [43].

The most serious clinical manifestations of hyperkalemia include muscle weakness, paralysis, respiratory difficulty or failure, cardiac conduction abnormalities, and malignant arrhythmias [43, 50]. These manifestations are generally associated with serum K greater than 7 mmol/L [64]. Some patients may present with only one or more of the characteristics of ECG features even with significantly increased serum K, which is greater than 9 mmol/L [65].

Hyperkalemia has been associated with increased risk of short-term mortality, which has been attributed to ventricular fibrillation [38]. In a study of 245, 808 hospitalized US veterans, serum K levels greater than 5.5 mmol/L were associated with a significant increased risk in 1-day mortality [38].

25.3.4 Mechanisms of Development of Hyperkalemia

Several mechanisms have been postulated for the development of hyperkalemia single or in combination with different clinical conditions: (i) In patients with moderate to severe CKD, kaliuretic mechanisms fail to maintain K homeostasis, thus enhancing the development of hyperkalemia [43]. This situation appears to occur when the failing GFR reaches 40–45 ml/min/1.73m^2 [43]. (ii) In diabetes mellitus, hyperkalemia is related to deficiencies in insulin and aldosterone [66]. Chronic hyperkalemia in elderly diabetic patients is most often attributed to hyporeninemic/hypoaldosteronism [67]. Further, the reduced insulin levels favor the accumulation of glucose and hyperosmolarity in the extracellular space, preventing intracellular K shift, leading to further elevation of serum K levels [68]. In addition, the presence of CKD in diabetic patients contributes to hyperkalemia [68, 69]. (iii) Use of some classes of drugs that interfere with urinary K excretion (RAAS inhibitors, K sparing diuretics, and NSAIDS) particularly in patients with renal impairment favors the development of hyperkalemia [49, 69].

25.3.5 Principles of Management of Hyperkalemia

The following principles have been recommended for the treatment of hyperkalemia [36, 50]: (i) potassium restricted diet that is often employed as an initial therapy to reduce risk of hyperkalemia in patients with CKD receiving RAAS inhibitors, (ii) elimination of other sources of potassium such as supplements, (iii) withdrawal of prescribed or over the counter drugs that restrict urinary K excretion, (iv) bicarbonate administration to correct metabolic acidosis, and (v) the use of K binding agents that are well tolerated and are effective in maintaining plasma K concentration within the normal range without having to reduce dosing or discontinuing RAAS inhibitors.

References

1. Yusuf S, Joseph P, Rangarajan S, Islam S, Mente A, Hystad P, et al. Modifiable risk factors, cardiovascular disease, and mortality in 155 722 individuals from 21 high-income, middle-income, and low-income countries (PURE): a prospective cohort study. Lancet. 2020;395:795–808.
2. Libianto R, Batu D, MacIsaac RJ, Cooper ME, Ekinci EI. Pathophysiological links between diabetes and blood pressure. Can J Cardiol. 2018;34:585–94.

3. Laffin LJ, Bakris G. Diabetes mellitus and hypertension. In: Berbari AE, Mancia G, editors. Disorders of blood pressure regulation. Springer International Publishing AG, Switzerland; 2018. p. 695–704.
4. Burnier M, Lin S, Ruilope L, Bader G, Durg S, Brunel P. Effect of angiotensin receptor blockers on blood pressure and renal function in patients with concomitant hypertension and chronic kidney disease: a systematic review and meta-analysis. Blood Press. 2019;28:358–74.
5. Wheeler DC, Becker GV. Summary of KDIGO guideline. What do we really know about management of blood pressure in patients with chronic kidney disease? Kidney Int. 2013;83:377–83.
6. Williams B, Mancia G, Spiering W, Agabiti Rosei E, Azizi M, Burnier M, et al. 2018 ESC/ESH Guidelines for the management of arterial hypertension: The Task Force for the management of arterial hypertension of the European Society of Cardiology and the European Society of Hypertension: The Task Force for the management of arterial hypertension of the European Society of Cardiology and the European Society of Hypertension. J Hypertens. 2018;36:1953–2041.
7. Whelton PK, Carey RM, Aronow WS, Casey DE, Collins KJ, Himmelfarb CD. 2017 ACC/AHA/AAPA/ABC/ACPM/AGS/APhA/ASH/ASPC/NMA/PCNA Guideline for the Prevention, Detection, Evaluation, and Management of High Blood Pressure in Adults: Executive Summary: A Report of the American College of Cardiology/American Heart Association Task Force on Clinical Practice Guidelines. J Am Coll Cardiol. 2018;71:2199–269.
8. Ryan MJ, Tuttle KR. Elevations in serum creatinine with RAAS blockade: why isn't it a sign of kidney injury? Curr Opin Nephrol Hypertens. 2008;17:443–9.
9. Bakris GL, Weir MR. Angiotensin-converting enzyme inhibitor-associated elevations in serum creatinine: is this a cause for concern? Arch Intern Med. 2000;160:685–93.
10. Kvam FI, Ofstad J, Iversen BM. Effects of antihypertensive drugs on autoregulation of RBF and glomerular capillary pressure in SHR. Am J Phys. 1998;275(4 part2):F576–84.
11. Bakris GL, Agarwal R. Creatinine bump following antihypertensive therapy. Think before you act. Hypertension. 2018;72:1274–6.
12. Suissa S, Hutchinson T, Brophy JM, Kezouh A. ACE-inhibitor use and the long-term risk of renal failure in diabetes. Kidney Int. 2006;69:913–9.
13. Liamis G, Milionis H, Elisaf M. Blood pressure drug therapy and electrolyte disturbances. Int J Clin Pract. 2008;62:1572–80.
14. Palmer BF, Clegg DJ. Electrolyte and acid-base disturbances in patients with diabetes mellitus. N Engl J Med. 2015;373:548–59.
15. Derezo C, Ruilope LM. The long-term effects of RAAS blockade in renal function. In: Berbari AE, Mancia G, editors. Special issues in hypertension. Springer-Verlag Italia; 2012. p. 467–75.
16. Schmidt M, Mansfield KE, Bhaskaran K, Nitsch D, Sørensen HT, Smeeth L, et al. Serum creatinine elevation after renin-angiotensin system blockade and long term cardiorenal risks: cohort study. BMJ. 2017;356:j791.
17. Palmer BF. Angiotensin-converting enzyme inhibitors and angiotensin receptor blockers: what to do if the serum creatinine and/or serum potassium concentration rises. Nephrol Dial Transplant. 2003;18:1973–5.
18. Weir MR. Acute changes in glomerular filtration rate with renin-angiotensin system (RAS) inhibition: clinical implications. Kidney Int. 2017;91:529–31.
19. Ku E, Bakris G, Johansen KL, Lin F, Sarnak MJ, Campese VM, et al. Acute declines in renal function during intensive BP lowering: implications for future ESRD risk. J Am Soc Nephrol. 2017;28:2794–801.
20. Levey AS, Inker LA, Matsushita K, Greene T, Willis K, Lewis E, et al. GFR decline as an end point for clinical trials in CKD: a scientific workshop sponsored by the National Kidney Foundation and the US Food and Drug Administration. Am J Kidney Dis. 2014;64:821–35.
21. Apperloo AJ, de Zeeuw D, de Jong PE. A short-term antihypertensive treatment-induced fall in glomerular filtration rate predicts long-term stability of renal function. Kidney Int. 1997;51:793–7.

22. Fu EL, Trevisan M, Clase CM, Evans M, Lindholm B, Rotmans JI, et al. Association of acute increases in plasma creatinine after renin-angiotensin blockade with subsequent outcomes. Clin J Am Soc Nephrol. 2019;14:1336–45.
23. Sanidas E, Papadopoulos D, Chatzis M, Velliou M, Barbetseas J. Renin angiotensin aldosterone system inhibitors in chronic kidney disease: a difficult equation. Am J Cardiovasc Drugs. 2021;21:619–27.
24. Onuigbo MAC, Onuigbo NTC. Late onset renal failure from angiotensin blockade (LORFFAB): a prospective thirty-month Mayo Health System clinic experience. Med Sci Monit. 2005;11:462–9.
25. Toto RD, Mitchell HC, Lee HC, Milam C, Pettinger WA. Reversible renal insufficiency due to angiotensin converting enzyme inhibitors in hypertensive nephrosclerosis. Ann Intern Med. 1991;115:513–9.
26. Shah R, Sparks MA. Renin-angiotensin system inhibition in advanced chronic kidney disease: how low can the kidney function go? Curr Opin Nephrol Hypertens. 2019;28:171–7.
27. Hou FF, Zhang X, Zhang GH, Xie D, Chen PY, Zhang WR, et al. Efficacy and safety of benazepril for advanced chronic renal insufficiency. N Engl J Med. 2006;354:131–40.
28. Weir MR, Lakkis JI, Jaar B, Rocco MV, Choi MJ, Kramer HJ, et al. Use of renin-angiotensin system blockade in advanced CKD: an NKF-KDOQI controversies report. Am J Kidney Dis. 2018;72:873–84.
29. Ruggenenti P, Perna A, Gherardi G, Gaspari F, Benini R, Remuzzi G. Renal function and requirement for dialysis in chronic nephropathy patients on long-term ramipril: REIN follow-up trial. Gruppo Italiano di Studi Epidemiologici in Nefrologia (GISEN). Ramipril Efficacy In Nephropathy. Lancet. 1998;352:1252–6.
30. Remuzzi G, Ruggenenti P, Perna A, Dimitrov BD, de Zeeuw D, Hille DA, et al. Continuum of renoprotection with losartan at all stages of type 2 diabetic nephropathy: a post hoc analysis of the RENAAL trial results. J Am Soc Nephrol. 2004;15:3117–25.
31. Oh YJ, Kim SM, Shin BC, Kim HL, Chung JH, Kim AJ, et al. The impact of renin-angiotensin system blockade on renal outcomes and mortality in pre-dialysis patients with advanced chronic kidney disease. PLoS One. 2017;25(12):e0170874.
32. Ahmed AK, Kamath NS, El Kossi M, El Nahas AM. The impact of stopping inhibitors of the renin-angiotensin system in patients with advanced chronic kidney disease. Nephrol Dial Transplant. 2010;25:3977–82.
33. Burnier M. Renin-angiotensin system blockade in advanced kidney disease: stop or continue? Kidney Med. 2020;2:231–4.
34. Weir MR, Rolfe M. Potassium homeostasis and renin-angiotensin-aldosterone system inhibitors. Clin J Am Soc Nephrol. 2010;5:531–48.
35. Truhlář A, Deakin CD, Soar J, Khalifa GA, Alfonzo A, Bierens JJLM, et al. European resuscitation council guidelines for resuscitation 2015: section 4. Cardiac arrest in special circumstances. Resuscitation. 2015;95:148–201.
36. Valdivielso JM, Balafa O, Ekart R, Ferro CJ, Mallamaci F, Mark PB, et al. Hyperkalemia in chronic kidney disease in the new era of kidney protection therapies. Drugs. 2021;81:1467–89.
37. Collins AJ, Pitt B, Reaven N, Funk S, McGaughey K, Wilson D, et al. Association of serum potassium with all-cause mortality in patients with and without heart failure, chronic kidney disease, and/or diabetes. Am J Nephrol. 2017;46:213–21.
38. Kovesdy CP. Epidemiology of hyperkalemia: an update. Kidney Int Suppl. 2016;6:3–6.
39. Fleet JL, Shariff SZ, Gandhi S, Weir MA, Jain AK, Garg AX. Validity of the international classification of diseases 10th revision code for hyperkalaemia in elderly patients at presentation to an emergency department and at hospital admission. BMJ Open. 2012;2:e002011.
40. Einhorn LM, Zhan M, Hsu VD, Walker LD, Moen MF, Seliger SL, et al. The frequency of hyperkalemia and its significance in chronic kidney disease. Arch Intern Med. 2009;169:1156–62.
41. Kovesdy CP. Management of hyperkalemia: an update for the internist. Am J Med. 2015;128:1281–7.

42. Drawz PE, Babineau DC, Rahman M. Metabolic complications in elderly adults with chronic kidney disease. J Am Geriatr Soc. 2012;60:310–5.
43. Vijayakumar S, Butler J, Bakris GL. Barriers to guideline mandated renin–angiotensin inhibitor use: focus on hyperkalaemia. Eur Heart J Suppl. 2019;21(Suppl A):A20–7.
44. Palmer BF, Clegg DJ. Renal considerations in the treatment of hypertension. Am J Hypertens. 2018;31:394–401.
45. Kunau RT, Stein JH. Disorders of hypo- and hyperkalemia. Clin Nephrol. 1977;7:173–90.
46. Gennari FJ, Segal AS. Hyperkalemia: an adaptive response in chronic renal insufficiency. Kidney Int. 2002;62:1–9.
47. Lazich I, Bakris GL. Prediction and management of hyperkalemia across the spectrum of chronic kidney disease. Semin Nephrol. 2014;34:333–9.
48. Jarman PR, Mather HM. Diabetes may be independent risk factor for hyperkalaemia. BMJ. 2003;327:812.
49. Thomsen RW, Nicolaisen SK, Adelborg K, Svensson E, Hasvold P, Palaka E, et al. Hyperkalaemia in people with diabetes: occurrence, risk factors and outcomes in a Danish population-based cohort study. Diabet Med. 2018;35:1051–60.
50. Hundemer GL, Sood MM. Hyperkalemia with RAAS inhibition: mechanism, clinical significance, and management. Pharmacol Res. 2021;172:105835.
51. Adelborg K, Nicolaisen SK, Hasvold P, Palaka E, Pedersen L, Thomsen RW. Predictors for repeated hyperkalemia and potassium trajectories in high-risk patients - a population-based cohort study. PLoS One. 2019;14:e0218739. https://doi.org/10.1371/journal.pone.0218739.
52. Reardon LC, Macpherson DS. Hyperkalemia in outpatients using angiotensin-converting enzyme inhibitors. How much should we worry? Arch Intern Med. 1998;158:26–32.
53. Park I-W, Sheen SS, Yoon D, Lee S-H, Shin G-T, Kim H, et al. Onset time of hyperkalaemia after angiotensin receptor blocker initiation: when should we start serum potassium monitoring? J Clin Pharm Ther. 2014;39(1):61–8.
54. Nilsson E, Gasparini A, Ärnlöv J, Xu H, Henriksson KM, Coresh J. Incidence and determinants of hyperkalemia and hypokalemia in a large healthcare system. Int J Cardiol. 2017;245:277–84.
55. Jun H-R, Kim H, Lee S-H, Cho JH, Lee H, Yim HW, et al. Onset of hyperkalemia following the administration of angiotensin-converting enzyme inhibitor or angiotensin II receptor blocker. Cardiovasc Ther. 2021;2021:5935149. https://doi.org/10.1155/2021/5935149.
56. Weinberg JM, Appel LJ, Bakris G, Gassman JJ, Greene T, Kendrick CA, et al. African American study of hypertension and kidney disease collaborative research group. Risk of hyperkalemia in nondiabetic patients with chronic kidney disease receiving antihypertensive therapy. Arch Intern Med. 2009;169:1587–94.
57. Sarafidis PA, Memmos E, Alexandrou ME, Papagianni A. Mineralocorticoid receptor antagonists for nephroprotection: current evidence and future perspectives. Curr Pharm Des. 2018;24:5528–36.
58. Perazella MA. Drug-induced hyperkalemia: old culprits and new offenders. Am J Med. 2000;109:307–14.
59. Rimmer JM, Horn JF, Gennari FJ. Hyperkalemia as a complication of drug therapy. Arch Intern Med. 1987;147:867–9.
60. McNay JL, Oran E. Possible predisposition of diabetic patients to hyperkalemia following administration of potassium-retaining diuretic, amiloride (MK 870). Metabolism. 1970;19:58–70.
61. The RALES Investigators. Effectiveness of spironolactone added to an angiotensin-converting enzyme inhibitor and a loop diuretic for severe chronic congestive heart failure (the Randomized Aldactone Evaluation Study [RALES]). Am J Cardiol. 1996;78:902–7.
62. Lehnhardt A, Kemper MJ. Pathogenesis, diagnosis and management of hyperkalemia. Pediatr Nephrol. 2011;26:377–84.
63. Altabas K, Altabas V, Gulin T. Nebivolol induced hyperkalemia: case report. Acta Clin Croat. 2016;55:663–6.
64. Montford JR, Linas S. How dangerous is hyperkalemia? J Am Soc Nephrol. 2017;28:3155–65.

65. Szerlip HM, Weiss J, Singer I. Profound hyperkalemia without electrocardiographic manifestations. Am J Kidney Dis. 1986;7:461–5.
66. Perez GO, Lespier L, Knowles R, Oster JR, Vaamonde CA. Potassium homeostasis in chronic diabetes mellitus. Arch Intern Med. 1977;137:1018–22.
67. Uribarri J, Oh MS, Carroll HJ. Hyperkalemia in diabetes mellitus. J Diabet Complications. 1990;4:3–7.
68. Brown RS. Potassium homeostasis and clinical implications. Am J Med. 1984;77:3–10.
69. Rastogi A, Arman F, Alipourfetrati S. New agents in treatment of hyperkalemia: an opportunity to optimize use of RAAS inhibitors for blood pressure control and organ protection in patients with chronic kidney disease. Curr Hypertens Rep. 2016;18:55. https://doi.org/10.1007/s11906-016-0663-4.

Diabetogenic Effects of Antihypertensive Drugs and Statins

26

Giuseppe Mancia, Gino Seravalle, and Guido Grassi

Hypertension, dyslipidemia, and type 2 diabetes are frequently present together in the same patient [1]. This depends not only on the casual concomitance of three highly prevalent conditions but also on the existence of common mechanisms and pathophysiological links. A clear illustration is offered by the quantitative relationship between diabetes, hypertension, and dyslipidemia that has been found in the PAMELA population. That is, on the observation that in this population, the prevalence of diabetes and dyslipidemia increased progressively from the quartile with the lowest to the quartile with the highest office, home, or ambulatory blood pressure (BP) (Fig. 26.1) [2].

Regardless the mechanisms and factors responsible for the above interrelationship, the concomitant presence of the above conditions markedly increases the risk of cardiovascular morbidity and mortality, which in hypertensive, dyslipidemic, and diabetic people has been found to be (1) greater than the sum of their individual contributions [3] and (2) raise the absolute risk value to its high range, i.e., more than 20% risk of a cardiovascular event within 10 years [4].

In the last two decades, evidence has also been obtained that the risk of developing diabetes increases with the use of antihypertensive drugs that majorly contribute to the effectiveness of antihypertensive treatment [5]. This may have profound negative clinical consequences because the prevalence of hypertension is increasing all over the world, the increase being particularly steep in developing countries [6, 7]. Because the prevalence of diabetes shows an even steeper increase [8], this means

G. Mancia (✉)
University Milano-Bicocca, Milano, Italy
e-mail: giuseppe.mancia@unimib.it

G. Seravalle
Cardiology Department, Istituto Auxologico Italiano, IRCCS S. Luca Hospital, Milan, Italy

G. Grassi
Clinica Medica, S. Gerardo Hospital, University Milano-Bicocca, Monza, Italy

A. E. Berbari, G. Mancia (eds.), *Blood Pressure Disorders in Diabetes Mellitus*, Updates in Hypertension and Cardiovascular Protection,
https://doi.org/10.1007/978-3-031-13009-0_26

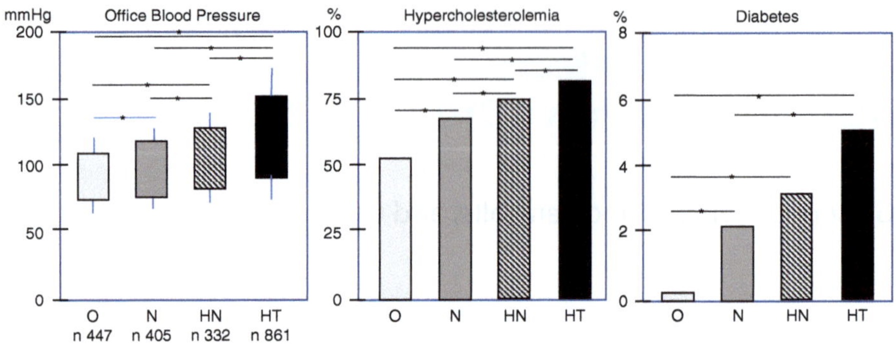

Fig. 26.1 Prevalence of hypercholesterolemia (:2'. 200 mg/dl) and diabetes (blood glucose:2'. 126 mg/dl) in the general population of the PAMELA study divided on the basis of office blood pressure categories according to the European Societies of Hypertension and Cardiology guidelines criteria. *O* optimal (office SBP/DBP < 120/80 mmHg), *N* normal (office SBP/DBP 120–129/80–84 mmHg), *HN* high-normal (office SBP/DBP 130–139/85–89 mmHg), *HT* hypertension (office SBP/DBP:2'.140/90 mmHg), *SBP* systolic blood pressure, *DBP* diastolic blood pressure. Data expressed as means±SD or %. **P* < 0.05. Modified from Ref [2]

that in the future, the number of diabetic hypertensive patients will exhibit a disproportional rise, with a marked increase in the need of implementing the use of antihypertensive agents, including those with a diabetogenic effect. Aim of this chapter is to analyze the impact of current antihypertensive and lipid-lowering treatment on new-onset diabetes (NOD) and the implications this may have for the management of hypertensive and dyslipidemic patients.

26.1 Effects of Antihypertensive Drugs on NOD

Longtime evidence is available that hypertension itself is an independent risk factor for the development of diabetes [9]. Evidence is now strong, however, that this phenomenon is worsened by the long-term use of some antihypertensive drugs that are regarded as first choice for BP-lowering treatment strategies. Hypertension guidelines recommend diuretics, angiotensin receptor blockers (ARBs), angiotensin-converting enzyme inhibitors (ACEIs), calcium channel blockers (CCBs), and, in some instances, beta-blockers (BBs) for the treatment of hypertension, mentioning drugs such as a-blockers, mineralocorticoid receptor antagonists and central agents for particular conditions and diseases [10, 11]. As shown in Table 26.1 [12–36] in post hoc analyses of comparison trials an increase in the risk of NOD has been usually found with the long-term use of thiazide diuretics, thiazide-like diuretics or BBs compared with ACEIs or ARBs. The risk of NOD has been found to be less in ARB-treated than in placebo individuals also in randomized trials on patients with an impaired fasting glucose condition (and thus an increased risk of type 2 diabetes) in which NOD was the primary end-point [36]. In contrast, CCBs and thiazide or thiazide-like diuretics have usually been found to be associated with a risk of NOD,

Table 26.1 Relative risk of developing NOD from studies with different antihypertensive therapies

Study	Ref.	Treatment	Relative risk of NOD	Study duration (years)
Comparison with placebo				
SHEP	[13]	D vs. pi	1.20	3.0
HOPE	[14]	ACEi vs. pi	0.66	4.5
SOLVD	[15]	ACEi vs. pi	0.26	2.9
EWPHE	[16]	D vs. pi	1.50	4.7
SCOPE	[17]	ARB vs. pi	0.81	3.7
FEVER	[18]	CCB vs. pi	1.20	3.3
PEACE	[19]	ACEi vs. pi	0.83	4.8
CHARM	[20]	ARB vs. pi	0.78	3.1
DREAM	[21]	ACEi vs. pi	0.99	3.0
TRASCEND	[22]	ARB vs. pi	0.86	4.7
Comparison with diuretics/beta blockers				
ALLHAT	[23]	ACEi vs. D	0.70	4.0
		CCB vs. D		
ALPINE	[24]	ARB vs. D	0.13	1.0
INSIGHT	[25]	CCB vs. D	0.77	3.5
AASK	[26]	ACEi vs. 88	0.53	3.8
LIFE	[27]	ARB vs. 88	0.75	4.8
INVEST	[28]	CCB vs. 88	0.85	2.7
STOP-2	[29]	ACEi vs. BB/D	0.96	4.0
		CCB vs. BB/D		
CAPPP	[30]	ACEi vs. BB/D	0.86	6.1
NORDIL	[31]	CCB vs. BB/D	0.87	4.5
ASCOT -BPLA	[32]	CCB vs. BB/D	0.70	5.5
ELSA	[36]	CCB vs. 88	0.96	4.0
Comparison with calcium channel blockers				
STOP-2	[29]	ACEi vs. CCB	0.98	4.0
VALUE	[33]	ARB vs. CCB	0.77	4.2
AASK	[26]	ACEi vs. CCB	0.49	3.8
ANBP2	[34]	D vs. CCB	1.45	4.1
Miscellaneous studies				
ONTARGET	[35]	ARB vs. ACEi	1.12	4.7
		ARB + ACEi vs. ACEi	0.91	
NAVIGATOR	[37]	ARB vs. D/statins	1.23	5.0

Legend: *ACEi* angiotensin-converting enzyme inhibitor, *ARB* angiotensin -receptor blocker, *BB* beta blocker, *CCB* calcium channel blocker, *D* diuretic, *pi* placebo, *NOD* new-onset diabetes, *AASK* African American Study of Kidney Disease and Hypertension, *ALLHAT* antihypertensive and lipidlowering treatment to prevent heart attack trial, *ALPINE* Antihypertensive Treatment and Lipid Profile in a North of Sweden Efficacy Evaluation, *ANBP2* Second Australian National Blood Pressure Study, *ASCOT BPLA* Anglo-Scandinavian Cardiac Outcomes Trial-Blood Pressure Lowering Arm, *CAPPP* Captopril Prevention Project, *CCB* calcium channel blocker, *CHARM* Candesartan in Heart failure Assessment of Reduction in Mortality and Morbidity, *DREAM* Diabetes Reduction Assessment with Ramipril and Rosiglitazone Medication, *ELSA* European Lacidipine Study on Atherosclerosis, *EWPHE* European Working Party on High Blood Pressure in the Elderly, *FEVER* felodipine event reduction, *HOPE* heart outcomes prevention evaluation, *INSIGHT* intervention as a goal in hypertension treatment, *INVEST* International Verapamil-Trandolapril Study, *LIFE* Losartan Intervention for Endpoint Reduction, *NAVIGATOR* Nateglinide and Valsartan in Impaired Glucose Tolerance Outcomes Research, *NORDIL* Nordic Diltiazem Study, *ONTARGET* ongoing telmisartan alone and in combination with ramipril global endpoint

(continued)

Table 26.1 (continued)
trial, *PEACE* prevention of events with angiotensin-converting enzyme inhibition trial, *SCOPE* study on cognition and prognosis in the elderly, *SHEP* systolic hypertension in the elderly program, *SOLVD* studies of left ventricular dysfunction, *STOP-2* Swedish Trial in Old Patients with Hypertension-2, *TRANSCEND* Telmisartan Randomized Assessment Study in ACE-lntolerant Subjects with Cardiovascular Disease, *VALUE* valsartan antihypertensive long-term use evaluation

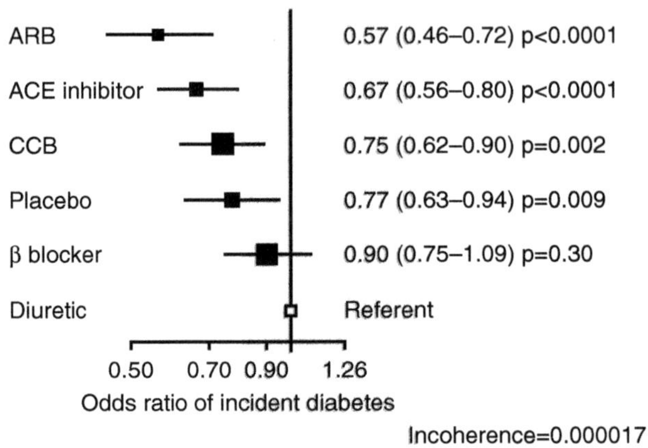

Fig. 26.2 Results of network meta-analysis of 22 clinical trials (143, 153 patients). Initial diuretic used as referent agent (open box at odds ratio = 1.00). Size of squares (representing the point estimate for each class of antihypertensive drugs) is proportional to number of patients who developed incident diabetes. Horizontal lines indicate 95% Cl. Odds ratios to the left of the vertical line at unity denote a protective effect (compared with initial diuretic). *ACEi* angiotensin-converting-enzyme inhibitors, *ARBs* angiotensin receptor blockers; CCB, calcium channel blockers. From Ref [42], with permission

respectively, similar or superior to that of placebo patients. Similar conclusions have been reached with the use of these drugs in conditions other than hypertension, i.e., in obesity, coronary disease, and heart failure [37, 38]. This has received full confirmation from the results of a number of reviews and meta-analyses [39–43].

In a network meta-analysis on more than 140,000 patients, for example, ARBs and ACEIs on one side and BBs and diuretics on the other have been found to, respectively, reduce and increase NOD compared with placebo, the use of CCBs exhibiting a neutral effect (Fig. 26.2) [42]. This evidence allows to conclude that antihypertensive drugs differ for their influence on the risk of developing type 2 diabetes. Because the evidence is also based on placebo-controlled studies, it also suggests that while CCBs appear to be neutral, diuretics and BBs may exert a diabetogenic influence in contrast with RAS blockers, which may exert an antidiabetogenic effect. In this context, however, it is also important to mention that this conclusion is somewhat weakened by the fact that, to control blood pressure, diuretics and BBs were used in the placebo arm of the relevant trials, possibly increasing the risk of NOD compared with the RAS blocker arm. This possibility is supported by the analysis of the Study on Cognition and Prognosis in the Elderly [44] in which the subgroup of patients who did not receive any therapy showed a risk of NOD similar to that of patients treated with candesartan (3.6 vs. 3.2%, $P = 0.29$).

Hypertension guidelines have since long recommended the use of more than one antihypertensive drug in the vast majority of the hypertensive population [45]. Furthermore, more recent guidelines recommendations support the use of dual drug combinations already from the beginning of treatment [10]. This makes information on the effects of different combinations on the risk of NOD of critical importance. Unfortunately, however, data on the effects of antihypertensive drug combinations on the risk of NOD are limited. While it seems clear that the risk of NOD is amplified by BB-thiazide diuretic combinations, no safe conclusion can be drawn about whether adding an ACEI or ARB to a diuretic (or a BB) may abolish the diuretic-related increase of NOD and preserve the renin angiotensin blocker-related antidiabetogenic effect. It is also unclear whether the effect on NOD is different for the combination of a CCB with a RAS blocker vs. a CCB combined with a diuretic. In this context, an interesting finding has been obtained by Brown et al. [46] who have shown that, at variance from thiazide diuretics, the diuretic amiloride does not adversely affect the blood glucose response to a glucose load. This has been regarded as a possible consequence of the potassium retaining properties of this drug because of the favorable effect of potassium on insulin sensitivity and secretion.

The implications of the above data are a matter of continuous debate because diuretics and BBs represent fundamentally important drugs against a condition that represents the first cause of death worldwide [47], their use in combination with other agents being necessary to control an elevated BP in perhaps 80% of the hypertensive population. The options under discussion are whether physicians should (1) disregard the above metabolic inconveniences, given the excellent BP lowering effect of thiazide diuretics and BBs and their ability to preferentially protect hypertensive patients from cardiovascular disease in several specific conditions [48, 49], (2) give importance to these inconveniences and refrain from any large use of these drugs, or (3) privilege a "flexible" attitude and use diuretics and BBs in some but not in other conditions. One possibility, for example, is to pose no limits to the use of diuretics and BBs when patients are at high cardiovascular risk, thereby requiring a timely BP reduction to the target values that maximize cardiovascular protection [10] while using these drugs with caution in other conditions. For example, caution may be desirable when, as in younger or mild hypertensive patients, the more limited benefit to be expected from a BP reduction may be neutralized or superseded by the increased cardiovascular risk associated with the occurrence of diabetes [50]. Furthermore, diuretics and beta-blockers may be avoided, unless strictly necessary, in patients with a high risk of developing diabetes such as those with an impaired fasting glucose condition or a metabolic syndrome. In the PAMELA population, the 10 year risk of developing type 2 diabetes was five to six times greater in subjects than in those without a metabolic syndrome (Fig. 26.3) [51]

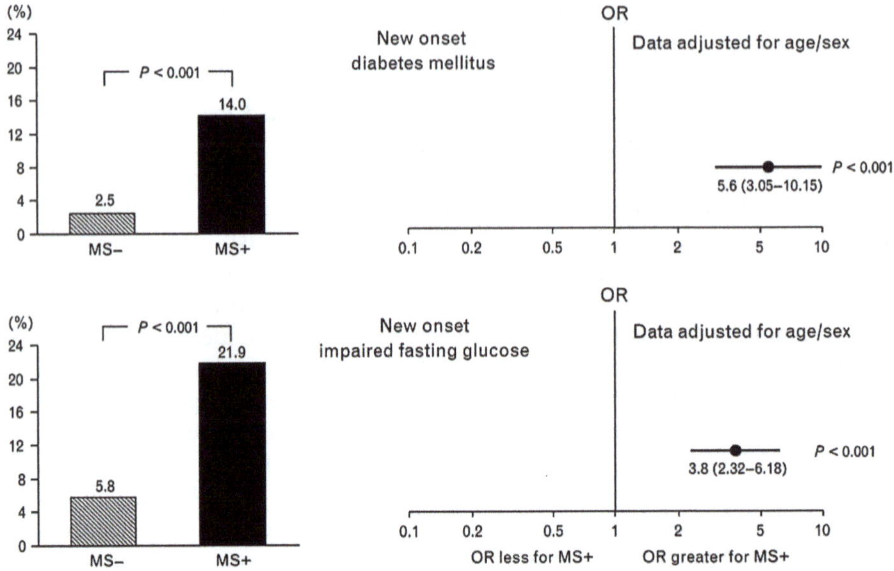

Fig. 26.3 Rate (%) of new onset diabetes or impaired fasting glucose in individuals without (−) and with (+) metabolic syndrome (MS) who did not display these condition at the first examination 10 years before. Right panels: age-adjusted and sex-adjusted odds ratio of new onset diabetes or impaired fasting glucose in MS- vs. MS+. Odds ratios (with 95% confidence intervals) are also shown as numbers. Modified from Ref [53], with permission

26.2 Effects of Statin on NOD

Statin therapy has been shown to increase the incidence and risk of NOD in several trials on the protective effect of lipid-lowering treatment on cardiovascular events. Observational data have been consistently supportive of these findings [52–55], suggesting that when statin is employed in medical practice, incidence of NOD may not be marginal. A systematic review and meta-analysis of 90 observational studies published from 1988 to 2012 reported an increased risk of NOD of 31% (odds ratio, 1.31; 95%Cl, 0.99–1.73) in patients exposed to statins [56]. Corrao and colleagues [53] investigated the relationship between adherence to statin therapy and the risk for developing diabetes in a cohort of 11, 5708 Italian individuals who started statins treatment during 2003–2004 and were followed for 6 years. Adherence to statin was assessed by the proportion of days covered by statins based on pharmacy refill records. During follow-up, 11, 154 subjects were diagnosed with diabetes. Compared with patients with low adherence (<25% of the follow-up time covered by statin), those with low (26–50%), intermediate (51–75%), and high (>75%) adherence to statin therapy showed a progressive increase in risk for developing diabetes (HR: 1.12 (95%Cl: 1.06–1.18), 1.22 (1.14–1.27), and 1.32 (1.26–1.39), respectively). Both trials and observational studies have also shown that there is a greater risk of NOD with the use of higher intensity statins [57]. This has been clearly documented in eight population-based cohort studies and a meta-analysis from six Canadian provinces and two international databases [54] in which the increase in NOD associated with higher versus lower intensity statins was measured in 136, 966 secondary prevention patients during a 14 years follow-up. In the first two years of regular statin use, there was a significantly greater increase in the risk of NOD with administration of higher intensity compared with lower intensity statins (fixed effect rate ratio 1.15; 95%CI, 1.05–1.26).

26.3 Increased NOD by Antihypertensive Drugs and Statins: Mechanisms

Several considerations and studies suggest that the variable risk of NOD associated with different antihypertensive drugs may have a predominant hemodynamic basis, i.e., that the responsible factor for the increased risk of NOD may be a reduction of skeletal muscle blood flow, because this reduction is associated with (1) a reduction of capillary network that increases the distance that blood transported insulin has to travel through to reach and act on the cell membrane and (2) this is followed by insulin resistance, which is the precursor and main actual mechanism of type 2 diabetes [58]. In line with this suggestion, glucose-clamp studies have shown that drugs that reduce skeletal muscle blood flow (diuretics and BBs) increase insulin resistance while the opposite is the case for drugs that cause skeletal muscle vasodilatation (ACEIs, ARBs, and CCBs) [59–61]. Furthermore, insulin resistance has been shown to occur when reflex skeletal muscle vasoconstriction is induced by deactivation of vagally innervated cardiopulmonary volume receptors [60, 61]. Finally, little or no increase in insulin resistance has been shown to occur with BBs, which do not cause or even increase skeletal muscle blood flow because an added vasodilator effect due to alpha blockade (carvedilol) or an increased secretion of endothelial relaxing factors (nebivolol) [62, 63]. The above may not be the only responsible mechanism, however. The lower incidence of NOD seen with valsartan and lisinopril compared with amlodipine, a drug with much greater vasodilator properties, suggests that mechanisms other than vasodilatation and maintenance or increase in peripheral blood flow may be involved [32]. Drugs interfering with the renin-angiotensin system may exert favorable effects on insulin sensitivity by direct effects at the membrane and intracellular level [64, 65]. These effects can be summarized as follows: (a) removal of the oxidative influence of angiotensin Il on cell membranes [66], (b) stimulation of insulin secretion from pancreatic islets via potassium retention [67], (c) peroxisome proliferator-activated receptor gamma agonist action [68] that can make ARBs similar to insulin sensitizers [69, 70], and (d) effect on adipocytes that can lead to a different mobilization of fatty acids [71].

The mechanisms responsible for an increased risk of NOD in patients treated with statins are unclear. Evidence is available that statins may both increase insulin resistance and reduce insulin secretion [72], although in some studies, an increase in plasma insulin has been reported probably in response to the increase of insulin resistance [73]. This effect has been ascribed to a variety of factors, i.e., weight gain increase of intracellular cholesterol, suppression of intracellular isoprenoids, perturbation of insulin signaling, increase in free fatty acids, and mitochondrial dysfunction [73], thereby probably having a multifactorial nature.

An additional interesting mechanism is a defect in the ability of pancreatic beta cells to provide sufficient insulin to maintain normal blood glucose levels [74, 75]. The reduction of the activity of hydroxymethylglutaryl coenzyme A reductase (HMG-CoAR) and, as a consequence, of cholesterol synthesis (the target of statin therapy) may also be directly involved because an association has been documented between reduced HMG-CoAR levels, lower LDL-Cholesterol levels, and increased risk of type 2 diabetes [76]. As mentioned above, the concomitant presence of an increased body mass index may also contribute [77] together with statin-induced changes in the regulation of isoprenoid metabolism and beta-cell-cholesterol contents.

Finally, statins are involved in the inflammatory processes as shown by its association with an increase of interleukin-1 secretion from macrophages, which has in turn been found to (1) activate the NLRP3 inflammasome that promotes insulin resistance [78, 79], (2) down-regulate the insulin receptor substrate 1 [80], and (3) decrease circulating adiponectin levels [81]. Adiponectin levels show a negative correlation with visceral fat distribution, dyslipidemia and insulin resistance, and higher adiponectin levels exhibiting a significant lower risk of type 2 diabetes [82]. Some single-nucleotide polymorphisms of the adiponectin gene have also been shown to predict low adiponectin levels and increased risk of diabetes [83, 84]. While statin-induced NOD is probably a class effect, pravastatin and pitavastatin have been recognized as having no effect on glycemic values in patients with and without diabetes [85].

The results from the Improved Reduction of Outcomes: Vytorin Efficacy International Trial (IMPROVE-IT) study have shown that on the background of statin treatment, the lipid lowering effect of the Niemann-Pick C1-Like 1 protein inhibitor ezetimibe also reduces cardiovascular events in patients surviving a myocardial infarction [86]. The statin-ezetimibe combination did not increase the risk of diabetes. Thus, adding ezetimibe to a statin may be a reasonable alternative to intensification of statin therapy, especially in patients with a high risk of developing type 2 diabetes (Fig. 26.4).

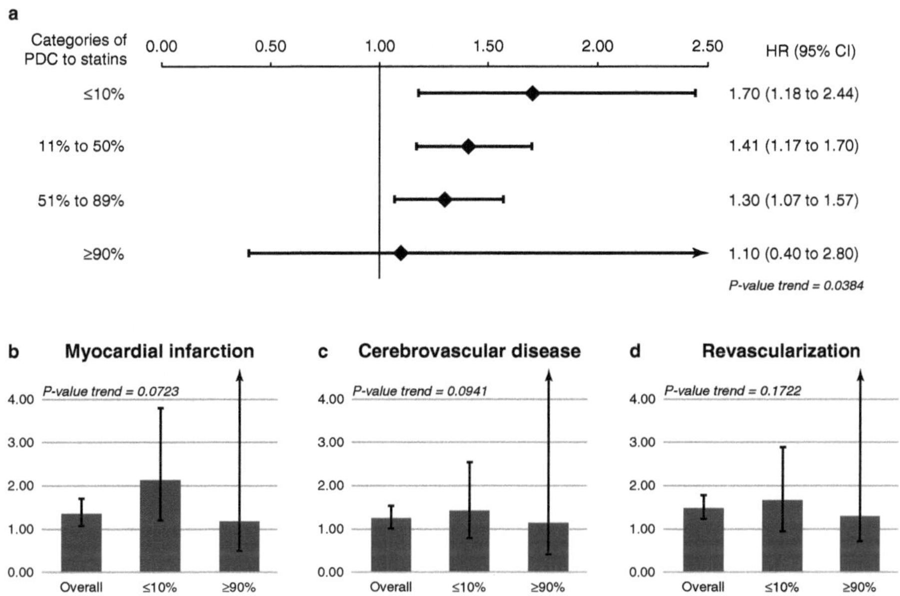

Fig. 26.4 Effect of diabetes on the hazard ratio (HR) of hospitalization for macrovascular complications according to adherence with statin therapy. Macrovascular complications on the whole and specific macrovascular outcomes (i.e., myocardial infarction, cerebrovascular disease, and myocardial revascularization) are shown in top and bottom panel, respectively (**a–d**). Hazard ratio (HR) of hospitalization for macrovascular complications and 95% Cl was estimated according to the Cox proportional hazard model. Adjustments were made for age (continuous), gender, type of statin therapy, concomitant use of other drugs, history of CV disease, and categories of Charlson comorbidity index score. *PDC* proportion of days covered From Ref [85], with permission

26.4 Drug-Induced NOD and Cardiovascular Risk

Despite the increase of NOD, trials on antihypertensive or lipid lowering drugs treatments were invariably associated with a reduction of cardiovascular outcomes, indicating that this adverse effect does not prevent the cardiovascular protection associated with these therapeutic interventions. This does not entirely answer the question, however, whether drug-induced NOD has an adverse cardiovascular effect similar to that of native type 2 diabetes or its consequences on the cardiovascular system are more benign or even devoid of an increased cardiovascular risk. This hypothesis has been raised because in ALLHAT and other trial patients under antihypertensive treatment developing NOD almost never showed a greater risk of diabetic related complications compared with no NOD patients. This has been explained by a few year duration of the trials, i.e., by the fact that NOD cases that occur within a 4 or 5 year period before the end of the trial may not allow complications to develop in a clinically detectable form. However, follow-ups of trials that doubled or tripled the original trial duration have provided inconsistent and somewhat difficult to interpret results, which leaves the issue of whether drug-induced NOD is a true diabetes or the observed increase in blood glucose has, at least in part, a cosmetic component still unanswered. In this context, some observational data have been obtained by Corrao et al. [87] via analysis of patients under statin treatment included in the Lombardy database. In 84, 828 patients, a progressive increase of adherence to statin treatment was associated with a progressive increase in NOD. Prolonged follow-up of these NOD patients showed that diabetic complications were maximal in the group, which had shown a very low adherence to statin treatment (<10% of the follow-up time) than in those in which adherence to statin treatment was very high (>90% of the follow up time) in which the risk was not significantly different from controls. Based on the assumption that, compared with native NOD, statin-induced NOD was much more frequent in patients with a very high adherence to statin treatment than in those with very low adherence to statin treatment; these results suggest that statin-dependent NOD may be prognostically more favorable than native NOD. This suggestion should be verified by controlled investigations.

26.5 Future Studies

Many more questions need to be answered to understand what a diabetic condition induced by antihypertensive drugs and statins mean for cardiovascular preventive strategies. In particular, we need to know whether (1) the increased risk of developing diabetes with diuretics and BBs becomes progressively greater with the increased exposure to these drugs; (2) the drug-related effect just anticipates the inevitable, i.e., it uncovers diabetes in individuals who will develop this condition few years later anyway; (3) diuretics or BBs have any diabetogenic effect when employed at low doses; (4) this effect can be entirely or partially counteracted by the antihypertensive agents with which diuretics and BBs are usually combined, and (5) the risk of drug-dependent NOD can be predicted based on demographic, clinical, genetic, and ethnic characteristics. It would also be important to obtain more clear data on differences between drugs from the same class and on the most proper timing of screening for NOD after treatment initiation. More research on the risk of complications of drug-induced NOD will also be highly desirable.

References

1. Barnett K, Mercer SW, Norbury M, Watt G, Wyke S, Guthrie B. Epidemiology of multimorbidity and implications for health care, research, and medical education: a cross-sectional study. Lancet. 2012;380:37–43.
2. Mancia G, Facchetti R, Bombelli M, Friz HP, Grassi G, Giannattasio C, et al. Relationship of office, home, and ambulatory blood pressure to blood glucose and lipid variables in the PAMELA population. Hypertension. 2005;45:1072–7.
3. Asia Pacific Cohort Studies Collaboration. Joint effects of systolic blood pressure and serum cholesterol on cardiovascular disease in the Asia Pacific region. Circulation. 2005;112:3384–90.

4. Pearle CA, Furberg CD, O'Meara ES, Psaty BM, Kuller L, Powe NR, et al. Characteristics and baseline clinical predictors of future fatal versus nonfatal coronary heart disease events in older adults: the Cardiovascular Health Study. Circulation. 2006;113:2177–85.
5. Taylor EN, Hu FB, Curhan GC. Antihypertensive medications and the risk of incident type 2 diabetes. Diabetes Care. 2006;29:1065–70.
6. Pradeepa R, Mohan V. Prevalence of type 2 diabetes and its complications in India and economie costs to the nation. Eur J Clin Nutr. 2017;71:816–24.
7. Zhang H, Qi D, Gu H, Wang T, Wu Y, Li J, et al. Trends in the prevalence, awareness, treatment and control of diabetes in rural areas of northern China from 1992 to 2011. J Diabetes lnvest. 2020;11:241–9.
8. Deshpande AD, Harris-Hayes M, Schootman M. Epidemiology of diabetes and diabetes-related complications. Phys Ther. 2008;88:1254–64.
9. Zhou M, Schulman HI. Prevention of diabetes in hypertensive patients: results from the VALUE trial. Vasc Health Risk Manag. 2009;5:361–8.
10. Williams B, Mancia G, Spiering W, Agabiti Rosei E, Azizi M, Burnier M, et al. 2018 Practice guidelines for the management of arterial Hypertension of the European Society of Hypertension and the European Society of Cardiology: ESH/ESC task force for the Management of Arterial Hypertension. J Hypertens. 2018;36:2284–309.
11. James PA, Oparil S, Carter BL, Cushman WC, Dennison-Himmelfarb C, Handler J, et al. 2014 evidence based guideline for the management of high blood pressure in adults: report from the panel members appointed to the Eight Joint National Committee (JNC8). JAMA. 2014;311:507–20.
12. Savage PJ, Pressel SL, Curb JD, Schron EB, Applegate WB, Blacket HR, et al. lnfluence of long-term, low-dose, diuretic-based, antihypertensive therapy on glucose, lipid, urie acid, and potassium levels in older men and women with isolated systolic hypertension: the Systolic Hypertension in the Elderly Program. SHEP Cooperative Research Group. Arch lntern Med. 1998;158:741–51.
13. Yusuf Y, Gerstein H, Hoogwerf B, Pogue J, Bosch J, Wolffenbuttel BH, et al. Ramipril and the development of diabetes. JAMA. 2001;286:1882–5.
14. Vermes E, Ducharme A, Bourassa MG, Lessard M, White M, Tardif J, et al. Enalapril reduces the incidence of diabetes in patients with chronic heart failure: insight from the studies of left ventricular dysfunction (SOLVD). Circulation. 2003;107:1291–6.
15. Fletcher A, Amery A, Birkenhager W, Bulpitt C, Clement D, de Leeuw P, et al. Risks and benefits in the trial of the European working party on high blood pressure in the elderly. J Hypertens. 1991;9:225–30.
16. Lithell H, Hansson L, Skoog I, Elmfeldt D, Hofman A, Olofsson B, et al. The study on cognition and prognosis in the elderly (SCOPE): principal results of a randomized double-blind intervention trial. J Hypertens. 2003;21:875–86.
17. Liu L, Zhang Y, Liu G, Li W, Zhang X, Zanchetti A, et al. The Felodipine event reduction (FEVER) study: a randomized long-term placebo-controlled trial in Chinese hypertensive patients. J Hypertens. 2005;23:2157–72.
18. Braunwald E, Domanski MJ, Fowler SE, Geller NL, Gersh BJ, Hsia J, et al. Angiotensin-converting-enzyme inhibition in stable coronary artery disease. N Engl J Med. 2004;351:2058–68.
19. Pfeffer MA, Swedberg K, Granger CB, Held P, McMurray JJV, Michelson EL, et al. Effects of candesartan on mortality and morbidity in patients with chronic heart failure: the CHARM-overall programme. Lancet. 2003;362:759–66.
20. DREAM Trial lnvestigators. Effect of ramipril on the incidence of diabetes. N Engl J Med. 2006;355:1551–62.
21. The Telmisartan Randomised AssessmeNt Study in ACE iNtolerant subjects with cardiovascular Disease (TRANSCEND) lnvestigators. Effects of the angiotensin-receptor blocker telmisartan on cardiovascular events in high-risk patients intolerant to angiotensin-converting enzyme inhibitors: a randomized controlled trial. Lancet. 2008;372:1174–83.

22. ALLHAT Officers and Coordinators for the ALLHAT Collaborative Research Group. Major outcomes in high-risk hypertensive patients randomized to angiotensin-converting enzyme inhibitor or calcium channel blocker vs diuretic: The Antihypertensive and Lipid-Lowering Treatment to Prevent Heart Attack Trial (ALLHAT). JAMA. 2002;288:2981–97.
23. Lindholm LH, Persson M, Alaupovic P, Carlberg B, Svensson A, Samuelssonet O. Metabolic outcome during 1 year in newly detected hypertensives: results of the Antihypertensive Treatment and Lipid Profile in a North of Sweden Efficacy Evaluation (ALPINE study). J Hypertens. 2003;21:1563–74.
24. Mancia G, Brown M, Castaigne A, de Leeuw P, Palmer CR, Rosenthal T, et al. Outcomes with nifedipine GITS or coamilozide in hypertensive diabetics and non-diabetics in Intervention as a Goal in Hypertension (INSIGHT). Hypertension. 2003;41:431–6.
25. Thornley-Brown D, Wang X, Wright JT Jr, Randall OS, Miller ER, Lash JP, et al. Differing effects of antihypertensive drugs on the incidence of diabetes mellitus among patients with hypertensive kidney disease. Arch Intern Med. 2006;166:797–805.
26. Dahlof B, Devereux RB, Kjeldsen SE, Julius S, Beevers G, de Faire U, et al. Cardiovascular morbidity and mortality in the Losartan Intervention For Endpoint reduction in hypertension study (LIFE): a randomized trial against atenolol. Lancet. 2002;359:995–1003.
27. Pepine CJ, Handberg EM, Cooper-DeHoff RM, Marks RG, Kowey P, Messerli FH, et al. A calcium antagonist vs a noncalcium antagonist hypertension treatment strategy for patients with coronary artery disease. The International Verapamil-Trandolapril Study (INVEST): a randomized controlled trial. JAMA. 2003;290:2805–16.
28. Hansson L, Lindholm LH, Ekbom T, Dahlöf B, Lanke J, Scherstén B, et al. Randomised trial of old and new antihypertensive drugs in elderly patients: cardiovascular mortality and morbidity the Swedish Trial in Old Patients with Hypertension-2 study. Lancet. 1999;354:1751–6.
29. Hansson L, Lindholm LH, Niskanen L, Lanke J, Hedner T, Niklason A, et al. Effect of angiotensin-converting-enzyme inhibition compared with conventional therapy on cardiovascular morbidity and mortality in hypertension: the captopril prevention project (CAPPP) randomised trial. Lancet. 1999;353:611–6.
30. Hansson L, Hedner T, Lund-Johansen P, Kjeldsen SE, Lindholm LH, Syvertsen JO, et al. Randomised trial of effects of calcium antagonists compared with diuretics and beta-blockers on cardiovascular morbidity and mortality in hypertension: the Nordic Diltiazem (NORDIL) study. Lancet. 2000;356:359–65.
31. Dahlof B, Sever PS, Poulter NR, Wedel H, Beevers DG, Caulfieldet M, et al. Prevention of cardiovascular events with an antihypertensive regimen of amlodipine adding perindopril as required versus atenolol adding bendroflumethiazide as required, in the Anglo-Scandinavian cardiac outcomes trial-blood pressure lowering arm (ASCOT BPLA): a multicentre randomized controlled trial. Lancet. 2005;366:895–6.
32. Kjeldsen SE, Julius S, Mancia G, McInnes GT, Hua T, Weber MA, et al. Effects of valsartan compared to amlodipine on preventing type 2 diabetes in high-risk hypertensive patients: the VALUE trial. J Hypertens. 2006;24:1405–12.
33. Chowdhury EK, Owen A, Ademi Z, Krum H, Johnston CI, Wing LMH, et al. Second Australian National Blood Pressure Study Management Committee. Short- and long-term survival in treated elderly hypertensive patients with or without diabetes: findings from the Second Australian National Blood Pressure study. Am J Hypertens. 2014;27:199–206.
34. ONTARGET Investigators. Telmisartan, ramipril, or both in patients at high risk for vascular events. N Engl J Med. 2008;358:1547–59.
35. Zanchetti A, Hennig M, Baurecht H, Tang R, Cuspidi C, Carugo S, et al. Prevalence and incidence of the metabolic syndrome in the European lacidipine study on atherosclerosis (ELSA) and its relation with carotid intima-media thickness. J Hypertens. 2007;25:2463–70.
36. Shen L, Shah BR, Reyes EM, Thomas L, Wojdyla D, Diem P, et al. Role of diuretics, beta blockers, and statins in increasing the risk of diabetes in patients with impaired glucose tolerance: reanalysis of data from the NAVIGATOR study. BMJ. 2013;347:f6745.

37. Low Wang CC, Hess CN, Hiatt WR, Goldfine AB. Atherosclerotic cardiovascular disease and heart failure in type 2 diabetes-mechanisms, management, and clinical considerations. Circulation. 2016;133:2459–502.
38. Kodama S, Fuijhara K, Horikawa C, Sato T, Iwanaga M, Yamada T, et al. Diabetes mellitus and risk of new-onset and recurrent heart failure: a systematic review and meta-analysis. ESC Heart Fail. 2020;7:2146–74.
39. Mancia G, Grassi G, Zanchetti A. New-onset diabetes and antihypertensive drugs. J Hypertens. 2006;24:3–10.
40. Padwal R, Laupacis A. AntihypJertensive therapy and incidence of type 2 diabetes: a systematic review. Diabetes Care. 2004;27:247–55.
41. Brunstrom M, Eliasson M, Nilsson PR, Carlberg B. Blood pressure treatment levels and choice of antihypertensive agent in people with diabetes mellitus: an overview of systematic reviews. J Hypertens. 2017;35:453–62.
42. Elliott WJ, Meyer PM. Incident diabetes in clinical trials of antihypertensive drugs: a network meta-analysis. Lancet. 2007;369:201–7.
43. Tocci G, Paneni F, Palano F, Sciarretta S, Ferrucci A, Kurtz T, et al. Angiotensin-converting enzyme inhibitors, angiotensin Il receptor blockers and diabetes: a meta-analysis of placebo-controlled clinical trials. Am J Hypertens. 2011;24:582–90.
44. Lithell H, Hansson L, Skoog I, Elmfeldt D, Hofman A, Olofsson B, et al. The study on cognition and prognosis in the elderly (SCOPE): outcomes in patients not receiving add-on therapy after randomization. J Hypertens. 2004;22:1605–12.
45. Mancia G, Fagard R, Narkiewicz K, Red6n J, Zanchetti A, Böhm M, et al. 2013 ESH/ESC guidelines for the management of arterial hypertension: the task force for the management of arterial hypertension of the European Society of Hypertension (ESH) and of the European Society of Cardiology (ESC). J Hypertens. 2013;31:1281–357.
46. Brown MJ, Williams B, Morant SV, Webb DJ, Caulfield MJ, Cruickshank JK, et al. Effect of amiloride, or amiloride plus hydrochlorothiazide, versus hydrochlorothiazide on glucose tolerance and blood pressure (PATHWAY-3): a parallel-group, double-blind randomized phase 4 trial. Lancet Diabetes Endocrinol. 2016;4:136–47.
47. Global Burden of Metabolic Risk Factors for Chronic Diseases Collaboration. Cardiovascular disease, chronic kidney disease, and diabetes mortality burden of cardiometabolic risk factors from 1980 to 2010: a comparative risk assessment. Lancet Diabetes Endocrinol. 2014;2:634–47.
48. Thomopoulos C, Bazoukis G, Tsioufis C, Mancia G. Beta-blockers in hypertension: overview and meta-analysis of randomized outcome trials. J Hypertens. 2020;38:1669–81.
49. Ettehad D, Emdin CA, Kiran A, Anderson SG, Callender T, Emberson J, et al. Blood pressure lowering for prevention of cardiovascular disease and death: a systematic review and meta-analysis. Lancet. 2016;387:957–67.
50. Ferrannini E, Kozakova M. Metabolic effects of antihypertensive treatment: long live the debate. J Hypertens. 2003;21:1459–62.
51. Mancia G, Bombelli M, Facchetti R, Madotto F, Corrao G, Trevano FQ, et al. Long-term risk of diabetes, hypertension and left ventricular hypertrophy associated with the metabolic syndrome in a general population. J Hypertens. 2008;26:1602–11.
52. Danaei G, Garcia Rodriguez LA, Fernandez Cantero O, Hernán MA. Statins and risk of diabetes: an analysis of electronic medical records to evaluate possible bias due to differential survival. Diabetes Care. 2013;36:1236–40.
53. Corrao G, Ibrahim B, Nicotra F, Soranna D, Merlino L, Catapano AL, et al. Statins and the risk of diabetes: evidence from a large population based cohort study. Diabetes Care. 2014;37:2225–32.
54. Dormuth CR, Filion KB, Paterson JM, James MT, Teare GF, Raymond CB, et al. Canadian network for observational drug effect studies investigators. Higher potency statins and the risk of new diabetes: multicenter, observational study of administrative databases. BMJ. 2014;348:g3244.

55. Macedo AF, Taylor FC, Casas JP, Adler A, Prieto-Merino D, Ebrahim S. Unintended effects of statins from observational studies in the general population: systematic review and meta-analysis. BMC Med. 2014;12:51.
56. Preiss D, Seshasai SR, Welsh P, Murphy SA, Ho JE, Waters DD, et al. Risk of incident diabetes with intensive-dose compared with moderate-dose statin therapy: a meta-analysis. JAMA. 2011;305:2556–64.
57. Jandeleit-Dahm KA, Tikellis C, Reid CM, Johnston CL, Cooper ME. Why blockade of the renin angiotensin system reduces the incidence of new-onset diabetes. J Hypertens. 2005;23:463–73.
58. Lind L, Pallare T, Berne C, Lithell H. Long-term metabolic effects of antihypertensive drugs. Am Heart J. 1994;128:1177–83.
59. Reaven GM. The role of insulin resistance and compensatory hyperinsulinemia in patients with essential hypertension. In: Oparil S, Weber MA, editors. Hypertension: a companion to Brenner and Rector's the kidney. Philadelphia, PA: Elsevier Saunders; 2005. p. 123–35.
60. Julius S, Gudbrandsson T, Jamerson K, Andersson O. The interconnection between sympathetic, microcirculation, and insulin resistance in hypertension. Blood Press. 1992;1:9–19.
61. Capaldo B, Lembo G, Napoli R, Rendina V, Albano G, Saccà L, et al. Skeletal muscle is a primarily site of insulin resistance in essential hypertension. Metabolism. 1991;40:1320–2.
62. McTavish D, Campoli-Richards D, Sorkin EM. Carvedilol. A review of its pharmacodynamic and pharmacokinetic properties, and therapeutic efficacy. Drugs. 1993;45:232–58.
63. Grassi G, Quarti Trevano F, Facchini A, Toutouzas T, Chanu B, Mancia G. Efficacy and tolerability profile of nebivolol vs atenolol in mild-to-moderate essential hypertension: results of a double-blind randomized multicentre trial. Blood Press Suppl. 2003;2:35–40.
64. Savage DB, Peterson KF, Shulman GI. Mechanisms of insulin resistance in humans and possible links with inflammation. Hypertension. 2005;45:828–33.
65. Shulman GI. Cellular mechanisms of insulin resistance in humans. Am J Cardiol. 1999;84:3–10.
66. Agarwal R, Campbell RC, Warnock DG. Oxidative stress in hypertension and chronic kidney disease: role of angiotensin II. Semin Nephrol. 2004;24:101–14.
67. Allon M, Takeshian A, Shaklin N. Effect of insulin-plus-glucose infusion with or without epinephrine on fasting hyperkaliemia. Kidney lnt. 1993;43:212–7.
68. Kurt TW, Pravenec M. Antidiabetic mechanisms of angiotensin-converting enzyme inhibitors and angiotensin Il receptor antagonists: beyond the renin-angiotensin system. J Hypertens. 2004;22:2253–61.
69. Schupp M, Janke J, Clasen R, Unger T, Kintscher U. Angiotensin type 1 receptor blockers induce peroxisome proliferator-activated receptor-gamma activity. Circulation. 2004;109:2054–7.
70. Uwaifo GI, Ratner RE. Novel pharmacologic agents for type 2 diabetes. Endocrinol Metab Clin N Am. 2005;34:155–97.
71. Trayhurn P, Wood IS. Adipokines: inflammation and the pleiotropic role of white adipose tissue. Br J Nutr. 2004;92:347–55.
72. Ward NC, Watts GF, Eckel RH. Statin toxicity. Circ Res. 2019;124:328–50.
73. Abbasi F, Lamendola C, Harris CS, Harris V, Tsai MS, Tripathi P, et al. Statins are associated with increased insulin resistance and secretion. Arterioscler Thromb Vasc Biol. 2021;41:2786–97.
74. DeFronzo RA. Banting lecture. From the triumvirate to the ominous octet: a new paradigm for the treatment of type 2 diabetes mellitus. Diabetes. 2009;58:773–95.
75. Mach F, Ray KK, Wiklund O, Corsini A, Catapano AL, Bruckert E, et al. Adverse effects of statin therapy; perception vs the evidence-focus on glucose homeostasis, cognitive, renal and hepatic function, haemorrhagic stroke and cataract. Eur Heart J. 2018;39:2526–39.
76. Swerdlow DI, Preiss D, Kuchenbaecker KB, Holmes MV, Engmann JEL, Shah T, et al. HMG-coenzyme A reductase inhibition, type 2 diabetes, and bodyweight: evidence from genetic analysis and randomized trials. Lancet. 2015;385:351–61.
77. Frayling TM. Statins and type 2 diabetes: genetic studies on target. Lancet. 2015;385:310–2.
78. Donath MY, Shoelson SE. Type 2 diabetes as an inflammatory disease. Nat Rev lmmunol. 2011;11:98–107.

79. Henriskbo BD, Lau TC, Cavallari JF, Denou E, Chi W, Lally JS, et al. Fluvastatin causes NLRP3 inflammosome-mediated adipose insulin resistance. Diabetes. 2014;63:3742–7.
80. Jager J, Gremeaux T, Commont M, Le Marchand-Brustel Y, Tanti J. lnterleukin-beta induced insulin resistance in adipocytes through down-regulation of insulin receptor substrate-1 expression. Endocrinology. 2007;148:241–51.
81. Chan DC, Pang J, Watts GF. Pathogenesis and management of the diabetogenic effect of statins: a role for adiponectin and coenzyme Q10? Curr Atheroscler Rep. 2015;17:472.
82. Li S, Shin HJ, Ding EL, van Dam RM. Adiponectin levels and risk of type 2 diabetes: a systematic review and meta-analysis. JAMA. 2009;302:179–88.
83. Kondo H, Shimomura I, Matsukawa Y, Kumada M, Takahashi M, Matsuda M, et al. Association of adiponectin mutation with type 2 diabetes: a candidate gene for the insulin resistance syndrome. Diabetes. 2002;51:2325–8.
84. Achari AE, Jain SK. Adiponectin, a therapeutic target for obesity, diabetes, and endothelial dysfunction. lnt J Mol Sci. 2017;18:1321.
85. Mita T, Watada H, Nakayama S, Abe M, Ogihara T, Shimizu T, et al. Preferable effect of pravastatin compared to atorvastatin on cell function in Japanese early-state type 2 diabetes with hypercholesterolemia. Endocr J. 2007;54:441–7.
86. Cannon CP, on behalf of the IMPROVE-IT investigators. IMPROVE-IT trial: a comparison of ezetimibe/simvastatin versus simvastatin monotherapy on cardiovascular outcomes after acute coronary syndromes. Late-breaking clinical trial abstracts and clinical science special reports abstract from the American Heart Association's Scientific Sessions 2014. Circulation. 2014;130:2105–26.
87. Corrao G, Compagnoni MM, Rea F, Merlino L, Catapano AL, Mancia G. Clinical significance of diabetes likely induced by statins: evidence from large population-based cohort. Diabetes Res Clin Prac. 2017;133:60–8.

Management of Diabetic Hypertensive Patient during Ramadan Fasting

27

Adel E. Berbari and Najla A. Daouk

27.1 Introduction

Ramadan is the ninth month of the Islamic Calendar and lasts 29–30 days depending on the visibility of the crescent moon [1].

Fasting during Ramadan, one of the five pillars of Islam, represents a model of intermittent fasting [1, 2]. It is characterized by daily cycles of fasting/refeeding and abstinence of all kinds of food, fluids, smoking, medications, and intravenous administration of all types of nutritional fluids during daylight [1, 2]. The duration of daily fasting varies from 12 to 20 h, according to the geographic location and season, whether falling in winter or summer [1, 3].

Meals are allowed after sunset to predawn, referred to as Iftar and Suhoor [2]. Although the frequency is reduced to two major meals, the total caloric intake often does not change [2, 3]. There is no restriction to the type and extent of food consumed [3]. However, in some populations, at fast breaking in the evening, the meal is heavier with a high meat content, than meals served in non-fasting periods in daily life [4–6].

Ramadan fasting is often associated with reduced physical activity, sleepiness, and changes in sleep patterns [4]. Fasters may wake up before sunrise for the predawn meal and return to sleep [4].

Studies that have evaluated the health effects of Ramadan fasting have reported opposing outcomes [3–6].

The aim of this chapter is to review the health effects and therapeutic approaches of Ramadan fasting in the following groups of subjects: (i) healthy normotensives, (ii) nondiabetic hypertensives, (iii) chronic renal nephropathies, and (iv) normotensive and hypertensive diabetics.

A. E. Berbari (✉) · N. A. Daouk
Department of Internal Medicine, American University of Beirut Medical Center, Beirut, Lebanon
e-mail: ab01@aub.edu.lb

A. E. Berbari, G. Mancia (eds.), *Blood Pressure Disorders in Diabetes Mellitus*, Updates in Hypertension and Cardiovascular Protection,
https://doi.org/10.1007/978-3-031-13009-0_27

27.2 Effects of Ramadan Fasting on Blood Pressure

27.2.1 Nondiabetic Normotensive/Hypertensive Subjects

Several studies that have evaluated the effects of Ramadan fasting on blood pressure (BP) in nondiabetic normotensive/hypertensive subjects have reported conflicting observations [2, 7, 8].

The effect of prolonged period of fasting for 12, 36, and 72 h was evaluated in 29 healthy normotensive volunteers [8]. Their systolic BP (SBP) increased during the 12–36 fast periods and returned to near prefasting values at 72 h [8]. Similar increases in SBP was also reported during Ramadan fasting. In a study that included 40 subjects with no previous history of hypertension fasting Ramadan and 55 nonfasters used as a control group, ambulatory BP monitoring demonstrated, in fasters, an increase of over 10% in SBP at 18 h, 19 h, and 20 h in respect to baseline determination at 0 h [9].

Conversely, several other studies indicated a fall in both systolic and diastolic BP levels during Ramadan [2]. London Ramadan Study (LORANS), which includes both an observational study of 85 healthy participants and a review and meta-analysis of published studies, evaluated the effect of Ramadan fasting on BP [2]. Among the 85 healthy participants, SBP and DBP fell by 7.29 and 3.42 mmHg, respectively, during Ramadan independently of weight, total body water, and fat mass [2]. Similarly, in the meta-analysis of 33 studies, which included 3213 participants, SBP and diastolic blood pressure (DBP) were lower by 3.19 and 2.26 mmHg, respectively, during the last 2 weeks of Ramadan [2].

In contrast, other studies have demonstrated no change in BP during Ramadan [2]. In a study of 89 healthy subjects, SBP remained unchanged in both genders during Ramadan, while DBP decreased significantly only in females [10].

In subjects with Grade 1 (mild) and well-controlled hypertension, Ramadan fasting does not appear to confer any adverse health effects, but even may be associated with favorable benefits [11–13].

Several studies indicate that during Ramadan fasting, BP levels remain unchanged or may even fall in hypertensives [10–13].

In a study of 99 hypertensive subjects, ambulatory BP monitoring (ABPM), performed before and during Ramadan, revealed no significant differences on the 24-h BP profile and SBP and DBP in the diurnal and nocturnal intervals between the fasting and nonfasting periods [14]. However, there was a delay of 2 h on the peak of the awakening BP and 1 h in the nocturnal trough during Ramadan [4, 14]. Likewise, in a study on 17-treated hypertensive patients, taking their prescribed medications once daily, ambulatory BP recorded twice, before and during the last 2 weeks of the fasting revealed no significant differences in the averages 24 h, awake and asleep BP levels during the two periods [4]. These results were confirmed in a study of treated grade 2 and 3 hypertension well controlled on combination therapy [15]. Again, there were no statistical differences in the ABPM recorded before and during Ramadan, except for a slight BP elevation before dawn, which coincided with the consumption of the morning meal [15]. Further, in a study of 21 well-controlled hypertensive patients, fasting did not alter the nocturnal dipping as evaluated by ABPM [16].

However, other studies demonstrated that Ramadan fasting may be associated with significant reduction in BP in well-controlled hypertensive patients [2]. In 20 subjects with well-controlled hypertension with medications administered at the break and before resumption of fast, ABPM revealed significant reduction in both daytime and nighttime BP levels [11]. However, these reductions in BP did not require changes in antihypertensive regimen [11]. Another observational study confirmed the fall in BP during Ramadan [17].

In terms of temporality, only one study that measures SBP/DBP in three different time points reported that a decline in BP occurred after the first week of Ramadan [2, 18].

27.2.2 Diabetic Normotensive/Hypertensive Subjects

Several studies have reported BP changes in both normotensive and hypertensive diabetic subjects [19–22].

In a large cohort of 1246 normotensive diabetic individuals, Ramadan fasting was associated with significant falls in both SBP and DBP [23]. Mean SBP and DBP decreased significantly and were from 135.4 ± 14.29/78.3 ± 8.70 mmHg to 128.5 ± 14.4/76.7 ± 9.9 mmHg [23]. Smaller studies confirmed the Ramadan associated fall in BP in normotensive diabetics [19, 20]. Further, the fall in BP appears to persist several weeks after the end of the fast [3]. In contrast, one study revealed an increase in SBP [24].

The effect of Ramadan fasting in diabetic subjects with untreated or poorly controlled hypertension has not well been evaluated [21, 25]. Further, the few studies that tackled this issue included only a small number of well-controlled diabetic participants, while others omitted to assess the outcome on BP indices [21, 26, 27].

In a prospective observational study of 68-treated diabetic hypertensive participants, a significant reduction both in BP (SBP/DBP) and body weight was documented in Ramadan fasters [27]. Smaller studies confirmed these observations [20].

Acute hypoglycemic reactions have been described during Ramadan fasting in diabetic subjects well controlled with antidiabetic medications [25]. Hypoglycemic reactions were evaluated in a study of 300 diabetic subjects with type 2 diabetes mellitus [19]. Ramadan fasting induced a significant fall in SBP/DBP in both normotensive and hypertensive diabetic subjects [19]. However, compared with normotensive diabetics, hypertensive diabetics were more prone to develop hypoglycemic reactions [19, 28]. Further, the hypoglycemic complications were higher in those receiving insulin or sulfonylureas [19, 28]. In contrast, a positive correlation was observed between the rate of hypoglycemia and BP changes in pre- and post-Ramadan periods [19]. The hypoglycemic reactions were associated with an increase in heart rate and SBP [19].

The incidence of hypoglycemic episodes in fasting diabetic type 2 patients has been described in 3–4% and appears to be attributed, in most cases to changes in doses of antidiabetic drugs or noncompliance with treatment and smoking [19, 29].

27.3 Liquorice and Blood Pressure Changes

Liquorice, a popular drink during Ramadan fasting in many Arab countries, has been shown to cause BP elevation and or hypertension [30].

Glycyrrhizic acid, the active ingredient of liquorice, inhibits the enzyme 11-beta-hydroxysteroid dehydrogenase type 2, leading to reduced conversion of the glucocorticoid cortisol to cortisone, with subsequent prolonged half-life of the former [31]. The glucocorticoid cortisol, which has similar affinity to mineralocorticoid receptors in target organs, promotes renal sodium (Na) retention and potassium (K) excretion with subsequent volume expansion, suppression of renin-angiotensin system (RAS), and hypokalemic hypertension [30, 31]. In addition, by promoting angiotensin II binding to vascular smooth muscles, cortisol mediates a direct pressor effect, further contributing to BP elevation and hypertension [30, 31].

In volunteers, liquorice administration, even in small doses, induces an increase in BP and even hypertension within 2 weeks [30–33].

No studies have evaluated the effect of liquorice on BP control in Ramadan fasting [33]. However, because of the uneven consumption and individual susceptibility, it has been recommended to avoid or at least reduce liquorice intake during Ramadan [33].

27.4 Effects of Blood Pressure Changes on Renal Function in Ramadan Fasting

Several studies have assessed the effects of BP changes on renal function in Ramadan fasting.

27.4.1 Normal Renal Function

27.4.1.1 Nondiabetes

In nondiabetic subjects, Ramadan fasting does not appear to have any deleterious effect on renal function.

In a study of 20 nondiabetic subjects with well-controlled hypertension on combination therapy, ambulatory BP monitoring revealed a significant fall in 24-h, daytime and nighttime average BP levels associated with preservation of renal function [34].

27.4.1.2 Diabetes

In contrast, in diabetic subjects, a deterioration of renal function has been described in Ramadan fasting.

A study of 90 subjects with type 2 diabetes mellitus was classified as group I with albuminuria and renal impairment, group II with albuminuria and normal renal function, and group III with normal renal function and no albuminuria [35]. Compared with groups II and III, subjects (with normal renal function), group I subjects had higher SBP, albuminuria, and lower glomerular filtration rate prior to Ramadan fasting [35]. In both groups II and III subjects, SBP and DBP decreased significantly lower at the 2 weeks post Ramadan [35]. Similarly, glomerular filtration rates also fell significantly (114 vs. 77.8 ml/min/1.73m^2 in group II and 112.7 vs. 97.5 ml/min/1.73m^2 in group III), although the values remain within the normal range [35]. Further, in group II, albuminuria as defined as albumin/creatinine ratio (UACR) was higher (UACR = 71.4 ± 21.1 vs. 112.3 ± 72.4 mcg/mg) [35].

27.4.2 Impaired Renal Function/Chronic Kidney Disease

Evaluation of the impact of Ramadan fasting on renal functional parameters in patients with impaired renal function has reported opposite observations [35, 36]. Some studies demonstrated that in patients with moderate to severe chronic kidney disease (CKD), Ramadan fasting did not provoke any adverse renal responses [36, 37].

In a prospective study of 31 patients with CKD stages 3/5 with a mean eGFR = 29 ± 16.3 ml/min/1.73m^2, hypertension in 71% of the patients, and diabetic kidney disease in 61%, Ramadan fasting was well tolerated as manifested by a tendency to weight loss, reduction in SBP/DBP, a significant increase in eGFR from 29.6 ± 6 to 30.9 ± 15.7 ml/min/1.73m^2, and persistence of these changes for 1 month postfasting [36]. However, age and use of diuretics increase the risk of deterioration of renal function in CKD during fasting [37].

Conversely, other studies indicated that fasting during Ramadan increases the risk of deterioration of renal function, which may become irreversible in moderate to severe CKD [38]. In a prospective observational study of 36 patients with moderate to severe renal insufficiency, fasting during Ramadan led to further deterioration of both biochemical profile and renal function, which persisted for 2 weeks after the end of Ramadan [39]. Calculated creatinine clearance decreased from a prefasting level of 17.1 ± 3.5 to 13.2 ± 2.2 and 13.7 ± 3.2 ml/min to the end of Ramadan and 2 weeks postfasting, respectively [39]. In nine patients of this study, there was also progressive fluid accumulation, weight gain, edema of the lower extremities, and poor BP control, requiring frequent adjustment of the management [39].

27.5 Impacts of Fasting/Refeeding Cycles on Blood Pressure Regulation

Studies in experimental animals have indicated that the mechanism (s) of BP control is (are) disrupted by repeated cycles of food restriction and refeeding [5]. Repeated cycles of food restriction and refeeding in a model of genetically obese spontaneously hypertensive rats (SHR) were characterized by loss and regain of baseline body weight, fluctuations in BP followed later by sustained hypertension despite food restriction periods [5]. The refeeding hypertension was attributed to over activity of the sympathetic nervous system [5]. According to the investigators, these observations suggested that repeated fluctuation in body weight associated with cycles of fasting/refeeding may provoke adverse health consequences [5].

In contrast, numerous studies have reported that Ramadan fasting, a model of daily intermittent cycles of fasting/refeeding, is safe and is associated with improvement in BP control and in several laboratory indices of the metabolic syndrome [34, 40].

Conversely, other investigators have demonstrated that Ramadan fasting may have deleterious and adverse health effects in patients with cardiorenal complications [41]. Caution has been recommended before undertaking this religious duty in certain groups of patients and in the elderly [41].

Certain factors in Ramadan may predispose to adverse health complications: 1) dehydration during fasting, especially when Ramadan falls in long summer days, 2) disruption of normal regular physical activities and sleep patterns, 3) alterations in the chronotherapy of drugs related to the treatment of hypertension and diabetes mellitus, 4) change in diet type, 5) consumption of hypertension inducing drinks such as liquorice [40, 41].

27.6 Management of Diabetic Hypertensive Fasting Subjects

27.6.1 General Principles

The management of diabetic hypertensive subjects observing fasting during the month of Ramadan represents a complex issue. Several factors have been postulated to alter basic homeostatic functions [25]. These variables include repeated daily cycles of fasting/refeeding, alterations in lifestyle patterns (physical activity, and sleep), physiologic function, and pharmacokinetic and pharmacodynamic properties of prescribed medications [25]. Further, the fasting subjects are prone to dehydration, extracellular fluid contraction, electrolyte abnormalities, hypotension, hypoglycemic and dysglycemic episodes, BP and renal functional dysregulation, and risk of cardiorenal complications [25].

Lack of adherence to dietary counseling and drug regimen recommendations often complicates the management of diabetic hypertensive patients during Ramadan fasting [25].

Proper management of these subjects requires dietary counseling and adjustment to the prescribed medications [25].

Due to the risk of dehydration, extracellular volume contraction and electrolyte imbalance, all classes of diuretics (thiazide diuretics, loop diuretics, and aldosterone antagonists), should be withdrawn or avoided [41]. In case their use is indicated, the dose of the diuretic should be reduced and should preferably be administered with predawn (Suhoor) meal to avoid sleep disturbances with sunset (Iftar) meals [41].

Taking medications immediately after large meals should be discouraged to prevent hypotension and orthostatic symptoms especially in the elderly [41].

Rigorous control of BP, glycemia, and lipid profile is essential in diabetic hypertensive subjects during fasting as in nonfasting periods to reduce the risk of cardiorenal complications [25].

27.6.2 Treatment of Hypertension

Mild to moderate hypertension well treated with monotherapy or combination therapy poses no health threat to diabetic hypertensive subjects observing fasting during the month of Ramadan [42]. BP levels remain unchanged or even fall [4]. These findings were confirmed in patients well controlled with grade 2/3 hypertension by ambulatory BP recordings [15]. Further, in numerous studies, ambulatory BP tracings revealed reduction in diurnal, nocturnal, and 24 h BP levels [34]. However, during the month of Ramadan, the peak of the awakening BP is delayed by 2 h and nocturnal trough was delayed by 1 h [14].

A study, which assessed BP changes during Ramadan fasting in subjects with untreated prehypertension or hypertension, revealed a significant reduction in BP levels on ambulatory BP recordings [41]. These studies suggest that fasting during the month of Ramadan appears to be safe and well tolerated in patients with essential hypertension [42–44].

Patients with severe and uncontrolled hypertension should be advised not to fast until the condition is well treated [41].

Fasting patients with hypertensive emergencies should be treated appropriately including by intravenous medications [41].

Hypertensive patients well controlled with antihypertensive medications should continue taking their prefasting drug regimen [4, 11, 45]. However, adjustment of their dosage schedules is advisable to avoid adverse reactions including hypotension [43].

In fasting subjects on monotherapy, the morning or day dose can be shifted to the predawn (Suhoor) period [43]. In cases of dual or combination therapy, it is recommended to use preparations with a long duration of action to reduce the number of prescribed pills [43].

27.6.3 Treatment of Diabetes Mellitus

Diabetes mellitus represents a high risk state characterized by a wide spectrum of clinicopathologic entities and laboratory disturbances that predispose to adverse cardiorenal events [25, 33]. Further, fasting itself carries a risk of serious comorbid events, which include hypo−/hyperglycemic episodes, hyperglycemic hyperosmolar syndrome, ketoacidosis, dehydration, extracellular volume contraction, hypotension, renal functional impairment, and a hypercoagulable state [3, 45, 46].

Management of the fasting diabetic subjects requires the following: (i) appropriate BP and blood glucose control and (ii) measures to prevent or reduce the risks of adverse cardiorenal outcomes, and (iii) interactions between different classes of prescribed medications [46].

Treatment of hypertension has been addressed in the previous paragraph.

Several therapeutic approaches have been used for the control of blood glucose/hyperglycemic levels by (i) dietary counseling, (ii) oral antidiabetic medications, and (iii) insulinotherapy [46].

Dietary counseling has been reported to control blood glucose levels in some fasting subjects without the need for medications [46]. Such subjects can observe fasting safely with minimal risk [46].

There are several classes of oral antidiabetic agents that are effective in the treatment of diabetes mellitus, either singly or in combination [25, 46]. However, in the fasting subjects, it has been recommended to preferably use those compounds associated with a reduced risk of hypoglycemia [46]. In general, oral antidiabetic drugs that act by increasing insulin sensitivity appear to be associated with a significantly lower risk of hypoglycemia than compounds that act by increasing insulin secretion [46]. The risk of hypoglycemic reactions have been reported to be lower with metformin, thiazolidinediones, short-acting insulin secretagogues, dipeptidyl peptidase-4 inhibitors, and glucagon-like peptide-1 receptor agonists [25].

The class of sodium-glucose cotransporters-2 (SGLT2) inhibitor recently introduced in the management of diabetes mellitus has been shown to be effective and safe in fasting diabetic subjects [25, 47]. These compounds control hyperglycemia by inhibition of renal tubular glucose reabsorption and afford cardiorenal and metabolic protection [47]. Further, their use is associated with low rate of hypoglycemic and renal adverse reactions [25, 47].

In contrast, sulfonylureas stimulate insulin secretion from pancreatic β-cells [25, 46]. However, the mechanism is glucose-independent resulting in a higher risk of hypoglycemia and making their use in Ramadan concerning [25, 46]. The newer generation of sulfonylureas is associated with a lower risk of hypoglycemia and is safer to be used during Ramadan [25].

Numerous studies have demonstrated that appropriate combination of antidiabetic agents can provide effective and safe glycemic control in fasting diabetic subjects [25, 46]. Further, several guidelines that have been published by scientific associations serve to recommend approaches for the use of antidiabetic drugs in the management of diabetes mellitus in the fasting diabetic subjects [25, 48, 49].

In order to reduce or prevent drug related adverse reactions, it is recommended to adjust dosage and timing of drug administration [25, 46, 49]. In general, for subjects receiving oral antidiabetic drugs, it is advisable that the higher dose be given in the evening reflecting the larger meal [49].

27.6.4 Drug–Drug Interactions

Diabetic hypertensive subjects who suffer from a wide spectrum of comorbidities require a multi-therapeutic regimen of drugs [50]. During Ramadan fasting, these medications have to be administered concomitantly within a short time period, extending from sunset to predawn when meals are allowed [50].

These medicinal compounds, which belong to different classes, may influence their therapeutic actions exposing the fasting diabetic subject to potentially serious adverse drug reactions referred to drug–drug interactions [50, 51].

A drug–drug interaction is defined as an increase or a decrease of a therapeutic action of a specific drug caused by another drug [49].

Antidiabetic drugs have been reported to interact with medications of different classes [46, 51]. Further, the risk of a drug–drug interaction is enhanced by the number of drugs administered and by aging [51]. In general, the greater the number of drugs is taken, the more frequent a clinically relevant drug–drug interaction is expected to occur [50]. Further, the decrease in hepatic and renal functions in the elderly increases the risk of drug–drug interactions requiring dose adjustment of the medications in this age group [50].

The most clinically relevant specific drug–drug interactions with antidiabetic agents occur with sulfonylureas, thiazolidinedione, and metformin [50].

27.6.4.1 Sulfonylureas

Hypoglycemia represents a major and serious adverse reaction occurring in about 20% of fasting diabetic subjects receiving sulfonylureas [25, 49].

Hypoglycemia predisposes to an increased risk of hypotension, falls, and fractures especially in the elderly [25, 50]. Hypoglycemia is independent of the glucose lowering action of sulfonylureas but is enhanced by elevated plasma concentrations of the drug, impaired renal function, changes in gastric pH, and coadministration with dipeptidyl peptidase-4 (DPP-4) inhibitors, glucagon-like peptide-1 (GLP-1) analogs, angiotensin-converting enzyme inhibitors (ACEI), nonsteroidal anti-inflammatory drugs (NSAID), and salicylates [50].

Dosage and administration of timing of prescribed sulfonylureas are advisable during Ramadan fasting to reduce the risk of hypoglycemia [49, 50].

27.6.4.2 Thiazolidinediones

Thiazolidinedione, also known as glitazones, a class of insulin sensitizers, increases the sensitivity to insulin of certain tissues without altering pancreatic insulin secretion [50]. Their adverse reactions are related to salt and fluid retention especially when coadministered with other antidiabetic compounds [50]. When dispensed in combination with sulfonylureas, insulin, and NSAID, thiazolidinediones enhance the risk of cardiovascular complications and hypoglycemia [50].

27.6.4.3 Metformin

Metformin is considered one of the safest antidiabetic drugs [49, 50]. However, lactic acidosis, a rare but health threatening adverse drug reaction, may occur with metformin therapy, especially in subjects with impaired renal function [49, 50].

Administration of metformin with medicinal compounds that alter glomerular filtration may precipitate lactic acidosis [50].

The risk of metformin-associated hypoglycemia is minimal [49, 50].

Metformin absorption rate is delayed when the drug is administered simultaneously with food ingestion [50].

27.6.4.4 Cardiovascular Drugs

Diabetic hypertensive patients receive a large number of medications that may interact with antidiabetic drugs [50]. However, only few of the adverse drug reactions are relevant to the fasting diabetic subjects.

Antihypertensive medications, which are frequently comedicated with antidiabetic drugs either enhance the hypoglycemic effect as with ACEI or impair the antidiabetic drug efficacy as with thiazide diuretics [50].

Further, patients with type 2 diabetes mellitus are comedicated with vitamin K antagonists such as warfarin for associated cardiovascular comorbidities [50]. Comedication of vitamin K with sulfonylureas has been reported to enhance hypoglycemic reactions and bleeding tendency in diabetic hypertensive subjects [50].

References

1. Alsafadi H, Wilson J, Patel V. Managing diabetes in people fasting during Ramadan. Diabetes Primary Care. 2011;13:152–9.
2. Al-Jafar R, Themeli MZ, Zaman S, Akbar S, Lhoste V, Khamliche A, et al. Effect of religious fasting in Ramadan on blood pressure: results from LORANS (London Ramadan study) and a meta-analysis. J Am Heart Assoc. 2021;10:e021560.
3. M'guil M, Ragala MA, El Guessabi L, Fellat S, Chraibi A, Chabraoui L, et al. Is Ramadan fasting safe in type 2 diabetic patients in view of the lack of significant effect of fasting on clinical and biochemical parameters, blood pressure, and glycemic control? Clin Exp Hypertens. 2008;30:339–57.
4. Perk G, Ghanem J, Aamar S, Ben-Ishay D, Bursztyn M. The effect of the fast of Ramadan on ambulatory blood pressure in treated hypertensives. J Hum Hypertens. 2001;15:723–5.
5. Ernsberger P, Koletsky RJ, Baskin JS, Foley M. Refeeding hypertension in obese spontaneously hypertensive rats. Hypertension. 1994;24:699–705.
6. de Cabo R, Mattson MP. Effects of intermittent fasting on health, aging, and disease. N Engl J Med. 2019;381:2541–51.
7. Krakoff LR. Fasting and ambulatory blood pressure monitoring. Blood Press Monit. 2017;22:258.
8. Webber J, Macdonald IA. The cardiovascular, metabolic and hormonal changes accompanying acute starvation in men and women. Br J Nutr. 1994;71:437–47.
9. Seker A, Demirci H, Ocakoglu G, Aydin U, Ucar H, Yildiz G, et al. Effect of fasting on 24-h blood pressure values of individuals with no previous history of hypertension. Blood Press Monit. 2017;22:247–52.
10. Sijavandi MSA, Shahsavan F, Askarizadeh F, Nematy M, Heravian J, Mahmodi Z, et al. Effects of Ramadan fasting on blood pressure and lipid profile. J Fasting Health. 2015;3:126–31.
11. Alinezhad-Namaghi M, Salehi M. Effects of Ramadan fasting on blood pressure in hypertensive patients: a systematic review. J Fasting Health. 2016;4:17–21.
12. Shehab A, Abdulle A, El Issa A, Al Suwaidi J, Nagelkerke N. Favorable changes in lipid profile: the effects of fasting after Ramadan. PLoS One. 2012;7:e47615.

13. Norouzy A, Daloee MH, Khoshnasab AH, Khoshnasab A, Farrokhi J, Nematy M, et al. Trend of blood pressure in hypertensive and normotensive volunteers during Ramadan fasting. Blood Press Monit. 2017;22:253–7.
14. Habbal R, Azzouzi L, Adnan K, Tahiri A, Chraibi N. Variations of blood pressure during the month of Ramadan. Arch Mal Coeur Vaiss. 1998;91:995–8.
15. Ural E, Kozdag G, Kilic T, Ural D, Sahin T, Celebi O, et al. The effect of Ramadan fasting on ambulatory blood pressure in hypertensive patients using combination drug therapy. J Hum Hypertens. 2008;22:208–10.
16. Khosropanah S, Ashraf F, Handjani AM. The effect of one-day Ramadan fast on blood pressure of hypertensive patients. Iranian Heart J. 2003;4:39–43.
17. Aslan S, Demir AR, Kahraman S, Memiç K, Avci Y, Gürbak I, et al. The effect of Ramadan fasting on ambulatory blood pressure in treated hypertensive patients using diuretics. Blood Press Monit. 2020;25:195–200.
18. Mansi KMS. Study the effects of Ramadan fasting on the serum glucose and lipid profile among healthy Jordanian students. Am J Applied Sci. 2007;4:565–9.
19. Ismail AAE, Megallaa MH, Badrah MH, Farghaly MAA. Study of the metabolic effects of Ramadan fasting on patients with type 2 diabetes. Relation to glycemic control, hypoglycemic events and diabetic complications. Clin Diabetol. 2021;10:161–8.
20. Alnasir FA. Effect of Ramadan fasting on hypertension and diabetes. Qatar Medical J. 1999;8:53–7.
21. Almulhem M, Susarla R, Alabdulaali L, Khunti K, Karamat MA, Rasiah T, et al. The effect of Ramadan fasting on cardiovascular events and risk factors in patients with type 2 diabetes: a systematic review. Diabetes Res Clin Pract. 2020;159:107918.
22. Bener A, Yousafzai MT. Effect of Ramadan fasting on diabetes mellitus: a population-based study in Qatar. J Egypt Public Health Assoc. 2014;89:47–52.
23. Bener A, Al-Hamaq AOAA, Öztürk M, Çatan F, Haris PI, Rajput KU, et al. Effect of ramadan fasting on glycemic control and other essential variables in diabetic patients. Ann Afr Med. 2018;17:196–202.
24. Traoré M, Lemieux S, Galibois I. Metabolic and clinical profiles before, during and after Ramadan in Malians with type 2 diabetes (French). Nutr Clin Métab. 2014;28:83–9.
25. Ahmed SH, Chowdhury TA, Hussain S, Syed A, Karamat A, Helmy A, et al. Ramadan and diabetes: a narrative review and practice update. Diabetes Ther. 2020;11:2477–520.
26. Hassanein M, Al Awadi FF, El Hadidy KE, Ali SS, Echtay A, Djaballah K, et al. The characteristics and pattern of care for the type 2 diabetes mellitus population in the MENA region during Ramadan: an international prospective study (DAR-MENA T2DM). Diabetes Res Clin Pract. 2019;151:275–84.
27. Shao Y, Lim GJ, Chua CL, Wong YF, Yeoh ECK, Low SKM, et al. The effect of Ramadan fasting and continuing sodium-glucose co-transporter-2 (SGLT2) inhibitor use on ketonemia, blood pressure and renal function in Muslim patients with type 2 diabetes. Diabetes Res Clin Pract. 2018;142:85–91.
28. Ba-Essa EM, Hassanein M, Abdulrhman S, Alkhalifa M, Alsafar Z. Attitude and safety of patients with diabetes observing the Ramadan fast. Diabetes Res Clin Pract. 2019;152:177–82.
29. Pinelli NR, Jaber LA. Practices of Arab American patients with type 2 diabetes mellitus during Ramadan. J Pharm Pract. 2011;24:211–5.
30. Sigurjónsdóttir HA, Franzson L, Manhem K, Ragnarsson J, Sigurdsson G, Wallerstedt S. Liquorice-induced rise in blood pressure: a linear dose-response relationship. J Hum Hypertens. 2001;15:549–52.
31. Farese RV Jr, Biglieri EG, Shackleton CH, Irony I, Gomez-Fontes R. Licorice-induced hypermineralocorticoidism. N Engl J Med. 1991;325:1223–7.
32. Latif SA, Conca TJ, Morris DJ. The effects of the licorice derivative, glycyrrhetinic acid, on hepatic 3 alpha- and 3 beta-hydroxysteroid dehydrogenases and 5 alpha- and 5 beta-reductase pathways of metabolism of aldosterone in male rats. Steroids. 1990;55:52–8.
33. Berbari AE, Daouk NA, Mallat SG, Jurjus AR. Ramadan fasting in health and disease. In: Berbari AE, Mancia G, editors. Special issues in hypertension. Springer-Verlag Italia; 2012. p. 331–46.

34. Aktürk IF, Biyik I, Kosas C, Yalcin AA, Ertürk M, Uzun F. Effects of Ramadan fasting on blood pressure control, lipid profile, brain natriuretic peptide, renal functions and electrolyte levels in hypertensive patients taking combination therapy. Nobel Med. 2013;9:43–6.
35. Abushady MM, Samy M, Bekhet M, Abdullah A. Effect of Ramadan fasting on renal function in patients with type 2 diabetes. Diabetes Res Clin Pract. 2019;153:176–83.
36. Bernieh B, Al Hakim MR, Boobes Y, Abu Zidan FM. Fasting Ramadan in chronic kidney disease patients: clinical and biochemical effects. Saudi J Kidney Dis Transpl. 2010;21:898–902.
37. Kara E, Sahin OZ, Kizilkaya B, Ozturk B, Pusuroglu G, Yildirim S, et al. Fasting in Ramadan is not associated with deterioration of chronic kidney disease: a prospective observational study. Saudi J Kidney Dis Transpl. 2017;28:68–75.
38. El-Wakil HS, Desoky I, Lotfy N, Adam AG. Fasting the month of Ramadan by Muslims: could it be injurious to their kidneys? Saudi J Kidney Dis Transpl. 2007;18:349–54.
39. Al Muhanna FA. Ramadan fasting and renal failure. Saudi Med J. 1998;19:319–21.
40. Salim I, Al Suwaidi J, Ghadban W, Alkilani H, Salam AM. Impact of religious Ramadan fasting on cardiovascular disease: a systematic review of the literature. Curr Med Res Opin. 2013;29:343–54.
41. Alper AT, Akboğa MK, Özcan KS, Tengiz I, Türk UO, Yıldız M, et al. Recommendations for Ramadan fasting to patients with cardiovascular diseases; Turkish Society of Cardiology consensus report. Anatol J Cardiol. 2021;25:284–93.
42. Soltani MH, Namayandeh SM, Latifeh J, Moghadam B, Maleknaz, Hadiani L. The effect of fasting during Ramadan on blood pressure in patients with controlled and mild hypertension. J Hypertens. 2016;5:227. https://doi.org/10.4172/2167-1095.1000227.
43. Aadil N, Houti IE, Moussamih S. Drug intake during Ramadan. BMJ. 2004;329:778–82.
44. Chamsi-Pasha M, Chamsi-Pasha H. The cardiac patient in Ramadan. Avicenna J Me. 2016;6:33–8.
45. Bejar MA, Zairi I, Echaieb W, Ben Mrad I, Kamoun S, Ben Moussa F, et al. Effects of Ramadan fasting on blood pressure in hypertensive patients. Archiv Cardiovasc Dis Suppl. 2020;12:215.
46. Barroso WKS, Jardim PCBV, Jardim TSV, Souza CTS, Magalhes ALA, Ibrahim FM, et al. Hypertensive diabetic patients: guidelines for conduct and their difficulties. Arq Bras Cardiol. 2003;81:143–7.
47. Al-Arouj M, Bouguerra R, Buse J, Hafez S, Hassanein M, Ibrahim MA, et al. Recommendations for management of diabetes during Ramadan. Diabetes Care. 2005;28:2305–11.
48. Hassanein M, Bashier A, Randeree H, Abouelmagd M, AlBaker W, Afandi B, et al. Use of SGLT2 inhibitors during Ramadan: an expert panel statement. Diabetes Res Clin Pract. 2020;169:108465.
49. Gilani A. Ramadan: a practical guide for the care of people with type 2 diabetes. Diabesity Pract. 2020;1:63–8.
50. May M, Schindler C. Clinically and pharmacologically relevant interactions of antidiabetic drugs. Ther Adv Endocrinol Metab. 2016;7:69–83.
51. Freeman JS, Gross B. Potential drug interactions associated with treatments for type 2 diabetes and its comorbidities: a clinical pharmacology review. Expert Rev Clin Pharmacol. 2012;5:31–42.

Part IX

Other Therapeutic Modalities

Control of Blood Glucose and Cardiovascular Risk Profile

28

Stefano Ciardullo and Gianluca Perseghin

28.1 Introduction

The most recent report from the International Diabetes Federation estimated that the global diabetes prevalence was 9.3% in 2019 (463 million people) and that it will rise to 10.9% (700 million) by 2045. Type 2 diabetes (T2D) accounts for approximately 90% of the cases, with other forms, including type 1 diabetes (T1DM) and gestational diabetes (GDM) representing less than 10% [1]. This epidemic has serious public health consequences. A large body of evidence supports the notion that patients with diabetes have a higher risk of dying from cardiovascular events compared with normoglycemic individuals even after other traditional risk factors are taken into account [2]. In particular, a large meta-analysis from the Emerging Risk Factors Collaboration, including data for 698,782 people from 102 prospective studies, showed that after adjustment for age, sex, smoking, systolic blood pressure, and body mass index (BMI), patients with diabetes had adjusted hazard ratios (aHR) of 2.0 for coronary artery disease (CAD), 2.3 for ischemic stroke, and 1.7 for the aggregate of other vascular deaths [3]. It has also been repeatedly demonstrated that among patients with T2DM, worse glycemic control is associated with higher risk of cardiovascular events and microvascular complications [4]. In the present chapter, we will discuss evidence on the effect of achieving a better glycemic control per se on the incidence of cardiovascular events in patients with diabetes and whether the use of specific medications has an impact on this endpoint. To minimize confounding, we based our considerations on evidence obtained from randomized controlled trials (RCTs) or meta-analyses of RCTs [5].

S. Ciardullo · G. Perseghin (✉)
Department of Medicine and Rehabilitation, Policlinico di Monza, Monza, Italy

Department of Medicine and Surgery, University of Milano Bicocca, Milan, Italy
e-mail: gianluca.perseghin@unimib.it

A. E. Berbari, G. Mancia (eds.), *Blood Pressure Disorders in Diabetes Mellitus*, Updates in Hypertension and Cardiovascular Protection,
https://doi.org/10.1007/978-3-031-13009-0_28

28.2 Glycemic Control and Cardiovascular Complications

Approximately 50 years after its discovery by Samuel Rahbar in the 1960s [6], in 2010, hemoglobin A1c (HbA1c) was added to the diagnostic criteria for diabetes mellitus. More importantly, it has become the universally accepted standard for assessing diabetes control and its levels served as the primary endpoint for most trials evaluating the effect of glycemic control on cardiovascular events.

Five large randomized clinical trials were designed to test the hypothesis that more stringent glycemic control reduces the incidence of micro- and macrovascular complications in diabetes. In these trials, the number of events occurring in the so-called standard treatment group (aiming at HbA1c levels between 7.3% and 9% in the different studies) was compared with those occurring in the intensive treatment group (aiming at HbA1c levels below 6.0–6.5%). Main results of these trials are summarized in Table 28.1 and discussed in detail in the present section in chronological order.

28.2.1 Diabetes Control and Complications Trial (DCCT)

The DCCT was performed in 1441 patients with T1DM of 1–15 years duration and a low rate of complications at baseline. It evaluated whether near-normal glycemic control obtained through multiple daily insulin injections or continuous insulin pump would prevent micro- and macrovascular complications [7]. The intensive treatment group was treated to obtain an HbA1c < 6.0%, whereas no specific target was defined for the control group. Nonetheless, achieving and maintaining this outcome was difficult, with less than half patients in the intensive group reaching the goal at least once and less than 5% maintaining this target for the entire duration of the trial (6.5 years). As a result, mean HbA1c levels in the intensive and conventional treatment groups were 7.0% and 9%, respectively. There was a significant reduction in the incidence of all microvascular complications in the intensive group, with no difference in the incidence of macrovascular events or mortality. It should be noted that patients in the intensive treatment arm had more severe hypoglycemic events and experienced significant weight gain. At the end of the trial, all patients were advised to follow the intensive treatment arm and were reevaluated for up to 30-years of follow-up. During this observational study, called EDIC (Epidemiology of Diabetes Interventions and Complications), HbA1c levels converged to approximately 8.0% in both groups [8]. Intensive therapy reduced the incidence of any cardiovascular disease by 30% (95% CI 7, 48; $P = 0.016$), and the lower HbA1c levels during the DCCT/EDIC statistically accounted for all of the observed treatment effect.

Table 28.1 Main results of trials evaluating the effect of intensive glycemic control on micro- and macrovascular complications

Study	Year	Diabetes type	Target - intensive group	HbA1 achieved—intensive group	HbA1c achieved—control group	Microvascular complications	Macrovascular events	Mortality
DCCT [7]	1993	T1DM	HbA1c < 6.05%	7.4%	9.1%	Retinopathy: RRR 76% (62–85%) Microalbuminuria: RRR 34% (2–56%) Neuropathy: RRR 69% (24–86%)	No significant difference	No significant difference
UKPDS 33 (SU, basal insulin) [10]	1998	T2DM	FPG < 110 mg/dl	7.0%	7.9%	RRR 25% (7–40%)	No significant difference	No significant difference
UKPDS 34 (metformin) [11]	1998	T2DM	FPG < 110 mg/dl	7.4%	8.0%	RRR 32% (13–47%)	MI: RRR 39% Composite: RRR 30% (5–48%)	RRR 36% (9–55%)
ACCORD [12]	2008	T2DM	HbA1c < 6.0%	6.4%	7.5%	No significant difference	MACE: No significant difference MI: No significant difference CV death: HR 1.35 (1.04–1.76)	HR 1.22 (1.01–1.46)

(continued)

Table 28.1 (continued)

Study	Year	Diabetes type	Target - intensive group	HbA1 achieved—intensive group	HbA1c achieved—control group	Microvascular complications	Macrovascular events	Mortality
ADVANCE [14]	2008	T2DM	HbA1c < 6.5%	6.5%	7.3%	Major: HR 0.86 (0.77–0.97) Renal: HR 0.79 (0.66–0.93) Neuropathy and retinopathy: No significant difference	No significant difference	No significant difference
VADT [16]	2009	T2DM	HbA1c reduction of 1.5%	6.9%	8.4%	Albuminuria: RR 0.66 ($p = 0.01$)	No significant difference	No significant difference

Abbreviations: *HbA1c* hemoglobin A1c, *RRR* relative risk reduction, *T1DM* type 1 diabetes mellitus, *T2DM* type 2 diabetes mellitus, *DCCT* Diabetes Control and Complication Trial, *UKPDS* United Kingdom Prospective Diabetes Study, *SU* sulfonylurea, *FPG* fasting plasma glucose, *ACCORD* Action to Control Cardiovascular Risk of Diabetes trial, *ADVANCE* Action in Diabetes and Vascular Disease: Preterax and Diamicron Modified Release Controlled Evaluation, *VADT* Veteran Affairs Diabetes Trial, *RR* relative risk, *HR* Hazard Ratio, *MI*, myocardial infarction, *MACE* major adverse cardiovascular events

28.2.2 The UK Prospective Diabetes Study (UKPDS)

The UKPDS recruited 5100 newly diagnosed patients with T2DM [9]. The conventional arm was advised to continue diet and weight control, whereas the intensive arm was treated to achieve a fasting plasma glucose (FPG) lower than 108 mg/dl with the use of sulfonylureas (SUs) or basal insulin. In both groups, rescue therapy with insulin was introduced with FPG levels >270 mg/dl. The intensively treated group achieved an HbA1c level < 6.0% in the first year, but a progressive increase was found with longer follow-up [10]. Again, a significant reduction in microvascular complications was present in the intensively treated patients, but no significant differences were found for cardiovascular endpoints and all-cause mortality. A UKPDS substudy, involving 342 overweight patients, randomized participants to a metformin arm, or to a SUs/basal insulin arm. Although probably not adequately powered to evaluate specific complications, the study showed lower all-cause mortality and cardiovascular complications in the metformin arm [11]. These results highlighted how the use of specific drugs might in part modulate the effect of glycemic control on cardiovascular complications.

28.2.3 Action to Control Cardiovascular Risk of Diabetes (ACCORD)

This trial recruited 10,251 patients with T2DM with either established cardiovascular disease or additional cardiovascular risk factors [12]. The intensive and standard treatment groups targeted an HbA1c level below 6.0% or between 7.0 and 7.9%, respectively. Major adverse cardiovascular events (MACE), comprising nonfatal myocardial infarction, nonfatal stroke, or death from cardiovascular causes, served as the primary study endpoint. Several classes of drugs including metformin, SUs, thiazolidinediones (TZDs), exenatide, and insulin were used in both groups, and the achieved Hba1c levels were 6.4% and 7.5%. The trial was stopped early as an increased risk of all-cause mortality was found in the intensively treated group (HR: 1.22; 95% CI, 1.01–1.46; $P = 0.04$). On the other hand, a nonsignificant trend for lower incidence of MACE was present. Similar results were obtained with long-term follow-up [13].

28.2.4 Action in Diabetes and Vascular Disease: Preterax and Diamicron Modified Release Controlled Evaluation (ADVANCE)

This trial enrolled 11,140 patients with a long history of T2DM and at high cardiovascular risk. Intensive glycemic control was defined by the use of gliclazide modified release plus other drugs as required to achieve an HbA1c value of 6.5% or less [14]. The two groups achieved HbA1c levels of 6.5% and 7.3%, respectively. A significant reduction of new-onset nephropathy was achieved by stricter glycemic control, whereas the incidence of macrovascular complications or death did not differ between groups. Also in this case, incidence of macrovascular events was similar between the groups in the long-term follow-up study [15]. On the other hand, there was no sign of an increased risk of all-cause mortality.

28.2.5 The Veteran Affairs Diabetes Trial (VADT)

The VADT investigators recruited 1791 military veterans with long-standing, poorly controlled T2DM and a high rate of complications to evaluate the impact of intensive glycemic control on MACE. The goal in the intensive therapy group was an absolute reduction of 1.5% in the HbA1c level, as compared with the standard therapy group [16]. This was achieved, as the two groups reached HbA1c levels of 6.9% and 8.4%, respectively. The rate of events was lower than predicted in both groups. No difference in the primary endpoint was present at the end of the trial between the treatment arms, whereas a lower risk of progression to microalbuminuria was evident in the intensively treated group. Once more, hypoglycemic episodes were more frequent in patients in the intensively treated arm. At 10-year follow-up, there was a statistically significant reduction in MACE in the intensively treated arm, which could suggest a potential legacy effect [17]. Recently, 15-year follow-up data from the study have been reported, showing no difference in the incidence of the primary outcome between the two treatment arms as HbA1c levels converged with time [18].

28.2.6 Meta-Analytic Assessment and Interpretation

Several aspects should be taken into account when trying to summarize results from these large RCTs. First, there was significant heterogeneity among study participants on diabetes subtype, disease duration, the rate of complications and comorbidities at baseline, glycemic targets, achieved HbA1c levels, and duration of follow-up. Second, antidiabetic drugs used in the trials differed, as did the method of therapy escalation and the incidence of hypoglycemic events, which were consistently higher in the intensively treated arms. These aspects fuel the never-ending debate on the optimal HbA1c target to be achieved in clinical practice.

A quite consistent finding across the trials is the reduction in the incidence of microvascular complications, even though not all of them were reduced in each study. This is not surprising as glucose levels represent the major pathogenic mechanism underlying the development of these complications. On the other hand, as summarized above, data on macrovascular events and mortality were not consistent, even though most studies suggested that longer follow-up time might be necessary to detect a beneficial effect of diabetes control.

As limited statistical power might also have affected results, trials performed in patients with T2DM were pooled to obtain meta-analytic evidence on the topic. Kelly et al. reviewed data on early (UKPDS-33 and UKPDS-34) and more recent trials (ACCORD, ADVANCE, and VADT) [19]. The evaluation of 27,802 patients showed that intensive control reduced the risk for cardiovascular disease (RR 0.90 [95% CI, 0.83–0.98]) but not cardiovascular death (RR, 0.97 [CI, 0.76–1.24]) or all-cause mortality (RR, 0.98 [CI, 0.84–1.15]). Conversely, intensive glucose control increased the risk for severe hypoglycemia (RR, 2.03 [CI, 1.46–2.81]).

While the cause of increased mortality in the ACCORD trial is still a matter of debate, it seems reasonable to speculate that it was not directly related to the achieved HbA1c level, but to the specific methods and drugs used to achieve it [20]. This is also supported by the results of the UKPDS-34 trial, in which metformin use was associated with lower mortality compared with insulin/SUs. A possible confounder of the association between glycemic control and cardiovascular events is represented by the occurrence of serious hypoglycemic events. A large body of evidence has demonstrated that hypoglycemia is one of the strongest predictors of macrovascular events, adverse clinical outcomes, and death in people with T2DM [21, 22]. As an example, an analysis of the ADVANCE trial showed that severe hypoglycemia was associated with a significant increase in the adjusted risks of MACE (HR 2.88; 95% CI, 2.01–4.12), cardiovascular death (HR 2.68; 95% CI, 1.72–4.19), and all-cause mortality (HR 2.69; 95% CI, 1.97–3.67) [23].

In conclusion, compelling evidence supports a beneficial role of intensive glycemic control on microvascular diabetes complications. A significant heterogeneity exists across different studies on the effects of intensive treatment on cardiovascular events. Nonetheless, results with longer follow-up and meta-analytic evidence support a favorable effect of obtaining near-normal HbA1c levels on MACE, especially when these are achieved without the occurrence of hypoglycemic events [24].

28.3 Changing the Focus of Regulatory Agencies and Clinical Trials

In 2006, Nissen and colleagues published a meta-analysis of 42 trials with rosiglitazone, a peroxisome proliferator-activated receptor agonist that was frequently utilized in clinical practice to treat patients with T2DM. The primary endpoints considered were myocardial infarction and death from cardiovascular causes [25]. The incidence of both outcomes was higher among patients treated with rosiglitazone compared with the control group (OR for myocardial infarction: 1.43, 95% CI 1.03–1.98; $P = 0.03$; OR for death from cardiovascular causes: 1.64, 95% CI 0.98–2.74; $P = 0.06$). The authors concluded that a change was due to the regulatory pathways for the development of drugs to treat diabetes. Until then, the Food and Drug Administration (FDA) considered demonstration of a sustained reduction in blood glucose levels with an acceptable safety profile adequate for approval of antidiabetic agents. On the other hand, the authors claimed that the ultimate value of treatment is the reduction of the complications of diabetes, and improvement in glycemic control could not be considered a reliable predictor of a reduction in cardiovascular events, which are the most common cause of death in these patients. Although the results of this meta-analysis have been criticized and discredited [26], in 2008, the FDA started to require that manufacturers conduct additional studies to detect atherosclerotic cardiovascular risk for all prospective FDA-approved therapies for the treatment of T2DM [27]. Drugs could be approved or stay on the market only if these studies did not show concerns of an increased risk of MACE. As a result, a large number of cardiovascular safety/outcome trials (CVOTs) were performed recruiting patients at high CV risk, the primary endpoint being non-inferiority compared with placebo on the incidence of MACE. It should be emphasized that in order to differentiate the effect of the drug from the effect of a better glycemic control, all trials aimed at achieving the same HbA1c levels in the active drug arm and the placebo arm (glycemic equipoise). In the following section, we summarize evidence obtained from RCTs with a cardiovascular endpoint for different therapeutic modalities and how these results influenced recent clinical practice guidelines from international societies.

28.3.1 Lifestyle Intervention

Evidence on the long-term effects of weight loss achieved through physical exercise and diet on cardiovascular outcome is limited. The largest trial to date (Look AHEAD, sponsored by the National Institute of Health) randomized 5145 overweight or obese patients with T2DM to intensive lifestyle intervention (decreased caloric intake and increased physical activity) or diabetes support and education (control group). The intensive arm aimed to achieve significant weight loss (defined as ≥7% of baseline weight) and increase physical activity to ≥175 min/week. Weight loss was greater in the intensive lifestyle intervention group both at year 1 (8.6% versus 0.7%) and at the end of follow-up (9.6 years: 6.0% vs 3.5%). Patients in the intensive treatment group also achieved better glycemic control (especially in the first 3–4 years) and a reduction in most CV risk factors, apart from low-density lipoprotein cholesterol. Despite all these improvements, the trial was stopped early on the basis of a futility analysis as the incidence of MACE was similar between the two groups (HR 0.95, 95% CI 0.83–1.09) [28]. It should be stressed, however, that patients in the intensive arm had significant benefits on secondary outcomes including sleep apnea, renal disease, overall fitness, and depression [29–32].

28.3.2 Metformin

While no adequately powered randomized clinical trial with a primary CV endpoint was performed comparing metformin treatment with placebo, indirect evidence seems to suggest a protective role of this drug. Apart from data from the already described UKPDS-34 trial, two additional small randomized studies support this notion. In the HOME trial, 390 patients treated with insulin were randomly assigned to either metformin or placebo and followed for a median of 4.3 years [33]. While the incidence of the primary endpoint of combined microvascular events did not differ between groups, patients in the metformin arm had a lower incidence of the macrovascular endpoint (HR 0.61, 95% CI 0.40–0.94; $P = 0.02$), which included cardiac, cerebrovascular, and peripheral arterial events. The second trial (SPREAD-DIMCAD) randomized 304 patients with T2DM and CAD to treatment with metformin or glipizide for a median of 5 years [34]. The composite cardiovascular outcome occurred less frequently in patients receiving metformin (HR 0.54, 95% CI 0.30–0.90).

28.3.3 Insulin

Cardiovascular safety of insulin glargine was assessed in the ORIGIN trial. In the study, 12,537 patients with cardiovascular risk factors plus impaired fasting glucose, impaired glucose tolerance, or T2DM were randomized to receive insulin glargine or standard care [35]. No difference was found in the primary outcome of MACE (HR 1.04, 95% CI 0.97–1.11). When insulin degludec was compared with insulin glargine in the DEVOTE head-to-head CVOT, no difference in the primary endpoint was seen (HR 0.91, 95% CI 0.78–1.06) [36]. Taken together, these results suggest a neutral role of insulin on CV events.

28.3.4 Thiazolidinediones (TZDs)

This class comprises pioglitazone and rosiglitazone, which have different binding affinities for peroxisome proliferator-activated receptors. As previously discussed, a meta-analysis by Nissen et al. raised concerns on CV safety of rosiglitazone. With regard to MACE, these concerns were not confirmed in the RECORD trial, which showed no difference between the rosiglitazone and the placebo groups on the primary endpoint consisting in hospitalization or death from cardiovascular causes (HR 0.99, 95% CI 0.85–1.16) [26]. A significant increase in HF hospitalizations was evident (HR 2.10, 95% CI 1.35–3.27). In the PROACTIVE clinical trial, patients with T2DM randomized to pioglitazone had a similar incidence of the primary endpoint (MACEs plus PVD events) compared with placebo. Interestingly, when only MACE was considered as an outcome, a significant reduction was present in the active treatment arm (HR 0.84, 95% CI 0.72–0.98) [37]. Conversely, an increased risk for HF hospitalization was present.

28.3.5 Dipeptidyl Peptidase-4 Inhibitors (DPP4-I)

The DPP4 enzyme is a ubiquitously expressed endopeptidase involved in cleaving several peptides. Its role in T2DM is related to the degradation of glucagon-like peptide 1 (GLP1), an incretin hormone that mediates glucose-dependent insulin secretion in response to food intake [38]. Inhibition of this activity therefore leads to increased incretin activity and a higher insulin response to glucose, without causing hypoglycemia. Clinical features of patients included in CVOTs with this class of drugs, and results on the primary endpoint are summarized in Table 28.2. They

Table 28.2 Cardiovascular safety trials with dipeptidyl peptidase-4 inhibitors (DPP4-i)

Trial	SAVOR-TIMI 53 [39]	EXAMINE [40]	TECOS [42]	CARMELINA [43]	CAROLINA [44]
Drugs	Saxagliptin vs. placebo	Alogliptin vs. placebo	Sitagliptin vs. placebo	Linagliptin vs. placebo	Linagliptin vs. glimepiride
Number of participants	16,492	5400	14,671	6979	6033
Age (years)	65	61	66	65	64
DM duration (years)	10	7.2	9.4	14.7	6.2
HbA1c (%)	8.0	8.0	7.3	7.9	7.2
Inclusion criteria	Age 40 years and CVD or Age 55 years and at least one CV risk factor	Recent (<90 days) acute coronary syndrome	CAD, CVD, or PVD	CVD and/or CKD	CVD or Age 70 years, or At least two CV risk factors
Previous CVD (%)	78	100	100	57	42
Follow-up (years)	2.1	1.5	2.8	2.2	6.3
Primary endpoint	3-point MACE 1.00 (0.89–1.12)	Three-point MACE 0.96 (95% UL <1.16)	Four-point MACE 0.98 (0.89–1.08)	Three-point MACE 1.02 (0.89–1.17)	Three-point MACE 0.98 (0.84–1.14)
HF hospitalization	1.27 (1.07–1.51)	1.19 (0.90–1.58)	1.00 (0.83–1.20)	0.90 (0.74–1.08)	1.21 (0.92–1.59)

Abbreviations: *DM* diabetes mellitus, *CVD* cardiovascular disease, *CAD* coronary artery disease, *PVD* peripheral vascular disease, *CKD* chronic kidney disease, *MACE* major adverse cardiovascular events, *HF* heart failure

consistently showed cardiovascular safety of this class of drugs on MACE, with no sign of either harm or protection. On the other hand, a worrying signal was found in the SAVOR-TIMI 53 trial, in which patients randomized to saxagliptin had a higher incidence of heart failure (HF) hospitalizations (HR: 1.27, 95% CI 1.07–1.51) [39]. While a similar, although not statistically significant trend was found in the EXAMINE trial (evaluating alogliptin) [40] and an increase in left ventricular volumes with no effect on left ventricle ejection fraction was found with vildagliptin in comparison with placebo in the VIVIDD trial [41], results from the other trials performed with sitagliptin and linagliptin [42–44] were reassuring.

28.3.6 Sulfonylureas (SUs)

As previously described, although focused on achieving a better glycemic control, patients in the intensive treatment arm of the ADVANCE trial were prescribed gliclazide as a first line drug, with no significant impact on cardiovascular events. Furthermore, indirect evidence on SUs can be drawn from comparison with other drugs. As previously shown, SUs were associated with higher incidence of MACE in the SPREAD-DIMCAD and UKPDS-34 trials, when compared with metformin [34]. On the other hand, the CAROLINA trial, which compared the effects of glimepiride and linagliptin (see Table 28.2), showed no difference in the incidence of MACE between the two groups [44]. As linagliptin showed neutrality compared with placebo in the CARMELINA trial, it is reasonable to assume that glimepiride treatment is not associated with an increased CV risk. This is also supported by the results of the TOSCA.IT trial, in which SUs (mainly gliclazide) were compared with pioglitazone, showing no difference in MACE [45] and by a recent meta-analysis of RCTs showing neutral effects of SUs on CV mortality [46]. In this last study, however, important concerns of a possible increased risk in all-cause mortality were raised.

28.3.7 GLP1-Receptor Agonists (GLP1-RA)

This class involves a series of peptide hormones that directly bind and activate the GLP1 receptor. Compared with the native GLP1 hormone (which is rapidly degraded by DPP4), they have been chemically modified in different ways to gain resistance against the DPP4 enzyme activity, thereby increasing their half-life [47]. They lead to significant reductions in HbA1c levels without directly causing hypoglycemic events and are also associated with a blood pressure lowering effect [48]. This potent effect resulted in lower HbA1c levels obtained in the active treatment arm despite aiming to a glycemic equipoise. As shown in Table 28.3, most CVOTs with this class of drugs showed a protective effect on MACE and a neutral effect on HF hospitalizations. A recent meta-analysis pooling all these trials together showed that these agents lead to a 12% reduction in MACE, a 12% reduction in CV death, a 16% reduction in stroke, and a 9% reduction in MI [49]. Moreover, a significant reduction was present for all-cause mortality (HR 0.88, 95% CI 0.83–0.95) and HF hospitalizations (HR 0.91, 95% CI 0.83–0.99) [49]. Results were consistent in subgroup analysis stratified by sex, age, BMI, kidney function, and the presence or absence of CVD at baseline. Finally, data showed a significant reduction in albuminuria, whereas no difference was found in worsening of kidney function in terms of estimated glomerular filtration rate.

28.3.8 Sodium Glucose Transporter 2 Inhibitors (SGLT2-I)

SGLT-2 is a transporter expressed in the proximal convoluted tubule in the kidneys and responsible for the large part of glucose reabsorption, following filtration in the glomerulus [50]. Inhibition of this activity by this class of agents leads to glycosuria and therefore lowers circulating glucose levels. Notably, systolic blood pressure also decreases by 3–5 mmHg following treatment [51]. The first CVOT with this class of agents (EMPAREG-OUTCOME with empagliflozin) was reported in 2015 and showed great promise, as patients in the active treatment group had a lower

Table 28.3 Cardiovascular safety/outcome trials with glucagon-like peptide 1 receptor agonists (GLP1-RA)

Trial	ELIXA [71]	LEADER [72]	SUSTAIN-6 [73]	EXSCEL [74]	Harmony outcomes [75]	REWIND[76]	PIONEER 6 [77]
Drugs	Lixisenatide vs. placebo	Liraglutide vs. placebo	Semaglutide vs. placebo	Exenatide vs. placebo	Albiglutide vs. placebo	Dulaglutide vs. placebo	Oral semaglutide vs. placebo
Number of participants	6068	9340	3297	14,752	9463	9901	3182
Age (years)	60	64	64	62	64	66	66
DM (years)	9.3	12.8	13.9	12.0	14.1	10.5	14.9
HbA1c (%)	7.7	8.7	8.7	8.0	8.7	7.2	8.2
Previous CVD (%)	100	81	83	73	100	31	35
CV risk inclusion criteria	Recent ACS (<180 days)	Age 50 years and CVD or CKD, or age 60 years and at least one CV risk factor	Age 50 years and CVD or CKD, or age 60 years and at least one CV risk factor	CVD, 27% had no previous CV event	CVD or PVD	Age 50 years and CVD or CV risk factors	Age 50 years and CVD, or CKD, or age 60 years and CV risk factors
Follow-up (years)	2.1	3.8	2.1	3.2	1.6	5.4	1.3
Primary endpoint	Four-point MACE 1.02 (0.89–1.17)	Three-point MACE 0.87 (0.78–0.97)	Three-point MACE 0.74 (0.58–0.95)	Three-point MACE 0.91 (0.83–1.00)	Three-point MACE 0.78 (0.68–0.90)	Three-point MACE 0.88 (0.79–0.99)	Three-point MACE 0.79 (0.57–1.11)
HF hospitalization	0.96 (0.75–1.23)	0.87 (0.73–1.05)	1.11 (0.77–1.61)	0.94 (0.78–1.13)	0.85 (0.70–1.04)	0.93 (0.77–1.12)	0.86 (0.48–1.55)

Abbreviations: *DM* diabetes mellitus, *ACS* acute coronary syndrome, *CVD* cardiovascular disease, *PVD* peripheral vascular disease, *CKD* chronic kidney disease, *MACE* major adverse cardiovascular events, *HF* heart failure incidence of MACE compared with those assigned to placebo (HR 0.86, 95% CI 0.74–0.99) [52]. Even more promising were the results on CV mortality (HR: 0.62, 95% CI 0.49–0.77) and HF hospitalizations (HR: 0.65, 95% CI 0.50–0.85). These data were later confirmed in the CANVAS program with canagliflozin [53]. While the effect on MACE was neutral in the other two CVOTs (with dapagliflozin and ertugliflozin), a consistent effect on HF and on the incidence and progression of nephropathy was present in all trials (Table 28.4), when meta-analysis was performed [54]. Based on the results on these secondary endpoints in CVOTs, several clinical trials focused on patients with HF and chronic kidney disease (CKD) were performed, including patients with and without diabetes. The positive effects of empagliflozin and dapagliflozin on HF were confirmed in the EMPEROR-Reduced and DAPA-HF trials, respectively, which recruited patients with HF and a reduced ejection fraction (EF) [55, 56], and in the SOLOIST-WHF trial, which evaluated the use of sotagliflozin in patients recently hospitalized for worsening HF, independently from EF [57]. Two other trials (EMPEROR-Preserved and DELIVER) will evaluate the effect of empagliflozin and dapagliflozin in patients with HF and a preserved EF, a condition in which no drug yet demonstrated significant protection.

Finally, dedicated renal outcome trials have been performed. In CREDENCE, conducted in patients with T2DM and macroalbuminuria, treatment with

Table 28.4 Cardiovascular and renal safety/outcome trials with sodium-glucose transporter 2 inhibitors (SGLT2-i)

Trial	EMPA-REG OUTCOME [52]	CANVAS [53]	DECLARE-TIMI 58 [78]	VERTIS [79]
Baseline	Empagliflozin vs. placebo	Canagliflozin vs. placebo	Dapagliflozin vs. placebo	Ertugliflozin vs. placebo
Number of participants	7020	10,142	17,160	8246
Age (years)	63	63	63	64
DM duration (years)	57% >10	13.5	11.8	13
Baseline HbA1c (%)	8.1	8.2	8.3	8.2
Previous CVD (%)	99	65	40	99
CV risk inclusion criteria	CVD or PVD	CVD or PVD	CVD or at least one CV risk factor	CVD or PVD
Follow-up (years)	3.1	2.4	4.5	3.5
Primary endpoint	Three-point MACE 0.86 (0.74–0.99)	Three-point MACE 0.86 (0.75–0.97)	Three-point MACE 0.93 (0.84–1.03)	Three-point MACE 0.97 (0.85–1.11)
HF hospitalization	0.65 (0.50–0.85)	0.67 (0.52–0.87)	0.83 (0.73–0.95)	0.70 (0.54–0.90)

Abbreviations: *DM* diabetes mellitus, *ACS* acute coronary syndrome, *CVD* cardiovascular disease, *PVD* peripheral vascular disease, *CKD* chronic kidney disease, *MACE* major adverse cardiovascular events, *HF* heart failure canagliflozin led to a 30% reduction in the incidence of end-stage kidney disease (dialysis, transplantation, or a sustained eGFR of <15 ml/min) [53]. Results were confirmed in the DAPA-CKD trial, exploring the effect of dapagliflozin compared with placebo in 4304 patients with CKD with and without diabetes [58].

28.3.9 The Impact on International Guidelines

This large number of positive, and sometimes unexpected, results had a major impact on recommendations for treatment of T2DM from international societies. In particular in the *Standards for Medical Care in Diabetes* from the American Diabetes Association [59], while metformin remains the first line therapy, cardiovascular risk assessment became the first step in the treatment algorithm if further agents are to be introduced. Patients with known or at high risk for atherosclerotic CVD should be treated with either a GLP1-RA or an SGLT2-I with proven benefit. Moreover, if the patient suffers from HF or has CKD and proteinuria, an SGLT2-I is preferred. The 2019 Guidelines on diabetes, prediabetes, and cardiovascular disease from the European Society of Cardiology, developed in collaboration with the European Association for the Study of Diabetes, gave CVD risk assessment an even more important role. According to the proposed algorithm, SGLT2-I or GLP1-RA are considered first line treatment for drug naïve patients with T2DM and at high or very high CV risk, while metformin should be added to these agents if HbA1c remains above target [60]. Moreover, if patients at high or very high risk are already on metformin treatment, one of these agents should be added to the regimen, independently from HbA1c levels.

28.4 Additional Measures of Glycemic Control

HbA1c levels carry a strong predictive value for diabetes complications and are considered the primary tool for assessing glycemic control [61]. Furthermore, the A1c-Derived Average Glucose (ADAG) study showed a strong correlation between HbA1c levels and self-monitored blood glucose (SMBG) as well as continuous glucose monitoring (CGM) ($r = 0.92$) [62]. Nonetheless, HbA1c has some limitations. Apart from specific conditions affecting its performance in estimating mean blood glucose concentrations, such as conditions that affect red blood cell turnover (e.g., anemias, recent transfusions, and cirrhosis), end-stage kidney disease, and pregnancy, it cannot provide an estimate of hypoglycemic events and glycemic variability. Both conditions have been linked to CVD, even after adjustment for mean blood levels or HbA1c [63–65]. Especially in patients with T1DM and those prone to a significant glycemic variability, a CGM system may provide a more accurate picture of the glycemic status. Several parameters can be obtained from analysis of CGM data, such as the amount of time spent in hypoglycemia, the time in range (TIR), and the time above range [66]. While data on the relationship between TIR and the incidence of cardiovascular events in large studies is still lacking, this measure is associated with the risk of microvascular complications. Using seven-point blood glucose profiles obtained from patients with T1DM in the DCCT trial, Beck et al. reported that the incidence of diabetic retinopathy and microalbuminuria increased by 64% and 40%, respectively, for each 10% decrease in TIR [67]. Similarly, Lu et al. evaluated the association between TIR and diabetic retinopathy in 3262 patients with T2DM. Results showed that patients with retinopathy had a lower TIR (defined as time spent with blood glucose levels of 70–180 mg/dl) and that the prevalence of retinopathy decreased with increasing TIR [68]. While implementation of CGM systems in clinical practice is still low and highly variable across countries, data obtained with these technologies give a much more detailed description of glycemic control, similar to what occurs with ambulatory blood pressure monitoring compared with office blood pressure measurement. Whether higher glycemic variability detected through these systems impacts on the incidence of macrovascular complications independently from mean blood glucose levels is still to be proven. However, several studies using indirect biomarkers of endothelial dysfunction and subclinical atherosclerosis seem to suggest an important relationship [69].

28.5 Final Remarks

In conclusion, achieving a good glycemic control in patients with diabetes leads to a fairly rapid reduction in the incidence of microvascular complications (retinopathy, neuropathy, and nephropathy). Intensive treatment is associated with a reduction in macrovascular complications as well, even though this protective effect seems to become evident with longer follow-up (more than 10 years) and in particular in patients with short diabetes duration and no prevalent CVD [70]. Furthermore, the use of specific drugs for the treatment of T2DM plays a major role. A series of pivotal CVOTs showed that GLP1-RA and SGLT2-I reduce the incidence of cardiovascular and renal events through mechanisms that are at least in part independent from their blood glucose lowering effects. This exciting finding has revolutionized diabetes care and clinical practice guidelines, which now recommend the use of these drugs to reduce complications independently from glycemic control, particularly in patients with prevalent CVD, HF, and CKD.

References

1. Saeedi P, Petersohn I, Salpea P, Malanda B, Karuranga S, Unwin N, et al. Global and regional diabetes prevalence estimates for 2019 and projections for 2030 and 2045: results from the international diabetes federation diabetes atlas. Diabetes Res Clin Pract. 2019;157:107843.
2. Klein KR, Buse JB. The trials and tribulations of determining HbA 1c targets for diabetes mellitus. Nat Rev Endocrinol. 2020;16:717–30.
3. Emerging Risk Factors Collaboration. Diabetes mellitus, fasting blood glucose concentration, and risk of vascular disease: a collaborative meta-analysis of 102 prospective studies. Lancet. 2010;375:2215–22.

4. Khaw K-T, Wareham N, Bingham S, Luben R, Welch A, Day N. Association of hemoglobin A1c with cardiovascular disease and mortality in adults: the European prospective investigation into cancer in Norfolk. Ann Intern Med. 2004;141:413–20.
5. Evans D. Hierarchy of evidence: a framework for ranking evidence evaluating healthcare interventions. J Clin Nurs. 2003;12:77–84.
6. Rahbar S, Blumenfeld O, Ranney HM. Studies of an unusual hemoglobin in patients with diabetes mellitus. Biochem Biophys Res Commun. 1969;36:838–43.
7. Diabetes Control and Complications Trial Research Group. The effect of intensive treatment of diabetes on the development and progression of long-term complications in insulin-dependent diabetes mellitus. N Engl J Med. 1993;329:977–86.
8. Diabetes Control and Complications Trial. (DCCT)/Epidemiology of Diabetes Interventions and Complications (EDIC) Study Research Group. Intensive diabetes treatment and cardiovascular outcomes in type 1 diabetes: the DCCT/EDIC study 30-year follow-up. Diabetes Care. 2016;39:686–93.
9. UK Prospective Diabetes Study Group. UK prospective diabetes study (UKPDS). Diabetologia. 1991;34:877–90.
10. Turner RC, Holman RR, Cull CA, Stratton IM, Matthews DR, Frighi V, et al. Intensive blood-glucose control with sulphonylureas or insulin compared with conventional treatment and risk of complications in patients with type 2 diabetes (UKPDS 33). Lancet. 1998;352:837–53.
11. UK Prospective Diabetes Study (UKPDS) Group. Effect of intensive blood-glucose control with metformin on complications in overweight patients with type 2 diabetes (UKPDS 34). Lancet. 1998;352:854–65.
12. Gerstein HC, Miller ME, Byington RP, Goff DC Jr, Bigger JT, Buse JB, et al. Effects of intensive glucose lowering in type 2 diabetes. N Engl J Med. 2008;358:2545–59.
13. ACCORD Study Group. Nine-year effects of 3.7 years of intensive glycemic control on cardiovascular outcomes. Diabetes Care. 2016;39:701–8.
14. Patel A, MacMahon S, Chalmers J, Neal B, Billot L, Woodward M, et al. Intensive blood glucose control and vascular outcomes in patients with type 2 diabetes. N Engl J Med. 2008;358:2560–72.
15. Zoungas S, Chalmers J, Neal B, Billot L, Li Q, Hirakawa Y, et al. Follow-up of blood-pressure lowering and glucose control in type 2 diabetes. N Engl J Med. 2014;371:1392–406.
16. Duckworth W, Abraira C, Moritz T, Reda D, Emanuele N, Reaven PD, et al. Glucose control and vascular complications in veterans with type 2 diabetes. N Engl J Med. 2009;360:129–39.
17. Hayward RA, Reaven PD, Wiitala WL, Bahn GD, Reda DJ, Ge L, et al. Follow-up of glycemic control and cardiovascular outcomes in type 2 diabetes. N Engl J Med. 2015;372:2197–206.
18. Reaven PD, Emanuele NV, Wiitala WL, Bahn GD, Reda DJ, McCarren M, et al. Intensive glucose control in patients with type 2 diabetes—15-year follow-up. N Engl J Med. 2019;380:2215–24.
19. Kelly TN, Bazzano LA, Fonseca VA, Thethi TK, Reynolds K, He J. Systematic review: glucose control and cardiovascular disease in type 2 diabetes. Ann Intern Med. 2009;151:394–403.
20. Riddle MC, Ambrosius WT, Brillon DJ, Buse JB, Byington RP, Cohen RM, et al. Epidemiologic relationships between A1C and all-cause mortality during a median 3.4-year follow-up of glycemic treatment in the ACCORD trial. Diabetes Care. 2010;33:983–90.
21. Bedenis R, Price AH, Robertson CM, Morling JR, Frier BM, Strachan MW, et al. Association between severe hypoglycemia, adverse macrovascular events, and inflammation in the Edinburgh type 2 diabetes study. Diabetes Care. 2014;37:3301–8.
22. McCoy RG, Van Houten HK, Ziegenfuss JY, Shah ND, Wermers RA, Smith SA. Increased mortality of patients with diabetes reporting severe hypoglycemia. Diabetes Care. 2012;35:1897–901.
23. Zoungas S, Patel A, Chalmers J, De Galan BE, Li Q, Billot L, et al. Severe hypoglycemia and risks of vascular events and death. N Engl J Med. 2010;363:1410–8.
24. Holman RR, Paul SK, Bethel MA, Matthews DR, Neil HAW. 10-year follow-up of intensive glucose control in type 2 diabetes. N Engl J Med. 2008;359:1577–89.

25. Nissen SE, Wolski K. Effect of rosiglitazone on the risk of myocardial infarction and death from cardiovascular causes. N Engl J Med. 2007;356:2457–71.
26. Home PD, Pocock SJ, Beck-Nielsen H, Curtis PS, Gomis R, Hanefeld M, et al. Rosiglitazone evaluated for cardiovascular outcomes in oral agent combination therapy for type 2 diabetes (RECORD): a multicentre, randomised, open-label trial. Lancet. 2009;373:2125–35.
27. Food and Drug Administration. Guidance for industry: diabetes mellitus—evaluating cardiovascular risk in new antidiabetic therapies to treat type 2 diabetes. US Department of Health and Human Services. 2008.
28. Look AHEAD Research Group. Cardiovascular effects of intensive lifestyle intervention in type 2 diabetes. N Engl J Med. 2013;369:145–54.
29. Kuna ST, Reboussin DM, Borradaile KE, Sanders MH, Millman RP, Zammit G, et al. Long-term effect of weight loss on obstructive sleep apnea severity in obese patients with type 2 diabetes. Sleep. 2013;36:641–9.
30. Look AHEAD Research Group. Effect of a long-term behavioural weight loss intervention on nephropathy in overweight or obese adults with type 2 diabetes: a secondary analysis of the look AHEAD randomised clinical trial. Lancet Diabetes Endocrinol. 2014;2:801–9.
31. Jakicic JM, Egan CM, Fabricatore AN, Gaussoin SA, Glasser SP, Hesson LA, et al. Four-year change in cardiorespiratory fitness and influence on glycemic control in adults with type 2 diabetes in a randomized trial: the look AHEAD Trial. Diabetes Care. 2013;36:1297–303.
32. Look AHEAD Research Group. Impact of intensive lifestyle intervention on depression and health-related quality of life in type 2 diabetes: the look AHEAD Trial. Diabetes Care. 2014;37:1544–53.
33. Kooy A, de Jager J, Lehert P, Bets D, Wulffelé MG, Donker AJ, et al. Long-term effects of metformin on metabolism and microvascular and macrovascular disease in patients with type 2 diabetes mellitus. Arch Intern Med. 2009;169:616–25.
34. Hong J, Zhang Y, Lai S, Lv A, Su Q, Dong Y, et al. Effects of metformin versus glipizide on cardiovascular outcomes in patients with type 2 diabetes and coronary artery disease. Diabetes Care. 2013;36:1304–11.
35. ORIGIN Trial Investigators. Basal insulin and cardiovascular and other outcomes in dysglycemia. N Engl J Med. 2012;367:319–28.
36. Marso SP, McGuire DK, Zinman B, Poulter NR, Emerson SS, Pieber TR, et al. Efficacy and safety of Degludec versus Glargine in type 2 diabetes. N Engl J Med. 2017;377:723–32.
37. Dormandy JA, Charbonnel B, Eckland DJA, Erdmann E, Massi-Benedetti M, Kmoules IK, et al. Secondary prevention of macrovascular events in patients with type 2 diabetes in the PROactive study (PROspective pioglitAzone Clinical Trial In macroVascular Events): a randomised controlled trial. Lancet. 2005;366:1279–89.
38. Drucker DJ, Nauck MA. The incretin system: glucagon-like peptide-1 receptor agonists and dipeptidyl peptidase-4 inhibitors in type 2 diabetes. Lancet. 2006;368:1696–705.
39. Scirica BM, Bhatt DL, Braunwald E, Steg PG, Davidson J, Hirshberg B, et al. Saxagliptin and cardiovascular outcomes in patients with type 2 diabetes mellitus. N Engl J Med. 2013;369:1317–26.
40. White WB, Cannon CP, Heller SR, Nissen SE, Bergenstal RM, Bakris GL, et al. Alogliptin after acute coronary syndrome in patients with type 2 diabetes. N Engl J Med. 2013;369:1327–35.
41. McMurray JJ, Ponikowski P, Bolli GB, Lukashevich V, Kozlovski P, Kothny W, et al. Effects of vildagliptin on ventricular function in patients with type 2 diabetes mellitus and heart failure: a randomized placebo-controlled trial. JACC Heart Fail. 2018;6:8–17.
42. Green JB, Bethel MA, Armstrong PW, Buse JB, Engel SS, Garg J, et al. Effect of Sitagliptin on cardiovascular outcomes in type 2 diabetes. N Engl J Med. 2015;373:232–42.
43. Rosenstock J, Perkovic V, Johansen OE, Cooper ME, Kahn SE, Marx N, et al. Effect of Linagliptin vs placebo on major cardiovascular events in adults with type 2 diabetes and high cardiovascular and renal risk the CARMELINA randomized clinical Trial. JAMA. 2019;321:69–79.

44. Rosenstock J, Kahn SE, Johansen OE, Zinman B, Espeland MA, Woerle HJ, et al. Effect of Linagliptin vs glimepiride on major adverse cardiovascular outcomes in patients with type 2 diabetes: the CAROLINA randomized clinical Trial. JAMA. 2019;322:1155–66.
45. Vaccaro O, Masulli M, Nicolucci A, Bonora E, Del Prato S, Maggioni AP, et al. Effects on the incidence of cardiovascular events of the addition of pioglitazone versus sulfonylureas in patients with type 2 diabetes inadequately controlled with metformin (TOSCA.IT): a randomised, multicentre trial. Lancet Diabetes Endocrinol. 2017;5:887–97.
46. Mannucci E, Monami M, Candido R, Pintaudi B, Targher G. Effect of insulin secretagogues on major cardiovascular events and all-cause mortality: a meta-analysis of randomized controlled trials. Nutr Metab Cardiovasc Dis. 2020;30:1601–8.
47. Baggio LL, Drucker DJ. Glucagon-like Peptide-1 receptor co-agonists for the treatment of metabolic disease. Mol Metab. 2020;46:101090.
48. Wang B, Zhong J, Lin H, Zhao Z, Yan Z, He H, et al. Blood pressure-lowering effects of GLP-1 receptor agonists exenatide and liraglutide: a meta-analysis of clinical trials. Diabetes Obes Metab. 2013;15:737–49.
49. Kristensen SL, Rørth R, Jhund PS, Docherty KF, Sattar N, Preiss D, et al. Cardiovascular, mortality, and kidney outcomes with GLP-1 receptor agonists in patients with type 2 diabetes: a systematic review and meta-analysis of cardiovascular outcome trials. Lancet Diabetes Endocrinol. 2019;7:776–85.
50. Hediger MA, Rhoads DB. Molecular physiology of sodium-glucose cotransporters. Physiol Rev. 1994;74:993–1026.
51. Mancia G, Cannon CP, Tikkanen I, Zeller C, Ley L, Woerle HJ, et al. Impact of empagliflozin on blood pressure in patients with type 2 diabetes mellitus and hypertension by background antihypertensive medication. Hypertension. 2016;68:1355–64.
52. Zinman B, Wanner C, Lachin JM, Fitchett D, Bluhmki E, Hantel S, et al. Empagliflozin, cardiovascular outcomes, and mortality in type 2 diabetes. N Engl J Med. 2015;373:2117–28.
53. Perkovic V, Jardine MJ, Neal B, Bompoint S, Heerspink HJL, Charytan DM, et al. Canagliflozin and renal outcomes in type 2 diabetes and nephropathy. N Engl J Med. 2019;380:2295–306.
54. Zelniker TA, Wiviott SD, Raz I, Im K, Goodrich EL, Bonaca MP, et al. SGLT2 inhibitors for primary and secondary prevention of cardiovascular and renal outcomes in type 2 diabetes: a systematic review and meta-analysis of cardiovascular outcome trials. Lancet. 2019;393:31–9.
55. Packer M, Anker SD, Butler J, Filippatos G, Pocock SJ, Carson P, et al. Cardiovascular and renal outcomes with empagliflozin in heart failure. N Engl J Med. 2020;383:1413–24.
56. McMurray JJV, Solomon SD, Inzucchi SE, Kober L, Kosiborod MN, Martinez FA, et al. Dapagliflozin in patients with heart failure and reduced ejection fraction. N Engl J Med. 2019;381:1995–2008.
57. Bhatt DL, Szarek M, Steg PG, Cannon CP, Leiter LA, McGuire DK, et al. Sotagliflozin in patients with diabetes and recent worsening heart failure. N Engl J Med. 2021;384:117–28.
58. Heerspink HJL, Stefánsson BV, Correa-Rotter R, Chertow GM, Greene T, Hou F-F, et al. Dapagliflozin in patients with chronic kidney disease. N Engl J Med. 2020;383:1436–46.
59. American Diabetes Association - 9. Pharmacologic approaches to glycemic treatment: standards of medical care in diabetes—2021. Diabetes Care. 2021;44:S111–24.
60. Cosentino F, Grant PJ, Aboyans V, Bailey CJ, Ceriello A, Delgado V, et al. 2019 ESC guidelines on diabetes, pre-diabetes, and cardiovascular diseases developed in collaboration with the EASD: the task force for diabetes, pre-diabetes, and cardiovascular diseases of the European Society of Cardiology (ESC) and the European Association for the Study of diabetes (EASD). Eur Heart J. 2019;41:255–323.
61. Stratton IM, Adler AI, Neil HA, Matthews DR, Manley SE, Cull CA, et al. Association of glycaemia with macrovascular and microvascular complications of type 2 diabetes (UKPDS 35): prospective observational study. BMJ. 2000;321:405–12.
62. Nathan DM, Kuenen J, Borg R, Zheng H, Schoenfeld D, Heine RJ. Translating the A1C assay into estimated average glucose values. Diabetes Care. 2008;31:1473–8.

63. Di Flaviani A, Picconi F, Di Stefano P, Giordani I, Malandrucco I, Maggio P, et al. Impact of glycemic and blood pressure variability on surrogate measures of cardiovascular outcomes in type 2 diabetic patients. Diabetes Care. 2011;34:1605–9.
64. Okada K, Hibi K, Gohbara M, Kataoka S, Takano K, Akiyama E, et al. Association between blood glucose variability and coronary plaque instability in patients with acute coronary syndromes. Cardiovasc Diabetol. 2015;14:111.
65. Su G, Mi S, Tao H, Li Z, Yang H, Zheng H, et al. Association of glycemic variability and the presence and severity of coronary artery disease in patients with type 2 diabetes. Cardiovasc Diabetol. 2011;10:19.
66. Battelino T, Danne T, Bergenstal RM, Amiel SA, Beck R, Biester T, et al. Clinical targets for continuous glucose monitoring data interpretation: recommendations from the international consensus on time in range. Diabetes Care. 2019;42:1593–603.
67. Beck RW, Bergenstal RM, Riddlesworth TD, Kollman C, Li Z, Brown AS, et al. Validation of time in range as an outcome measure for diabetes clinical trials. Diabetes Care. 2019;42:400–45.
68. Lu J, Ma X, Zhou J, Zhang L, Mo Y, Ying L, et al. Association of time in range, as assessed by continuous glucose monitoring, with diabetic retinopathy in type 2 diabetes. Diabetes Care. 2018;41:2370–6.
69. Lu J, Ma X, Shen Y, Wu Q, Wang R, Zhang L, et al. Time in range is associated with carotid intima-media thickness in type 2 diabetes. Diabetes Technol Ther. 2020;22:72–8.
70. Prattichizzo F, de Candia P, De Nigris V, Nicolucci A, Ceriello A. Legacy effect of intensive glucose control on major adverse cardiovascular outcome: systematic review and meta-analyses of trials according to different scenarios: Metabolism. 2020;110:154308.
71. Pfeffer MA, Claggett B, Diaz R, Dickstein K, Gerstein HC, Kober LV, et al. Lixisenatide in patients with type 2 diabetes and acute coronary syndrome. N Engl J Med. 2015;373:2247–57.
72. Marso SP, Daniels GH, Brown-Frandsen K, Kristensen P, Mann JFE, Nauck MA, et al. Liraglutide and cardiovascular outcomes in type 2 diabetes. N Engl J Med. 2016;375:311–22.
73. Marso SP, Bain SC, Consoli A, Eliaschewitz FG, Jódar E, Leiter LA, et al. Semaglutide and cardiovascular outcomes in patients with type 2 diabetes. N Engl J Med. 2016;375:1834–44.
74. Holman RR, Bethel MA, Mentz RJ, Thompson VP, Lokhnygina Y, Buse JB, et al. Effects of once-weekly exenatide on cardiovascular outcomes in type 2 diabetes. N Engl J Med. 2017;377:1228–39.
75. Hernandez AF, Green JB, Janmohamed S, D'Agostino RB Sr, Granger CB, Jones NP, et al. Albiglutide and cardiovascular outcomes in patients with type 2 diabetes and cardiovascular disease (harmony outcomes): a double-blind, randomised placebo-controlled trial. Lancet. 2018;392:1519–29.
76. Gerstein HC, Colhoun HM, Dagenais GR, Diaz R, Lakshmanan M, Pais P, et al. Dulaglutide and cardiovascular outcomes in type 2 diabetes (REWIND): a double-blind, randomised placebo-controlled trial. Lancet. 2019;394:121–30.
77. Husain M, Birkenfeld AL, Donsmark M, Dungan K, Eliaschewitz FG, Franco DR, et al. Oral semaglutide and cardiovascular outcomes in patients with type 2 diabetes. N Engl J Med. 2019;381:841–51.
78. Wiviott SD, Raz I, Bonaca MP, Mosenzon O, Kato ET, Cahn A, et al. Dapagliflozin and cardiovascular outcomes in type 2 diabetes. N Engl J Med. 2019;380:347–57.
79. Cannon CP, Pratley R, Dagogo-Jack S, Mancuso J, Huyck S, Masiukiewicz U, et al. Cardiovascular outcomes with ertugliflozin in type 2 diabetes. N Engl J Med. 2020;383:1425–35.

Part X

Hypotensive Disorders

Orthostatic Hypotension and Diabetes

29

Cesare Cuspidi, Elisa Gherbesi, Carla Sala,
and Marijana Tadic

29.1 Introduction

Diabetes mellitus (DM) is associated with the development of premature cardiovascular disease, which relates to the clustering of risk factors such as hyperglycemia in the presence of insulin resistance, hypertension, dyslipidemia, obesity, and subclinical systemic inflammation [1, 2]. In particular, hypertension is known to be highly prevalent among patients with DM. Similarly, it is known that the prevalence of DM in hypertensive patients is markedly higher than in the general population. The ipertensione diabetes (IPERDIA) study, a multicenter cross-sectional surveys.

performed in a cohort of 1397 patients with hypertension referred to 30 hospital outpatient clinics for the treatment of hypertension, revealed that DM was present in a high percentage of participants (17%) [3]. Patients with DM were older and had higher values of body mass index (BMI), systolic blood pressure (BP), and lower high-density lipoprotein cholesterol as well as higher triglyceride levels and microalbuminuria than individuals without it. The close association between hypertension and DM has been further confirmed over time by the growing diffusion of BP measurement techniques outside the clinical setting. An altered circadian rhythm of BP (i.e., nondipping and reverse dipping pattern) has been documented to be highly prevalent in patients with long-lasting type 2 DM [4]. In a study from our group, carried out in a carefully selected sample of patients with a history of type 2 DM of

C. Cuspidi (✉)
Department of Medicine and Surgery, University of Milano-Bicocca, Milan, Italy
e-mail: cesare.cuspidi@unimib.it

E. Gherbesi · C. Sala
Department of Clinical Sciences and Community Health, University of Milano and Fondazione Ospedale Maggiore IRCCS Policlinico di Milano, Milan, Italy

M. Tadic
University Clinical Hospital Centre "Dragisa Misovic", Belgrade, Serbia

A. E. Berbari, G. Mancia (eds.), *Blood Pressure Disorders in Diabetes Mellitus*, Updates in Hypertension and Cardiovascular Protection,
https://doi.org/10.1007/978-3-031-13009-0_29

more than 10 years, a reproducible nocturnal nondipping profile, as assessed by two 24-h periods of ambulatory BP monitoring within a 4-week period, was found in 58% of cases [5]. A cross-sectional analysis of 567 participants in the Jackson Heart Study, a population-based study of African Americans, taking antihypertensive medication, showed that patients with DM were more likely to have day-time hypertension, masked hypertension, and masked isolated nocturnal hypertension [6]. However, the spectrum of BP alterations in DM not only is limited to a variety of hypertensive phenotypes (i.e. sustained, masked, nocturnal, and white coat hypertension) but also includes the opposite phenomenon represented by hypotension, and in particular, orthostatic hypotension (OH) [7, 8]. OH is a dangerous condition whose failure to identify leads to an underestimation of the global cardiovascular risk in the general population and in the hypertensive and diabetic setting. Symptomatic OH is regarded as the most disabling features of autonomic dysfunction and a strong predictor of adverse cardiovascular outcomes [9]. Importantly, it should be noted that even asymptomatic OH shares the same unfavorable clinical and prognostic significance as the symptomatic one [10]. Nonetheless, in clinical practice, attention to postural hypotension is largely neglected, resulting in a suboptimal prevention and treatment of its harmful consequences.

Thus, this present chapter will review a number of issues concerning OH and its association to DM with particular attention to: (I) pathogenetic mechanisms, (II) prevalence and clinical correlates, (III) prognostic significance, (IV) impact of drugs on orthostatic regulation of BP, and (V) clinical aspects and therapeutic interventions.

29.1.1 Pathigenetic Mechanisms

The healthy individual is able to minimize the orthostatic BP drop thanks to a normal plasma volume, intact baroreflexes, and efficient venomotor tone [11]. Therefore, OH occurs when one or more mechanisms involved in the regulation of BP postural changes fail. The upright position determines in the majority of healthy individuals a pooling of 500–750 ml blood from the thorax into splanchnic circulation and lower extremities. This large shift in blood volume leads a rapid fall in venous return, stroke volume, and systemic BP. The BP drop immediately triggers the activation of the baroreceptors, which in coordination with the central autonomic network allow to maintain cardiovascular homeostasis by modulating cardiac output and peripheral vascular resistance [12, 13]. OH can be classified in relation to the prevalent underlying mechanism in non-neurogenic and neurogenic [14] (Fig. 29.1). Non-neurogenic causes are generally associated with episodic and reversible clinical manifestations of OH. Circulating volume depletion due to fever-induced dehydration and/or gastrointestinal disorders associated with vomiting and diarrhea is a common cause of hypotension and clinical symptoms of OH in the general population. Hypovolemia, with or without hyponatremia caused by diuretics, often causes OH in treated hypertensives and patients with chronic heart failure. In addition to, or independently of hypovolemia, numerous drugs that interfere at

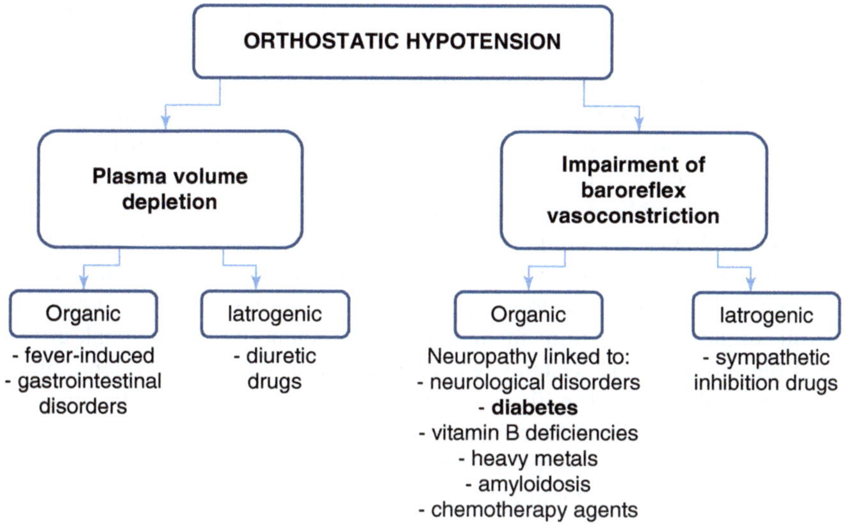

Fig. 29.1 Pathogenetic mechanisms of orthostatic hypotension

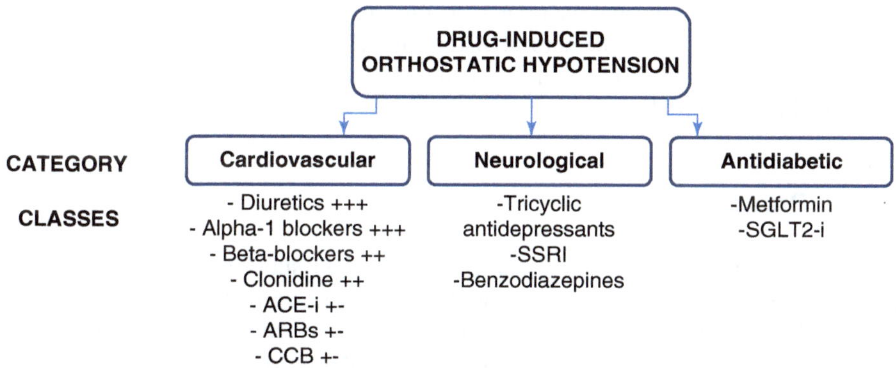

Fig. 29.2 Drug-induced orthostatic hypotension. Abbreviations: *ACE-i* ACE inhibitors, *ARBs* angiotensin receptor blockers, *CCB* calcium channel blockers, *SSRI* selective serotonin reuptake inhibitors, *SGLT2-I* sodium-glucose cotransporter-2 inhibitors

different levels of the orthostatic BP reflex pathway (i.e., sympathetic inhibition, cardioinhibitory effects, and vasodilation) prescribed for conditions such as hypertension, type 2 DM, urological pathologies, and depression carry an increased risk of OH [15] (Fig. 29.2). As for neurogenic OH, the underlying key mechanism is the impairment of baroreflex-mediated vasoconstriction of the skeletal muscle and splanchnic circulation due to damage or dysfunction at central and/or peripheral sites in the baroreflex afferent pathway. The severity and natural history of neurogenic OH largely depends on the subtype of degenerative disorder such as Parkinson's disease, dementia and multiple system atrophy, and pure autonomic failure [16]. It has been reported that in these conditions, there is a marked impairment in norepinephrine release during standing in over 70% of patients [17]. The deficiency in norepinephrine release mirrors an inability of sympathetic vasoconstrictor neurons to activate properly, which is responsible for a blunted peripheral vasoconstriction and consequent postural hypotension. Among the peripheral neuropathies, DM is the most common cause worldwide (particularly frequent in developed countries) capable of profoundly altering the normal BP and HR response to standing [18]. Other causes of peripheral neuropathy associated to OH include vitamin B deficiencies, exposure to heavy metals, amyloidosis, and some chemotherapy agents (i.e., platinum-based drugs) [19]. Diabetic autonomic neuropathy affects numerous organs and functions including cardiovascular, gastrointestinal, urogenital, and thermoregulatory systems resulting in OH as well as neurogenic bladder and bowel involvement. The Toronto Consensus [20] defined diabetic autonomic neuropathy as "a disorder of the autonomic nervous system in the setting of diabetes or metabolic derangements of pre-diabetes after the exclusion of other causes" and diabetic cardiovascular autonomic neuropathy as "the impairment of autonomic control of the cardiovascular system."

There is a wide spectrum of subtypes of diabetic neuropathies that differ from each other based on the type of fibers (i.e., myelinated and unmyelinated) and nerves involved. OH is mainly related to progressive involvement of autonomic unmyelinated fibers [21]. The natural history of OH in DM patients is characterized by progressive worsening over time related to the underlying metabolic control and associated risk factors [22].

29.2 Prevalence

The prevalence of OH can vary markedly depending substantially on the demographic and clinical characteristics of the sample examined (Table 29.1). Age, comorbidities, and drugs that alter BP homeostasis are among the most important factors linked to OH. Beyond these variables, the definition used for the diagnosis of OH must be also taken into account [15]. Postural changes in BP for unmasking OH are determined in clinical practice by taking the difference between seated BP and standing. Both measurements, however, can be derived from a different number

Table 29.1 Prevalence of orthostatic hypotension in various clinical settings

Setting	Number	Prevalence (%)	Reference
General geriatric population	5465	29	Tran et al. [26]
Community based			
Prediabetes	452	17.7	Wu et al. [27]
Type 2 diabetes	157	25.5	
Mild to moderate CKD	3939	4.6	Rouabhi et al. [28]
Type 2 diabetes	4266	20	Fleg et al. [27]
Type 1 diabetes	440	16.1	Hirai et al. [30]

Abbreviations: *CKD* chronic kidney disease

of recordings (i.e., the average of 2–3 measurements, sometimes excluding the first measurement) and the timing of standing (i.e., close to 1 min, 2 min, within 3 min, or at 1 and 3 min). Beyond these differences, there is a general consensus in defining OH as a sustained reduction of at least 20 mm Hg of systolic BP or 10 mm Hg of diastolic BP within 3 min of standing [23].

The prevalence of OH increases with age, as a consequence of the physiological decline in baroreceptor sensitivity, as well as the increased prevalence of neurodegenerative diseases related to aging per se and comorbidities in the elderly. As a result, OH is relatively rare in young and middle-aged individuals.

A recent meta-analysis by Tran et al. [24], based on 13 studies, mainly carried out in community-based cohorts (76% of the pooled population) and including a total of 5465 adults aged >65 years, showed that pooled prevalence of OH was 29.0%. The prevalence of OH appears, however, to be a very limited phenomenon when evaluated in healthy elderly, as suggested by a study on a selected sample of 80 nonhypertensive, nondiabetic elderly individuals aged 60 years [25]. Evidence on this topic in the diabetes setting comes from both cross-sectional population-based studies and prospective randomized trials. In a community-based study of 1638 participants classified as having normal glucose tolerance ($n = 1069$), prediabetes ($n = 452$), and diabetes ($n = 157$), prevalence rates of OH were 13.8%, 17.7%, and 25.5%, respectively [26]. Hypertension was significantly associated to OH in all subgroups. In addition, age and glucose control were the main correlates of OH in prediabetic and diabetic participants. In the Action to Control Cardiovascular Risk in Diabetes (ACCORD BP) trial, OH, defined by a decline in systolic BP ≥20 mm Hg or a decline in diastolic BP ≥10 mm Hg, was diagnosed at one or more of the three visits in 20% of participants. Independent factors associated with OH were female sex, white race, higher baseline systolic BP and hemoglobin A1c, and use of alpha-blockers, beta-blockers, insulin, and current smoking [27].The Chronic Renal Insufficiency Cohort (CRIC) study, including 3939 patients with mild to moderate CKD aged 21–74 years and prevalent DM (48%) documented that OH (i.e., a reduction in systolic BP > 20 mmHg on standing) occurred in 180 participants (4.6%) [28]. The most important factors independently associated with OH were DM, reduced body mass index (BMI), and beta-blocker use. The increased risk of OH in individuals with reduced BMI has been reported in previous studies based on different methods including beat-to-beat technology or the head-up tilt test to assess OH. Among the 882 participants from Maracaibo Aging Study (19% with DM), BMI showed an inverse association in both sexes that presented a similar prevalence of this altered BP pattern (18.5% women and 20.9% men) [29].

Finally, the data on the high prevalence of OH in patients with type 1 DM deserve mention, despite coming from cohorts with a significantly lower mean age than those of type 2 DM. The Wisconsin Epidemiologic Study of Diabetic Retinopathy investigating the frequency of OH and associations with risk factors in a cohort of 440 persons with long-term type 1 DM (45 ± 10 years, 51% men) showed a prevalence of 16.1% [30]. Heart rate variability and supine systolic BP were independently associated to postural BP abnormalities after controlling for the confounders.

29.3 Prognostic Significance

OH is associated with a broad spectrum of unhealthy outcomes, such as the risk of falls and consequent trauma, the development of subclinical organ damage, and cardiovascular events. Most of cross-sectional and prospective studies that have investigated this topic have been conducted in elderly people. A meta-analysis performed on six of prospective observational studies investigating the relationship between OH and falling including individual data of 1022 elderly patients, in whom the prevalence of OH ranged from 11% to 82% and the prevalence of one or more fall incidents ranged from 51% to 62% showed a clear and significant relationship between OH and time to first fall incident [31].

A large prospective observational cohort study including 1997 individuals over 60 years old (425 with OH) assessed the relationship between several markers of target organ damage such as carotid intima-media thickness (IMT), brachial-ankle pulse wave velocity (baPWV), clearance of creatinine, and microalbuminuria [32]. After adjustment, IMT per one-SD increment (OR = 1.38, CI 95%:1.05–1.82; $p = 0.02$), baPWV (OR = 1.63, 95% CI: 1.04–2.54; $p = 0.03$), and microalbuminuria (OR = 1.40, 95% CI: 1.00–1.96; $p = 0.04$) were still associated with OH.

The Hypertension in the Very Elderly Trial (HYVET) examined the relationship between orthostatic fall and subsequent cognitive decline or dementia in an older adult hypertensive population with a prevalence of type 2 DM of almost 10% [33]. In that study, 538 out 3121 patients (17%) fulfilled the diagnostic criteria of OH (a fall of $\geq$15 mmHg in systolic and or $\geq$7 mmHg in diastolic BP after 2 min standing from a sitting position), which was independently associated with increased risk of cognitive decline and dementia.

A growing body of evidence is also accumulating on the impact of OH on the risk of cardiovascular events in different clinical settings. Among the 9139 middle aged participants (9% with DM) to the Atherosclerosis Risk in Communities (ARIC) Study, OH, diagnosed during the first visit, was a robust predictor of myocardial infarction (OR = 1.88; 95% CI, 1.44–2.46), congestive heart failure (OR = 1.65; 95% CI, 1.34–2.04), stroke (OR = 1.83; 95% CI, 1.35–2.48), fatal coronary heart disease (OR = 2.77; 95% CI, 1.93–3.98), and all-cause death (OR = 1.68; 95% CI, 1.45–1.95) [34].

As for heart failure (HF), a meta-analysis based on a total of 51,270 individuals and 3603 incident chronic HF cases from four prospective cohorts indicated that the presence of OH at baseline was significantly associated with an increased risk for future chronic HF outcomes (adjusted OR = 1.30, 95% CI: 1.09–1.55; $p = 0.004$) [35]. Interestingly, results of subgroups analysis showed that the association between OH and chronic incident HF was significant in middle-age individuals or patients with hypertension and DM at baseline; this was not the case in the pooled elderly subgroup.

The relationship between OH and recurrent stroke was addressed by Secondary Prevention of Small Subcortical Strokes (SPS3) trial [36]. To this purpose, a total of 2275 patients were included with a mean follow-up time 3.2 years. In a fully adjusted model, the 881 patients with OH at some point during their follow up (12% with DM) had a 1.8 times higher risk of recurrent stroke than those without OH (6%

with DM). Not in line with the individual studies and meta-analyses cited above, were the results obtained from the Systolic Blood Pressure Intervention Trial (SPRINT) study [37]. During the follow-up period (median 3 years), the incidence of OH was 5.7% among those assigned a standard BP goal, and 5.0% among those assigned the intensive BP goal. Of note, OH was not associated with higher risk of nonfatal and fatal cardiovascular events (primary outcome: OR = 1.06; 95%CI: 0.78–1.44) as well as of syncope, electrolyte abnormalities, injurious falls, or acute renal failure. Whether this was related to the fact that in the SPRINT study DM was one of the exclusion criteria, together prior stroke, dementia, symptomatic, or severe heart failure, remains a matter of debate.

The ACCORD BP study represented a unique opportunity for understanding the relationship between OH and cardiovascular complications in the DM setting [27]. In that study, 4266 participants with both hypertension and type 2 DM at high cardiovascular risk were randomly assigned to either intensive (<120 mmHg) or standard (<140 mmHg) systolic BP control, and orthostatic BP change was assessed at baseline 12 and 48 months. Over a median follow-up of 47 months, OH was associated with increased risk of total death (OR = 1.61, 95% CI: 1.11–2.36) and heart failure death/hospitalization (OR = 1.85, 95% CI: 1.17–2.93), with no difference in risk between intensive and standard BP lowering treatment.

29.4 Drug-Induced OH

Drug-induced OH is common in the general population, and even more so in DM, and its resulting in brain hypoperfusion may increase the risk of adverse events including falls, transitory ischemic attacks, strokes, cognitive impairment, and death [38]. In addressing this complex topic, it may be useful to distinguish drugs that can interfere with orthostatic pressure in patients with DM into three categories: cardiovascular medications (mainly BP lowering drugs), drugs acting on central nervous system, and antidiabetic drugs.

29.4.1 Antihypertensive Drugs

Reports on antihypertensive drugs and risk of OH in current literature are controversial. The association of diuretics, beta-blockers, alpha-blockers, and ACE-inhibitors with OH emerged in some studies but not confirmed by others.

In a recent secondary analysis of the 23,964 participants of the Antihypertensive and Lipid-Lowering Treatment to Prevent Heart Attack Trial (ALLHAT) study, no differences in risk of fall, syncope, and OH between principal classes of antihypertensives was observed during the trial period with the only exception of amlodipine, which was associated to an increased risk of fall in the short term [39]. Altogether, these results showed that among older adults with prevalent DM (approximately 40%), antihypertensive class was not an important determinant of risk of falls, syncope, or OH. A meta-analysis of Bhanu et al. [14], based on 69 randomized controlled trials comprising 27.079 participants suggested that compared with placebo, beta-blockers were associated with increased risk of OH (OR = 7.76; 95%: CI:2.51–24.03). On the contrary, there was no statistically significant difference in odds of OH with calcium antagonists, ACE-inhibitors, and angiotensin II receptor antagonists compared with placebo. A further meta-analysis targeting the impact of intensive versus less intensive antihypertensive treatment on OH provided reassuring information on the risk of hypotension in patients achieving optimal BP targets [39]. Among 18,466 hypertensive patients enrolled in five randomized trials, a lower BP treatment goal decreased the odds of OH. The odds of OH were even lower in patients without DM but not significantly influenced by age and sex suggesting that a more intensive BP treatment regimen does not increase risk for OH. Despite this evidence, it should be emphasized that in patients with DM the use of antihypertensive drugs that could interfere with orthostatic regulatory mechanisms should be carefully evaluated. From this point of view diuretics (excessive reduction of circulating volume), alpha-1 blockers (impaired vasoconstriction from vascular smooth muscle alpha-1 receptor blockade) and beta-blockers (reduced heart rate and contractility) should require a more careful monitoring than other classes of BP lowering drugs (i.e., ACE-inhibitors and angiotensin II receptor antagonists).

29.4.2 Drugs Acting on Central Nervous System

Tricyclic antidepressants exert their effects on postural BP through combined sympathetic inhibition and reduced vascular resistance. OH is a common cardiovascular unfavorable effect of tricyclic antidepressants occurring in approximately 30% of the patients [40]. The meta-analysis of three controlled trials comprising a total of 261 patients with major depressive disorder showed that tricyclic antidepressants were associated with higher odds of OH compared with placebo (OR = 6.30, 95% CI:2.86–13.91) [14]. Although serotonin reuptake inhibitors cause peripheral vasodilation through inhibition of calcium channels and, in some cases, slight reduction in heart rate, OH is generally regarded as a relatively uncommon adverse effect. The meta-analysis of six trials including 2333 patients comparing a selective serotonin reuptake inhibitors or serotonin modulator with placebo failed to find this adverse association [14]. Subgroup analysis on trials comparing low with high dose, as well as on those performed in older patients, showed similar results. Benzodiazepines can also alter the physiological adaptation of upright BP through multiple though not fully elucidated mechanisms (i.e., reduced the sympathetic tone and norepinephrine response to postural changes and vascular myorelaxation, leading to increase in venous capacitance and lower-body venous pooling) [41, 42].

29.4.3 Antidiabetic Drugs

Metformin has been reported to impair absorption of vitamin B12 leading to reduced level of circulating B12, which in turn is a well-known risk factor for cardiovascular autonomic neuropathy [43]. Starting from this background, the Copenhagen Insulin and Metformin Therapy (CIMT) substudy assessed in 442 patients with type 2 DM the effect of 18 months intervention with metformin versus placebo, each in combination with one of three different insulin regimens, on measures of cardiovascular autonomic neuropathy [44]. At the end of the follow-up, early fall in orthostatic BP (30 s after standing) was significantly increased in the metformin group compared with placebo (3.4 mmHg for systolic and 1.3 mmHg for diastolic BP, respectively).

OH can occur during the course of therapy with sodium-glucose cotransporter 2 inhibitors (SGLT2i). This is because the inhibition of the cotransporters in the proximal tubule leading to a mild increase of sodium urine excretion, osmotic diuresis due enhanced glucose excretion, and blunted sympathetic nervous activity can cause a reduction in BP and increase the likelihood of OH [45]. However, in this regard, it should be remarked that the available evidence is quite conflicting. A meta-analysis based on 27 randomized controlled trials (n = 12,960 participants) showed that SGLT2i had no significant effect on the incidence of OH [46]. In contrast, the previously cited meta-analysis by Bhanu et al. [14], based on 10 studies totaling 9641 patients, suggested that SGLT2i use was associated with increased odds of OH compared with placebo (OR = 1.24; 95% CI: 1.08–1.43).

29.5 Clinical Aspects and Treatment

Patients with symptomatic OH may have complaints of increasing intensity, which include generalized weakness, dizziness, visual disturbance, headache pre-syncope, and occasionally syncope. Typically, symptoms should only occur upon assuming upright posture, become more severe with ongoing stand, markedly less frequent when seated, and resolve in supine position [47].

Some individuals, however, are surprisingly asymptomatic, despite systolic BPs <90 mmHg. This may be ascribed, in part, to cerebral autoregulation, in which patients are able to maintain cerebral perfusion pressures despite critically low systemic BP.

The identification and replacement of medications that predispose to OH is the initial intervention of choice to treat this condition. In order to prevent OH in the setting of DM associated with hypertension and particularly in the elderly with a long history of diabetes, diuretics, alpha-blockers, and clonidine should be avoided, whenever possible, preferring calcium antagonists, ACE inhibitors, and angiotensin receptor II antagonists.

There are many non-pharmacologic interventions that can be used not only alone but also in combination with pharmacologic agents. In this section, we will briefly report the main non-pharmacological indications useful for reducing the risk of OH and the severity of its clinical manifestations. Patients with OH should be educated about simple behavioral measures in order to avoid situations that can exacerbate the orthostatic drop in BP (i.e., insufficient water intake, excessive temperature of the rooms, hot baths, and sudden passage from lying to standing position, abundant meals, and Valsalva maneuver). Regular physical activity and exercise should be recommended to avoid deconditioning, which is well recognized to aggravate orthostatic symptoms. The use of stockings and elastic bands applied to the lower limbs and abdomen reduce peripheral blood pooling in the lower extremities consequently mitigating the orthostatic pressure drop. It has also been suggested that sleeping in the head-up position may reduce the risk of OH. This is based on observation that the supine position at night-time is accompanied by a rise in BP, which in turn determines an increase in urinary volume and sodiuria [48]. Thus, the head-up position may decrease nocturnal water and sodium excretion, thus reducing the risk of morning orthostatic intolerance associated to nocturnal hypertension [49].

29.6 Conclusions

OH represents one of the main manifestations of the cardiovascular autonomic neuropathy of patients with DM that may be precipitated by acute or chronic factors. Indeed, the clinical picture in this setting is made more complex by the fact that the neurogenic damage underlying this pathological condition can be aggravated by numerous concomitant risk factors [50]. Of particular importance is the potentially unfavorable role of a series of commonly used drugs that interfere with orthostatic regulation such as diuretics, hypotensive, oral hypoglycemic agents, antidepressants, and alpha-adrenoreceptor antagonists to treat benign prostatic as well as anti-Parkinsonian agents.

Therefore, it should never be forgotten that medical therapy is one of the most common causes of OH. This is particularly true in the DM setting whose comorbidities require multiple therapies that can frequently have negative synergistic effects on orthostatic BP. From a clinical perspective to avoid identifying OH, it is mandatory that healthcare professionals implement the recommendations of the hypertension guidelines [51]. Supine and standing BP measurements should be performed in all patients at the first visit to exclude OH, and this procedure should also be applied in subsequent visits in older people, patients with DM, and people with other conditions in which OH may frequently occur. Thus, the early identification of OH in the setting can allow to reach important therapeutic goals such as improvement of the quality of life and cardiovascular prognosis through the optimization of the pharmacological treatment of the associated conditions (hypertension, depression, and urological pathologies) and of glucose metabolism whose amelioration can lead to an improvement of the cardiovascular autonomic failure [52].

Disclosure
The authors report no conflicts of interest.

Funding None.

Data Availability Statement Nonapplicable, the paper is a review.

References

1. Yandrapalli S, Malik AH, Namrata F, Pemmasani G, Bandyopadhyay D, Vallabhajosyula S, et al. Influence of diabetes mellitus interactions with cardiovascular risk factors on post-myocardial infarction heart failure hospitalizations. Int J Cardiol. 2022;348:140–6.
2. Liu Y, Li J, Dou Y, Ma H. Impacts of type 2 diabetes mellitus and hypertension on the incidence of cardiovascular diseases and stroke in China real-world setting: a retrospective cohort study. BMJ Open. 2021;11:e053698.
3. Lonati C, Morganti A, Comarella L, Mancia G, Zanchetti A. IPERDIA Study Group. Prevalence of type 2 diabetes among patients with hypertension under the care of 30 Italian clinics of hypertension: results of the (Iper)tensione and (dia)bete study. J Hypertens. 2008;26:1801–8.
4. Cuspidi C, Vaccarella A, Leonetti G, Sala C. Ambulatory blood pressure and diabetes: targeting non-dipping. Curr Diabetes Rev. 2010;6:111–5.
5. Cuspidi C, Meani S, Lonati L, Fusi V, Valerio C, Sala C, et al. Short-term reproducibility of a non-dipping pattern in type 2 diabetic hypertensive patients. J Hypertens. 2006;24:647–53.
6. Bromfield SG, Shimbo D, Bertoni AG, Sims M, Carson AP, Muntner P. Ambulatory blood pressure monitoring phenotypes among individuals with and without diabetes taking antihypertensive medication: the Jackson Heart Study. J Hum Hypertens. 2016;30:731–6.
7. Chang J, Hou YP, Wu JL, Fang XY, Li SL, Liu MB, et al. Blood pressure circadian rhythms and adverse outcomes in type 2 diabetes patients diagnosed with orthostatic hypotension. J Diabetes Investig. 2018;9:383–8.
8. Lyhne JM, Laugesen E, Høyem P, Cichosz S, Christiansen JS, Knudsen ST, et al. Morning blood pressure surge and target organ damage in newly diagnosed type 2 diabetic patients: a cross sectional study. BMC Endocr Disord. 2015;15:77.
9. Rose KM, Eigenbrodt ML, Biga RL, Couper DJ, Light KC, Sharrett AR, et al. Orthostatic hypotension predicts mortality in middle-aged adults: the atherosclerosis risk in communities (ARIC) study. Circulation. 2006;114:630–6.
10. Fagard RH, De Cort P. Orthostatic hypotension is a more robust predictor of cardiovascular events than night-time reverse dipping in elderly. Hypertension. 2010;56:56–61.
11. Low PA, Tomalia VA. Orthostatic hypotension: mechanisms, causes, management. Clin Neurol. 2015;11:220–6.
12. Thomas GD. Neural control of the circulation. Adv Physiol Educ. 2011;35:28–32.
13. Barman SM. 2019 Ludwig lecture: rhythms in sympathetic nerve activity are a key to understanding neural control of the cardiovascular system. Am J Physiol Regul Integr Comp Physiol. 2020;318:R191–205.
14. Bhanu C, Nimmons D, Petersen I, Orlu M, Davis D, Hussain H, et al. Drug-induced orthostatic hypotension: a systematic review and meta-analysis of randomised controlled trials. PLoS Med. 2021;18:e1003821.
15. Freeman R, Abuzinadah AR, Gibbons C, Jones P, Miglis MG, Sinn DI. Orthostatic hypotension: JACC state-of-the-art review. J Am Coll Cardiol. 2018;72:1294–309.
16. Freeman R. Diabetic autonomic neuropathy. Handb Clin Neurol. 2014;126:63–79.
17. Loavenbruck A, Sandroni P. Neurogenic orthostatic hypotension: roles of norepinephrine deficiency in its causes, its treatment, and future research directions. Curr Med Res Opin. 2015;31:2095–104.
18. Arora RR, Bulgarelli RJ, Ghosh-Dastidar S, Colombo J. Autonomic mechanisms and therapeutic implications of postural diabetic cardiovascular abnormalities. J Diabetes Sci Technol. 2008;2:645–57.
19. Teng C, Cohen J, Egger S, Blinman PL, Vardy JL. Systematic review of long-term chemotherapy-induced peripheral neuropathy (CIPN) following adjuvant oxaliplatin for colorectal cancer. Support Care Cancer. 2022;30:33–47.
20. Sasaki H, Kawamura N, Dyck PJ, Dyck PJB, Kihara M, Phillip A, et al. Spectrum of diabetic neuropathies. Diabetol Int. 2020;11:87–96.

21. Kaufmann H, Norcliffe-Kaufmann L, Palma JA, Biaggioni I, Low PA, Singer W, et al. Autonomic Disorders Consortium. Natural history of pure autonomic failure: a United States prospective cohort. Ann Neurol. 2017;81:287–97.
22. Budyono C, Setiati S, Purnamasari D, Rumende CM. The proportion of orthostatic hypotension and its relationship with HbA1c levels in elderly patients with diabetes. Acta Med Indones. 2016;48:122–8.
23. Gibbons CH, Schmidt P, Biaggioni I, Frazier-Mills C, Freeman R, Isaacson S, et al. The recommendations of a consensus panel for the screening, diagnosis, and treatment of neurogenic orthostatic hypotension and associated supine hypertension. J Neurol. 2017;264:1567–82.
24. Tran J, Hillebrand SL, Meskers CGM, Iseli RK, Maier AB. Prevalence of initial orthostatic hypotension in older adults: a systematic review and meta-analysis. Age Ageing. 2021;50:1520–8.
25. Baliga R, Prabhu G. Orthostatic hypotension in healthy elderly: is it a myth? N Am J Med Sci. 2010;2:416–8.
26. Wu JS, Yang YC, Lu FH, Wu CH, Wang RH, Chang CJ. Population-based study on the prevalence and risk factors of orthostatic hypotension in subjects with pre-diabetes and diabetes. Diabetes Care. 2009;32:69–74.
27. Fleg JL, Evans GW, Margolis KL, Barzilay J, Basile JN, Bigger JT, et al. Orthostatic hypotension in the ACCORD (Action to Control Cardiovascular Risk in Diabetes) Blood Pressure Trial: prevalence, incidence, and prognostic significance. Hypertension. 2016;68:888–95.
28. Rouabhi M, Durieux J, Al-Kindi S, Cohen JB, Townsend RR, Rahman M. Orthostatic hypertension and hypotension and outcomes in CKD: the CRIC (Chronic Renal Insufficiency Cohort) Study. Kidney Med. 2021;3:206–15.
29. Méndez AS, Melgarejo JD, Mena LJ, Chávez CA, González AC, Boggia J, et al. Risk factors for orthostatic hypotension: differences between elderly men and women. Am J Hypertens. 2018;31:797–803.
30. Hirai FE, Moss SE, Klein BE, Klein RJ. Postural blood pressure changes and associated factors in long-term Type 1 diabetes: Wisconsin Epidemiologic Study of Diabetic Retinopathy. Diabetes Complications. 2009;23:83–8.
31. Hartog LC, Schrijnders D, Landman GWD, Groenier K, Kleefstra N, Bilo HJG, et al. Is orthostatic hypotension related to falling? A meta-analysis of individual patient data of prospective observational studies. Ageing. 2017;46:568–75.
32. Chi HJ, Feng HJ, Chen XJ, Zhao XT, Zhang EX, Fan YF, et al. The association between orthostatic blood pressure changes and subclinical target organ damage in subjects over 60 years old. Geriatr Cardiol. 2019;16:387–94.
33. Peters R, Anstey KJ, Booth A, Beckett N, Warwick J, Antikainen R, et al. Orthostatic hypotension and symptomatic subclinical orthostatic hypotension increase risk of cognitive impairment: an integrated evidence review and analysis of a large older adult hypertensive cohort. Eur Heart J. 2018;39:3135–43.
34. Juraschek SP, Daya N, Appel LJ, Miller ER 3rd, McEvoy JW, Matsushita K, et al. Orthostatic hypotension and risk of clinical and subclinical cardiovascular disease in middle-aged adults. Am Heart Assoc. 2018;7:e008884.
35. Xin W, Lin Z, Li X. Orthostatic hypotension and the risk of congestive heart failure: a meta-analysis of prospective cohort studies. PLoS One. 2013;8:e63169.
36. Mehta T, McClure LA, White CL, Taylor A, Benavente OR, Lakshminarayan KJ. Effect of postural hypotension on recurrent stroke: secondary prevention of small subcortical strokes (SPS3) Study. Stroke Cerebrovasc Dis. 2019;28:2124–31.
37. Juraschek SP, Taylor AA, Wright JT Jr, Evans GW, Miller ER 3rd, Plante TB, et al. SPRINT Research Group. Orthostatic hypotension, cardiovascular outcomes, and adverse events: results from SPRINT. Hypertension. 2020;75:660–7.
38. Rivasi G, Rafanelli M, Mossello E, Brignole M, Ungar A. Drug-related orthostatic hypotension: beyond anti-hypertensive medications. Drugs Aging. 2020;37:725–38.

39. Juraschek SP, Simpson LM, Davis BR, Beach JL, Ishak A, Mukamal KJ. Effects of antihypertensive class on falls, syncope, and orthostatic hypotension in older adults: the ALLHAT Trial. Hypertension. 2019;74:1033–40.
40. Calvi A, Fischetti I, Verzicco I, Belvederi Murri M, Zanetidou S, Volpi R, et al. Antidepressant drugs effects on blood pressure. Front Cardiovasc Med. 2021;8:704281.
41. Rivasi G, Kenny RA, Ungar A, Romero-Ortuno R. Effects of benzodiazepines on orthostatic blood pressure in older people. Eur J Intern Med. 2020;72:73–7.
42. Shi SJ, Garcia KM, Meck JV. Temazepam, but not zolpidem, causes orthostatic hypotension in astronauts after spaceflight. J Cardiovasc Pharmacol. 2003;41:31–9.
43. Reinstatler L, Qi YP, Williamson RS, Garn JV, Oakley GP Jr. Association of biochemical B12 deficiency with metformin therapy and vitamin B12 supplements: the National Health and Nutrition Examination Survey, 1999-2006. Diabetes Care. 2012;35:327–33.
44. Hansen CS, Lundby-Christiansen L, Tarnow L, Gluud C, Hedetoft C, Thorsteinsson B, et al. CIMT study group. Metformin may adversely affect orthostatic blood pressure recovery in patients with type 2 diabetes: sub-study from the placebo-controlled Copenhagen Insulin and Metformin Therapy (CIMT) trial. Cardiovasc Diabetol. 2020;19:150.
45. Mancia G, Cannon CP, Tikkanen I, Zeller C, Ley L, Woerle HJ, et al. Impact of empagliflozin on blood pressure in patients with type 2 diabetes mellitus and hypertension by background antihypertensive medication. Hypertension. 2016;68:1355-64.
46. Baker WL, Smyth LR, Riche DM, Bourret EM, Chamberlin KW, White WB. Effects of sodium-glucose co-transporter 2 inhibitors on blood pressure: a systematic review and meta-analysis. J Am Soc Hypertens. 2014;8:262–75.
47. Lei LY, Chew DS, Raj SR. Differential diagnosis of orthostatic hypotension. Auton Neurosci. 2020;228:102713.
48. Ohishi M, Kubozono T, Higuchi K, Akasaki Y. Hypertension, cardiovascular disease, and nocturia: a systematic review of the pathophysiological mechanisms. Hypertens Res. 2021;44:733–9.
49. Wieling W, Raj SR, Thijs RD. Are small observational studies sufficient evidence for a recommendation of head-up sleeping in all patients with debilitating orthostatic hypotension? MacLean and Allen revisited after 70 years. Clin Auton Res. 2009;19:8–12.
50. Grassi G, Biffi A, Dell'Oro R, Quarti Trevano F, Seravalle G, Corrao G, et al. Sympathetic neural abnormalities in type 1 and type 2 diabetes: a systematic review and meta-analysis. J Hypertens. 2020;38:1436–42.
51. Williams B, Mancia G, Spiering W, Agabiti Rosei E, Azizi M, Burnier M, et al. 2018 ESC/ESH guidelines for the management of arterial hypertension. The task force for the management of arterial hypertension of the European Society of Cardiology and the European Society of Hypertension: the task force for the management of arterial hypertension of the European Society of Cardiology and the European Society of Hypertension. J Hypertens. 2018;36:2284–309.
52. Jun JE, Lee SE, Choi MS, Park SW, Hwang YC, Kim JH. Clinical factors associated with the recovery of cardiovascular autonomic neuropathy in patients with type 2 diabetes mellitus. Cardiovasc Diabetol. 2019;18:29.

Correction to: Diabetes and Microcirculation

Adel E. Berbari, and Giuseppe Mancia

Correction to:
A. E. Berbari, G. Mancia (eds.), *Blood Pressure Disorders in Diabetes Mellitus*,
https://doi.org/10.1007/978-3-031-13009-0_11

The first name of the series editor was omitted from the front matter and chapter 11 of the book. In the revised version, the series editor's full name Enrico Agabiti Rosei has been corrected.

The updated original version of the book can be found at
https://doi.org/10.1007/978-3-031-13009-0_11

A. E. Berbari, G. Mancia (eds.), *Blood Pressure Disorders in Diabetes Mellitus*,
Updates in Hypertension and Cardiovascular Protection,
https://doi.org/10.1007/978-3-031-13009-0_30

MIX
Papier aus verantwortungsvollen Quellen
Paper from responsible sources
FSC® C105338

If you have any concerns about our products,
you can contact us on
ProductSafety@springernature.com

In case Publisher is established outside the EU,
the EU authorized representative is:
Springer Nature Customer Service Center GmbH
Europaplatz 3, 69115 Heidelberg, Germany

Printed by Libri Plureos GmbH
in Hamburg, Germany